Advanced Assessment

Interpreting Findings and Formulating Differential Diagnoses

FIFTH EDITION

Mary Jo Goolsby, EdD, MSN, NP-C, FAANP
Principal, Institute for NP Excellence, LLC
Augusta, GA

Laurie Grubbs, PhD, ARNP-C
Professor of Nursing
Florida State University
College of Nursing
Tallahassee, Florida

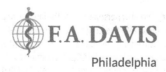
F.A. DAVIS
Philadelphia

F.A. Davis Company
1915 Arch Street
Philadelphia, PA 19103
www.fadavis.com

Printed in the United States of America

Last digit indicates print number: 10 9 8 7 6 5 4 3 2 1

Editor-in-Chief, Nursing: Jean Rodenberger
Publisher: Susan Rhyner
Manager of Project and eProject Management: Cathy Carroll
Content Project Manager: Sean West
Design Manager: Carolyn O'Brien

As new scientific information becomes available through basic and clinical research, recommended treatments and drug therapies undergo changes. The author(s) and publisher have done everything possible to make this book accurate, up-to-date, and in accord with accepted standards at the time of publication. The author(s), editors, and publisher are not responsible for errors or omissions or for consequences from application of the book, and make no warranty, expressed or implied, in regard to the contents of the book. Any practice described in this book should be applied by the reader in accordance with professional standards of care used in regard to the unique circumstances that may apply in each situation. The reader is advised always to check product information (package inserts) for changes and new information regarding dose and contraindications before administering any drug. Caution is especially urged when using new or infrequently ordered drugs.

Library of Congress Cataloging-in-Publication Data

Names: Goolsby, Mary Jo, editor. | Grubbs, Laurie, 1951- editor.
Title: Advanced assessment : interpreting findings and formulating
    differential diagnoses / [edited by] Mary Jo Goolsby, Laurie Grubbs.
Description: Fifth edition. | Philadelphia, PA : F.A Davis Company, [2023] |
    Includes bibliographical references and index.
Identifiers: LCCN 2022029058 (print) | LCCN 2022029059 (ebook) |
    ISBN 9781719645935 (paperback) | ISBN 9781719648301 (ebook)
Subjects: MESH: Nursing Assessment--methods | Diagnosis, Differential |
    Diagnostic Errors--prevention & control | Nurse Practitioners.
Classification: LCC RC71.5 (print) | LCC RC71.5 (ebook) | NLM WY 100.4 |
    DDC 616.07/5--dc23/eng/20220819
LC record available at https://lccn.loc.gov/2022029058
LC ebook record available at https://lccn.loc.gov/2022029059

Preface

A growing body of literature addresses the risks associated with clinical decision making, with diagnostic error described as the "blind spot" in health-care delivery (National Academy of Medicine, 2015). The original idea for this book arose from our recognition that the many health assessment texts available lacked an essential component—content on how to narrow a differential diagnosis when a patient presents with one of the almost endless possible complaints. The response to earlier editions of this text supported our belief in the need for a text that addressed the lack of content designed to support expertise in the assessment and diagnostic process. We hope that this significantly updated edition will continue to aid advanced practice students, new practitioners, and experienced practitioners faced with new presentations.

In spite of the growth in available diagnostic technology and studies, expertise in correctly performing assessment skills, obtaining valid data, and interpreting the findings accurately remains fundamental to the provision of the safe, high-quality, patient-centered, and cost-effective practice for which NPs are known. Even once these skills are accomplished, accurate diagnosis remains a difficult aspect of practice. Novice practitioners often spend much energy and time narrowing their differential diagnosis when they have no clear guidance that is driven by the patient or complaint. For this reason, our aim was to develop a guide in the assessment and diagnostic process that is broad in content and suitable for use in varied settings.

Advanced Assessment: Interpreting Findings and Formulating Differential Diagnoses is designed to serve as both a textbook during advanced health assessment course work and subsequent clinical courses and as a quick reference for practicing clinicians. We believe that studying the text will help students develop proficiency in performing and interpreting assessments, recognizing the range of conditions that can be indicated by specific findings. Once in practice, we believe that the text will aid individualized assessment and narrowing of differential diagnosis.

The book consists of three parts. Part I provides a summary discussion of assessment and some matters related to clinical decision making. In addition to discussing the behaviors involved in arriving at a definitive diagnosis, each chapter in Part I and in subsequent sections covers some pitfalls that clinicians often experience and the types of evidence-based resources that are available to assist in the diagnostic process.

This edition introduces a unique chapter on issues related to integrating laboratory and imaging studies into clinical decision-making. Knowledge regarding selecting, ordering, and interpreting diagnostic studies are critical skills for clinicians.

This section also includes a chapter on conducting a genetic assessment. This component of health assessment has great potential, with recent advances in the information and technology related to genetics and genomics. It is critical that clinicians be able to address the potential of hereditary diseases and genetic variations that may affect their patients. This chapter, like the one on clinical decision-making, is relevant to the content of all subsequent chapters.

Part II serves as the core of the book and addresses assessment and diagnosis using a system and body region approach. Each chapter in this part begins with an overview of the comprehensive history and physical examination of a specific system, as well as a discussion of common diagnostic studies. The remainder of the chapter is then categorized by chief complaints commonly associated with that system. For each complaint, there is a description of the focused assessment relative to that complaint, followed by a list of the conditions that should be considered in the differential diagnosis, along with the symptoms, signs, or diagnostic findings that would support each condition.

Figures within chapters are provided to better depict examination techniques or expected findings. This edition introduces a number of diagnostic algorithms to assist in the differential diagnosis and also includes a number of additional complaints and conditions in several differential diagnosis sections.

Finally, Part III addresses the assessment and diagnosis of specific populations, such as those at either extreme of age (young and old) and pregnant women. This section also includes content on the assessment of transgender individuals and of persons with physical disabilities, placing a heavy emphasis on the assessments that allow clinicians to evaluate the special and cultural needs of individuals in the populations addressed in these chapters.

To aid the reader, we have tried to follow a consistent format in the presentation of content so that information can be readily located. This format is admittedly grounded on the sequence we have found successful as we presented this content to our students. However, we have a great appreciation for the expertise of the contributors in this edited work, and some of the content they recommended could not consistently fit our "formula." We hope that the organization of this text will be helpful to all readers.

REFERENCE
National Academies of Science. (2015). Consensus Study Report: Improving diagnosis in health care. Retrieved February 4, 2022, from https://www.nap.edu/catalog/21794/improving-diagnosis-in-health-care

Acknowledgments

We want to express our sincere appreciation for the support and assistance provided by so many in the development of this book. Their contributions have made the work much richer.

Particular mention goes to all at F.A. Davis for their enthusiasm, support, and patience throughout the history of this text. Special thanks to F.A. Davis staff; Susan Rhyner, publisher; Sean West, Content Project Manager; Cathy Carroll, eProject Manager; and Carolyn O'Brien, Design Manager.

We are immensely grateful to the contributors to this edition, who shared their expertise and knowledge to enhance the content. They were a pleasure to work with. We also acknowledge those who contributed content to an earlier edition: JoEllen Wynne, Quanetta Edwards, Saundra Turner, Randolph Rasch, Karen Koozer-Olson, Diane Mueller, Phillip Rupp, Patricia Hentz, Casey Jones, Charon Pierson, Christine Aramburu Alegra, and Susan Havel. In addition to the contributors, we also want to thank the many reviewers of this and previous editions for their timely and thoughtful feedback.

Personal Acknowledgments from Laurie Grubbs

Most of all, I would like to thank my friend and coauthor, Mary Jo, for providing the impetus to write this book—an often talked about aspiration that became a reality—and to F.A. Davis for their enthusiasm, support, and patience during the process for each edition.

I would also like to thank my children, Jennifer and Ashley, for their support and for being themselves—intelligent, talented, beautiful daughters.

Personal Acknowledgments from Mary Jo Goolsby

I whole-heartedly express thanks to my dear friend and colleague, Laurie. After serving together as faculty for several years, I have had the pleasure and honor or working with Laurie for almost 20 years on this project.

Above all else, I also thank my husband, H. G. Goolsby. He continues to offer constant support and encouragement, without which this and other professional achievements would not have been possible.

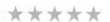

Contributors

Sara F. Barber, MSN, APRN-BC
Pediatric Nurse Practitioner, Psychiatric/Mental Health
  Nurse Practitioner
Capital City Psychiatry
Tallahassee, Florida

James T. Blackwell, DNP, FNP-BC
Nurse Practitioner
WG (Bill) Hefner VA Medical Center
Charlotte, NC

Lisa Byrd APRN, PhD, FNP-BC, GNP-BC,
  Gerontologist
Nurse Practitioner
Devoted Medical Group
Tampa, Florida
Assistant Professor
University of South Alabama
Mobile, Alabama

Maria Colandrea, NP-C, CORLN, CCRN, FAANP
Clinical Consulting Faculty, Duke University
Durham, North Carolina
Nurse Practitioner
Durham Veterans Affairs Medical Center
Cary, North Carolina

Leslie L. Davis, PhD, RN, ANP-BC, FAANP, FACC,
  FAHA, FPCNA
Associate Professor
University of North Carolina at Chapel Hill
School of Nursing

Janatha S. Grant, DNP, CRNP, FNP-BC
Nurse Practitioner, Division of Maternal & Fetal
  Medicine
The University of Alabama at Birmingham
Birmingham, Alabama

Aimee C. Holland DNP, CRNP, WHNP-BC,
  NP-C, FAANP
Associate Professor and Assistant Dean for Graduate
  Clinical Education
University of Alabama at Birmingham
Birmingham, AL

Anna R. Jessup, DNP, APRN, FNP-C
Assistant Professor and Nursing Program Director
South University
Round Rock, TX

Michelle Lajiness, APRN, FNP-BC
Nurse Practitioner
University of Toledo Medical Center
Department of Urology
Toledo, Ohio

Karen D. Lipford, PMHNP-C, FNP, EdD, DNP
Teaching Faculty, Florida State University,
  College of Nursing
Tallahassee, FL
Psychiatric Nurse Practitioner, Florida Therapy
  Services, Inc.
Chattahoochee, FL

Ann Maradiegue, PhD, RN, FNP-BC, FAANP
Consultant, Genetics Education and Patient Advocacy
Washington, DC

Vanessa Pomarico-Denino, Ed.D, APRN,
  FNP-BC, FAANP
Lead Clinician, Diversity, Inclusion & Diversity
Northeast Internal Medical Group
Hamden, CT
Part-time Clinical Assistant Professor
Quinnipiac University School of Nursing
North Haven, CDT

Susanne Quallich, PhD, ANP-BC, NP-C,
     CUNP, FAANP
Andrology Nurse Practitioner
Division of Andrology and Microsurgery
Department of Urology
University of Michigan Health System
Ann Arbor, Michigan

Diane Seibert, PhD, RN, ANP, WHNP-BC,
     FAANP
Professor
Associate Dean for Academic Affairs
Daniel K. Inouye Graduate School of Nursing
Uniformed Services University
Bethesda, Maryland

Kelley Stallworth Borella, DNP, MSN,
     WHNP-BC
Assistant Professor, Co-Specialty Track Coordinator
University of Alabama at Birmingham
Birmingham, Alabama

Ashton T. Strachan, DNP, FNP-C, WHNP-BC
Nurse Practitioner
Georgia Institute of Technology
Atlanta, GA
Adjunct Faculty
University of Alabama at Birmingham
Birmingham, AL

Brandy Tanner, DNP, WHNP-BC
Lead APP
UAB OB Complications Clinic
Birmingham, Alabama

Karen J. Whitt, PhD, AGN-BC, FNP-C, FAANP
Associate Professor
George Washington University School of Nursing
Washington, DC

Michael E. Zychowicz, DNP, ONP, ANP, FAAN,
     FAANP
Professor; Lead Faculty Orthopedic NP Specialty
Co-Director, Duke-Durham VA Primary Care Residency
Duke University
Durham, NC

Reviewers

Margaret Rose Benz, MSN(R), APRN, ANP-BC, FAANP
Assistant Professor
Trudy Busch Valentine, Saint Louis University School of Nursing
Saint Louis, MO

Jordon D. Bosse, PhD, RN
Assistant Professor
Northeastern University, School of Nursing
Boston, MS

Angie Thomure, MPH, MSN, APRN-CRN
Nurse Practitioner
Cincinatti, OH

MaryAnn Troiano, DNP, APN-C
Associate Professor
Monmouth University
West Long Branch, NJ

Contents

PART

I

The Art of Assessment and Clinical Decision Making

Chapter 1

Clinical Decision Making: Assessment and Differential Diagnosis

Mary Jo Goolsby ·

Laurie Grubbs ·

C linical decision making is often fraught with uncertainties. According to a recent report (Bernstein, 2017), in one facility more than 20% of persons presenting for second opinions had been misdiagnosed. Croskerry (2013) estimates that the overall diagnostic failure rate is as high as 15%. Estimates from a recent study specific to U.S. outpatient diagnostic errors suggests that about 5% of outpatient adults had a diagnostic error (Singh et al., 2014).

Croskerry (2013) describes two major types of clinical diagnostic decision making: intuitive and analytical. Intuitive decision making (i.e., fast system) is consistent with the "Augenblick diagnosis," that is, one made in "the blink of an eye," because the clinician relies on experience and intuition and the diagnosis occurs rapidly and with little effort (Croskerry, 2013, p. 2445). However, while experienced diagnosticians' intuitions are often correct, this process can result in dangerous errors. Intuitive decision making is less reliable and is paired with fairly common errors. In contrast, analytical decision making (i.e., slow system) is based on careful consideration, takes more time and effort, and has greater reliability with fewer errors. Because practice settings present a number of distractors and competing demands, it is critical that diagnosticians step back, assess their processes and the data they are gathering, and attend to the possibilities.

Diagnostic reasoning involves a complex process that can be quickly clouded by first impressions. The need to ensure necessary "data" requires a measured approach, even when faced with common complaints such as chest pain. This requires a consistent and deliberate approach to symptom analysis, physical assessment, and data analysis. Expert diagnosticians are more able to maintain a degree of suspicion throughout the assessment process, consider a range of potential explanations, and then generate and narrow their differential diagnosis on the basis of their previous experience, familiarity with the evidence related to various diagnoses, and understanding of their individual patient. Through the process, clinicians perform assessment techniques involving both the history and the physical examination in an effective, purposeful, and reliable manner and then select appropriate diagnostic studies to support their assessment.

The importance of diagnostic reasoning and expertise is gaining recognition. The Society to Improve Diagnosis in Medicine (improvediagnosis.org) and the Society of Bedside Medicine (bedsidemedicine.org) offer a number of resources for clinicians and educators, designed to enhance clinical decision making and address diagnostic error.

Cultural Sensitivity in Assessment and Differential Diagnosis

In discussing health assessment and differential diagnosis, it is essential to consider the importance of maintaining awareness of the broad range of ways in which cultural, geographic, linguistic, and other factors impact health and outcomes. While clinician cultural sensitivity and cultural competence often are mentioned as specific constructs, in fact they are entwined with many factors affecting a given patient's ability to receive high-quality and appropriate care (AHRQ, 2014).

A couple of overarching objectives promote cultural sensitivity to the patients and families we serve—knowing ourselves and knowing our patients. First, clinicians must consider their own background and experiences as they relate to our personal values and biases, recognizing that these are not shared by all we encounter. Next, they must strive to individuate each patient (i.e., to be open to knowing each patient as an individual rather than an aggregate representation of a specific culture, religion, community, or other component with which the patient may identify). This means asking our patients about any beliefs, habits, or concerns they as individuals have and how they prefer to receive information, discuss their health, and so on. Achieving these objectives requires knowing ourselves and knowing our patients in a way that allows us to practice the "platinum rule," which is often mentioned related to cultural sensitivity—treating our patients as *they* would like to be treated.

There are many resources available to clinicians to promote culturally sensitive care. One resource available from the CMS Office of Minority Health (CMS, 2016) identifies standards and relevant resources for providing culturally and linguistically appropriate services (CLAS) for a range of populations, including patients with disabilities, limited English proficiency and/or low health literacy, and patients of racial and ethnic or sexual and gender minorities. The principal CLAS standard is the provision of "effective, equitable, understandable, and respectful quality care and services that are responsive to diverse cultural health beliefs and practices, preferred languages, health literacy, and other communication needs" (CMS, 2016, p. 9); in other words, truly patient-centered care and communication. While a myriad of resources exist to promote CLAS, this guide provides a list and summary of relevant resources, specific to different populations. Resources include papers with background information, tools, and forms that can be used in practice, training materials, and resources to share with patients.

This book includes specific chapters on persons with disabilities (mobility and sensory), transgender patients, and groups such as older adults. Within the assessment and differential diagnosis, key information specific to unique groups is noted. For instance, this chapter describes the use of translators and interpreters for written and verbal communication when patients speak a language different from that of the clinician. Chapter 2 stresses the importance of discussing diagnostic test options with each patient to determine their acceptance, limitations, or concerns related to the plan. Chapter 3 describes populations at heightened genetic risk for specified conditions. Chapter 4 notes populations who often have delayed diagnosis of skin cancer and resultant worsened outcomes. Other examples are embedded in each chapter. However, the content is generally provided with the expectation that the reader will strive toward cultural competence as they engage in obtaining a history, conducting a physical examination, considering diagnostic options, and so on.

History

The ability to perform a fact-finding history is essential to a valid diagnosis. To obtain adequate history, providers must be well organized, attentive to the patient's verbal and nonverbal language, and able to accurately interpret the patient's responses to questions. Rather than reading into the patient's statements, providers clarify any areas of uncertainty. The expert history, like the expert physical examination, is informed by the knowledge of a wide range of conditions, their physiological bases, and their associated signs and symptoms.

The ability to draw out descriptions of patients' symptoms and experiences is important because only patients can tell their own story. To assist patients in describing a complaint, a skilled interviewer asks salient and focused questions to gather necessary information without straying (i.e., avoiding a shotgun approach that lacks focus). The provider should know, based on the chief complaint and any preceding information, what other questions are essential to the history. It is important to determine why the symptom brought the patient to the office—that is, the significance of this symptom to the patient, which may uncover the patient's anxiety and the basis for the patient's concern. It may also help to determine severity in a stoic patient who may underestimate or underreport symptoms.

Throughout the process of taking the history, it is important to recognize that patients may forget details, so probing questions may be necessary. Patients sometimes have trouble finding the precise words to describe their complaint; they may be apprehensive about using the wrong term. However, good descriptors are necessary to isolate the cause, source, and location of symptoms. Often, patients must be encouraged to use common language and terminology. For instance, encourage patients to describe the problem just as they would describe it to a relative or neighbor, using common terms. Additionally, neophyte providers can be led down the wrong path by patients who have already diagnosed themselves prior to their visit.

The history should include specific components (summarized in Table 1.1) to ensure that the problem is comprehensively evaluated. The questions to include in each component of the history are described in detail in subsequent chapters.

Table 1.1

Components of History

Component	Purpose
Chief complaint	Provides "title" for the encounter. To determine the reason patient seeks care. Important to consider using the patient's terminology. For instance, why the patients made the specific appointment, what led them to seek care.
History of present illness	To provide a thorough description of the chief complaint and current problem. Suggested format: **P-Q-R-S-T**, detailed below.
• **P:** precipitating and palliative factors	To identify factors that may have triggered the symptom, make it better or worse, and any response to previously prescribed or self-treatment.
• **Q:** quality and quantity descriptors	To quantify patient's rating of symptom (e.g., pain on a 1–10 scale) and obtain descriptors (e.g., numbness, burning, stabbing).
• **R:** region and radiation	To identify the exact location of the symptom, as well as any area of radiation.
• **S:** severity and associated symptoms	To identify the symptom's severity (e.g., how bad at its worst) and any associated symptoms (e.g., presence or absence of nausea and vomiting associated with chest pain).
• **T:** timing and temporal descriptions	To identify when complaint was first noticed; how it has changed/progressed since onset (e.g., remained the same or worsened/improved); whether onset was acute or chronic; whether it has been constant, intermittent, or recurrent.
Past medical history	To identify the patient's past and concurrent diagnoses, surgeries, hospitalizations, injuries, allergies, immunizations, current medications.
Habits	To describe any use of tobacco, alcohol, drugs, and to identify patterns of sleep, exercise, etc.
Sociocultural	To identify occupational and recreational activities and experiences, living environment, financial status/support as related to health-care needs, travel, lifestyle, etc.
Family history	To identify relevant potential sources of hereditary diseases; a genogram is helpful. The minimum includes first-degree relatives (i.e., parents, siblings, children), although second and third orders are helpful.
Review of systems	To review a list of possible symptoms that the patient may have noted in each of the body systems.

Content on communicating with patients who have physical communication deficits is provided in Chapter 23. However, clinicians may encounter patients who communicate using languages different from those of the provider. In these instances, alternative communication methods such as using an interpreter for spoken language or a translator for written content are critical in obtaining a necessary health history to support a valid assessment and diagnosis.

When the patient speaks a different language from the interviewer, an interpreter who is fluent in the languages of both the patient and the provider must be called upon. The interpreter should be impartial, have experience in interpreting health-related information, and understand the importance of confidentiality and of accurately conveying each party's communication. The patient's permission is needed prior to involving an interpreter.

When using an interpreter, questions should be as succinct as possible and understanding should be validated by the interpreter. The clinician should face and speak to the patient, rather than to the interpreter, being sensitive to body language and expressions.

Physical Examination

The expert diagnostician must also be able to accurately perform a purposeful or hypothesis-driven (Garibaldi & Olson, 2018) physical assessment. For instance, each chief complaint and history should trigger to plan for which areas to examine, using a focused approach rather than a head-to-toe physical.

Extensive, repetitive practice; exposure to a range of normal variants and abnormal findings; and keen observation skills are required to develop physical examination proficiency. Each component of the physical examination must be performed correctly to ensure that findings are as valid and reliable as possible. In addition to referring to the accuracy of each maneuver, optimal performance also requires that the body part being examined be visible in order to fully examine it. In other words, the skin over the chest should be visible during palpation, percussion, and auscultation, and the skin over the knee should be visible during palpation, percussion, and any stress maneuvers. Otherwise, the examiner risks missing physical deformity or scars relevant to the diagnosis. Examination through clothing is a dangerous habit and can result in missed examination findings. Chapter 23 describes assessment of patients with physical disabilities.

While performing the physical examination, the examiner must be able to

- tailor the examination to the individual and history.
- differentiate between normal and abnormal findings.
- recall knowledge of a range of conditions, including their associated signs and symptoms.
- recognize how certain conditions affect the response to other conditions in ways that are not entirely predictable.
- distinguish the relevance of varied abnormal findings.
- notate findings accurately.

The aspects of physical examination are summarized in the following chapters using a systems approach. Each chapter also reviews the relevant examination for varied complaints. Along with obtaining an accurate history and performing a physical examination, it is crucial that the clinician consider the patient's vital signs, general appearance, and condition when making clinical decisions.

Diagnostic Studies

The history and physical assessment findings help to guide the selection of diagnostic studies. For instance, diagnostic studies often assist when a diagnosis remains uncertain after the history or physical examination, when the severity or degree of the condition is uncertain, or when a critical diagnosis must be ruled out. Just as the history should be relevant and focused, the selection of diagnostic studies should be judicious and directed toward specific conditions under consideration. Content on selection of diagnostic studies is provided in Chapter 2.

Clinical Decision Resources

Depending on the amount of experience in assessing patients with a presenting complaint, a diagnostician uses varied systems through which information is processed and decisions are made. However, experience is not always adequate to support accurate clinical decision making, and memory is not perfect. To assist in clinical decision making, a number of evidence-based resources have been developed to assist the clinician. Resources such as algorithms and clinical practice guidelines assist in clinical reasoning when properly applied.

Algorithms are formulas or procedures for problem-solving and include both decision trees and clinical prediction rules. Decision trees provide a graphical depiction of the decision-making process, showing the pathway based on findings at various steps in the process. A decision tree begins with a chief complaint or physical finding and then leads the diagnostician through a series of decision nodes. Each decision node or decision point provides a question or statement regarding the presence or absence of some clinical finding. The response to each of these decision points determines the next step. (An example of a decision tree is provided in Fig. 14.5, which illustrates a decision-making process for amenorrhea.) These decision trees are helpful in identifying a logical sequence for the decisions involved in narrowing the differential diagnosis and providing cues to questions that should be answered and/or tests that should be performed through the diagnostic process. A decision tree should be accompanied by a description of the strength of the evidence on which it has been developed as well as a description of the settings and/or patient population to which it relates.

Clinical decision (or prediction) rules provide another support for clinical reasoning. Clinical decision rules are evidence-based resources that provide probabilistic statements regarding the likelihood that a condition exists if certain variables are met with regard to the prognosis of patients with specific findings. Decision rules use mathematical models and are specific to certain situations, settings, and/or patient characteristics. They are used to express the diagnostic statistics described earlier. The number of decision, or predictive, rules is growing, and select examples are included in this text. For instance, the Ottawa ankle and foot rules are described in the discussion of musculoskeletal pain in Chapter 15. The Gail Model, a well-established rule relevant to screening for breast cancer, is discussed in Chapter 10. Many of the rules involve complex mathematical calculations, but others are simple. In addition to discussions of tools, this text provides several sources of electronic "calculators" based on rules. Box 1.1 includes a limited list of sites with clinical prediction calculators. These resources should be accompanied by information describing the methods by which the rule was validated.

Clinical practice guidelines have also been developed for the assessment and diagnosis of various conditions. They are typically developed by national advisory panels of clinical experts who base the guidelines on the best available evidence. Like decision trees and diagnostic rules, guidelines should be accompanied by a description of their supporting evidence and the situations in which they should be applied.

These resources are not without limitations, and it is essential that they be applied in the situations for which they were intended. In applying these tools to clinical situations, it is essential that the diagnostician determine the population for which the tool was developed, ensure the tool is applicable to the case at hand, and have accurate data to consider in the tool's application. For instance, a clinical prediction rule based on a population of young adult college students is not valid if applied to an older patient. The provider must also recognize that these resources are intended to assist in the interpretation of a range of clinical evidence relevant to a particular problem, but they are not intended to take the place of clinical judgment, which rests with the provider.

BOX 1.1

Online Sources of Medical Calculators

Essential Evidence Plus

www.essentialevidenceplus.com

MedCalc 3000 Online Clinical Calculators

www.calc.med.edu/cc-idx.htm

Medical Algorithms Project

medicalalgorithms.com

Note: Sites active as of January 27, 2021. Most require subscriptions.

The Differential Diagnosis

Clinical decision making begins when the patient first voices the reason for seeking care. Expert clinicians immediately compare their patients' complaints with the "catalog" of knowledge that they have stored about a range of clinical conditions and then determine the direction of their initial history and symptom analysis. However, as mentioned earlier, it is crucial that the provider not jump to conclusions or be biased by one particular finding; information is continually processed to inform decisions that guide further data collection and to begin to detect patterns in the data.

As data are collected through the history and physical examination, providers tailor their approach to subsequent data collection. They begin to detect patterns that guide the development of a differential diagnosis that is based on an understanding of probability and prognosis. This means that conditions considered are those that most commonly cause the perceived cluster of data (probability) as well as conditions that may be less common but would require urgent detection and action (prognosis). This leads to the development of a differential diagnosis, which is "a list of possible diagnoses ranked from the most probable to least probable, based on the available information" (National Academies of Sciences, 2015, p. 166).

Differential diagnosis goes beyond the more rapid diagnostic thinking to involve analytical consideration. Here, the diagnostician contemplates the likelihood of each condition being considered and determines what further information is needed to refine the differential. Care is required to consider a range of options, as a condition that does not "make the cut" for inclusion in the differential diagnosis is usually not explored, thus its omission may result in a missed or wrong diagnosis.

Memorable adages are frequently used to encourage novice diagnosticians to always consider clinical explanations that are most likely to explain a patient's situation. For instance, students often are told, "Common diseases occur commonly." Using the term *zebra* to refer to less likely or rare explanations for a presentation, another adage suggests, "When you hear hooves in Central Park, don't look for zebras." Both adages direct novices to consider the most likely explanation for a set of findings. This text is designed to enhance the process of differential diagnosis. Each chapter identifies common conditions to be considered in the differential diagnosis of common complaints, as well as some less common but potentially urgent possibilities. With the emergence of conditions, "zebras" may well be responsible for findings, and providers must always maintain some level of suspicion for these less common explanations.

Thus, even though it is appropriate that conditions with high probabilities be considered in the differential diagnosis, it is also vital in the diagnostic process to consider conditions that put the patient at highest risk. To do otherwise places the patient in jeopardy of life-threatening or disabling complications. Indications of these life-threatening situations are often referred to as *red flags*, which are clues signaling the high likelihood of an urgent situation requiring immediate identification and management. This text includes red flags for the various systems to promote their recognition in clinical practice. Chapter 3, on genomic assessment, describes genetic patterns to promote identification of patients at higher risks of certain hereditary conditions.

Development of a differential diagnosis is not a "one and done" process. It is iterative. As new information is gathered, the list of possible conditions may be narrowed or expanded. As the potential list of conditions in the differential diagnosis develops, the provider determines what, if any, further history, physical examination, or diagnostic studies are warranted to confirm or rule out specific diagnoses. Knowledge of the specificity and sensitivity of different maneuvers or tests for given diagnoses is helpful in the selection process. The diagnostician combines the knowledge gained through the history and physical assessment with the findings from any diagnostic studies to assess the probability for the conditions remaining in the differential diagnosis.

The development and narrowing of a differential diagnosis also require the clinician to be present, or mindful and aware of, the mental process involved. It is important to establish a routine through which to confirm that an adequate assessment and analysis has occurred, free of distraction, and that the differential diagnosis does include those items that must be considered and ruled in or out, based on the likelihood that they are responsible for the presentation and the potential for serious harm if excluded too early.

The following case study illustrates the diagnostic process, including the initial differential diagnosis.

CASE 1.1. Jon, a relatively new nurse practitioner, encounters Marge, who is a new patient to his practice. Their encounter is summarized below:

CC and HPI: Marge is 58 years old and presents with fatigue and difficulty catching her breath. The history of present illness reveals that she has coughed frequently for months, which she thought might be allergies, but the fatigue and shortness of breath have come on over the past 2 months. Asked about any previous symptoms in the past, she responds, "Not exactly," and then says she was treated twice for bronchitis in the last 12 or 13 months. Both bouts included a severe cough accompanied by shortness of breath, but they also included yellow sputum and fever each time. She was prescribed antibiotics both times, and by the time the prescription was completed, the shortness of breath resolved and she was doing fine until recently. She is not a current smoker. She was able to quit successfully on her 58th birthday, after a 40-year history of smoking one pack per day.

Past Medical History: Marge's past medical history is negative for asthma and any respiratory conditions other than the ones mentioned. She does have T2 diabetes, hypertension, and elevated lipids, all of which are treated and fairly controlled. Her surgical history includes a hysterectomy at age 45 due to uterine fibroids, bilateral cataract removals 2 years ago, and an appendectomy at age 16.

Current Medications: She lists the following medications: metformin 500 mg bid, HCTZ 25 mg daily, enalapril 10 mg daily, atenolol 25 mg daily, and atorvastatin 10 mg daily.

Psychosocial History

Marge says she routinely works 2 days a week as a sales associate in a local department store and volunteers 1 day a week at the local library. However, she has recently taken a leave from her volunteer role and decreased from 8-hour to 4-hour workdays at the store because of the fatigue. She used to walk daily but has not felt like it lately. She says, "It is all I can do to make the bed some days!"

Physical Examination

The physical examination findings reveal:

- Vital signs: T 98, BP 138/86, HR 92, RR 34, HT 64, WT 155 lb.
- General: Appearance in no acute distress. Alert and oriented. Well groomed. Articulate and seems to be a good historian. Fluid movements.
- HEENT: Normal.
- CV: RR&R. S1/S2 without audible extra sounds or murmurs.
- Respiratory: Initially some crackles, which cleared with forceful cough. Decreased breath sounds, slight wheeze noted. Slight increased AP/lateral ratio.
- Skin: Intact, pink, resilient. No rashes or lesions noted.
- MS/Extremities: Full ROM, non-pitting edema ankles/feet bilaterally. Pulses 2+ bilaterally.

As Jon interviews and examines Marge, he begins mentally to formulate a differential diagnosis. He takes a couple of minutes to review his history and the list of potential diagnoses. The differential diagnosis includes the following conditions:

- Chronic obstructive pulmonary disease (COPD) seems the most likely, as Marge is a former smoker with 40-pack-a-year history, history of infectious bronchitis, chronic cough, increased AP/lateral ratio, decreased breath sounds.
- Heart failure is also included with the history of recent onset fatigue, cough, and shortness of breath; mild edema; history of hypertension and hyperlipidemia.
- Bronchiectasis should be considered due to recent onset shortness of breath and cough, fatigue; recent infectious bronchitis.
- Malignancy is one of the "urgencies" he chooses as Marge is a former smoker with 40-pack-a-year history.
- Asthma is low on the list. She does have recent onset shortness of breath and cough; unlikely, but it is listed as a remote cause.
- Angiotensin-converting enzyme (ACE) inhibitor–induced cough is noteworthy, but seems unlikely with symptoms beyond the cough.

As he reviews his list, Jon recognizes that he needs some more details that he omitted.

First, he elaborates in the history, asking about the following:

- **Presence of sputum, then the amount and color:** Marge admits some sputum although hard to quantitate and it varies. However, she says it is not yellow like before.
- **When cough is worst, when the shortness of breath is worst, and any triggers:** The cough is intermittent and can be very severe, to the point she feels she might not be able to catch her breath. The shortness of breath is worst with activity. Both are not as noticeable while resting.
- **Whether she is able to sleep flat or has to sit or elevate her head to sleep:** Says she uses one pillow, as she has for years.
- **Details regarding her current medications, focusing on any recent additions or dosage changes:** She has had no recent change in the drugs or dosages in at least 2 years.
- **Any hobbies or situations in which she is exposed to dust, chemicals, irritants, strong odors:** She denies all of these.
- **Family history of chronic lung disease, heart disease, or cancers:** Her family history of chronic lung disease is negative. Her aunt had breast cancer in middle age. Her parents had high blood pressure, but no known heart attacks or heart failure.

Next Jon checks a few additional items on the physical examination:

- Checking her neck for jugular distention or bruits reveals neither.
- Her PMI is not displaced.
- No abdominal organomegaly detected.
- A brief neurological exam is normal.
- Her nailbeds are pink with prompt refill, and there is no clubbing.

While Jon is not ready to significantly narrow or alter his differential diagnosis, he decides that drug-induced cough is very unlikely, as is asthma. He still ranks COPD as the most likely cause and orders an in-clinic chest x-ray, spirometry, and laboratory CBC and chemistry panel. The chest x-ray reveals a flattened diaphragm; no masses, cardiac enlargement, or other abnormalities are detected. The spirometry results measure FEV_1: 58% of predicted, FVC: 70% of predicted, and FEV_1/FVC: 54%. Both the CBC and chemistry panels are within normal limits.

At this point, the working diagnosis is COPD, Stage II.

Notes: This case depicts the process of working through clinical decision making with a new patient. By creating a differential diagnosis, Jon was able to recognize some gaps in the data initially obtained and was able to complete the history and physical to arrive at the likely diagnosis. He also would be able to document significant negatives to support his decision making and to serve as future reference.

While this case study was resolved during one visit, there are times when urgent explanations have been ruled out, yet a definitive diagnosis is not confirmed. In these situations, options include moving forward with additional diagnostic measures, including further history, physical examination, diagnostic studies, and/or referral or consultation. Another option, depending on the patient's condition, involves waiting briefly before further diagnostic studies are performed in order to see whether the condition declares itself. In this case, serial assessments should be scheduled over a period of days or weeks in order to arrive at a diagnosis. An important factor involved in the decision to wait is the patient's ability and willingness to return for follow-up at the specified intervals. In situations such as emergency department or urgent care visits, the clinician has no long-term relationship with the patient, and the likelihood of the patient returning for follow-up is greatly decreased. A plan should be in place to complete the assessment and diagnosis, and the patient should be informed of and should verbalize understanding of the plan as well as what symptoms would warrant reconsideration. Missed diagnosis and delayed diagnosis are among the most common causes of malpractice complaints, particularly the failure to diagnose myocardial infarctions and breast cancer.

Although not always to the patient's advantage, patient expectations often play a part in clinical decision making. Some patients are less willing to wait; others are less willing to be treated. This can be the cause for errors, and clinicians should be aware that they should try to accommodate patients' wishes without putting them at risk.

Box 1.2 includes a list of common diagnostic errors. Although the list is far from exhaustive, avoidance of these errors will improve clinical decision making.

BOX 1.2

Common Diagnostic Errors

- Failure to take "time out" to consider the diagnostic process
- Failure to develop differential diagnoses, comparing each with presentation
- Jumping to conclusions or being biased by an early finding (e.g., something in the patient's medical history or recheck from a previous visit)
- Accepting previous diagnosis/explanation without exploring other possible explanations (e.g., diagnosis of chronic bronchitis as explanation of chronic cough in patient on ACE inhibitor)
- Using a "shotgun approach" to assessment without adequate focus
- Focusing solely on the most obvious or likely explanation
- Relying solely on memory, which limits the diagnostician's knowledge and options to only what is memorized or readily recalled
- Using the wrong rule, decision tree, or other resource to guide analysis or using the correct device incorrectly

BOX 1.2—cont'd

Common Diagnostic Errors

- Performing skills improperly
- Misinterpreting or using wrong data
- Allowing the patient to make diagnosis (e.g., "I had sinusitis last year, and the symptoms are exactly the same.")
- Allowing other health-care professionals to lead the diagnosis in the wrong direction
- Accepting the "horses" without contemplating the "zebras"; contemplating "zebras" without adequately pursuing the possibility of a more common condition
- Accommodating patient wishes against clinician judgment
- Ignoring basic findings, such as vital signs
- Failing to consider medical conditions as the source of "psychiatric" symptoms and psychiatric conditions as the source of "medical" symptoms

Summary

The content of this book is directed toward assisting clinicians to adequately assess presenting complaints and then to consider reasonable explanations for the complaint and findings. For each complaint, a summary of the relevant history and physical assessment is provided, along with a list of conditions that should be considered in the differential diagnosis. The lists of conditions are not exhaustive. However, by noting the possibility of those included, clinicians will consider various potential etiologies and, by weighing the likelihood of these options, begin to develop critical-thinking skills necessary for clinical decision making. Very brief descriptions of the possible findings for each of the conditions are listed to help guide the reader in recognizing definitive clusters of signs and symptoms.

Above all, practice and experience provide the skills necessary for accurate diagnosis. These skills are supported by lifelong learning through which clinicians maintain an awareness of the highest level of evidence relative to assessment and diagnosis.

REFERENCES

Agency for Healthcare Research and Quality (July 9, 2014). Improving cultural competence to reduce health disparities for priority populations. www.effectivehealthcare.ahrq.gov

Bernstein, L. (2017). 20 percent of patients with serious conditions are first misdiagnosed, study says. *The Washington Post.* https://www.washingtonpost.com/national/health-science/20-percent-of-patients-with-serious-conditions-are-first-misdiagnosed-study-says/2017/04/03/e386982a-189f-11e7-9887-1a5314b56a08_story.html?utm_term=.b0775c60f376

Centers of Medicare and Medicaid Services (CMS), Office of Minority Health (OMH) (2016). A practical guide to implementing the national CLAS standards: For racial, ethnic and linguistic minorities, people with disabilities and sexual gender minorities. https://www.cms.gov/About-CMS/Agency-Information/OMH/Downloads/CLAS-Toolkit-12-7-16.pdf.

Croskerry, P. (2013). From mindless to mindful practice—Cognitive bias and clinical decision making. *New England Journal of Medicine 368*(26), 2445–2448. https://doi.org/10.1056/NEJMp1303712

Garibaldi, B., & Olson, A. (2018). The hypothesis-driven physical examination. *Medical Clinics of North America, 102*(3), 433–442. https://doi.org/10.1016/j.mcna.2017.12.005

National Academies of Sciences, Engineering, and Medicine (2015). Diagnostic team members and tasks: Improving patient engagement and health care professional education and training in diagnosis. In *Improving diagnosis in health care* (pp 136–216). The National Academies Press. https://doi.org/10.17226/21794

Singh, H., Meyer, A., & Thomas, E. (2014). The frequency of diagnostic errors in outpatient care: Estimations from three large observational studies involving US adult populations. *BMJ Quality & Safety, 23*(9), 727–731. https://doi.org/10.1136/bmjqs-2013-002627

Chapter 2

Diagnostic Studies

Mary Jo Goolsby •
Laurie Grubbs •

C hapter 1 introduced issues related to clinical decision making. One source of potential clinical decision problems involves selecting, ordering, and interpreting diagnostic studies. Although laboratory and imaging studies are commonly ordered in clinical practice, most academic training programs offer limited content on their selection and interpretation. Yet in refining a differential diagnosis, judiciously and appropriately choosing and interpreting diagnostic tests are key skills for clinicians.

Reasons Diagnostic Studies Are Ordered

As part of a hypothesis-driven examination, it is essential to be purposeful in ordering diagnostic tests such as laboratory studies and imaging. This starts with knowing how each test ordered will be used and ensuring that the right study is selected for that purpose. In general, the uses of diagnostic studies fall into three broad categories: screening, diagnosis, and management, as described in Table 2.1.

Beyond the purpose for which diagnostic studies may be indicated, the literature identifies a number of other issues clinicians must consider when ordering diagnostic studies such as laboratory tests. These are summarized in Table 2.2.

Test Accuracy and Validity

The accuracy and validity of a given diagnostic test often is reflected by statistics on the test's sensitivity and specificity, positive and negative predictive values, and likelihood ratio. These contribute differently to a clinician's understanding of clinical or physical examination findings and to clinical decision making.

Sensitivity and specificity statistics are calculated exclusively from actual results of individuals either with a disease (sensitivity) or without a disease (specificity), not from results of the general population. They do not reflect the prevalence of a disease in a community or setting. Furthermore, there is a trade-off between sensitivity and specificity. If the diagnostic set point is altered

Table 2.1

Uses of Laboratory Tests

Purpose	Example
Screening	As part of preventive care, screening tests are used to identify risk factors, as well as occult disease. Screening recommendations are established by clinical experts and organizations using the best available evidence. Examples include screening for prostate cancer (PSA), diabetes (glucose), breast cancer (mammogram), and colon cancer (colonoscopy).
Diagnosis	As part of the diagnostic process, tests are used to either rule out or confirm conditions included in a differential diagnosis. They often contribute to staging or determining severity of a condition. Examples include heterophile antibody test (Monospot) for mononucleosis or thyroid-stimulating hormone (TSH) for thyroid disorders.
Management	For established conditions, tests contribute to disease management by providing information on response to treatment, progression, remission, or recurrence. Examples include periodic lipid panels for hypercholesterolemia or complete blood count (CBC) following treatment of iron-deficiency anemia.

Table 2.2

Issues to Consider in Diagnostic Study Selection

Issues	Explanation
Purpose of Study	See Table 2.1.
Accuracy and predictive value of test for individual patient	A general awareness of how statistics such as specificity and sensitivity for various studies relate to a specific patient is important. These are important in establishing the validity of diagnostic studies. See Box 2.1.
Availability of safe and effective treatment	If the purpose of a test is to diagnose a condition, consider whether safe or effective treatments exist for the suspected condition. Comorbidities may make the potential for treatment ineffective or require additional testing to determine how, if at all, one condition may impact the other.
Clinician's ability to accurately interpret	The clinician's ability to interpret the results affects a test's contribution to decision making. Some tests require highly specialized knowledge and experience for accurate interpretation. As needed, consulting with or referring to a specialist may be warranted to assist with the workup.
Explanation of test and potential treatment to patient	Consider the patient's perspective, providing information on the study's purpose, related procedure, and anticipated application, allowing time for questions.
Cost and convenience	Determine whether alternative options are available at a lower cost or if previous test results are adequate. Determine whether completing the test is feasible for the patient.

so that if either sensitivity or specificity is strengthened, the other is decreased. Sensitivity and specificity are briefly described in Box 2.1.

Positive predictive values (PPVs) and negative predictive values (NPVs) are based exclusively on populations who either tested positive (i.e., PPV) or tested negative (i.e., NPV). They often better reflect the value of a positive or negative finding in a general population. Furthermore, if a community s disease

Box 2.1

Sensitivity and Specificity

Sensitivity: The percentage of patients who have the disease or condition who will test positive with the test. The more sensitive the test, the greater is the probability that a patient with the disease will test positive and the better the test is at identifying persons with the disease (i.e., true positives). The higher the sensitivity, the less likely it is that the test will have false negatives for the condition. Out of a population of subjects who have the disease, a test with 0.95 sensitivity will detect 95% of them, with false negatives resulting for the remaining 5%. Thus, the higher the sensitivity, the more likely that a negative value reflects a subject without the disease.

   Specificity: The percentage of patients without the disease or condition who will test negative. The more specific a test, the greater is the probability that a patient without the disease will test negative and the better it detects those without the disease (i.e., true negatives). A high-specificity test is helpful in confirming a diagnosis because false positives are less likely. Out of a population of subjects without the disease, a test with 0.95 specificity will result in negative findings for 95% of those without the disease, with 5% false positives among those without the disease. Thus, the higher the specificity, the more likely it is that a positive test reflects one with the disease.

Examples of sensitivity and specificity:

1. *A rapid strep test is described as being 95% sensitive and 98% specific for streptococcus. Your patient with a sore throat has self-diagnosed as having "strep throat" but tests negative to a rapid strep screen. The decision to treat could be influenced by the knowledge that false negatives are rare combined with your overall assessment. If the test were positive, the specificity for streptococcal infection paired with your findings would influence the decision to treat, recognizing that the risk of false positives is low. However, when dealing with high-risk conditions such as strep throat, which could have sequelae, a confirmatory test (such as culture) is often advisable, as even a 5% likelihood (1 in 20) of a false negative may be unacceptable.*

2. *A 35-year-old woman presents with a palpable breast mass. The ACR Appropriateness Criteria notes that ultrasound has a higher sensitivity than mammogram in this age group (95.7% and 60.9%, respectively). Specificity is 89.2% for ultrasound and 94.4% for mammogram. The recommendation is for ultrasound as the first image, unless risk factors or clinical examination suggest otherwise (ACR, 2016). It is important to recognize that about 4% will have false-positive findings and 11% false negatives.*

Box 2.2

Positive and Negative Predictive Values

Positive Predictive Value	The percentage of patients with a positive test result who have the condition of interest. The higher the PPV, the less likely the test results in a false positive. Out of a population of subjects with a positive test result with a 0.95 PPV, 95% will have been correctly identified; the remaining 5% will be false positives.
Negative Predictive Value	The percentage of patients testing as negative who do not have the condition of interest. A NPV of 0.95 indicates that 95% of those testing negative will have been correctly ruled out; the remaining 5% will be false negatives (i.e., have a negative result while having the condition).

Examples of Predictive Values

1. The PPV and NPV of a rapid influenza test are dependent on the prevalence of influenza in a specific community. If the prevalence is "moderate," then the rapid test PPV ranges from 38% to 56%, meaning that up to 62% of the positive results may be false positives. The NPV will range from 86% to 89%, so that as few as 11% of negative results may be false negatives. As the prevalence of influenza goes up, the PPV value will be higher (more true positives) and the NPV will be lower (fewer false negatives).

2. A recent study conducted in France (Herpe et al. 2020) demonstrated calculated PPV and NPV of chest CT for diagnosing COVID-19. With 28.6% prevalence of COVID-19, a chest CT had a PPV of 66.2% and a NPV of 93.6%, higher than previously estimated. While 34% of positive findings may be false positives, only 6% of false negatives would be expected.

---

prevalence is quite high or low, or testing was performed in a high-prevalence population (e.g., adolescents for mononucleosis), the results will be skewed. Box 2.2 describes PPV and NPV.

Decision to Test

The decision to order diagnostic studies should be judicious, based on a testing threshold (i.e., a value-based judgment of how the results will inform or contribute to your assessment). A relevant consideration is the pretest likelihood.

A pretest likelihood may be based on the odds gleaned from one's own clinical experience and knowledge. For instance, if interpretation of a patient's signs, symptoms, and risk factors places the likelihood of a specific condition as low (below 20% or 10%, depending on the clinician's comfort level), there is limited value to ordering tests to uncover that condition. The exception might be a red flag condition that must be ruled out (e.g., troponin for chest pain). Alternatively, when a patient presents with textbook findings indicating a high likelihood of having a specific condition (80% or 90% or higher), it is often prudent to treat the patient based on the other findings rather than to order and wait for a test result (e.g., antibiotics before confirming urinary tract infection). A confirmatory laboratory test may still be helpful if there is a need to confirm the diagnosis, if response to treatment is not as expected, and so on. But the clinical value of a laboratory test is probably limited.

While a number of sources contribute to developing a likelihood of a disease, perhaps the best sources are evidence-based clinical prediction (or decision) tools. These often provide a list of findings, with points associated with the number of potential problems present so that the sum indicates the likelihood of a given diagnosis.

When these evidence-based clinical decision tools are not available, other resources are helpful. Prevalence statistics for your community from the department of health or other sources help when considering likelihood. For instance, if you know that measles has been diagnosed in your community or that the rate of influenza is high, that information will inform your thought processes. Of course, clinical textbooks and articles that identify key diagnostic findings are important to consider.

Laboratory tests and imaging are among the most commonly ordered diagnostic studies. The following section addresses some specific issues related to ordering and interpreting diagnostic laboratory tests versus diagnostic imaging.

Laboratory Studies

■ Selecting the Right Test

Clinicians commonly order and interpret a large number of laboratory tests daily. However, as the complexity and nomenclature of laboratory tests grow, it becomes more difficult to select the right test and easier to select the wrong one—often because one test can be labeled by several names. Passiment et al. (2012) describe the various ways in which tests are named (based on the developer, reagent, or associated disease) and then often abbreviated in varied ways, contributing to confusion and inappropriate ordering. Thus, part of learning about laboratory tests includes becoming familiar with the tests as they are available and named in a given setting, as well as what resources are available to assist in test selection. When in doubt, ask or investigate using local resources, whether they be evidence-based clinical decision rules, algorithms, textbooks, guidelines, or clinical specialists and laboratory professionals.

Cadamuro et al. (2019) estimate that 5% to 95% of laboratory tests are used inappropriately, with variability dependent on the criteria used by researchers. Inappropriate use is defined as falling within three broad categories: overuse (ordering unnecessary or wrong tests), underuse (failing to order necessary tests), and

Box 2.3

Considerations Before Ordering Laboratory Studies

Contribution to diagnosis, prognosis, and treatment
Impact on patient care
Absence of other sufficient results in current or previous order
Order appropriate given any retesting intervals
Test acknowledged by clinicians as significant
Tests consistent with guidelines and recommendations

From Cadamuro et al. (2019).

incorrect interpretation of ordered tests. Contributing factors include the increasing ease of ordering tests, the practice of defensive medicine, and a lack of awareness of clinicians' part in the consequences associated with inappropriate usage.

Overuse can be minimized by thoughtfully considering the purpose and value of a test and avoiding duplication, using the points listed in Box 2.3. This also means determining when one test or a few targeted tests are needed, rather than ordering preset test panels even if these options are highlighted: in other words, "using a rifle, not a shotgun." For instance, various "metabolic profile" options may include 15 or more tests, when only one or a few tests are relevant to a given patient's situation.

Conversely, efforts to avoid test underuse require familiarity with relevant guidelines and laboratory diagnostic algorithms, which identify an evidence-based direction of diagnostic testing by specifying the pathway. Absent a relevant decision tool, a laboratory professional can identify the appropriate test for a specified indication (Cadamuro et al., 2019).

The Choosing Wisely initiative is designed to minimize resource utilization, specifically for costly and overused tests and treatments. This program provides dozens of evidence-based laboratory recommendations submitted by numerous specialty organizations. These range from not ordering red blood cell folate levels for microcytic anemia, starting with thyroid-stimulating hormone (TSH) before expanding testing for thyroid disease, and not ordering low-risk human papillomavirus (HPV) testing (Baird, 2019).

■ Interpreting Results

Once a test is ordered, results must be interpreted specific to the patient. Interpreting laboratory test results involves knowledge of how a result compares to established reference ranges, which are usually provided along with a test result. Even when textbook reference ranges are available, the range specified by the laboratory performing the test should be used as the comparison as it is specific to the instruments and reagents used in that setting. When available, use the range based on the patient's sex or age. Standard reference ranges are established with healthy individuals. Thus, when applying an evidence-based clinical guideline to a patient with a known condition (i.e., using adult treatment guidelines for cholesterol management), the ranges indicating treatment goals should be considered, as they may be more or less restrictive than a laboratory's general reference range.

Normal ranges are based on and distributed along a bell curve representing 95% of the healthy population's results, with false negatives and false positives possible. False negatives may also occur in early states of a condition (e.g., with mononucleosis, an early false-negative result is more likely as antibodies increase for 3–4 weeks into the infection and then begin to decline). Always consider any diagnostic results as part of the full picture—treat your patient, not the laboratory value.

Other laboratory values are ordered to determine whether treatment is within a therapeutic range (i.e., whether a concentration of some drug or surrogate measure is in the therapeutic, subtherapeutic, or toxic range). While most medications are not monitored by laboratory studies, a few examples include certain antibiotics, digitoxin, lithium, and valproic acid. At other times, another value is measured as a surrogate or proxy in monitoring a drug's therapeutic value. For instance, when treating a patient with warfarin, an international normalized ratio (INR) is ordered. An understanding of how to consider therapeutic ranges for a specific patient is important.

On occasion, it is necessary to compare a patient's current and previous values, noting the direction or velocity of change over time. Interpretation of prostate-specific antigen (PSA) results provides an example of this, where the rate of doubling or increase in PSA is monitored over time when predicting potential for prostate cancer.

While laboratory results are often included among the criteria for establishing a diagnosis, they must be considered as just one data point among others. Fortunately, clinicians have access to a variety of point-of-care resources, both electronic and in print, that help in applying knowledge of test features, such as specificity and sensitivity related to a condition. Clinical guidelines and clinical decision rules help clinicians incorporate their laboratory findings in decision making. Even with these resources, clinicians need a basic level of understanding of test validity, etc., in order to make informed evidence-based interpretations of the findings.

Imaging Studies

Just as with diagnostic laboratories, the importance of understanding why and how diagnostic images are ordered and the need to apply results to your patient's overall status are critical. In constructing and refining a differential diagnosis, judiciously and appropriately choosing and interpreting diagnostic tests are key skills for clinicians. While the points in Box 2.3 refer to laboratory studies, they are equally relevant to knowing when a diagnostic image is needed. While the content of Tables 2.1 and 2.2 applies to any diagnostic study, an added consideration in selecting among diagnostic image options includes the amount of radiation exposure associated with each. This is important not only for a one-time diagnostic image but also as patients' aggregate exposure over time.

■ Selecting the Right Imaging Test

Unlike laboratory tests, the nomenclature for diagnostic imaging is generally consistent, regardless of the setting. However, it is confusing to select one image that is most appropriate for a specific patient's age, gender, history, and immediate complaint. As the term *diagnostic imaging* implies, all diagnostic imaging options do provide some type of image of body structures. However, clinicians often are uncertain regarding which test to choose from the available options, such as radiography, computed tomography (CT), magnetic resonance imaging (MRI), or ultrasound. And for some, there is the further option of with or without contrast.

However, in contrast to laboratory tests, there is one recognized resource designed to help clinicians identify the best option for their patients. The American College of Radiology (ACR) Appropriateness Criteria (ACR-AC) provides a wealth of resources to support appropriate ordering of images. The ACR-AC has provided evidence-based guidance on the selection of diagnostic images for almost 30 years. Each recommendation is regularly reviewed and updated by an expert panel. The accompanying guidance and rating of options makes this an important resource when ordering diagnostic images for a variety of clinical problems. In 2021, ACR-AC included 216 topics covering almost 2,400 diagnostic clinical scenarios (ACR, n.d.). The online portal provides for intuitive search by both filters and index.

As an example, one topic is right lower quadrant pain, which includes three variants, one of which involves a pregnant patient. There is a rating table for each variant, listing 10 procedure options, including radiography, CT of abdomen/pelvis with or without contrast, MRI of abdomen/pelvis with or without contrast, ultrasound of the abdomen or pelvis, fluoroscopy contrast enema, and white blood cell scan of abdomen/pelvis. Each option is rated as "usually appropriate," "may be appropriate," or "usually not appropriate," along with the associated radiation exposure for each. A reader may select only the rating table or may include the evidence-based narrative, which includes a summary of the literature and the recommendations. The narrative summarizes the sensitivity and specificity for given presentations, as available, as well as the rationale for recommendations.

If access to the ACR-AC is unavailable or questions remain after that information is reviewed, a radiologist at the relevant imaging department or center should be contacted. Radiologists are prepared to provide consultation when the ordering clinician has questions.

An important part of ordering the right imaging test is ensuring that the request includes adequate history to support the request. This is critical information for the radiologist who interprets the image.

■ Interpreting Results

Another difference between most laboratory and imaging studies is that the imaging report includes the radiologist's interpretation of the film. However, the way that a radiologist and a referring clinician interpret particular wording in reports may vary, leading to confusion. For instance, a description noting a finding as "suspicious for cancer" or "consistent with cancer" may be downplayed by the ordering clinician, who interprets a higher level of uncertainty than the radiologist intended, and this interpretation can contribute to delayed or misdiagnosis (Gunn et al., 2016). For this reason, the ordering clinician should follow up with the radiologist if questions or uncertainty remain based on the results received.

Summary

As discussed in Chapter 1, diagnostic reasoning involves a complex process that is optimized when all necessary "data" are available (e.g., history, physical, diagnostic studies) and carefully considered. Appropriate use of diagnostic studies contributes to making an accurate diagnosis when results are incorporated with the "whole picture." Box 2.4 provides a list of evidence-based resources to assist in selecting appropriate diagnostic studies.

Box 2.4	
Recommended Resources	
Site and URL	Description
Choosing Wisely https://www.choosingwisely.org/	Choosing Wisely promotes conversations between clinicians and patients by providing evidence-based information from a number of professional societies.
Choosing Wisely: American Society for Clinical Pathology (ASCP) https://www.choosingwisely.org /societies/american-society-for-clinical -pathology/	The ASCP has specifically published "35 Things Physicians and Patients Should Question" on Choosing Wisely.
ACR Appropriateness Criteria (ACR-AC) https://www.acr.org/Clinical-Resources /ACR-Appropriateness-Criteria	The ACR-AC provide evidence-based guidance to optimize selection of the most appropriate imaging for specific presentations.
Image Wisely https://www.imagewisely.org/	The Image Wisely campaign is aimed at lowering the amount of radiation used in medically necessary imaging, as well as eliminating procedures deemed unnecessary.
Image Gently Imagegently.org	The Image Gently alliance aims to promote improved practices in adjusting radiation when dosing children.

It is imperative to consult resources (particularly for inexperienced providers) in order to obtain results that are complete and accurate. The "shotgun approach" is expensive for the patient and the health-care system, and repetitive, inaccurate testing can cause harm to the patient in some cases. Additionally, new diagnostic testing methods are added to the list of possible choices on a frequent basis, and it is necessary to keep current regarding cutting-edge technology.

REFERENCES

ACR. (2016). Palpable breast masses. https://acsearch.acr.org/docs/69495/Narrative/

ACR. (n.d). About the ACR appropriateness criteria. https://www.acr.org/Clinical-Resources/ACR
-Appropriateness-Criteria/About-the-ACR-AC

Baird, G. (2019). The Choosing Wisely initiative and laboratory test stewardship. *Diagnosis, 6*(1), 15–23.
https://doi.org/10.1515/dx-2018-0045

Cadamuro, J., Ibarz, M., Cornes, M., Nybo, M., Haschke-Becher, E., von Meyer, A., Lippi, G., & Simundic,
A. (2019). Managing inappropriate utilization of laboratory resources. *Diagnosis, 6*(1), 5–13. https:doi
.org/10.1515/dx-2018-0029

Gunn, A. J., Tuttle, M. C., Flores, E. J., Mangano, M. D., Bennett, S. E., Sahani, D. V., Choy, G., &
Boland, G. W. (2016). Differing interpretations of report terminology between primary care physicians
and radiologists. *Journal of the American College of Radiology, 13*(12PA), 1525–1529.

Herpe, G., Lederlin, M., Tasu, J. P. (2020). Positive predictive value of chest CT compared to RT-PCR in
COVID-19 diagnosis, from the estimated to the calculated. Radiology Brief Communications Blog.
https://pubs.rsna.org/page/radiology/blog/2020/4/brief_communications_201809

Passiment, E., Meisel, J. L., Fontanesi, J., Fritsma, G., Aleryani, S., & Marques, M. (2012). Decoding laboratory test names: A major challenge to appropriate patient care. *Journal of General Internal Medicine,
28*(3), 453–458. https://doi.org://10.1007/s11606-12-2253-8

Genomic Assessment: Interpreting Findings and Formulating Differential Diagnoses

Ann Maradiegue ·
Diane Seibert ·
Karen Whitt ·

Advances in the field of genetics/genomics and the associated technologies have rapidly evolved, enabling new discoveries such as monoclonal antibody development, faster testing, and targeted drug and vaccine development such as the COVID-19 vaccine (National Human Genome Institute, 2021). Technology has allowed medicine to harness accurate, personal, clinically relevant information leading to a shift toward *precision medicine*, defined by the Institute for Precision Medicine as an approach to health care "to prevent and treat disease based upon a person's unique genetic makeup and their lifestyle habits," in order to implement and deliver personalized care (Institute for Precision Medicine, 2021). Precision medicine adds genomic information to the standard history, physical examination, and diagnostic findings to select more effective therapies or inform prevention strategies for an individual, rather than using only the symptom model of care. Developments in genomic information continue to transform the way health care is delivered. Studies were completed to examine how parents, clinicians, and health-care systems managed genomic information when a baby's entire genomic profile was sequenced shortly after birth, and the implications of this effort are still being evaluated (National Human Genome Institute, 2020).

Identifying the cause of common chronic diseases such as coronary artery disease, cancer, stroke, and diabetes is difficult because most common conditions are influenced by a combination of multifactorial, polygenic, and environmental factors (van Rheenen et al., 2019). Nurses and nurse practitioners (NPs) play a key role in the integration of genetics and genomics into the health-care setting. The original essential competencies for advance practice nurses were established in 2011 (Greco et al., 2012). Since that time, many advancements within this specialized field have occurred. Genetics/genomics has broad practice implications that are accelerating at a rapid pace. Therefore, all nurses must have the knowledge and skills to conduct an adequate genomic assessment, including obtaining and interpreting data, to identify individuals who are at increased risk or have symptoms of an inherited genetic disorder. NPs in collaboration with other clinicians should be able to gather a complete family health history (FHH), provide education and information about genetic inheritance patterns and conditions, offer genetic testing information based on clinical practice settings, make appropriate referrals to genetic professionals, and tailor care based on genetic/genomic information, including the use of pharmacogenomics/pharmacogenetics (Regan et al., 2019; Tully et al., 2020).

Several terms commonly used when conducting a genomic assessment or when referring patients to genetic professionals are defined here, as these terms are rapidly evolving (additional terms are described in Tables 3.1 and 3.2). The term *genetics* refers to the study of heredity and a particular gene and *genomics* to the study of the entire genome and its functions, noting that the primary difference between the two terms is that *genomics* describes the interaction of *many genes* and how their combined actions influence the growth and development of the organism. *Genomic medicine* includes the use of genomic data when making diagnostic, prognostic, prevention, or therapeutic decisions as well as the use of a wide array of sequencing and laboratory techniques (Brody, n.d.; Roberts & Littleton, 2018). Genomic science, often referred to as *omics-based medicine*, includes the genome as well as concepts such as *polymorphisms* (small, and often silent, genetic "spelling differences"), the *interactome* (the totality of molecular interactions in an organism), and *proteome* (all the proteins) to name a few (Biopharmaceutical Glossaries & Taxonomies, 2021). Using omics-based medicine increases understanding of disease processes; advances disease prediction, prognosis, drug response (pharmacogenetic/pharmacogenomics); and offers the opportunity to personalize care (Manolio et al., 2020). Omics-based platforms such as proteomics are used in the development of monoclonal antibody treatments for cancer, and more recently for COVID-19 (National Cancer Institute [NCI], n.d., [a]).

This chapter emphasizes assessment techniques such as collecting and interpreting the FHH and using risk assessment to help NPs more rapidly and effectively identify patients who might be at increased risk for a genetic condition. Early recognition of hereditary conditions and complex conditions influenced by genomic variations is critical to promptly initiating primary and secondary preventive measures and implementing appropriate surveillance, referral, diagnostic, and management strategies. Better understanding of the relationship between genes and an individual's response to disease and the pharmacotherapeutic agents

Table 3.1

Selected Definitions Commonly Used in Genetics and Genomics

Genetic/Genomic Term	Definition
Affected[a]	Individual who manifests the disorder.
Allele	One version of a gene at a given location (locus) along a chromosome.
Consanguinity[a]	Related in descent by a common ancestor.
De novo mutations[a]	A new, spontaneous mutation (noninherited); alteration in a gene resulting from a germ cell mutation present for the first time in the family member.
Expressivity (variable)[b]	The range of clinical features observed in individuals with a particular disorder. Variable expressivity applies to disorders following all patterns of inheritance.
Genes[a]	The functional and physical unit of heredity passed from parent to offspring. There are approximately 20,000 to 25,000 genes in each cell of the human body.
Genetics[a]	The study of heredity, the process in which a parent passes certain genes onto their children, and how particular qualities of traits are transmitted from parents to offspring; the study of single genes and their effects. A person's appearance (e.g., height, hair color, skin color, eye color) is determined by genes. Other characteristics, such as mental abilities, natural talents, and susceptibility to develop certain diseases, are also affected by heredity.
Genome[a]	All the DNA contained in an organism or a cell, which includes both the chromosomes within the nucleus and the DNA in mitochondria.
Genomics[b]	The study of the functions and interactions of all the genes in the genome.
Mutation[a]	A permanent structural alteration in DNA. In most cases, DNA changes either have no effect or cause harm, but occasionally a mutation can improve an organism's chance of surviving and passing the beneficial change on to its descendants.
Pedigree[a]	A graphic illustration of a FHH using standardized symbols. A genetic representation of a family tree that diagrams the inheritance of a trait or disease through several generations and shows relationships between members.
Penetrance[a, b]	The proportion of individuals with a mutation causing a particular disorder who exhibit clinical symptoms of that disorder.
Phenotype[a]	Observable traits or characteristics.
Proband[a]	The affected individual by whom a family with a genetic disorder is ascertained.

[a]U.S. National Library of Medicine (2020e); [b]U.S. National Library of Medicine (2021[b]).

used as treatments has become increasingly important in clinical practice. In June 2020, the U.S. Food and Drug Administration (FDA) reported that pharmacogenomic information was included in the labeling of over 300 drugs (FDA, 2021). Selecting the right drug based on the way an individual absorbs, distributes, metabolizes, or excretes a particular drug is becoming a more common practice (FDA, 2021).

Table 3.2

Definitions and Characteristics of Single-Gene Patterns of Inheritance

Term	Definition	Characteristics
Autosomal dominant (AD)	A gene on one of the autosomes that may be expressed even if only one copy is present.	50% chance of parental transmission; males and females affected; phenotype is observed in multiple or every generation with each affected person having an affected parent (vertical transmission on pedigree). NOTE: Exceptions may be de novo variable expressivity; penetrance family structure, early onset of deaths, and conditions related to sex assigned at birth (e.g., breast and ovarian cancer syndromes) may not be observed in families with limited size or small number of females.
Autosomal recessive (AR)	A genetic disorder that appears only in a patient who has received two copies of a gene mutation, one from each parent. Two genetic mutations on the autosomes.	50% chance of the offspring inheriting one gene mutation carrier; 25% chance of inheriting disease/phenotype; horizontal transmission on the pedigree proband may have affected siblings; none in parents (carriers), offspring, or other relatives; males and females affected equally.
X-linked dominant	Genetic mutations located on the X chromosome requires only one copy for phenotype or disease in males or females.	Disorders are rare, but most disorders are lethal in pregnancy with male fetus; no male-to-male transmission; there is no carrier state; affected males transmit to affected daughters only.
X-linked recessive	Genetic mutation located on the X chromosome requires both X chromosomes to be affected in females; males with affected gene will have the disorder.	Typically males are affected (rare in females) with transmission from the mother (carrier); 50% of females will inherit the gene from their father and are unaffected carriers; no male-to-male transmission.
Mitochondrial mtDNA	Mutations located in the mitochondria inherited by the mother.	All offspring of affected females; none of the offspring of affected males.

Risk Assessment

Risk assessment is part of the comprehensive health assessment process and has an important role in the health-care continuum to address preventable and non-preventable illnesses. Conducting a risk assessment puts the focus on disease mitigation, known as *precision health*. Health assessment includes a physical status evaluation, health history, symptoms, a comprehensive FHH, and a physical examination as key components of overall health, wellness, and risk assessment. The risk assessment process takes into account all known relevant factors in order to determine the probability of developing a disease, both common chronic illnesses (e.g., diabetes, hypertension, high serum cholesterol) and genetic/genomic disorders (Bylstra et al., 2021; Ginsburg et al., 2019; Risk Assessment, n.d.).

Health risks or threats can be multifaceted and may involve genetic/genomic (e.g., genetic test results, phenotype), physiological, biological (e.g., age, race/ethnicity), behavioral, psychosocial, and environmental factors. Quantifying disease burden that is caused by different risks informs prevention by providing an account of the potential for disease development and loss of health (Ginsburg et al., 2019). Risk assessment includes two important elements: (1) identification of a hazard or threat that may lead to harm, injury, illness/disease, or death and (2) determination of the *probability of occurrence* of the event (harm, injury, illness/disease) as a result of the identified hazard or threat identified from data collection (Ginsburg et al., 2019).

The first step in the process of risk assessment is to identify potential threats or hazards by collecting and interpreting data on the individual/family thought to be at increased risk. The acronym *RAPID*—**R**isk **A**ssessment using **P**robability and **I**dentification through **D**ata collection (Fig. 3.1)—can facilitate the assessment. Assessing and interpreting an individual's risk for potential adverse outcomes requires a complete personal history and FHH and pertinent laboratory, ancillary, and/or diagnostic test data. Recognition of individuals/families at increased risk due to ethnic heritage is part of the FHH data because certain ethnic groups are at increased risk for some illnesses; for example, Ashkenazi Jews are at increased risk for *BRCA* mutations (University of Pennsylvania, 2020), and African Americans are at increased risk for Alzheimer's disease (Alzheimer's Association, 2020). In some cases, an environmental assessment may also be warranted because some diseases are a result of environmental exposures—for example, Agent Orange exposure in Vietnam Veterans (American Cancer Society, 2020). Through effective and appropriate risk assessment, *risk communication* and *risk management* can be implemented, enabling preventive measures to reduce risk through early surveillance measures and to implement risk-reduction strategies before disease occurrence.

Obtaining a risk probability or risk estimate is the second step and is crucial to risk assessment. Establishing probability of risk provides an estimate for the individual's risk for developing a disease compared to that of the general population. Although risk probability may be conducted using quantitative or qualitative measures (e.g., average, moderate, or high risk), quantitative estimation is preferred because it provides a valuable measure to apply against a known benchmark or standard. It is necessary to have accurate data to enable individual and family decision making. Several evidence-based tools are currently being used to estimate risk probabilities. A well-known and long-established evidence-based tool was obtained from the Framingham Study to assess the 10-year risk of having a heart attack (Lloyd-Jones et al., 2019; U.S. Preventive Services Task Force [USPSTF], 2018). This tool provides a quantitative probability risk estimate to predict the risk of having a heart attack for an individual without a history of heart disease or diabetes.

Another example is the Gail Model, an empiric risk assessment tool for women age 35 and older who meet specific criteria; it is designed to be used by healthcare providers (HCPs) to estimate the quantitative probability for a woman's risk

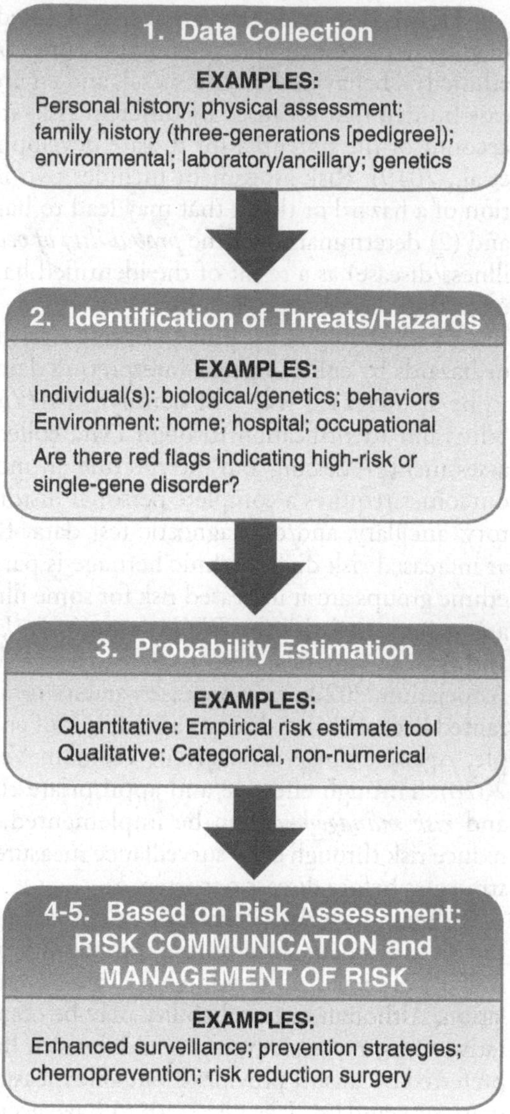

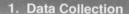

1. Data Collection

EXAMPLES:
Personal history; physical assessment;
family history (three-generations [pedigree]);
environmental; laboratory/ancillary; genetics

2. Identification of Threats/Hazards

EXAMPLES:
Individual(s): biological/genetics; behaviors
Environment: home; hospital; occupational

Are there red flags indicating high-risk or
single-gene disorder?

3. Probability Estimation

EXAMPLES:
Quantitative: Empirical risk estimate tool
Qualitative: Categorical, non-numerical

4-5. Based on Risk Assessment: RISK COMMUNICATION and MANAGEMENT OF RISK

EXAMPLES:
Enhanced surveillance; prevention strategies;
chemoprevention; risk reduction surgery

Figure 3.1 Risk Assessment Using Probability and Identification of Risk from Data Collection (RAPID) approach: (1) data collection; (2) identification of data to assess hazards or threats for disease occurrence; (3) estimation of probability; (4) communication of risk; and (5) risk management if applicable.

of developing breast cancer (NCI, n.d.[b]). The Gail Model assesses several risk elements: age, family history (first-degree relative with breast cancer), personal history (history of ductal hyperplasia), ethnicity, and surgical history (breast biopsy) to estimate a patient's 5-year and lifetime (to age 90) risk of developing invasive breast cancer (NCI, n.d.[b]). The model is useful in determining which individuals are at risk for developing breast cancer, *excluding* those with hereditary breast cancer syndromes or high risk due to other reasons (e.g., prior thoracic radiation to treat Hodgkin's lymphoma), so that risk-reduction and enhanced surveillance strategies such as chemoprevention (e.g., tamoxifen, raloxifene) can be communicated and considered by patients based on their personal history and mutually agreed-upon decision making (National Comprehensive Cancer Network [NCCN], 2021). Additionally, other risk models for breast cancer and other gynecological cancers are available on the NCI Web site (NCI, n.d.[b]).

It is important to note that there are limitations with any risk model and using the correct model that accounts for the patient's individual characteristics is an important consideration. Risk interpretation is a continuous process based on established science (McClintock et al., 2020).

Family History—The First Genetic Test

A critical first step in any health assessment is collecting and interpreting the FHH. Family history is key because it reflects shared genetic susceptibilities, shared environment, and common behaviors (Centers for Disease Control and Prevention [CDC], 2020b) and can provide information that (1) facilitates diagnosis; (2) identifies at-risk family members; (3) highlights risk for potential disease; (4) prevents disease through increased surveillance, lifestyle changes, and prophylactic measures such as chemoprevention and/or surgery; (5) promotes individualized treatment strategies; and (6) suggests referral when appropriate. A comprehensive FHH highlights and facilitates the diagnosis and identification of individuals and family members at increased risk for inheriting certain conditions.

The role of nurses in collecting (and for graduate nurses, interpreting) a FHH is clearly articulated in *Genetic/Genomics Nursing: Scope and Standards of Practice*, competencies developed to guide the nursing workforce (Consensus Panel, 2016).

A complete and accurate FHH is the key to an accurate risk/health assessment, and several tools have been created to facilitate obtaining this information (Table 3.3). Regardless of which FHH tool is used, a minimum of three generations on both the maternal and the paternal sides should be included. Whenever possible, this information should be recorded in the form of a *pedigree*, which is a graphic representation of the FHH that illustrates relationships and highlights traits that cluster in families and across generations (Bennett et al., 2008; Jorde et al., 2020). Pedigrees are low-cost, effective tools that highlight risk for genetic/genomic conditions and facilitate accurate diagnosis, but standardized symbols must be used when recording information to improve understanding and support interpretation (Bennett et al., 2008; Bennett, 2010). Pedigrees can help establish a diagnosis, illuminate inheritance patterns, identify at-risk family members, differentiate genetic from other risk factors, and support management decisions (Bennett, 2010). Pedigrees can also aid in establishing rapport, facilitate decision making, and clarify misconceptions, serving both as a valuable diagnostic tool and as an important educational tool (Bennett, 2010). There has been no change in the pedigree symbols since they were established and refined in 2008 (Bennett et al., 2008). Current discussions are ongoing to establish symbols related to gender identity and disorders of sex differentiation (Tuite et al., 2020).

Table 3.3

Resources for Family History Tools, Genetic Referral Consultation, and Genetic Education for Nurses

Resource	Purpose	Web Site
Family History Resources		
American Medical Association, Collecting a Family History	Prenatal providers; prenatal genetic screening; adult family history. Provides forms for data collection, links to policy statements and information for patients.	www.ama-assn.org/delivering-care/precision-medicine/collecting-family-history
Center for Disease Control and Prevention Surgeon General's Family History Initiative	To encourage all American families to learn more about their FHH. Site has broad information on genomic medicine and precision health knowledge.	www.phgkb.cdc.gov/FHH/html/index.html
March of Dimes, Medical Resources	Information on pregnancy and genetic prenatal screening, health profile/risk assessment, pocket facts, and family history form.	www.marchofdimes.org/profes-sionals/medical-resources.aspx www.marchofdimes.org/family-health-history-form.pdf
Jackson Laboratory	Standard pedigree nomenclature and information; a tool to draw a three-generation pedigree.	www.jax.org/education-and-learning/clinical-and-continuing-education/cancer-resources/pedigree-tool
Genetic Referral Consultation Resources		
National Society of Genetic Counselors, Healthcare Providers	Information for HCPs; resources for finding a genetic counselor.	www.geneticcounselors.org
National Comprehensive Cancer Network	Guidelines on risk reduction for selected cancers and hereditary cancers (e.g., colorectal, breast).	www.nccn.org
National Cancer Institute, Physician Data Query	Expert-reviewed information summary of hereditary cancer and other cancer genetics; expert-reviewed information summary, including cancer risk perception, risk communication, and risk counseling.	www.cancer.gov/cancertopics/pdq
Boston Children's Hospital	Provides pediatric genetic programs and referral services for families.	www.childrenshospital.org/centers-and-services/departments/genetics/programs-and-services
Nursing Genetic Resources		
International Society of Nurses in Genetics (ISONG)	Global nursing specialty organization dedicated to fostering the scientific and professional growth of nurses in human genetics and genomics worldwide.	www.isong.org
Summer Genetic Institute	Provides genetic education and training for accepted applicants for use in research, teaching, and clinical practice.	www.ninr.nih.gov/training/summergeneticsinstitute
Omics Nursing Science & Education Network (ONSEN)	A Web site to support nurse scientists, investigators, and educators both nationally and internationally, by facilitating collaborations, mentoring, and access to training opportunities to advance nursing participation in omic science.	https://www.ninr.nih.gov/researchandfunding/onsen

Constructing the Pedigree for Genetic Assessment

The following guidelines can help HCPs construct an accurate FHH using a pedigree:

1. *Use standardized pedigree symbols and nomenclature* (Table 3.4). Standardization helps to avoid misinterpretation of the pedigree data, which may improve the quality of care provided. Standardized symbols enhance quality control and make family events (births and deaths) as well as social and biological relationships (including consanguinity) more apparent.

2. *Document who recorded the history, who provided the information, and what date the FHH was collected/updated.* The FHH is dynamic and continually changing. Collecting a detailed FHH at the initial visit is important as a baseline, but updating it on subsequent patient/client visits is equally important to ensure an accurate picture of risk.

3. *Begin the pedigree with the individual whose history is being assessed.* The person whose history is being assessed may be the *consultand* or *proband*, and the FHH is built around that individual. The *consultand*, who is often (but not always) healthy, is the person presenting for counseling or testing and/or through whom a family comes to medical attention (Bennett, 2010; Pagon et al., 1993–2021). A *proband* is a family member who manifests symptoms of a particular condition and/or who brings the family to medical attention (Bennett, 2010). It is not uncommon for an individual to be both a consultand and a proband. For example, a white woman presenting with a history of breast cancer diagnosed at age 35 may have genetic testing that reveals she has inherited a hereditary breast cancer syndrome (*BRCA)* mutation. In this case, her pedigree would display an arrow designating her as the proband, with the letter *P* at the end of the arrow (Figs. 3.2 and 3.3).

4. *Collect a three-generation history.* To be complete, the pedigree should include the client/patient, siblings, children, parents, aunts/uncles, nieces, nephews, and grandparents so that a family history of at least three generations from both maternal and paternal lineage is represented. Assessment should include:

   a. *Ethnic background or ancestry of each grandparent* because some disorders have a higher incidence among certain populations. For example, sickle cell disease is diagnosed more frequently among individuals of African descent, and Tay-Sachs is more common among Ashkenazi Jewish individuals.

   b. *Age of each family member*, using the symbol "?" if unknown, or indicate an approximate age (e.g., age ~50s, 60s). Recording actual or approximate (e.g., ~1952) birth year is often more helpful when reviewing the pedigree at later dates.

   c. *Relevant medical information to include age of diagnosis* (e.g., maternal aunt, age 40, diagnosed with breast cancer at age 37; maternal cousin,

Table 3.4

Examples of Commonly Used Standardized Pedigree Symbols and Nomenclature

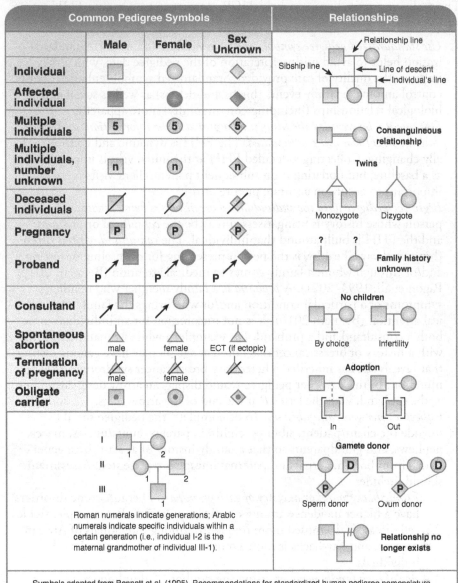

	Common Pedigree Symbols		
	Male	**Female**	**Sex Unknown**
Individual	□	○	◇
Affected individual	■	●	◆
Multiple individuals	5	5	5
Multiple individuals, number unknown	n	n	n
Deceased individuals	⊘	⊘	⊘
Pregnancy	P	P	P
Proband	P↗	P↗	P↗
Consultand	↗□	↗○	
Spontaneous abortion	△ male	△ female	△ ECT (if ectopic)
Termination of pregnancy	◺ male	◺ female	◺
Obligate carrier	⊡	⊙	◈

Roman numerals indicate generations; Arabic numerals indicate specific individuals within a certain generation (i.e., individual I-2 is the maternal grandmother of individual III-1).

Relationships

Relationship line
Sibship line
Line of descent
Individual's line

Consanguineous relationship

Twins
Monozygote   Dizygote

? ?
Family history unknown

No children
By choice   Infertility

Adoption
In   Out

Gamete donor
D   D
P   P
Sperm donor   Ovum donor

Relationship no longer exists

Symbols adopted from Bennett et al. (1995). Recommendations for standardized human pedigree nomenclature. *Am J Genet* 56:745-52.

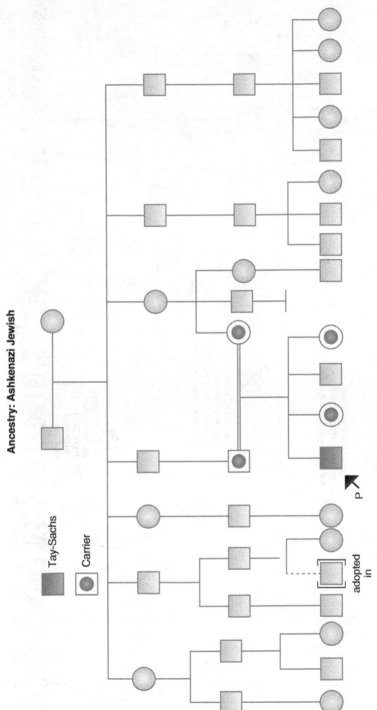

Figure 3.2 Fictitious four-generation pedigree depicting an autosomal recessive inheritance pattern of Tay-Sachs disease in family of Ashkenazi ancestry with a consanguineous relationship.

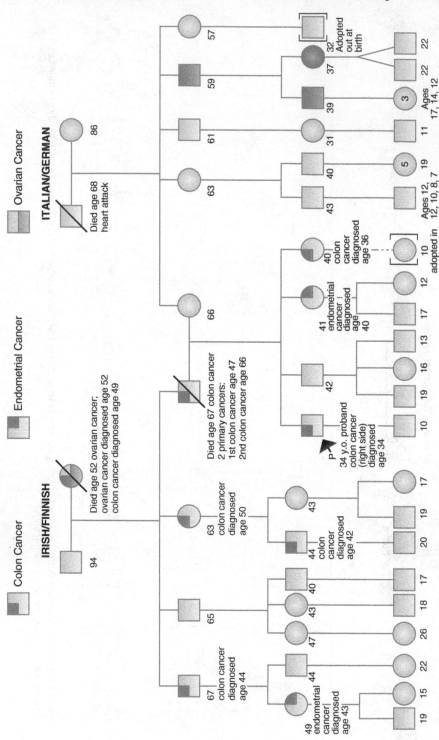

Figure 3.3 Fictitious four-generation pedigree depicting an autosomal dominant inheritance pattern due to Lynch syndrome on the paternal lineage.

age 38, diagnosed with ovarian cancer at age 37), and *pertinent surgical history*, including age and reason for surgery (e.g., mother with hysterectomy for fibroids at age 52) (CDC, 2020a).

d. *Age and cause of death of each family member* (e.g., father died at age 38 of massive heart attack; sister, age 40, died of motor vehicle accident).

e. *Consanguinity* using two horizontal lines between the male and female partners (Table 3.4 and Fig. 3.2).

f. *Adoption* in or out of the family using bracket symbols (Table 3.4 and Fig. 3.3).

g. *History of infertility and pregnancy complications*, including gestational age, miscarriage, stillbirth, pregnancy termination, or ectopic pregnancy (e.g., a proband with a history of three spontaneous abortions at 8 weeks of gestation).

h. *History of intellectual disability or severe learning problems, mental illness, or depression* (Bennett et al., 2008; Bennett, 2010).

Include a legend or key to provide family members and other providers with a guide to interpreting the pedigree and to improve visualization of conditions and how they cluster in the family (Figs. 3.2, 3.3, and 3.4). The completed pedigree is now ready to be analyzed for risk for inheritance of Mendelian (single gene), chromosomal, complex, or multifactorial conditions (e.g., cardiovascular disease, rheumatologic conditions, mental health disorders).

■ Pedigree Interpretation

The human body contains 46 chromosomes: 22 pairs (44 chromosomes) known as *autosomes* and 1 pair (2 chromosomes: X and Y) known as *sex chromosomes*. A female has no Y chromosome but normally has two copies of X, while males normally have one X and one Y chromosome. While the sex chromosomes are different depending on sex, both males and females have exactly the same 22 pairs of autosomes (except in chromosomal abnormalities). The basic unit of heredity, consisting of a segment of DNA arranged in a linear manner along a chromosome, is known as a *gene* (Pagon et al., 1993–2021). Each gene has a specific location on the chromosome known as a *locus*. The genes located on the chromosomes provide the code for specific proteins or segments of protein that determine particular characteristics or body functions (Pagon et al., 1993–2021). After the human genome was first sequenced, the initial estimate of protein-coding genes was 40,000 to 100,000; this number has been revised downward with more recent estimates of just 19,000 to 20,000 protein-coding genes in the human genome (Piovesan et al., 2019).

Inheritance Patterns Due to Single-Gene Disorders

Individuals inherit their genes from each of their parents. Single-gene disorders are a result of an alteration in the gene or a permanent heritable change in the sequence or arrangement of DNA, commonly called a *mutation* (Nussbaum, McInnes, & Willard, 2016). Somatic cells are all the cells that compose the body except for sperm and ova. Sperm and ova are known as germline cells.

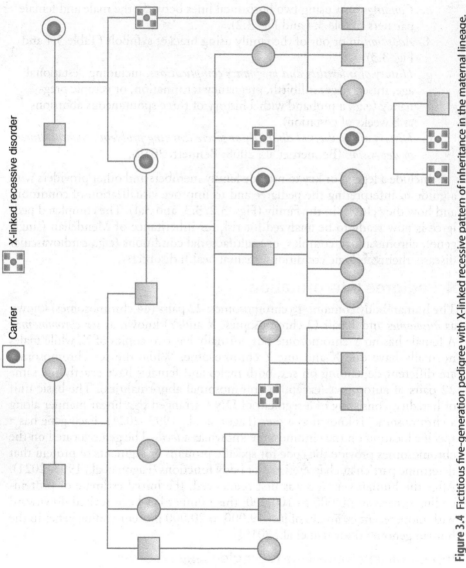

Figure 3.4 Fictitious five-generation pedigree with X-linked recessive pattern of inheritance in the maternal lineage.

Mutations that occur in somatic cells are not passed on to offspring. However, mutations that occur in germline cells can be passed on to offspring (Jorde et al., 2020). Mutations often result in an alteration or absence of protein function, which contributes to the pathophysiology and symptoms related to single-gene disorders. A single-gene mutation may occur on an autosome, on the X or Y sex chromosome, or in the mitochondria. Genetic testing for single-gene disorders often involves evaluating single nucleotide polymorphisms (SNPs), which are variations in a single base pair on the DNA strand. Genetic tests for single-gene disorders are designed to detect SNPs at certain gene loci that are highly correlated with the disease phenotype (Jorde et al., 2020). Single-gene disorders usually have unique patterns of inheritance that can be identified in a family pedigree. Because the mutations in single-gene disorders are inherited in a predictable pattern, they are often classified as dominant or recessive, or as autosomal or X-linked. See Table 3.5 for more information on single-gene inheritance.

Autosomal Dominant Inheritance

Autosomal dominant (AD) inheritance is a result of a gene mutation in one of the 22 autosomes. In AD disorders, gene mutations are transmitted from either the father or the mother, with each offspring having a 50% chance of inheriting the mutation. Offspring need to inherit only one copy of the gene mutation to outwardly manifest an AD disorder. Unless the mutation originates spontaneously during conception (called a *de novo mutation*; see Table 3.1), individuals with an AD disorder have one parent (either a mother or father) who also has the mutation. Pedigrees associated with AD disorders typically reveal multiple affected family members with evidence of the disease or syndrome appearing in each generation. When analyzing the pedigree for AD disorders or syndromes, it is common to see a "vertical" pattern denoting several generations of affected members. Figure 3.3 denotes a four-generation pedigree with multiple family members with colon cancer on the paternal lineage. Note that each of the four generations has at least one member with colon cancer. The presence or absence of affected members in a given family with an AD condition depends on the family structure, such as familial size, sex concentrations (e.g., lots of males but few females), early age of death from other causes (e.g., accidents), and features of the disease (e.g., age of onset at which the gene typically expresses symptoms or clinical features).

Not all genetic disorders are observed at birth. For example, women with a *BRCA* mutation that predisposes them to hereditary breast and ovarian cancer are not born with breast or ovarian cancer but are at risk for developing these cancers in adulthood. Additionally, physical expression of some single-gene disorders depends on exposure to certain environmental conditions. Sex assigned at birth may also influence the presence of affected members in a family with a genetic mutation. For instance, in a limited family structure with few women older than age 50, paternal inheritance of a *BRCA* mutation may be missed or the probability of a familial *BRCA* mutation underestimated (Edwards et al., 2007; Weitzel et al., 2007). Table 3.5 lists examples of AD conditions.

Table 3.5

Examples of Single-Gene Disorders With Chromosome Location, Estimated Prevalence, and Clinical Features

Inheritance Pattern Disorder	Estimated Prevalence	Clinical Features
Autosomal Dominant		
Polycystic kidney disease[a,c]	1/500 to 1/1,000[b]	Progressive renal failure characterized by bilateral renal cysts; cysts in other organs, (e.g., hepatic, pancreatic, ovarian, splenic); mitral valve prolapse; intracranial saccular aneurysms; hypertension[a]
Marfan syndrome[c,d]	1/10,000[e] (25% to 35% de novo)	Multisystem: skeletal, ocular, cardiovascular, skin, pulmonary, and ductal abnormalities[e]
Familial hypercholesterolemia[c]	1/500[e]	Hypercholesterolemia; atherosclerosis; xanthomas
Autosomal Recessive		
Hemochromatosis[g]	1/200 to 1/400 (Northern European ancestry); 1/7,000 (rare in African Americans)	High absorption of iron in excessive storage in liver, skin, pancreas, heart, joints, and testes
X-Linked Recessive		
Fragile X[c,f]	1/4,000 (males); 1/8,000 (females)	Moderate mental retardation (males); mild mental retardation (females); characteristic physical features (e.g., long, narrow face); behavioral issues; usually males more severely affected than females
Duchenne muscular dystrophy[c,f]	1/3,500 (males)	Progressive myopathy leading to muscle degeneration and weakness
Mitochondria (mtDNA)		
Leber hereditary optic neuropathy[e]	Varies: 1/10,000; 1/8,500 (Northeast England)[h]	Rapid central field vision loss due to optic nerve death

[a]Harris & Torres (2018); [b]U.S. National Library of Medicine (2020d); [c]OMIM (n.d.); [d]U.S. Department of Health and Human Services, National Institutes of Health, National Heart, Lung and Blood Institute (2019); [e]Nussbaum et al. (2016); [f]U.S. National Library of Medicine (2020e); [g]Jorde et al. (2020b); [h]U.S. National Library of Medicine (2020d).

Penetrance and variable expressivity are two terms that are important to understand when interpreting pedigrees for AD conditions. The proportion of individuals with a particular genotype who develop the disease phenotype is known as penetrance. The penetrance of a genetic condition influences gene expression and development of the disease phenotype. For example, a disease-causing gene mutation is said to have 100% penetrance if individuals with the gene mutation always express the disease phenotype. Huntington's disease is a condition with near 100% penetrance (Jorde et al., 2020). A gene mutation is said to have incomplete or reduced penetrance if less than 100% of individuals with the mutation develop the disease phenotype.

Variable expressivity refers to differences in clinical features among individuals with the same genotype (Patel et al., 2017). For example, individuals with the AD connective tissue disorder Marfan syndrome all have mutations in the *FBN1* gene that encodes fibrillin. However, there is wide variation in the outward symptoms of the disease among family members, with some individuals having mild clinical features, such as tall thin stature, and other family members with a more severe phenotype having involvement of the heart and blood vessels (Aubart et al., 2015).

Autosomal Recessive Inheritance

In autosomal recessive (AR) disorders, the offspring inherits the condition by receiving one copy of the gene mutation from each of the parents. *AR disorders must be inherited through both parents* (Nussbaum et al., 2016). Individuals who have an AR disorder have two mutated genes, one on each locus of the chromosome. Parents of an affected person are called *carriers* because each parent carries one copy of the mutation on one chromosome and a normal gene on the other chromosome. Carriers typically are not affected by the disease because one gene usually produces enough normal protein to sustain cellular function.

Because an AR disorder affects the autosomes rather than the sex chromosomes, the disease can manifest in either males or females who receive two copies of the mutated genes. The offspring of two parents who are both carriers of an AR condition have a 50% chance of being a carrier and receiving one mutated gene (like the parents), a 25% chance of receiving two copies of the mutation (one from each parent) and having the AR disorder, and a 25% chance of having two normal genes. It is important that parents understand that if they both carry a mutation, the risk to each of their offspring (each pregnancy) is an independent event: 25% disease free, 25% affected, and 50% carrier.

In pedigrees with an AR inheritance pattern, *males and females will be equally affected* because the gene mutation is on the autosome. In addition, the pedigree will have a "horizontal" presentation (many unaffected generations followed by an affected generation). If more than one family member is affected by an AR disorder, the pedigree will usually show disease in the proband and in the siblings, *not* in the parents (who are carriers) or other relatives, as noted in Figures 3.2 and 3.4 (Nussbaum et al., 2016). Ancestry of origin and ethnicity are also important in evaluating patients and families for AR disorders, since some ethnic groups have a higher incidence of AR disorders (Table 3.6; see Fig. 3.2).

Genetic testing for AR disorders often evaluates SNPs, sometimes at different loci within a gene that correlate with a disease phenotype. Disease phenotypes in AR disorders can be the result of inheriting two copies (alleles) (one from each parent) of a mutation at the same loci within the gene, which is known as being *homozygous* for the condition. It is also important to note that AR disease phenotypes can manifest as a result of being a *compound heterozygote*. An individual is considered a compound heterozygote if they inherit alternate alleles from each parent with disease-associated mutations at different gene loci (Jorde et al., 2020).

Table 3.6

Examples of Genetic Conditions Commonly Seen Among Certain Racial/Ethnic Groups or by Ancestry of Origin

Genetic Condition Pattern of Inheritance	Race/Ethnicity Ancestry of Origin	Estimated Prevalence	Carrier Frequency
Sickle cell anemia (AR)[b]	African American	1/400 to 1/600[a]	1/12[a]
Tay-Sachs disease (AR)[b]	Ashkenazi Jewish	1/3,600[c]	1/30[a]
	American non-Jewish	1/360,000	1/300[c]
Cystic fibrosis (AR)[b]	White, Northern European	1/2,500[a,c,d]	1/25[a,c]
	African American	1/17,000[d]	1/65[e]
	Asian American	1/31,000[d]	1/90[e]
Alpha-thalassemia (AR)[a,b]	Southeast Asian and Chinese	1/2,500	1/25[a]
Beta-thalassemia (AR)[a,b]	Mediterranean (Greek, Italian)	1/3,600	1/30[a]
Gaucher disease (AR)[b,f]	Ashkenazi Jewish	1/500 to 1/1,000[f]	1/10[g]
	General population	1/50,000 to 1/100,000[d]	1/200[g]
Hemochromatosis (AR)[a,b]	White, Northern European	1/200 to 1/400	1/10

[a]Jorde et al. (2020b); [b]Online Mendelian Inheritance in Man (n.d.); [c]Center for Jewish Genetics (n.d.); [d]U.S. National Library of Medicine (2020a); [e]March of Dimes (2019); [f]U.S. National Library of Medicine (2020c); [g]National Gaucher Foundation (n.d.); AR = autosomal recessive.

An example of compound heterozygosity can be seen in the AR condition hereditary hemochromatosis. Hereditary hemochromatosis is an iron metabolism disorder, more common in white men and in postmenopausal women, in which mutations in the *HFE* gene result in lower levels of the iron-regulating protein hepcidin. Lower levels of hepcidin in turn lead to symptoms of iron overload. Several *HFE* gene mutations, including the *C282Y* and *H63D* mutations, are commonly tested for in suspected hereditary hemochromatosis. Homozygous individuals inherit two copies of the *C282Y* mutation, which is often associated with a more severe iron overload phenotype with clinical symptoms of cardiomyopathy, diabetes, and arthropathy. An individual who inherits one copy of the *C282Y* and one copy of *H63D HFE* gene mutations is considered a compound heterozygote and may experience a milder hemochromatosis phenotype compared with the *C282Y* homozygote (Hollerer, Bachmann, & Muckenthaler, 2017). It is important for HCPs to have an understanding of these terms in order to provide appropriate assessment, screening, and follow-up for individuals with homozygous or compound heterozygous genotypes for AR conditions.

Consanguineous families are at increased risk for genetic disorders, in particular AR and multifactorial disorders (Bhinder et al., 2019; Jorde et al., 2020; Shawky et al., 2013), so it is important to denote consanguinity on the pedigree (see Fig. 3.2). A consanguineous family is related by descent from a common ancestor and is defined as a "union between two individuals who are related as second cousins or closer" (Bhinder et al., 2019; Hamamy, 2012, p. 2). Consanguinity is practiced in one-tenth of the world population (Alkuraya, 2013), and in many populations, such as in North Africa, West Asia, and South India, it is culturally and socially favored (Bhinder et al., 2019; Hamamy, 2012).

X-Linked Patterns of Inheritance

The X and Y chromosomes determine one's sex assigned at birth. Females have two X chromosomes, and males have an X and Y chromosome. An estimated 1,100 genes are thought to be located on the X chromosome, and 40% of them are known to be associated with a genetic phenotype (Jorde et al., 2020; Nussbaum et al., 2016; Ross et al., 2005). X-linked diseases may be dominant (expressed with only one X chromosome) or recessive (requiring both X chromosomes affected).

X-Linked Dominant Pattern

Only one X chromosome mutation is required for an X-linked dominant disorder to occur, and fortunately, these disorders are extremely rare. Everyone born with an X-linked dominant disorder will be affected with the disease. However, transmission of the disorder to the next generation varies by sex. A woman will transmit the mutation to 50% of all her offspring (male or female), while a man will transmit the mutation to 100% of his daughters (they receive his X chromosome) and none of his sons (they receive his Y chromosome). The pedigree of a family with an X-linked dominant disorder would reveal *all the daughters and none of the sons affected with the disorder if the father has an X-linked disorder.* Some X-linked dominant inheritance disorders are characterized by male lethality before birth (multiple miscarriages) or reduced male viability; as a result, one striking feature of these X-linked dominant disorders is a relative absence of male family members (Bennett, 2010; Franco & Ballabio, 2006; Migeon, 2020; Nussbaum et al., 2016). For example, incontinentia pigmenti, an extremely rare X-linked dominant disorder affecting the skin, hair, teeth, nails, eyes, and central nervous system, causes a very low survival rate for male fetuses (Bennett, 2010; Franco & Ballabio, 2006; Migeon, 2020). Females with one copy of an X-linked dominant mutation survive because they have a second healthy X chromosome capable of producing normal protein. Pedigrees of a family with an X-linked dominant disorder will be markedly different depending on which parent carries the mutation, but they follow the general rule for dominant pedigrees, demonstrating a vertical pattern of inheritance. A pedigree with X-linked dominant inheritance will demonstrate a vertical pattern of inheritance, observed in every generation, but it differs from that of AD due to the lack of male-to-male transmission (Bennett, 2010). A pedigree may also be helpful in ruling out an X-linked dominant disorder. If a father is suspected of having an X-linked genetic disorder, but the pedigree shows unaffected daughters or affected sons, the inheritance pattern does not conform to an X-linked pattern. The mutation must therefore be on an autosome and not a sex chromosome (Nussbaum et al., 2016).

X-Linked Recessive Pattern

Some X-linked disorders are recessive, which means that in a woman both X chromosomes must have the mutation if she is to be affected. If only one X chromosome carries the mutation and the other is normal, she will be a carrier and typically unaffected. Because males have only one copy of the X chromosome, they will be affected if their X chromosome carries the mutation. Because of the rarity of X-linked recessive disorders, it is unusual for a female to have two affected X chromosomes unless her father had an X-linked disorder and her mother was either a carrier or was also affected with the disorder. Thus, *X-linked recessive disorders occur typically in males.* There is no male-to-male transmission because the father with an X-linked disorder can transmit the Y chromosome only to his male offspring. *All daughters of affected fathers with an X-linked recessive disorder will be carriers.* Female carriers have a 50% chance of transmitting the gene mutation to their sons, who will all be affected (see Fig. 3.4). An example of an X-linked recessive disorder is hemophilia A; additional X-linked disorders are listed in Table 3.5.

Chromosomal Disorders

In addition to single-gene mutations, entire chromosomes or large sections of chromosomes can be affected, resulting in disease. Abnormalities of any of the chromosomes (autosomes and/or sex chromosomes) can be a consequence of numerical or structural problems. There can be too few (less than 46) or too many (more than 46) chromosomes. An individual with an abnormal number of chromosomes has a condition called *aneuploidy*, which is frequently associated with mental problems or physical problems or both (Nussbaum et al., 2016). The normal structural appearance of the chromosome may be altered due to deletions, duplications, inversions, translocations, rearrangements, insertions, or other changes of segments of chromosomes. These structural alterations can result in positional changes of the gene, leading to nonfunctional genes, excessive or inadequate protein production, or the development of cancer (Jorde et al., 2020).

Chromosomal disorders have also been associated with mental retardation, failure to thrive, developmental delay, low birth weight, infertility, and histories of frequent spontaneous abortions or stillbirths. Approximately 50% of spontaneous abortions have chromosomal abnormalities (Nussbaum et al., 2016; van den Berg et al., 2012). An estimated 1 in 160 newborns have a chromosomal abnormality (Nussbaum et al., 2016). For instance, a newborn with trisomy 21 (Down's syndrome) has an extra chromosome 21 and therefore has a total of 47 chromosomes instead of the usual 46. A complete family history includes inquiring about prior pregnancy outcomes such as spontaneous abortions, stillbirths, and neonatal deaths. In addition, maternal age is important because Down's syndrome and other trisomies have been associated with maternal age older than 35 years at time of delivery. Although most aneuploidy conditions involve autosomes (particularly chromosomes 21, 13, and 18), sex chromosomes may also be duplicated or omitted, resulting in disorders such as Turner's and Klinefelter's syndromes.

Chromosomal alterations affecting the sex chromosomes may not be apparent until later in life. Individuals with Klinefelter's syndrome have too many sex chromosomes (47 XXY) and may show no indications of the syndrome until adolescence, when signs of hypogonadism become apparent. Individuals with Turner's syndrome (45 X) are missing a sex chromosome and may be identified at birth (clinical features of webbed neck and lymphedema of hands and feet) or later because of primary amenorrhea (Jorde et al., 2020; Nussbaum et al., 2016). Although there is still much to learn about the role of paternal age and birth defects, there is some evidence that this, too, plays a role in chromosomal abnormalities, complex disease, and reproductive outcomes (Brandt et al., 2019; Janeczko et al., 2020). In addition to the relationship between paternal age, DNA mutations, and chromosomal abnormalities, increased paternal age has also been suggested to have an association with epigenetic changes and an increased incidence of multifactorial inheritance disorders such as autism, schizophrenia, bipolar disorders, and leukemia in offspring (Sharma et al., 2015). *Epigenetics* refers to changes in phenotype related to the way that genes are expressed (U.S. National Library of Medicine, 2021b). These changes are not caused by altered DNA sequence or chromosome structure but rather by how well the genes are expressed or able to carry out processes such as transcription to mRNA.

Mitochondrial DNA (mtDNA) Disorders

The majority of genetic mutations are located in nuclear DNA within the cell nucleus; however, disease due to genetic mutations can also occur in the mitochondria. Mitochondria are oblong-shaped organelles found in the cytoplasm of most cells in the body and are involved in producing energy for the cell, known as cellular respiration. The number of mitochondria found in each cell varies depending on the metabolic activity and type of cell. Mitochondria have their own circular DNA that can reproduce and divide independently of the cell where they reside (Cooper & Hausman, 2018). The circular mitochondrial DNA contains 37 genes, which can carry mutations causing disease (Nussbaum et al., 2016). Because mitochondrial mutations involve oxidative phosphorylation and metabolic energy, mitochondrial abnormalities often involve the central nervous and musculoskeletal systems; however, they can also be multisystem (Jorde et al., 2020; Nussbaum et al., 2016). Over 250 pathogenic mtDNA mutations have been identified (Larsson & Wedell, 2020).

Mitochondrial inherited disorders have a distinct *maternal inheritance* because, at conception, the sperm contributes only the nuclear content (chromosomes) while the ovum provides mitochondria and all the cellular structures (Nussbaum et al., 2016). Fathers therefore cannot transmit a mitochondrial condition to their offspring. The pedigree of a family with an mtDNA disorder is unique in that *all offspring (regardless of sex) of an affected female will have disease, and none of the offspring from an affected male will have disease*. Because mutations may be present in all mtDNA (homoplasmy) or in some (heteroplasmy), the risk and severity of mtDNA diseases often vary widely among family members. One example of an mtDNA disorder is Leber hereditary optic neuropathy (see Table 3.5).

Special Consideration in Genetic/Genomic Assessment

■ Preconception Counseling

The goal of preconception care is to "reduce the risk of adverse health effects for the woman, fetus, and neonate by working with the woman to optimize health, address modifiable risk factors, and provide education about healthy pregnancy" (American College of Obstetricians and Gynecologists [ACOG] Committee, 2019). One of the core preconception considerations is gathering a complete and accurate family history with a minimum of a three-generation pedigree to help identify hereditary conditions so that appropriate information, education, genetic testing, and referral for genetic counseling can be implemented (Maradiegue & Edwards, 2016).

Some individuals or couples have unique identifiable risks that should be discussed prior to conception whenever possible. For example, women who will be age 35 years or older at delivery (advanced maternal age) are at increased risk for aneuploidy, and certain racial/ethnic groups are at higher risks for specific genetic conditions (see Table 3.6). Prior adverse pregnancy outcomes such as congenital birth defects, pregnancy loss, or fetal death may offer important information about future reproductive risks or may be a red flag for parental chromosomal abnormalities. ACOG recommends that every pregnant patient be offered information about carrier screening prior to conceiving so that patients and their partners can make informed decisions about their reproductive risks and options. Currently, ACOG recommends that all patients be offered screening for spinal muscular atrophy, cystic fibrosis, and hemoglobinopathies (Edwards et al., 2015). Patients with intellectual disability or family history of fragile X–related disorders should be offered fragile X syndrome screening, and couples of Ashkenazi Jewish descent should be counseled regarding their risk for carrying a Tay-Sachs mutation (ACOG, 2017). Table 3.3 contains online resources for preconception and prenatal assessment.

■ Hereditary Cancer Syndromes

A cancer diagnosis is often found in one or more family members when conducting a three-generation pedigree and are usually AD. While most hereditary cancers are rare, approximately 5% to 10% of all cancers are due to a single-gene mutation or a germ line mutation. These hereditary mutations often possess a loss of heterozygosity. This means that the individual has inherited a loss of a normal copy of a particular gene or group of genes, unlike the individual who is homozygous. Homozygous individuals have inherited two normal copies of a gene or group of genes from their parents (Dutra, n.d). The majority of cancers are considered polygenic or multifactorial due to a combination of genetic and environmental factors. Approximately 5% to 10% of all cancers are due to a single-gene mutation (NCI, 2017). The FHH in the form of a pedigree is a key tool in the recognition of individuals who are suspect for hereditary cancer so that genetic counseling, informed decision making for genetic testing if available, and management of care strategies can be implemented. Several professional guidelines are available to assist HCPs in understanding genetic risk assessment. For instance, in 2019 the USPSTF issued updated guidelines for genetic risk assessment and *BRCA* mutation testing to determine susceptibility for breast and ovarian cancer; these recommendations and guidelines continue to be reviewed and updated at regular intervals (USPSTF, 2019). The current draft recommends that primary care providers screen women who have a personal history, family history, or ancestry associated with breast or ovarian cancer with one of several screening tools designed to identify a family history that may be associated with an increased risk for potentially harmful mutations in breast cancer susceptibility genes (*BRCA1* or *BRCA2*). Women and men with a positive screen should receive genetic counseling and, if indicated after counseling, genetic testing and other treatment options (USPSTF, 2019). Women with a *BRCA* mutation are at a high risk for developing breast and ovarian cancers (NCCN, 2021; Peshkin & Isaacs, 2020; Samadder et al., 2019). Appropriate measures for women diagnosed with a *BRCA* mutation might include enhanced surveillance, possible chemoprevention, or optional surgery to reduce their risk for developing the disease. Though most guidelines do not address genetic testing among postmenopausal women, genetic screening may be warranted in this age group to guide treatment regimens and notify other family members (Kurian et al., 2020).

Most hereditary cancer syndromes like that of *BRCA* mutations are AD, and thus multiple family members with a specific cancer and early age of onset are among the red flags associated with an inherited predisposition to the disease. Some hereditary cancer syndromes are associated with several different cancers or other diseases. Lynch syndrome, for example, is an AD inherited disorder that increases the risk of colon cancer and other extracolonic cancers, including that of the endometrium, ovary, stomach, small bowel, pancreas, hepatobiliary tract, ureter/renal pelvis, and skin (Dominguez-Valentin et al., 2020; Tanakaya et al., 2019). Lynch syndrome is not considered a rare disorder, and estimates indicate that mutations responsible for Lynch syndrome may be as prevalent as 1 in every 300 people (American Society of Clinical Oncology, 2021a). An example of a four-generation pedigree of a Lynch syndrome family is depicted in Figure 3.3. In Lynch syndrome, like many hereditary cancer syndromes, the cancers often present at an earlier than expected age and are considered red flags for the syndrome. The colon cancer genes are often part of a family of mismatch repair genes (MMR). Specific guidelines for cancer and hereditary cancer care can be found on the National Comprehensive Cancer Network Web site.

Evaluation of those at high risk for hereditary cancers is continually changing as scientific advancements continue to evolve. There is often shared genetic susceptibility for a variety of cancers among family members, requiring complex evaluation and referral to genetic specialists in order to adequately assess the patient. Single-gene analysis was used in the past to identify a genetic cause for disease. In this case, gene selection was based on the personal history and FHH, including the more commonly known genes (i.e., *BRCA* and MMR).

Next generation sequencing (NGS) has ushered in multigene or panel testing, an approach that simultaneously tests multiple genes at once, and is the preferred method for those whose personal or family history is suggestive of hereditary cancer (Tsaousis et al., 2019). While *BRCA* and Lynch syndrome are the more common hereditary cancer syndromes, there are multiple hereditary cancer syndromes complicating the genetic evaluation process (American Society of Clinical Oncology, 2021b). Multigene panels include genes of high and moderate penetrance, and in some cases, genes of low penetrance or unknown significance. This data is leading to more accurate diagnosis (Tsaousis et al., 2019). NGS is currently being used in large swaths of the population through sponsored programs like All of Us. This research program has a goal of collecting and analyzing data from more than 1 million Americans; more information can be found on the NIH All of Us Website. Researchers are using this as an opportunity to evaluate the clinical and economic implications of NGS, as well as to identify future challenges and appropriate uses (Phillips, Douglas, & Marshall, 2020).

■ Genomics, Polygenic, and Multifactorial Conditions

Genetics/genomics impacts all aspects of health and illness across the life span. Most disease-causing conditions are not due to a single-gene disorder but are due to *multifactorial inheritance*, a result of genomics and environmental or behavioral influences. In fact, the leading causes of mortality in the United States—heart disease, cerebrovascular disease, diabetes, and cancer—all have a strong genomic component. Most congenital malformation, hypertension, arthritis, asthma, obesity, epilepsy, Alzheimer's, and mental health disorders are also multifactorial (Jorde et al., 2020). Ongoing research is under way to better understand the contribution of the genome to these disorders and to behavioral conditions such as alcoholism.

The use of personal, behavioral, and environmental history coupled with a three-generation family history is important in assessing an individual's risk for multifactorial disease. In general, first-degree relatives (parents, children, siblings) have 50% shared genes, second-degree relatives (aunts, uncles, grandparents) have 25% shared genes, and third-degree relatives (cousins, great-grandparents) have 12.5% shared genes (Children's Wisconsin, 2021; Hill & White, 2013; Jorde et al., 2020). The family history is important since risk occurrence is higher if more than one family member is affected with the disease/disorder and is lower with a remote degree of family relationship (e.g., history of first-degree relative compared to third-degree relative). The use of evidence-based risk assessment tools, where applicable and if available, also enables HCPs to assess the risk for disease occurrence, which can lead to preventive measures to reduce disease risk. In addition, future genomic research will continue to advance the discovery of susceptibility genes and provide opportunities of genetic profiling for personalizing medicine to predict common complex diseases (Collins et al., 2021).

Significance of common disease conditions noted within families is indicative of the occurrence of some heritability. Genome-wide association studies

(GWAS) have shown many single polymorphic variants, which has changed the field of multifactorial inheritance. Hundreds of susceptible loci have been identified across cancers, autoimmune diseases, and other common disease conditions (polygenicity). While further research is needed to clarify the role of polygenicity in the clinical setting, GWAS may provide important information for multifactorial disease management in the future (Lello et al., 2019; Roberts et al., 2019).

Analyzing and Interpreting Family History Findings

Once completed, the family history must be evaluated for patterns of inheritance that may indicate a genetic disorder. Key points to look for include the presence of consanguinity, male-to-male transmission and female-to-male transmission, and whether males and females are affected in equal numbers or if only males are affected, all of which can aid in distinguishing autosomal versus X-linked disorders. Pedigrees can sometimes be difficult to evaluate, and errors in interpretation can occur for many reasons. Therefore, it is important that all HCPs take as careful, thorough, and detailed a family history as possible. Even if an accurate family history is obtained, other difficulties can arise in interpreting the pedigree. Several common problems include the following:

1. A new or de novo disorder. The proband is the first person to have the disease. New mutations are a not-infrequent cause of dominant and X-linked diseases (Nussbaum et al., 2016). For example, over 80% of children born with achondroplasia, an AD disorder, have a de novo mutation and are born to parents of normal stature (Pauli, 2012).
2. Nonpaternity. The person identified as the father on the pedigree is not the biological father.
3. The family is very small (limited in structure) or limited by sex assigned at birth. This is particularly important when assessing for sex-associated conditions. For example, if a *BRCA* mutation occurs in the paternal lineage with mostly male members, a vertical pattern of the disease may not be noted on the pedigree. The sole family member, a female daughter with newly diagnosed breast cancer at age 35, might be the red flag that is indicative of a *BRCA* mutation that she inherited from the paternal lineage.
4. The person providing the history is not aware of all the details of the family history, has inaccurate information (e.g., ovarian cancer was actually cervical cancer), or is deliberately withholding information (perhaps from fear of discrimination).
5. Early death of a family member from other causes (e.g., in a war or an accident) limits the family structure, particularly when there are genetic diseases that express symptoms in adulthood (Weitzel et al., 2007).
6. Disorders are inherited from an individual who does not typically express the disorder. For example, color blindness, an X-linked recessive disorder, is not usually seen in women because they are typically carriers and unaffected.

It is difficult to assess for color blindness in a family with many females but few males or in families in which males died early of other causes or never mentioned having any visual problems. In these situations, color blindness can appear to be a new condition, when in fact it may have been present in the family for many generations. Most AR disease carriers do not generally have disease symptoms; however, it is possible for them to have a milder version of the disease.

7. Some disorders have a range of expression from mild to severe. For example, patients with neurofibromatosis (NF1), an AD disorder of the nervous system, may manifest with many forms of the disease (*variable expressivity*). The diagnosis may be further complicated by the variability in symptoms. For instance, some patients with NF1 may have mild symptoms like café au lait spots or freckling on the axillary or skin, while others may have life-threatening spinal cord tumors or malignancy (Jorde et al., 2020; Nussbaum et al., 2016).

8. Some gene mutations are more penetrant than others. In mutations of varying penetrance, some individuals will have the gene mutation but will never develop the disease (Jorde et al., 2020). Some genetic disorders are not 100% penetrant. For example, a woman with a *BRCA* mutation is at a 50% to 85% risk of developing breast cancer and a 35% to 50% risk of developing ovarian cancer (American Society of Clinical Oncology, 2021b; Kuchenbaecker et al., 2017). While these risks are higher than the population risk for developing the disease (estimated at 12.4% for women in the United States), the mutation is not 100% penetrant. Reduced penetrance may be attributed to a combination of genetic, lifestyle, and environmental factors (NCI, 2017).

While pedigree interpretation may be at times difficult to ascertain, assessing the family history for red flags may lead to recognition of hereditary disorders (Table 3.7). Also, clinicians should continuously examine their own competence of practice on a regular basis, identifying areas of strength and areas where professional development related to genetics/genomics would be beneficial. The *Essential Genetic and Genomic Competencies for Nurses With Graduate Degrees* provides an excellent resource for the competencies required for nurses to deliver competent genomic care.

■ Questionable Medical History

Critical family medical information may be missing that could be important in determining whether a family member is at risk for a genetic/genomic condition. If a hereditary condition is being considered but family medical information is unclear or unknown, requesting medical records and pathology or autopsy reports may be warranted. For instance, the cause of early death (age 35) of a parent's mother might be unknown. However, the death certificate or an autopsy report may reveal that the cause of death thought to be a stomach problem was actually metastatic ovarian cancer diagnosed at age 34. Coupling this

Table 3.7

Example of Family History Red Flags

Hereditary Cancer Syndromes
- Early-age onset (e.g., breast cancer at age 50 or younger; colon cancer at age 45 to 50 years or younger)
- Occurrence of cancer in the less-often-affected sex (e.g., male breast cancer)
- Multiple family members with cancer, especially if age of onset is earlier than usual
- Autosomal dominant pattern of inheritance
- Known hereditary cancer gene mutation in the family (e.g., *BRCA* mutation)
- Family member with multiple primary cancers
- Clustering of syndromes associated with a hereditary cancer (e.g., breast and ovarian cancer; colon cancer and endometrial cancer)
- Two or more unusual cancers in the same person or close relative

Medical Disorders
- Heart disease before age 40 to 50 years
- Dementia before age 60
- Hearing loss before age 50 to 60
- Three or more pregnancy losses
- Several family members with the same condition
- Multisystem, bilateral or multisystem occurrences (e.g., deafness and nephritis suggestive of Alport's syndrome)

Family GENES mnemonic[a]
G Group of congenital anomalies
E Extreme or exceptional presentation of common conditions (e.g., multiple primary cancers seen with hereditary cancer syndromes such as *BRCA* mutation)
N Neurological delays or degeneration (e.g., early-age onset Alzheimer's or dementia)
E Extreme or exceptional pathology (e.g., medullary thyroid cancer; multiple adenomatous polyps in familial adenomatous polyposis)
S Surprising laboratory values (e.g., familial hypercholesterolemia, cholesterol greater than 500)

Other[b]
- Ethnic predisposition to certain genetic disorders
- Close biological relationship between parents (i.e., consanguinity)

Table adapted from information from American College of Obstetricians and Gynecologists, 2011; American Medical Association, 2021; Bennett, 2010.
[a]Family GENE mnemonic taken from Whelan et al., 2004; [b]Genetics in Primary Care Institute, 2013.

information with the FHH reveals a red flag for a hereditary cancer syndrome, leading to the patient's (consultand) genetic referral, testing, and diagnosis of a *BRCA* mutation.

Importance of Physical Examination

A physical examination should be conducted on all patients suspected of having a genetic/genomic condition or who, based on FHH, may be at risk for a medical problem. Physical examination should be focused on the characteristics of the disease and the system(s) needed to aid in diagnosing or excluding the genetic/genomic condition (Tables 3.8 and 3.9). Special attention to height and weight, head circumference, and physical development, to include hearing, vision, motor skills, language, linguistics, behavior, and social skills, are important components when assessing for genetic disorders in infants and children (Jorde et al., 2020).

Table 3.8

Examples of Genetic Single-Gene Disorders by Body Systems

System	Medical Condition and Frequency	Inheritance Pattern	Characteristics
Skin	Neurofibromatosis type 1 (1/3,000 to 1/4,000)[a]	AD; 80% de novo	Variable expression; skin café au lait spots; axial or inguinal freckling; neurofibromas; Lisch nodules on retina; optic gliomas; malignant tumors of peripheral nerve sheath
Ear	Deafness (1/500 to 1/1,000 neonates)[b]	AR	Congenital hearing impairment or deafness (nonsyndromic); congenital in AR
Respiratory	α[1]-antitrypsin deficiency (1/5,000 to 1/3,500 Northern European descent)[b]	AR	Increased risk of chronic obstructive lung disease, emphysema, and liver cirrhosis
Cardiovascular	Familial hypercholesterolemia (1/500 whites)[b]	AD	Hypercholesterolemia, atherosclerosis; xanthomas; arcus corneae
	Long QT syndrome (~1/5,000 to 1/7,000)[b]	AD	Tachyarrhythmias; syncope episodes; QT prolongation; sudden death
Genitourinary	Polycystic kidney disease, adult type 1[b]	AD	Progressive renal failure; see Table 3.5
Musculoskeletal	Huntington's disease (3–7/100,000 European descent)[a]	AD	Progressive movement, cognitive and psychiatric abnormalities
Neurological	Alzheimer's disease, type 1[a] (10% to 15% of early disease)[b]; Alzheimer's disease, type 3[a] (30% to 70% of early disease)[b]	AD	Early-age onset disease; progressive dementia with family occurrence before age 60 to 65 years and often before age 55

[a] U.S. National Library of Medicine (2021d); [b]Online Mendelian Inheritance in Man (n.d.); Bird (2012).

Assessing for dysmorphic features may enable identification of certain syndromes or genetic or chromosomal disorders (Jorde et al., 2020).

Dysmorphology is defined as "the study of abnormal physical development" (Jorde et al., 2020, p. 295). For example, epicanthal folds, up-slanted palpebral fissures, single transverse palmar crease, and a low nasal bridge are clinical findings found in trisomy 21 or Down's syndrome (Jorde et al., 2020). Enlarged head circumference, tongue and skin lesions, and/or thyroid nodules may suggest Cowden's syndrome if hereditary breast cancer syndrome is suspected. Individuals with Cowden's syndrome, a rare AD disease caused by a mutation in the *PTEN* gene, are at high risk for benign and malignant tumors of the breast, thyroid, and endometrium as well as other benign disorders such as multiple hamartomatous polyps and fibrocystic breast disease (Eng & Malhotra, 2018). Clinical signs suggestive of Cowden's syndrome often include macrocephaly (occipital

Table 3.9

Selected Hereditary Cancer Syndromes by Body Systems

Body System	Genetic Condition (Gene Mutation)	Inheritance Pattern	Characteristics/Associated Cancer
Skin	Malignant melanoma[a]	AD	Increased risk melanoma
Eye	Retinoblastoma[a]	AD	Bilateral disease usually presents in the first year of life; rare neoplasm of retina; strabismus; visual deterioration; other neoplasms (e.g., osteosarcomas, soft tissue sarcomas, melanomas)
Breast	Hereditary breast and ovarian[a]	AD	High-risk breast and ovarian cancer; multiple primary tumors; increased risk of other cancers (e.g., prostate, pancreatic)
	Li-Fraumeni syndrome[a]	AD	Breast; osteo and soft tissue sarcomas; leukemia, brain, and adrenocortical cancer
	Cowden's disease[a]	AD	Breast; associated cancers: thyroid (especially follicular), endometrial
	Peutz-Jeghers syndrome[a]	AD	Breast; associated cancers: gastrointestinal, ovarian, lung
	Partner and localizer of *BRCA2*[a]	AD	Breast and pancreatic
Gastrointestinal (colon)	Lynch syndrome (mismatch repair genes)[a]	AD	Extracolonic cancer: ovary, endometrium, stomach, small bowel, bile duct, urinary tract (sebaceous skin tumors, keratoacanthomas with Muir-Torre syndrome and brain tumors; Lynch variant); brain tumors (e.g., glioblastomas, Turcot Lynch variant)
	Familial adenomatous polyposis (FAP)[a]	AD	Colorectal adenomatous polyps greater than 100 (~10–100 in attenuated FAP): colon cancer; medulloblastoma; Gardner syndrome: desmoid tumors, osteomas, congenital hypertrophy of the retinal pigment epithelium
Genitourinary	von Hippel-Lindau[a]	AD	Clear cell renal cell carcinoma; multiple tumor types with great variability (e.g., retinal angiomas, cerebellar and spinal cord hemangioblastoma; pheochromocytoma, pancreatic cysts, islet cell/neuroendocrine tumors); endolymphatic sac tumor (inner ear); 70% of patients with CCRCC[b]
Neurological	Ataxia-telangiectasia[a]	AR	Progressive cerebellar ataxia; facial and conjunctiva telangiectasia; infant may appear normal at birth, symptoms occurring usually between 1 and 4 years; most wheelchair-bound by adolescence; humoral and cellular immune dysfunction; associated cancer: lymphoreticular malignancies (e.g., lymphosarcoma, leukemias), breast cancer, melanoma[c]
Endocrine	Multiple endocrine neoplasia (MEN)[a] type 2A/B	AD	MEN type 2A: medullary thyroid cancer (MTC), hyperparathyroidism and pheochromocytoma[d]; MEN type 2B: MTC pheochromocytoma, no hyperparathyroidism; Marfanoid appearance[d]

[a]Online Mendelian Inheritance in Man (n.d.); [b]Frantzen et al. (2015); Gatti & Perlman (2016); Jorde et al. (2020).
NOTE: Only selected hereditary cancer syndromes are presented; table is not all-inclusive.

frontal circumference in the 97th percentile or greater), facial trichilemmomas, acral keratoses, papillomatous papules, palmoplantar keratoses, cobblestone-like pattern of oral mucosa (especially the buccal and gingival mucosae), and/or a multinodular thyroid (Eng & Malhotra, 2018). In another example, assessment of the skin with noted lesions of café au lait spots, axillary freckling, or neurofibromas might meet the diagnostic criteria suggestive of NF1, formerly known as von Recklinghausen's disease (Friedman, 2012; Jorde et al., 2020).

Additional Medical and Social History

Assessment of the social, environmental, occupational, and medication history is important when caring for any patient, including those with genetic/genomic conditions. Individuals with an X-linked recessive disorder known as glucose-6-phosphate dehydrogenase (G6PD) deficiency, for example, may be impacted by numerous external factors such as drugs, viral and bacterial infections, toxins, and metabolic acidosis (Nussbaum et al., 2016). Individuals with G6PD have a genetic mutation that causes a defect in the glucose-6-phosphate dehydrogenase enzyme that can lead to premature hemolysis. For some individuals with G6PD, acute hemolytic anemia can occur when taking certain medications such as antimalarial primaquine, NSAIDs, aspirin, quinine, nitrofurans, and sulfonamides. Also, some people with G6PD may be sensitive to certain chemicals, such as mothballs, and must avoid eating fava beans (Nussbaum et al., 2016). G6PD occurs mainly in males, and symptoms can range from severe to mild, with some individuals unaware that they have the condition. Deep vein thrombosis is another condition for which many environmental factors, such as trauma, surgery, malignant disease, immobility, oral contraceptives, and advanced age, increase the risk. The risk for deep vein thrombosis is further enhanced in some patients with a genetic mutation in the factor V Leiden gene, illustrating the importance of assessing family history in combination with environmental, social, and occupational history.

Genetic Testing and Direct-to-Consumer Results

Genetic tests are used clinically in a variety of ways. Genetic tests can assist in making a diagnosis, identifying gene changes associated with disease, predicting disease severity, selecting the right drug to treat a condition, and presymptomatically, can identify an individual's risk for developing a disease, identify risk to future offspring, and rapidly identify newborns with genetic diseases. Because genomic science is still in its infancy, associations between the spelling of a particular stretch of DNA and a particular set of symptoms or a clinical disorder are still being discovered every day. This plays out clinically on a regular basis; a woman with a strong family history of breast cancer, for example, may have a genetic test and be told she does not carry a deleterious *BRCA1* or *BRCA2* mutation. That does not mean she does not have an increased genetic risk for breast cancer; it just means the test did not assess other risk alleles, or the gene associated with the family's increased risk is not yet known.

In addition to genetic tests ordered by providers, consumers can purchase many different types of direct-to-consumer (DTC) genetic tests. Consumers can buy DTC tests to explore their ancestry and athletic ability, as well as prenatal, microbiome (gut and vaginal flora), nutrigenomic (food and health), forensic (paternity testing), genetic relatedness, and health testing, to name but a few. One company, DNARomance.com, offers their participants the option of uploading genomic information from other DTC vendors (e.g., 23andMe, Ancestry.com, FamilyTreeDNA, MyHeritage) and then produces a "DNA romance profile" to determine compatibility. Some of these DTC services may offer some interesting insights, but others are more suspect. For example, companies offering "nutrigenomic" testing may also be selling nutritional supplements or fitness packages based on genetic profiles. Other issues, like surreptitious testing (taking a genetic sample from a straw or a hair sample, etc.) without the other person's knowledge or consent to expose infidelity or paternity, have already made their way into courtrooms (Strand, 2016). "The hazards associated with consumer tests extend well beyond cancer risk. These products also offer tests for diabetes, celiac disease, Parkinson's disease and others, meaning many people could be similarly lulled into a false sense of security about their health" (Cheng, 2020).

Genetic testing is likely to play a very important role in the future of health and health care. The COVID-19 pandemic offers a glimpse of the power that genomics has to influence health. From the rapid sequencing and publication of the viral gene sequence to the development of two mRNA-based vaccines and from the development of gene-based (polymerase chain reaction) tests to the mapping of the spread of COVID-19 variants to the identification of genetic factors that increase risk for disease severity, genomics is transforming health care around the globe.

Pharmacogenomics

Pharmacogenomics, defined as how genes affect a person's response to drugs, is important when conducting genetic/genomic assessment (U.S. National Library of Medicine, 2021c). Pharmacogenomics utilizes genetic information to predict both drug action and drug responses (Roden et al., 2019; Caudle et al., 2017; Madadi & Koren, 2012). Specifically, pharmacogenomics deals with the effects of *genetic variation* on a patient's response to specific drugs (Roden et al., 2019; Snozek et al., 2012). The objective of pharmacogenomics is to ascertain how genetic markers are associated with differences in pharmacokinetics, pharmacodynamics, and drug toxicity. Utilizing this genetic information is another measure toward personalized medicine to guide drug selection, optimize dosing to increase therapeutic benefits, and minimize toxicity to avoid adverse effects (Roden et al., 2019; Snozek et al., 2012). Pharmacogenomics may be useful in the management of a wide variety of drugs, including some antidepressants, immunosuppressants, cardioactive drugs, anesthetics, and analgesics (Lam & Guitierrez, 2020).

Research in pharmacogenomics looks to identify drug-gene pairs that have a high degree of clinical validity and utility with evidence to support clinical action. Oral medications must undergo biotransformation in order to be utilized by the body. Much of the process of biotransformation occurs in the liver in the cytochrome P450 (CYP450) system. Genetic variants in the CYP450 enzyme system have been the focus of much of the research in pharmacogenomics. For example, genetic variation in the *CYP2D6* gene has been widely studied and is thought to affect metabolism of over 25% of prescription drugs (Jorde et al., 2020).

Drug target polymorphisms are genetic variants, usually SNPs, that have a relationship with drug efficacy. One of the issues with drug target pharmacogenetics is that often there is an inability of just one single polymorphism to be highly predictive of drug response, since drug responses often involve a large number of proteins whose genes have several polymorphisms. This makes it unlikely that a single gene could predict drug variability. Drug metabolism pharmacogenomics refers to the relationship between multiple polymorphisms in genes encoding drug-metabolizing enzymes involved with drug response (Caudle et al., 2017). In drug-metabolizing pharmacogenetics, genetic testing is carried out on several genetic variants that code for enzymes such as the CYP450 family. By testing for groups of alleles or genetic variants in the CYP450 family, you can classify individuals as "poor," "intermediate," "extensive," or "ultrarapid" metabolizers based on the individual's genetic test results (Caudle et al., 2017). The results of this type of genetic testing can help to guide prescribing practices based on drug responses correlated with genetic variants that code for metabolizing enzymes.

Assessment of a patient's medication use is integral to managing the care and prevention of adverse drug outcomes and ensuring appropriate drug responses; this is particularly important when certain genotypes or variants in the individual's genome impact drug dosage and management. One example is the association of warfarin, the anticoagulant to prevent thromboembolic events, and the two gene variants: cytochrome P450 2C9 (*CYP2C9*) and vitamin K epoxide reductase (*VKORC1*) (Krasowki, 2012; Ruff, 2018). Variants in these genes have been found to influence warfarin dose requirements, warfarin resistance, and/or bleeding risk (Krasowski, 2012). Genetic testing is available to assess for variations in these genes, and a patient's *CYP2C9* and *VKORC1* genotype can be used to help determine the optimal starting dose of warfarin (Ruff, 2018).

Knowledge of pharmacogenomics is becoming increasingly important in clinical practice. Medicare and some insurance companies provide payment for pharmacogenomic testing for some genetic variants with evidence of their being involved in drug metabolism. The FDA has warnings in the drug inserts for over 200 medications with known genetic interactions (FDA, 2021). It is important for clinicians to know where to find authoritative information to guide decisions about using pharmacogenomic information to guide drug choice and dosage.

The Clinical Pharmacogenetics Implementation Consortium (CPIC, 2021) provides peer-reviewed, evidence-based guidelines for certain gene–drug pairs designed to help clinicians understand how available genetic test results should be used to optimize drug therapy (Caudle et al., 2017; Whirl-Carrillo et al., 2012). There are over 100 medications with clinically actionable CPIC guidelines. Table 3.10 lists some of the medications with clinically actionable CPIC guidelines along with their associated genetic markers. CPIC includes ratings of the quality of the evidence, indicated as "levels" for certain gene–drug pairs. Guidelines regarding drug use (e.g., codeine, simvastatin, mercaptopurine) and genetic testing are available and can be found at CIPC's Web site (CPIC, 2021) and in the journal *Clinical Pharmacology and Therapeutics*.

Table 3.10

Examples of Medications With Pharmacogenomic CPIC Guidelines

Clinical Specialty	Drug	Gene
Cardiology	Clopidogrel	*CYP2C19*
	Simvastatin	*SLCO1B1*
	Warfarin	*CYP2C9, VKORC1, CYP4F2*
Infectious Disease	Abacavir	*HLA-B*
	Atazanavir	*UGT1A1*
	Efavirenz	*CYP2B6*
	Voriconazole	*CYP2C19*
Rheumatology	Allopurinol	*HLA-B*
	Thiopurines	*TPMT*
Pain Management	Codeine	*CYP2D6*
	Tramadol	*CYP2D6*
Psychiatry	SSRIs	*CYP2D6, CYP2C19*
	TCAs	*CYP2D6, CYP2C19*
Neurology	Carbamazepine	*HLA-B, HLA-A*
	Oxcarbazepine	*HLA-B*
	Phenytoin	*HLA-B, CYP2C9*
Oncology	Thiopurines	*TPMT*
	Fluoropyrimidines	*DPYD*
	Tamoxifen	*CYP2D6*
	Ondansetron	*CYP2D6*

PharmGKB (2021); Clinical Pharmacogenetics Implementation Consortium (2021).

The PhamGKB database is another comprehensive source of information about genome–drug associations. The database annotates information according to FDA-approved drug levels categorized as "Genetic testing required," "Genetic testing recommended," "Actionable PGx," and "Informative PGx." This database is maintained by Stanford University and includes a search engine that allows clinicians and researchers to search by drug name for pharmacogenomic information, including dosing guidelines, drug labels, gene–drug associations, and genotype–phenotype relationships (PharmGKB, 2021).

Clinical Decision Making and Differential Diagnoses

When the family history is suspect for a hereditary condition, patients should be informed about options for expert genetic counseling and referred when necessary. Genetic counseling visits include the collection and validation of the family and medical history, further assessment of genetic risk, genetic education and testing options, management and screening recommendations if indicated, discussion of insurance and employment issues, post-test genetic test results disclosure and interpretation if ordered, treatments and options, and the implications of the results for the individual and family members, as well as anticipatory guidance and support (Bennett, 2010; Jorde et al., 2020). Genetic services should be given by individual genetic experts or a team of professionals that often includes physicians, geneticists, genetic counselors, and advanced practice nurses in genetics. Referral to a physician specialist may also be warranted for patients who require immediate medical consultation (e.g., a new obstetrical patient with an abnormal genetic test finding). Several online resources are available to assist in locating genetic counseling services (see Table 3.3).

Ethical, Legal, and Social Implications

On May 21, 2008, President George W. Bush signed the Genetic Information Nondiscrimination Act (GINA) after a 9-year effort to get some genomic protection into law. GINA was a first important step in providing some protection against health insurance and employment discrimination (National Human Genome Research Institute, 2017). Although passing GINA was critical to the continued progress of genomic health care, the law does have several significant limitations. First, GINA protects individuals from discrimination based on family history and/or genetic/genomic test results, but there is a gray area when considering when a "preexisting condition" turns into an "existing condition." Second, GINA protects against employer discrimination based on genetic findings, but once an individual receives a clinical diagnosis (e.g., abnormal EKG associated with a long QT mutation), that protection is gone (Green et al., 2015). GINA and other laws do not protect people from genetic discrimination in all situations; GINA does not apply when an employer has fewer than 15 employees, and it does not provide protection against discrimination based on genetics in life, disability, or long-term care insurance. It's also important to pay attention to policy changes because lawmakers continue to propose bills that would limit or eliminate GINA protections (Aron-Dine et al., 2017).

It is important to remember that the basic tenets of ethics (beneficence, nonmaleficence, patient respect, autonomy, and fairness) are as important in genomics as they are in any other area of medicine. The public expects NPs to know the major ethical issues that should be considered when providing care that involves genomics, and they want their health-care teams to provide privacy and confidentiality of information throughout the care experience. Ethical issues that often arise in genetics center around the topics of (1) genetic testing (e.g., risks, benefits, informed consent, who to screen, when, what age); (2) protection and privacy of genomic data for the individual being tested and, because genes are shared among family members, the issue of a "duty to warn" relatives; (3) misuse of genetic information by insurers; and (4) stigmatization associated with genetic test results (Nussbaum et al., 2016).

These issues are complex and nuanced, and NPs should be familiar with and comfortable discussing the issues before patients find themselves grappling with unexpected decisions and difficult conversations. Genetic information can cause anxiety, depression, anger, and/or guilt, and it may create tension among family members because results can reveal information about other family members. Results can also create a false sense of security (negative *BRCA* mutation does not mean a woman will not develop breast cancer) or result in stigma and bias (Bennett, 2010). Patients at increased risk for having hereditary conditions should be offered a genetic referral/consultation so that appropriate ethical, legal, and social implications can be addressed.

Genetic/Genomic Health Assessment: Putting It All Together

Time constraints are often the biggest barrier to collecting an in-depth, three-generation FHH. Asking the patient to complete a family history worksheet prior to an office visit can increase the accuracy of the information, save time, and also establish rapport. Several family history collection tools are available to assist in collecting this information, such as the U.S. Surgeon General's "My Family Portrait" Initiative and the American Medical Association tools (see Table 3.3).

In conclusion, NPs should be prepared to collect a comprehensive FHH, identify family members at increased risk for genomic conditions, educate clients/patients on genetic/genomic tests and therapies, provide informed consent, and refer at-risk individuals to appropriate health-care professionals, agencies, or other resources (Ginsburg et al. 2019). It is also important to continue learning about genomics (see Table 3.3) because the field is continually evolving, and knowledge becomes outdated quickly.

REFERENCES

Alkuraya, F. S. (2013). Impact of new genomic tools on the practice of clinical genetics in consanguineous populations: The Saudi experience. *Clinical Genetics, 84*(3), 203–208.

Alzheimer's Association. (2020). Alzheimer's disease facts and figures. Alzheimer's dementia. https://alz -journals.onlinelibrary.wiley.com/doi/full/10.1002/alz.12068

American Cancer Society. (2020). Agent orange and cancer risk. www.cancer.org/cancer/cancer-causes/agent -orange-and-cancer.html

American College of Obstetricians and Gynecologists. (2011). Family history as a risk assessment tool. Committee Opinion, 478. Retrieved March 9, 2022 from https://www.acog.org/clinical/clinical -guidance/committee-opinion/articles/2011/03/family-history-as-a-risk-assessment-tool

American College of Obstetricians and Gynecologists. (2017). Carrier screening for genetic conditions. ACOG Committee Opinion 691. https://www.acog.org/clinical/clinical-guidance/committee-opinion /articles/2017/03/carrier-screening-for-genetic-conditions

American College of Obstetricians and Gynecologists. (2019). Committee Opinion 762. Prepregnancy counseling. *Obstetrics & Gynecology, 133*(1), e7889. https://journals.lww.com/greenjournal/Fulltext /2019/01000/ACOG_Committee_Opinion_No__762__Prepregnancy.53.aspx

American Medical Association. (2021). Family medical history in disease prevention. https://www.ama-assn .org/delivering-care/precision-medicine/collecting-family-history

American Society of Clinical Oncology. (2021a). Lynch syndrome. From www.cancer.net/cancer-types /lynch-syndrome

American Society of Clinical Oncology. (2021b). Hereditary cancer related syndromes. www.cancer.net /navigating-cancer-care/cancer-basics/genetics/hereditary-cancer-related-syndromes

Aron-Dine, A., Park, E., & Leibenluft, J. (2017). Amendment to House ACA repeal guts protections for people with pre-existing conditions. Center on Budget and Policy Priorities. http://www.cbpp.org /research/health/amendment-to-house-aca-repeal-bill-guts-protections-for-people-with-pre-existing.

Aubart, M., Gross, M., Hanna, M., Zabot, M., Sznajder, M., Detaint, D., Gouya, L., Jondeau, G., Boileau, C., & Stheneur, C. (2015). The clinical presentation of Marfan syndrome is modulated by expression of wild-type *FBN1* allele. *Human Molecular Genetics, 24*(10), 2764–2770. https://doi.org/10.1093 /hmg/ddv037

Bennett, R. L. (2010). *The practical guide to the genetic family history* (2nd ed.). Wiley-Blackwell.

Bennett, R. L., French, K. S., Resta, R. G., & Doyle, D. L. (2008). Standardized human pedigree nomenclature: Update and assessment of the recommendations of the National Society of Genetic Counselors. *Journal of Genetic Counselors, 17*(5), 424–433. https://doi.org /10.1007/s10897-008-9169-9

Bhinder, M. A, Sadia, H., Mahmood, N., Qasim, M., Hussain, Z., Rashid, M. R., Zahoor, M. Y., Bhatti, R., Shehzad, W., Waryah A. M., & Jahan, S. (2019). Consanguinity: A blessing or menace at population level? *Annals of Human Genetics., 83*, 214–219. https://doi.org/10.1111/ahg.12308

Biopharmaceutical Glossaries & Taxonomies. (2021, January 9). Genomics glossary. http://www .genomicglossaries.com

Bird, T. D. (2012). Early-onset familial Alzheimer disease. In R. A. Pagon, M. P. Adam, T. D. Bird, et al. (Eds.). *GeneReviews* [Internet]. University of Washington, Seattle, 1993–2013. Retrieved from www.ncbi.nlm.nih.gov/books/NBK1236

Brandt, J. S., Cruz Ithier, M. A., Rosen, T., & Ashkinadze, E. (2019). Advanced paternal age, infertility, and reproductive risks: A review of the literature. *Prenatal Diagnosis. 39*: 81–87. https://doi.org/10.1002 /pd.5402

Brody, L. C. (n.d.). National Human Genome Research Institute—Talking Glossary of Genetic Terms. https://www.genome.gov/genetics-glossary/genomics

Bylstra, Y., Lim, W. K., Kam, S., Wan Tham, K. W., Wu, R. R., Teo, J. X., Davila, S., Kuan, J. L., Chan, S. H., Bertin, N., Yang, C. X., Rozen, S., Teh, B. T., Yeo, K. K., Cook, S. A., Jamuar, S. S., Ginsburg, G. S., Orlando, L. A., & Tan, P. (2021). Family history assessment significantly enhances delivery of precision medicine in the genomics era. Genome Medicine, 13(3), pg 1-11. DOI:10.1186/s13073-020-00819-1

Caudle, K. E., Dunnenberger, H. M., Freimuth, R. R., Peterson, J. F., Burlison, J. D., Whirl-Carrillo, M., Scott, S. A., Rehm, H. L., Williams, M. S., Klein, T. E., Relling, M. V., & Hoffman, J. M. (2017). Standardizing terms for clinical pharmacogenetic test results: Consensus terms from the clinical pharmacogenetics implementation consortium (CPIC). *Genetics in Medicine; Genet Med, 19*(2), 215–223. https://10.1038/gim.2016.87

Centers for Disease Control and Prevention. (2020). Knowing Is Not Enough—Act on Your Family Health History. www.cdc.gov/genomics/famhistory/knowing_not_enough.htm

Centers for Disease Control and Prevention. (2020). Breast and Ovarian Cancer and Family History Risk Categories. www.cdc.gov/genomics/disease/breast_ovarian_cancer/risk_categories.htm

Center for Jewish Genetics. (n.d.). Diseases common to all Jewish groups. Retrieved from https://www
.jewishgeneticdiseases.org/jewish-genetic-diseases/ (accessed May 5, 2021).

Cheng, H. (2020, March 10). The problem with direct-to-consumer genetic tests. *Scientific American*.
May 5, 2021 from https://blogs.scientificamerican.com/observations/the-problem-with-direct-to
-consumer-genetic-tests/

Children's Wisconsin. (2021). Multifactorial Inheritance. https://childrenswi.org/medical-care/genetics-
and-genomics-program/medical-genetics/multifactorial-inheritance

Clinical Pharmacogenetics Implementation Consortium. (2021). Guidelines. https://cpicpgx.org/guidelines/

Consensus Panel. (2016). *Genetics/Genomics Nursing: Scope and standards of practice* (2nd ed.). American
Nurses Association (ANA), International Society of Genetics (ISONG). Retrieved May 10, 2017 from
Genomes/EssentiCompetenciesandCurriculaGuidelinesforGeneticsandGenomics.pdf

Collins, F. S., Doudna, J. A., Lander, E. S., & Rotimi, C. N. (2021). Human molecular genetics and
genomics—Important advances and exciting possibilities. *The New England Journal of Medicine, 384*(1),
1–4. https://doi.org/10.1056/NEJMp2030694

Cooper, G., & Hausman, R. E. (2018). *The cell: A molecular approach* (8th ed.). Sinauer Associates, Inc.

Dominguez-Valentin, M., Sampson, J. R., Seppälä, T. T., Ten Broeke, S. W., Plazzer, J. P., Nakken, S.,
Engel, C., Aretz, S., Jenkins, M. A., Sunde, L., Bernstein, I., Capella, G., Balaguer, F., Thomas, H.,
Evans, D. G., Burn, J., Greenblatt, M., Hovig, E., de Vos Tot Nederveen Cappel, W. H., . . . Møller, P.
(2020). Cancer risks by gene, age, and gender in 6350 carriers of pathogenic mismatch repair variants:
findings from the Prospective Lynch Syndrome Database. *Genetics in Medicine, 22*(1), 15–25.
https://doi.org/10.1038/s41436-019-0596-9

Dutra, A. S. (n.d.). Heterozygous. National Human Genome Research Institute. Retrieved February 7,
2021, from www.genome.gov/genetics-glossary/heterozygous

Edwards, J., Feldman, G., Gregg, A., Norton. M., Rose, N., Schneider, A., Stoll, K., Wapner, R., Watson, M. S.
(2015). Expanded carrier screening in reproductive medicine—Points to consider. *Obstetrics & Gynecology,
125*(3), 653–662.

Edwards, Q. T., Seibert, D., Maradiegue, A., MacDonald, D., Jasperson, K., Lowstuter, K., & Weitzel, J.
(2007). Breast cancer and the family tree. *Advance for Nurse Practitioners, 15*(5), 34–41.

Eng, C., & Malhotra, S. (2018). *PTEN* hamartoma tumor syndrome. In NORD Rare Disease Database.
Retrieved on May 5, 2021, from https://rarediseases.org/rare-diseases/pten-hamartoma-tumor-syndrome/

Franco, B., & Ballabio, A. (2006). X-inactivation and human disease: X-linked dominant male-lethal disorders.
Current Opinions in Genetic Development, 16(4), 254–259.

Frantzen, C., Klasson, T. D., Links, T. P., & Giles, R. H. (2015). Von Hippel-Lindau disease. In R. A. Pagon,
M. P. Adam, T. D. Bird, et al. (Eds.). *GeneReviews* [Internet]. University of Washington, Seattle,
1993–2013.

Friedman, J. M. (2012). *Neurofibromatosis 1*. In R. A. Pagon, M. P. Adam, T. D. Bird, et al. (Eds.).
GeneReviews [Internet]. University of Washington, Seattle, 1993–2013. www.ncbi.nlm.nih.gov/books
/NBK1109.

Gatti, R., & Perlman, S. (2016). Ataxia-Telangiectasia. In R. A. Pagon, M. P. Adam, T. D. Bird, et al. (Eds.).
GeneReviews [Internet]. University of Washington, Seattle, 1993–2013. www.ncbi.nlm.nih.gov/books
/NBK26468.

Genetics in Primary Care Institute. (2013). Genetic red flags. Retrieved November 23, 2013, from www.
geneticsinprimarycare.org/YourPractice/Family-Health-History/Pages/Genetic%20Red%20Flags.aspx

Geoffrey, S., Ginsburg, R., Ryanne, Wu., Orlando, L. A. (2019) Family health history: underused for
actionable risk assessment. *The Lancet, 394*(10198), 596603. https://doi.org/10.1016/S0140
-6736(19)31275-9

Greco, K. E., Tinley, S., & Seibert, D. (2012). Essential genetic and genomic competencies for nurses
with graduate degrees. American Nurses Association and International Society of Nurses in Genetics.
Retrieved March 9, 2022 from https://www.genome.gov/Pages/Health/HealthCareProvidersInfo
/Grad_Gen_Comp.pdf

Green, R., Lautenbach, D., & McGuire, A. (2015). Perspective: GINA, genetic discrimination, and genomic
medicine. *New England Journal of Medicine, 372*(5), 397–399.

Hamamy, H. (2012). Consanguineous marriages. *Journal of Community Genetics, 3*(3), 185–192.

Harris, P. C., & Torres, V. E. (2018). Autosomal dominant polycystic kidney disease. In R. A. Pagon,
M. P. Adam, T. D. Bird, et al. (Eds.). *GeneReviews* [Internet]. University of Washington, Seattle,
1993–2013. https://www.ncbi.nlm.nih.gov/books/NBK1246/

Hill, W. G., & White, I. M. S. (2013). Identification of pedigree relationship from genome sharing. *G3, 3*(9),
1553–1571. doi: 10.1534/g3.113007500

Hollerer, I., Bachmann, A., & Muckenthaler, M. U. (2017). Pathophysiological consequences and benefits of
HFE mutations: 20 years of research. *Haematologica, 120*(5). doi: 10.3324/haematol.2016.160432

Institute for Precision Medicine. (2021). Definition of precision medicine. Institute for Precision Medicine—Definition of Precision Medicine. https://ipm.pitt.edu/definition-precision-medicine

Janeczko, D., Hołowczuk, M., Orzeł, A., Klatka, B., & Semczuk, A. (2020). Paternal age is affected by genetic abnormalities, perinatal complications and mental health of the offspring (Review). *Biomedical Reports*, 12, 83–88. https://doi.org/10.3892/br.2019.1266

Jorde, L. B., Carey, J. C., & Bamshad, M. J. (2020). *Medical genetics* (6th ed.). Mosby.

Krasowski, M. D. (2012). Pharmacogenomics aspect of warfarin therapy. In L. J. Langman & A. Dasgupta (Eds.). *Pharmacogenomics in clinical therapeutic.* Wiley-Blackwell.

Kuchenbaecker, K. B., Hopper, J. L., Barnes, D. R., Phillips, K.-A., Mooij, T. M., Roos-Blom, M.-J., Jervis, S., van Leeuwen, F. E., Milne, R. L., Andrieu, N., Goldgar, D. E., Terry, M. B., Rookus, M. A., Easton, D. F., Antoniou, A. C., and the BRCA1 and BRCA2 Cohort Consortium. (2017). Risks of breast, ovarian, and contralateral breast cancer for *BRCA1* and *BRCA2* mutation carriers. *JAMA, 317*(23), 2402–2416. https//doi.org/10.1001/jama.2017.7112

Kurian, A.W., Bernhisel, R., Larson K., Caswell-Jin, J. L., Shadyab, A. H., Ochs-Balcom, H. & Stefanick, M. L. (2020). Prevalence of pathogenic variants in cancer susceptibility genes among women with postmenopausal breast cancer. *JAMA. 323*(10), 995–997. https://doi.org/10.1001/jama.2020.0229

Lam, J. T., & Guitierrez, M. A. (2020). *Pharmacogenomics: A primer for clinicians*. McGraw-Hill Professional.

Larsson, N.-G., & Wedell, A. (2020), Mitochondria in human disease. *J Intern Med, 287*: 589–591. https://doi.org/10.1111/joim.13088

Lello, L., Raben, T. G., Yong, S. Y., Tellier, L., & Tsu, S. (2019). Genomic Prediction of 16 Complex Disease Risks Including Heart Attack, Diabetes, Breast and Prostate Cancer. *Scientific Reports. 9*(15286). https://doi.org/10.1038/s41598-019-51258-x

Lloyd-Jones, D. M., Braun, L. T., Ndumele, C. E., Smith, S. C., Sperling, L. S., Virani, S. S., & Blumenthal, R. S. (2019). Use of Risk Assessment Tools to Guide Decision-Making in the Primary Prevention of Atherosclerotic Cardiovascular Disease: A Special Report From the American Heart Association and American College of Cardiology. *Circulation, 139*(25), e1162-e1177. https://doi.org/10.1161/CIR.0000000000000638

Madadi, P., & Koren, G. (2012). Pharmacogenomics principles: Introduction to personalized medicine. In L. J. Langman & A. Dasgupta (Eds.). *Pharmacogenomics in clinical therapeutics.* Wiley-Blackwell.

Manolio, T. A., Bult, C. J., Chisholm, R. L., Deverka, P. A., Ginsburg, G. S., Goldrich, M., Jarvik, G. P., Mensah, G. A., Relling, M. V., Roden, D. M., Rowley, R., Tamburro, C., Williams M. S., & Green, E. D. (2020). Genomic Medicine: A Year in Review 2020. *American Journal of Human Genetics*, 107(6), 1007–1010.

Maradiegue, A., & Edwards, Q. (2016). A primer: Risk assessment, data collection & interpretation for genomic clinical assessment. In D. Seibert, Q. Edwards, A. Maradiegue, & S. Tinley (Eds.), *Genomic essentials for graduate level nurses.* DesTech Publishing.

March of Dimes. (2019). Carrier screening for cystic fibrosis (CF). https://www.marchofdimes.org/complications/cystic-fibrosis-and-pregnancy.

McClintock, A. H., Golob, A. L., & Laya, M. B. (2020). Breast Cancer Risk Assessment: A Step-Wise Approach for Primary Care Providers on the Front Lines of Shared Decision Making. *Mayo Clinic Proceedings, 95*(6), 1268–1275.

Migeon, B. R. (2020). X-linked diseases: susceptible females. *Genetics in Medicine, 22*, 1156–1174. https://doi.org/10.1038/s41436-020-0779-4

National Cancer Institute. (n.d.-a). NCI dictionary of cancer terms. Retrieved January 31, 2021 from Definition of monoclonal antibody—NCI Dictionary of Cancer Terms.

National Cancer Institute. (n.d.-b). Breast cancer risk assessment tool. www.cancer.gov/bcrisktool/

National Cancer Institute. (2017). The genetics of cancer. www.cancer.gov/about-cancer/causes-prevention/genetics

National Comprehensive Cancer Network. (2021). NCCN Clinical Practice Guidelines in Oncology. Retrieved February 7, 2021 from www. www.cancer.gov/types/breast/hp/breast-treatment-pdq

National Gaucher Foundation. (n.d.). What is Gaucher disease? https://www.gaucherdisease.org/about-gaucher-disease/what-is/

National Human Genome Research Institute. (2017). Genetic Information Nondiscrimination Act (GINA) of 2008. Retrieved from https://www.genome.gov/10002077/

National Human Genome Research Institute. Newborn Sequencing in Genomic Medicine and Public Health. (December 7). http://www.genome.gov/Newborn Sequencing in Genomic Medicine and Public Health (NSIGHT) (genome.gov)

National Human Genome Research Institute. (2021). Division of Genomics in Medicine. http://www.genome.gov/about-nhgri/Division-of-Genomic-Medicine

Nussbaum, R. J., McInnes, R. R., & Willard, H. F. (2016). *Thompson & Thompson Genetics in Medicine* (8th ed.). Philadelphia: Saunders.

Online Mendelian Inheritance in Man. (n.d.). Retrieved March 9, 2022 from https://www.omim.org/

Pagon, R. A., Adam, M. P., Bird, T. D., et al. (Eds.). (1993–2021). Illustrated glossary. In R. A. Pagon, M. P. Adam, T. D. Bird, et al. (Eds.). *GeneReviews* [Internet]. University of Washington, Seattle. www.ncbi.nlm.nih.gov/books/NBK5191.

Patel, N., Khan, A. O., Al-Saif, M., Moghrabi, W. N., AlMaarik, B. M., Ibrahim, N., Abdulwahab, F., Hashem, M., Alshidi, T., Alobeid, E., Alomar, R. A., Al-Harbi, S., Abouelhoda, M., Khabar, K. S. A., & Alkuraya, F. S. (2017). A novel mechanism for variable phenotypic expressivity in Mendelian diseases uncovered by an AU-rich element (ARE)-creating mutation. *Genome Biology 18*(144). https://doi.org /10.1186/s13059-017-1274-3

Pauli, R. M. (2012). Achondroplasia. In R. A. Pagon, M. P. Adam, T. D. Bird, et al. (Eds.). *GeneReviews* [Internet]. University of Washington, Seattle. www.ncbi.nlm.nih.gov/books/NBK1152

Peshkin, B.N., & Isaacs, C. (2020). Genetic testing and management of individuals at risk of hereditary breast and ovarian cancer syndromes. *UpToDate*. www.uptodate.com/contents/genetic-testing-and -management-of-individuals-at-risk-of-hereditary-breast-and-ovarian-cancer-syndromes

PharmGKB. (2021). The Pharmacogenomics Knowledgebase. Retrieved March 9, 2022 from https://www .pharmgkb.org/

Phillips, K. A., Douglas, M. P., & Marshall, D. A. (2020). Expanding use of clinical genome sequencing and the need for more data on implementation. *JAMA, 324*(20), 2029–2030. doi:10.1001/jama.2020.19933

Piovesan, A., Antonaros, F., Vitale, L, Stippole, P., Pelleri, M. C., & Caracausi, M. (2019). Human protein-coding genes and gene feature statistics. *BMC Research Notes, 12* (315). https://doi.org/10.1186/s13104 -019-4343-8

Regan, M., Engler, M. B., Coleman, B., Daack-Hirsch, S., & Calzone, K. A. (2019). Establishing the genomic knowledge matrix for nursing science. *Journal of Nursing Scholarship, 51*(1), 50–57. doi: 10.1111 /jnu.12427

Risk assessment. (n.d.). In DOD dictionary of military terms. Retrieved February 2, 2021 from medicaldic-tionary.thefreedictionary.com/Risk+assessment

Roberts, M. R., Asgari, M. M., & Toland, A. E. (2019). Genome-wide association studies and polygenic risk scores for skin cancer: clinically useful yet? *British Journal of Dermatology, 181*(6), 1146–1155.

Roberts, J., & Littleton, A. (2018). Genetics in the 21st Century: implications for patients, consumers and citizens, Version 2. *F1000Research, 6*, doi: 10.12688/f1000research.12850.2

Roden, D. M., McLeod, H. L., Relling, M. V., Williams, M. S., Mensah, G. A., Peterson, J. F., & Van Driest, S. L., (2019). Pharmacogenomics. *The Lancet (British Edition); Lancet, 394*(10197), 521–532. https://10.1016/S0140-6736(19)31276-0

Ross, M. T., Grafham, D. V., Coffey, A. J., Scherer, S., McLay, K., Muzny, D., Platzer, M., Howell, G. R., Burrows, C., Bird, C. P., Frankish, A., Lovell, F. L., Howe, K. L., Ashurst, J. A., Fulton, R. S., Sudbrak, R., Wen, G., Jones, M. C., Hurles, M. E., Daniel, T., Andrews, . . . Bentley, D. R. (2005). The DNA sequence of the human X chromosome. *Nature, 434*(7031), 325–337.

Ruff, C. (2018). Pharmacogenetics of warfarin therapy. *Clinical Chemistry 64*(11), 1558–1559. https://doi .org/10.1373/clinchem.2017.284927

Sharma, R., Agarwal, A., Rohra, V. K., Assidi, M., Abu-Elmagd, M., & Turki, R. F. (2015). Effects of increased paternal age on sperm quality, reproductive outcome and associated epigenetic risks to offspring. *Reproductive Biology and Endocrinology, 13*(35). doi: 10.1186/s12958-015-0028-x

Shawky, R., Elsayed, S., Zaki, M., El-Din, S., & Kamal, F. (2013). Consanguinity and its relevance to clinical genetics. *The Egyptian Journal of Medical Human Genetics, 14*(2), 157–164.

Samadder, N. J., Giridhar, K. V., Baffy, N., Riegert-Johnson, D., & Couch, F.J. Hereditary cancer syndromes: A primer on diagnosis and management, Part 1: Breast-ovarian cancer syndromes. *Mayo Clinical Proceedings, 94*(6), 1084-1098. https://doi.org/10.1016/j.mayocp.2019.02.017 www.mayoclinicproceedings.org

Snozek, C. L. H., Langman, L. J., & Dasgupta, A. (2012). Traditional therapeutic drug monitoring and pharmacogenomics: Are they complementary? In L. J. Langman & A. Dasgupta (Eds.). *Pharmacogenomics in clinical therapeutics*. Wiley-Blackwell.

Strand, N. (2016) *AMA J Ethics, 18*(3), 264–271. doi: 10.1001/journalofethics.2017.18.3.pfor2-1603

Tanakaya, K. (2019). Current clinical topics of Lynch syndrome. *International Journal of Clinical Oncology, 24*(9), 1013–1019. https://doi.org/10.1007/s10147-018-1282-7

Tuite, A., Piazza, A. D., Brandi, K., & Pletcher, B. A. Beyond circles and squares: A commentary on updating pedigree nomenclature to better represent patient diversity. *Journal of Genetic Counseling, 29*(3), 435-439. https://doi.org/10.1002/jgc4.1234

Tully, L. A., Calzone, K. A., & Cashion, A. K. (2020). Establishing the Omics Nursing Science & Education Network. *Journal of Nursing Scholarship, 52*(2), 192–200. https://doi.org/10.1111/jnu.12541

Tsaousis, G. N., Papadopoulou, E., Apessos, A., Agiannitopoulos, K., Pepe, Kampouri, G., Diamantopoulos, S. N., Floros, T., Iosifidou, R., Katopodi, O., Koumarianou, A., Markopoulos, C., Papazisis, K., Venizelos, V., Xanthakis, I., Xepapadakis, G., Banu, E., Eniu, D. T., Negru, S., Stanculeanu, D.L., . . . Nasioulas, G. (2019). Analysis of hereditary cancer syndromes by using a panel of genes: novel and multiple pathogenic mutations. *BMC Cancer, 19*(535). https://doi.org/10.1186/s12885-019-5756-4

University of Pennsylvania. (2020). Ashkenazi Jewish heritage and genetic risk. www.oncolink.org/risk-and-prevention/genetics-family-history/ashkenazi-jewish-heritage-and-genetic-risk

U.S. Department of Health and Human Services, National Institutes of Health, National Heart, Lung and Blood Institute. (2019). What is Marfan syndrome? https://www.nhlbi.nih.gov/health-topics/marfan-syndrome

U.S. Food and Drug Administration. (2021). Table of pharmacogenomic biomarkers in drug labeling. Retrieved March 9, 2022 from https://www.fda.gov/drugs/science-and-research-drugs/table-pharmacogenomic-biomarkers-drug-labeling

U.S. National Library of Medicine. (2020a). Cystic fibrosis. https://medlineplus.gov/cysticfibrosis.html

U.S. National Library of Medicine. (2020b). Fragile X syndrome. https://medlineplus.gov/genetics/condition/fragile-x-syndrome

U.S. National Library of Medicine. (2020c). Genetics home reference: Leber hereditary optic neuropathy. https://medlineplus.gov/genetics/condition/leber-hereditary-optic-neuropathy

U.S. National Library of Medicine. (2020d). Genetics home reference: Polycystic kidney disease. https://medlineplus.gov/genetics/condition/polycystic-kidney-disease

U.S. National Library of Medicine. (2020e). MedlinePlus: Genetics. Retrieved January 31, 2021, from https://www.medlineplus.gov/genetics/understanding/inheritance/penetranceexpressivity

U.S. National Library of Medicine. (2021a). Gaucher disease. https://medlineplus.gov/gaucherdisease.html

U.S. National Library of Medicine. (2021b). Gene reviews. Retrieved January 31, 2021, from https://www.ncbi.nlm.nih.gov/books/NBK5191/#IX-C

U.S. National Library of Medicine. (2021c). MedlinePlus: What is pharmacogenomics? Retrieved March 9, 2022, from https://medlineplus.gov/genetics/understanding/genomicresearch/pharmacogenomics/

U.S. National Library of Medicine. (2021d). MedlinePlus: Genetics. Retrieved March 9, 2022 from https://medlineplus.gov/genetics/

U.S. Preventive Services Task Force. (2018, July, 17). Risk assessment for cardiovascular disease with nontraditional risk factors U.S. Preventive Services Task Force Recommendation statement. *JAMA, 320*(3), 272280. doi:10.1001/jama.2018.8359

U.S. Preventive Services Task Force. (2019). *BRCA* related cancer: Risk assessment, genetic counselling and genetic testing—recommendation statement. Retrieved February 8, 2021, from www.uspreventiveservicestaskforce.org/uspstf/document/ClinicalSummaryFinal/brca-related-cancer-risk-assessment-genetic-counseling-and-genetic-testing

van den Berg, M. M., van Maarle, M. C., van Wely, M., & Goddijn, M. (2012). Genetics of early miscarriage. *Biochimica et Biophysica Acta (BBA)—Molecular Basis of Disease, 1822*(12), 1952–1959.

van Rheenen, W., Peyrot, W. J., Schork, A. J., Lee, S. H., & Wray, S. H. (2019) Genetic correlations of polygenic disease traits: from theory to practice. *Nature Reviews Genetics, 20*(10), 567–581. https://doi.org/10.1038/s41576-019-0137-z

Weitzel, J. N., Lagos, V. I., Cullinane, C. A., Gambol, P. J., Culver, J. O, Blazer, K. R., Gambol, P. J., Culver, J. O., Blazer, K.R., Palomares, M. R., Lowstuter, K. J., & MacDonald, D. J. (2007). Limited family structure and *BRCA* mutation status in single cases of breast cancer. *Journal of the American Medical Association, 297*(23), 2587–2595.

Whelan, A. J., Ball, S., Best, L., Best, R. G., Echiverri, S. C., Ganschow, P., Hopkin, R. J., Mayefsky, J., & Stallworth, J. (2004). Genetic red flags: Clues to thinking genetically in primary care practice. *Primary Care, 31*(3), 497–508.

Whirl-Carrillo, M., McDonagh, E. M., Hebert, J. M., Gong, L., Sangkuhl, K., Thorn, C. F., Altman, R. B., & Klein, T. E. (2012). Pharmacogenomics knowledge for personalized medicine. *Clinical Pharmacology & Therapeutics, 92*(4), 414–417.

Advanced Assessment and Differential Diagnosis by Body Regions and Systems

Chapter 4
Skin

Kathleen Haycraft •

The skin is the largest organ. In addition to the obvious protective functions, the skin helps regulate body heat and moisture, has endocrine and immune functions, and is a major sensory organ. Even though many skin disorders are self-limiting, skin conditions can be extremely distressing. Not only is a large portion of the skin clearly visible, so that all can see any abnormality, but the skin is also an extremely sensitive organ, and its disorders invoke a wide range of symptoms, including pruritus, pain, burning, paresthesias, and stinging. However, in addition to minor, self-limited conditions, the skin serves as a barometer for overall health because it often exhibits changes occurring in response to serious systemic problems. Cutaneous manifestations of systemic disease are an important evolving field of knowledge.

Some dermatologically specific conditions, such as skin cancer, present significant risks to a patient's health. Skin cancer is the most common cancer in the United States, with 1 in 5 likely to develop a skin cancer during their lifetime. It is estimated that in 2021 almost 200,000 will be diagnosed with melanoma in the United States. Skin cancer can affect anyone. While skin cancer is less common among persons of color, these patients often are diagnosed in a late stage so that survival is lower (AAD, 2021).

The annual cost of treating skin cancer is more than $8.1 billion. The diagnosis of skin cancer has climbed 77% from 1994 through 2014. Ultraviolet rays are a group 1 carcinogen, with tanning beds emitting 10- to 15-fold of what the sun emits at maximum intensity. Efforts to reduce skin cancer include improvement in sunscreen and other skin protection and legislation to prohibit tanning in the youth and adolescent population (Skin Cancer Foundation, 2021).

Because the skin is such a large organ and exhibits changes in response to so many elements in the internal and external environments, the list of skin disorders is extensive. This chapter is organized to assist providers in making a definitive diagnosis for the most common conditions and some less-common conditions that mimic other disorders.

History

■ General Integumentary History

When a patient presents with a skin-related complaint, there is an inclination to immediately examine the skin, as the lesion or change is often readily observable. However, it is crucial to obtain a history before proceeding to the examination in order to understand the background of the problem. A thorough symptom analysis is essential and should include details regarding the onset and progression of the skin change; anything the patient believes may trigger, exacerbate, or relieve the problem; how it has changed since first noticed; and all associated symptoms, such as itching, malaise, and so on. When a patient has a skin complaint, it is important to include a wide range of other integumentary symptoms in the review of systems. For instance, ask about the following: dryness, pruritus, sores, rashes, lumps, unusual odor or perspiration, changes in warts or moles, lesions that bleed or do not heal, or areas of chronic irritation. Establish whether the patient has noticed any changes in the skin's coloration or texture. Consider the range of systemic conditions associated with skin changes. Determine what the patient believes caused or contributed to the problem, any self-treatment and the response, and any distress caused by the complaint.

■ Past Medical History

The medical history should include details on any previous dermatological illnesses. Ask about infectious diseases associated with skin changes, such as chickenpox, shingles, measles, impetigo, pityriasis rosea, methicillin-resistant staphylococcus aureus (MRSA), and others. Identify chronic skin problems, such as acne vulgaris or rosacea, psoriasis, and eczema. Ask about prior diagnoses of skin cancer. Determine the history of any previous skin treatments, biopsies, or procedures as well as general surgical history. Because disorders in other systems frequently affect the skin, ask about the history of cardiovascular, respiratory, hepatic, immunological, and endocrine disorders. Identify any recent exposures to others who have been ill or who have had obvious skin problems that might have been contracted. Many medications affect the skin, and a list of all prescribed and over-the-counter agents should be obtained, including herbal and nutritional supplements. Table 4.1 includes a nonexhaustive list of medications that can cause potential adverse skin effects. Finally, ask how the patient generally tolerates exposure to the elements, such as heat, cold, and sun, to determine whether environmental exposure is responsible for or may contribute to the patient's complaint.

■ Family History

The family history should include the occurrence of such skin diseases as eczema, psoriasis, and skin cancer as well as other disorders commonly associated with skin problems, such as cardiovascular, respiratory, hepatic, immunological, and endocrine disorders.

Table 4.1

Cutaneous Reactions From Medications

Type of Reaction	Appearance of Skin	Medications That May Cause Reaction
Acne-like reaction	Erythematous raised papules that are usually tender	Steroids, phenytoin, iodine, bromide
Toxic epidermal necrolysis/Stevens-Johnson syndrome	Inflamed red skin that will peel. May affect mucous membranes as well. May be fatal	Antibiotics, sulfa, anticonvulsants, phenytoin
Red-man syndrome	A profound overall flushing of the skin that may be associated with hypotension and may be serious	Vancomycin, ciprofloxin, cefepime, amphotericin B, rifampin, allopurinol
Fixed drug eruption	A patch or macule that reoccurs in the same area when the offending medication is administered	Antibiotics, NSAIDs; a wide range of medications can be involved
Drug allergy	Macular-papular rash that is usually symmetrical	Antibiotics, antihypertensives; a wide range of medications can be involved
Urticaria	A raised wheal that moves as the histamines are consumed by the lesion	Antibiotics and nearly any medication
Petechiae or purpura	Small to medium-sized purplish macules of patches (that may be raised)	Anticoagulants or diuretic
Photosensitivity	Appearance of sunburn-like rash on sun-exposed skin	Doxycycline, TNF inhibitors, ciprofloxin, sulfa, diuretics with a sulfa ring
Erythema nodosum	Nodules occurring on the lower extremities	Oral contraception
Telangiectasia, atrophy of skin, hypopigmentation	Skin folds, face, genitalia	High-potency topical steroids or too frequent application

Adapted with permission from Dillon, P. (2003). *Nursing health assessment: A critical thinking, case studies approach.* Philadelphia, PA: F.A. Davis, pp. 147–148.

■ Habits

Investigate habits related to skin, hair, and nail care. Identify any chemicals used in grooming as well as potential exposures encountered through work and recreational activities. Identify occupational, daily living, and recreational activities that could be responsible for lesions resulting from friction, infestations, environmental extremes (heat, cold, sun), and other variables. Dietary history is helpful for identifying the potential sources of allergic dermatitis.

Physical Examination

■ Order of the Examination

As the history is obtained, a general survey is performed to determine the patient's general status. Notice the posture, body habitus, obvious respiratory status, and whether the patient is guarding or protecting any area of the skin.

The general survey should provide an indication of the patient's overall skin condition, including color, visible lesions, moisture, and perspiration.

The progression for the skin examination can be completed in a systematic head-to-toe fashion or by region as other systems are being examined and are uncovered. Regardless of the sequence or system chosen, the examination of the skin consists of both inspection and palpation. During the general examination of the skin, compare side to side for symmetry of color, texture, temperature, and so on. Then look more closely at specific areas. Good lighting is essential. In many situations, additional equipment, such as a magnifier, dermatoscope, measuring device, flashlight or transilluminator, and Wood's (ultraviolet) lamp, is helpful.

Privacy is an important consideration because any area being examined must be completely exposed. Keep in mind the structures underlying the skin and the amount of exposure a particular area is likely to receive to explain any particular "wear-and-tear" patterns, scars, calluses, stains, and bruises. For instance, an eczematous rash on the area of the nipple and areola should always trigger consideration of Paget's disease, a malignant breast condition, or mycosis fungoides.

Basic considerations for each section of skin inspected and palpated include the skin's color, temperature, moisture, texture, turgor, and any lesions.

Color

Color is highly variable among individuals of all racial and ethnic backgrounds. The skin color is identified by the Fitzpatrick scale with phenotype 1–6. The lightest skin that always burns is classified as a 1, whereas a 6 represents very dark coloring and skin that never burns (Oakley, 2012). Color variation is even found among an individual's own various body regions, depending on several factors, including general exposure to the elements. For instance, coloring is typically darker in exposed areas, and calluses may be slightly darkened or have a yellow hue. Albinism is an inherited condition with little to no pigmentation in skin, hair, and eyes. Some patients develop a vascular flush over their face, neck, chest, and extremity flexor surfaces when they are exposed to warm environments or emotional disturbances.

Changes in color can also indicate a systemic disorder. For instance, cyanosis, which may indicate pulmonary or heart disease, a hemoglobin abnormality, or merely that the patient is cold, is looked for in the nailbeds, lips, and oral mucosa. Cold, pale, or blue fingers and toes may indicate Raynaud's disease. Jaundice indicates an elevation in bilirubin and often is evident in the sclera and mucous membranes before it is obvious in the skin. Pallor can indicate decreased circulation to an area or a decrease in hemoglobin. Like cyanosis, pallor is frequently first noticed in the face, conjunctiva, oral mucosa, and nailbeds. Redness of the skin may indicate a generalized problem associated with a fever or localized problems, such as sunburn, infection, or allergic response. Table 4.2 lists several alterations in coloring associated with specific conditions.

Table 4.2

Pigmentary Variations Associated With Systemic Conditions

Pigmentary Change	Associated Conditions
Bronze	Addison's disease (adrenal insufficiency) Hemochromatosis
Hyperpigmentation	Chloasma (pregnancy) Lupus Scleroderma Ichthyosis Sprue Tinea versicolor
Yellow	Renal failure Hepatic failure Carotenemia
Dusky blue	Arsenic poisoning Cyanosis Silver toxicity
Red	Polycythemia
Pallor	Anemia Vitiligo Albinism

Temperature

As each area is examined for visible changes, palpation helps to further explore the findings. Skin temperature is best assessed by the dorsal aspects of the hand and fingers. Situations that increase skin temperature include increased blood flow to the skin or underlying structures; thermal or chemical burns; local infections; and generalized, systemic infections and fever. Decreased skin temperature may result from arterial obstruction, pressure, atherosclerosis, or shock.

Moisture

The moisture of the skin varies among body parts and with changes in the environmental temperature, activity level, or body temperature. Skin is typically drier during winter months and moister in warm months. Dehydration, myxedema, genetic disorders, and chronic nephritis can all cause dry skin. Older patients tend to have drier skin than younger patients. The proper term for dry skin is xerosis. The skin's natural moisturizing factor is a cocktail of lipids, ceramides, and essential acids. This system is regulated by the filaggrin system in the skin.

Texture

Skin texture is an important variable. Coarseness may be a sign of chronic or acute irritation as well as hypothyroidism. Extremely fine or smooth texture may indicate hyperthyroidism. Aging results in marked thinning of the skin,

---

RED FLAG ◀ **Red Flags in the Skin Assessment**

- Fever
- Ill appearance
- Extreme of age (young or old)
- Purpura or petechiae
- Generalized or musculoskeletal pain
- Immunocompromised
- Lymphadenopathy
- Commonly offending drugs
- Nonhealing chronic lesion
- Chronic, irregular, and evolving lesion greater than 6 mm
- Oral lesions

---

which has difficulty in maintaining its integrity, and resultant "tissue paper" lacerations.

Turgor

Finally, skin turgor and elasticity are indications of several variables, including hydration and age. The skin should feel resilient, move easily, and return to place quickly after a fold is lifted. The skin overlying the forehead or dorsal hand is more likely to provide a false impression of tenting or decreased elasticity; therefore, turgor should be tested by gently pinching a fold of skin over the abdomen, forearm, or sternum. Some disorders, such as scleroderma, are associated with stiffening of the skin with reduced skin turgor.

■ Assessing Skin Lesions

All lesions must be assessed in detail for size, shape, configuration, color, and texture as well as whether they are a primary or secondary lesion. Primary lesions provide the key details for differential diagnosis. For instance, the primary lesion of eczema is a scale, usually associated with erythema. However, secondary infections can result in secondary changes, including bullae and drainage.

Determine whether any lesion is elevated, depressed, or pedunculated. The color, odor, amount, and consistency of any exudate should be determined. If multiple lesions are present, consider their pattern, location, and distribution.

In determining the distribution or area of skin involvement, the terms *lesion* and *rash* are commonly used. A skin lesion is a single area of altered skin, whereas a wider eruption of lesions is referred to as rash. Table 4.3 describes different characteristics of skin lesions/rashes.

All these variables, along with information obtained during the history and findings related to other systems, are important to making an accurate diagnosis. Take into consideration any changes in hair and nails, both of which can provide signs of cutaneous and systemic diseases. Specialized techniques such as magnification, diascopy, skin scrapings, biopsy, skin taping assessments, and use of the Wood's lamp are helpful in assessing skin lesions.

Table 4.3

Types of Lesions

Macule	Flat less than 10 mm	Patch	Flat greater than 10 mm
Papule	Raised solid less than 10 mm	Plaque	Raised solid greater than 10 mm
Nodule	Palpable solid found in dermis or below less than 10 mm	Tumor	Palpable solid greater than 10 mm in various levels (e.g., mass)
Erosion	Shallow superficial	Ulcer	Deep, including dermal loss of tissue
Vesicle	Fluid-filled blister less than 10 mm	Bulla	Fluid-filled blister greater than 10 mm
Excoriation	Linear usually from a scratch	Fissure	Tears in skin with an abrupt wall
Wheal	Transient patch or papule	Pustule	Pus-filled papule
Petechiae	1–2 mm nonblanchable blood-filled macule	Purpura	Bleeding into the skin that results in purplish discoloration; nonblanchable

Differential Diagnosis of Common Chief Complaints

■ Common Benign Lesions

FRECKLES

Freckles are benign lesions found on most individuals. They develop due to exposure to ultraviolet light. When adults receive lots of ultraviolet exposure, they develop lentigo (large freckles). If the exposure is intense enough, the melanocyte can be destroyed leaving behind small white patches.

Signs and Symptoms
Freckles are asymptomatic, tan to brown macules ranging from 1 to 5 mm in diameter. The color is usually consistent on an individual.

NEVI

Nevi are extremely common and have genetic predetermination for the number, distribution, and coloring among individuals. The term reflects "nests" of melanocytes with hyperpigmentation.

Signs and Symptoms
The lesions are usually less than 0.6 cm in diameter and are evenly pigmented. The margins are well demarcated, and the shape is round. The patient reports that the nevus has existed for a long period without change. The distribution is random.

Diagnostic Studies
None are necessary. Biopsy can be performed to rule out malignancy.

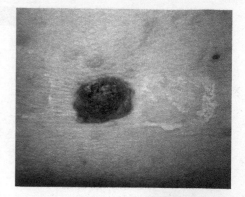

Figure 4.1 Seborrheic keratosis. Papules of varying size and pigmentation, with roughened surface and adhesive appearance commonly seen in older adults. These are benign tumors, and the cause is not known. (Barankin & Friemann, 2006.)

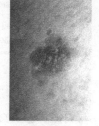

Figure 4.2 Seborrheic keratosis. Raised hyperpigmented lesion with keratotic surface and irregular border. (Copyright Kathleen Haycraft.)

SEBORRHEIC KERATOSIS

Seborrheic keratoses (SKs) are common benign skin changes found in older adults. They are the most common skin finding on a mature adult. Common distribution is on the face, back, under the bra area, and abdomen. SKs occur due to the failure of keratinocyte suppressor genes to control the amount of keratin, which results in a buildup of keratin on the skin. SKs are genetic in origin and not related to sun exposure (Figs. 4.1 and 4.2).

Signs and Symptoms

SKs are usually asymptomatic. If the keratoses are subjected to frequent trauma, by location and exposure, patients may complain of itching, tenderness, or irritation at their site. SKs appear as flat, light tan lesions that evolve to become raised and have keratotic surfaces, often with increased pigmentation. The mature lesion has a "stuck-on" appearance, and the keratotic cover can be scraped off.

Diagnostic Studies

None are warranted; however, some seborrheic keratosis can be visually misconstrued when it is a melanoma. If in doubt, do a shave biopsy.

WARTS

Warts are harmless skin tumors caused by the human papillomavirus (Figs. 4.3 and 4.4). Many subtypes of the human papillomavirus live on the skin and are usually kept in check by the immune system. However, warts typically occur at sites of trauma, recurrent wetness, or nail-biting.

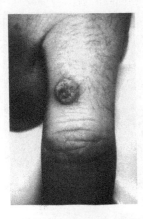

Figure 4.3 Close dorsal view of a proximal cutaneous lesion on right index finger determined to be a common wart. (Courtesy of CDC, Richard S. Hibbets.)

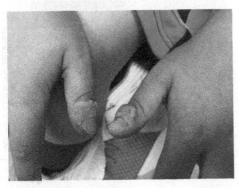

Figure 4.4 Warts. Raised, nonpigmented lesion with rough and irregular surface. (Copyright Kathleen Haycraft.)

Signs and Symptoms

Warts are raised lesions with no significant pigmentation, often paler than surrounding skin. The surface is irregular and may be rough or smooth. If the surface is scraped or pared, minute bleeding points appear. The most common sites include the hands and feet, face, and genitalia. Lesions often occur in clusters. What patients refer to as the seeds or roots of the wart are the vessels associated with the wart.

Diagnostic Studies

None are needed except in the case of recurrent genital warts where subtype evaluation may be important.

ACTINIC KERATOSES

Actinic keratoses, also called solar keratoses, are potentially premalignant lesions, although most do not convert to skin cancer. They appear in sun-exposed areas of skin. Actinic keratoses are typically found in individuals with fair skin and who have a history of developing sunburns without tanning (Figs. 4.5 and 4.6).

Signs and Symptoms

Typical sites include the face, ears, scalp, arms, and legs, although any area of chronic sun exposure is at risk. These scaly lesions may have margins that

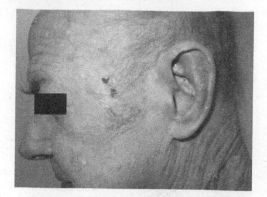

Figure 4.5 Actinic keratoses. Rough, scaly lesions on skin surfaces exposed to the sun. These are the most common precancerous lesions. (Barankin & Friemann, 2006.)

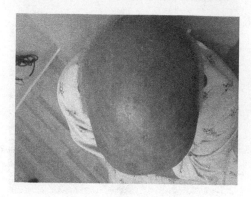

Figure 4.6 Actinic keratoses. Scaly lesion with irregular border on sun-exposed scalp. (Copyright Kathleen Haycraft.)

are irregular. The lesions vary in color and may be hypo- or hyperpigmented. If excess itching or pain occurs at the lesion, a biopsy should be performed to rule out squamous cell cancer.

Diagnostic Studies

Biopsy is indicated only to rule out suspected malignancy.

CORNS AND CALLUSES

A callus is an area of skin thickening at a site exposed to repetitive force and wear and tear. Calluses represent friction over a large patch of skin; a corn is a site of focal friction.

Signs and Symptoms

Both calluses and corns have varying levels of pain. Calluses have rather indistinct borders, while corns have very distinct borders. The sites include areas exposed to wear-and-tear pressures, often against bony prominences, such as on the hands and feet. Unlike warts, these lesions will not reveal pinpoint black dots and bleeding if pared or scraped.

Diagnostic Studies

None are needed.

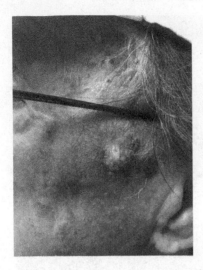

Figure 4.7 Epidermal cyst. Nodular, round and firm, subcutaneous lesion on face. (Copyright Kathleen Haycraft.)

EPIDERMAL CYST

Epidermal cysts are formed from epidermal hyperplasia. The cause is unknown. Some epidermal inclusion cysts develop malignancy. This is rare but is more likely in older persons and on sun-damaged skin (Fig 4.7).

Signs and Symptoms

The patient complains of a cystic lesion that produces cheesy discharge with foul odor. The lesion is sometimes tender or painful and is nodular, round, firm, and subcutaneous; thus, it is flesh-colored but may be erythematous if it is inflamed. The most common sites include the face, scalp, neck, upper trunk, and extremities. However, epidermoid cysts can involve the oral mucosa, breasts, and perineum.

Diagnostic Studies

Usually none are necessary. However, the contents can be cultured, and the lesion should be sent to pathology if excised. Encourage the patient not to squeeze the lesions if they are not removed.

MOLLUSCUM CONTAGIOSUM

Molluscum contagiosum is a skin lesion caused by the DNA poxvirus. It affects persons of all ages but usually presents in infants and youth. Similar to warts, the immune system controls the pox virus, and it must "learn them" (Figs. 4.8 and 4.9).

Signs and Symptoms

Although they are usually asymptomatic, patients occasionally present with the complaint of burning or pruritus at the site of the lesion. The lesion has a smooth surface with a central indentation. Although the lesion is skin-colored or pink, the area immediately surrounding the lesion may be red. If the surface over the

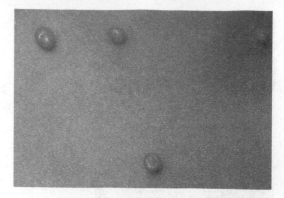

Figure 4.8 Molluscum contagiosum. Small, umbilicated, flesh-colored and dome-shaped lesions caused by infection with poxvirus. The contagious infection occurs mainly in children and immunocompromised patients. (Barankin & Friemann, 2006.)

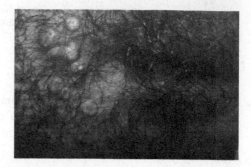

Figure 4.9 Molluscum contagiosum. Characteristic pearly papules that are umbilicated (i.e., depressed center). (CDC.)

center of the lesion is broken, pressure may express keratotic core material. The skin trunk and extremities are most often the site, although it can affect the face, genitals, inguinal area, and oral mucosa.

Diagnostic Studies

Molluscum are diagnosed by clinical exam. Because molluscum contagiosum is self-limited in healthy individuals, treatment may be unnecessary. To avoid scarring, physically removing the lesions is not often recommended in otherwise healthy individuals.

MILIA

Milia occur in infants and are like miniature epidermal inclusion cysts.

Signs and Symptoms

Milia consist of 1- to 2-mm pearl-colored lesions scattered over a newborn infant's face. They may involve the oral mucosa over the palate (Epstein's pearls). While they do not require treatment, they can present a cosmetic concern.

Diagnostic Studies

None are warranted.

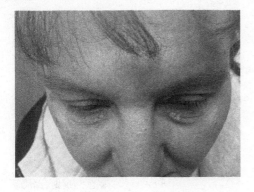

Figure 4.10 Xanthoma. Clusters of yellow, well-defined lesions near eyes. (Copyright Kathleen Haycraft.)

XANTHOMAS/XANTHELASMA

Xanthomas are reflective of abnormal lipid metabolism in the skin. They are caused by accumulation of lipid-laden macrophages in the skin (Fig 4.10).

Signs and Symptoms

There may be a family history of similar lesions and/or a history of hyperlipidemia or heart, thyroid, or liver disorders. The lesion is asymptomatic. The color ranges from flesh to yellow. The distribution includes the area surrounding the eyes and eyelids (xanthelasma) or the extensor areas of the knees and elbows (xanthomas). Xanthomas have a higher risk with lipid elevation. Regardless of the lipid level, administration of a statin may eliminate these lesions over time.

Diagnostic Studies

In some individuals, the lipid levels are elevated.

ACANTHOSIS NIGRICANS

Acanthosis nigricans may be a normal variant or associated with insulin resistance. It is most prevalent in individuals who are obese and of a higher Fitzpatrick skin color. Onset is usually in youths or young adults. If the lesion is very pruritic in a patient with a low body mass index, it may be associated with an underlying malignancy (Figs. 4.11 and 4.12).

Signs and Symptoms

There is a history of progressively growing hyperpigmented areas that may be associated with pruritus. The lesions have a velvety surface and are often located in the skin of the axilla, neck, and groin. In malignant acanthosis nigricans, the lesions develop more rapidly, often involve the mouth, and are associated with different forms of cancer.

Diagnostic Studies

The patient should be evaluated for diabetes. With late onset or rapid progression of lesions, the patient should be evaluated for potential malignancy.

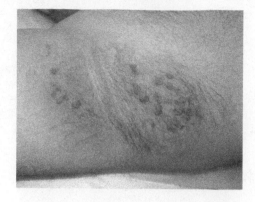

Figure 4.11 Acanthosis nigricans. Hyper-pigmented plaques with velvety surface, typically on the neck, axillae, or groin. This may be associated with endocrine disorders and obesity and with the use of certain drugs. It does run in families and can be seen with some malignancies. (Barankin & Friemann, 2006.)

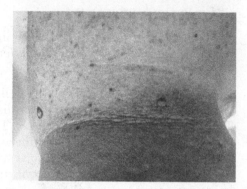

Figure 4.12 Acanthosis nigricans. Hyper-pigmentation in skin fold. (Copyright Kathleen Haycraft.)

Café Au Lait

Café au lait spots are caused by increased melanin content and are associated with neurofibromatosis. They vary in appearance and size, with color ranging from tan to brown (Fig. 4.13).

Signs and Symptoms

There frequently is a history of a variety of developmental and congenital conditions. The lesions are asymptomatic. They range in size from millimeters to over

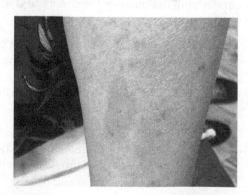

Figure 4.13 Café au lait. Flat, asymptomatic, hyperpigmented patch. (Copyright Kathleen Haycraft.)

10 cm and are usually flat macules or patches. Although the color varies, most are coffee colored. Physical findings include signs of accompanying conditions, such as neurofibromatosis or Fanconi anemia. Six or more café au lait patches are a concern, and a workup is warranted.

Diagnostic Studies

Clinical evaluation is diagnostic and rarely is a biopsy warranted.

CONGENITAL NEVUS

Congenital nevi are usually present at birth or appear in the first few years of life. They vary in size and have a low likelihood of becoming malignant unless they are large congenital nevi (greater than 20 cm). These patients should be referred to a dermatology specialist. Small congenital nevi should be monitored; routine excision is not recommended.

Signs and Symptoms

The lesions are typically round or oval and have an irregular surface. Giant pigmented lesions may have coarse hairs in approximately 50% of cases. There is usually a single lesion, and the color ranges from light to dark brown. The coloring may be speckled. The surface may be verrucous, smooth, or nodular. Typically, the lesion grows proportionally with the child.

Diagnostic Studies

Biopsy is warranted if there is a change in the lesion.

ANGIOMAS

Angiomas arise from dilated capillaries. They are the result of sun damage and genetic predisposition (Fig 4.14).

Signs and Symptoms

The patient may describe onset after age 30, with number and size increasing over time. The lesions are asymptomatic. The color is typically bright red, though they may be darker, including purple to black in coloring. They do not blanch.

Diagnostic Studies

None are warranted.

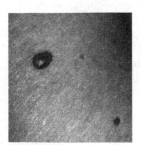

Figure 4.14 Angioma. Bright red, nonblanching papule. (Copyright Kathleen Haycraft.)

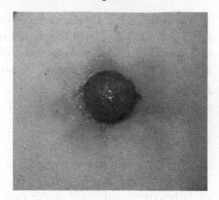

Figure 4.15 Pyogenic granulomas. A firm, red, isolated papule that may ulcerate and crust. This is a benign tumor often referred to as "proud flesh." (Barankin & Friemann, 2006.)

PYOGENIC GRANULOMAS

Pyogenic granulomas are benign lesions that stem from vascular proliferation. They often occur after a minor skin injury but also occur spontaneously and have a higher incidence during pregnancy. The cause is not well understood, although they are not caused by infection, as the name would imply (Fig. 4.15).

Signs and Symptoms

The 1- to 10-mm lesion initially appears as a bright red papule that consists of capillaries and collagen and quickly evolves over a period of a few weeks to become a duller shade of red with a roughened and friable surface. They often have a collarette (ring of keratin tissue) base. They open and bleed with mild trauma. The lesions may become pale, flesh-colored, and chronic, but they rarely resolve spontaneously. It is important to diagnose them early so they can be treated at a more manageable stage.

Diagnostic Studies

A shave biopsy is intended to be both curative and diagnostic; however, reoccurrence does happen, necessitating more definitive surgery.

FURUNCLES

Furuncles are commonly called boils. These lesions are usually staphylococcal infections of hair follicles or sebaceous glands. Multiple or clustered furuncles are called carbuncles.

Signs and Symptoms

Patients complain of pain, redness, and swelling at the affected site. The lesion may ooze pus. The most common sites are the axillae and groin. The patient's temperature may be elevated, and there is often lymphadenopathy. The size of lesion varies. There is significant tenderness.

Diagnostic Studies

None are generally indicated. Cultures should be performed.

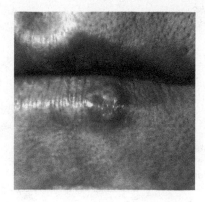

Figure 4.16 Herpes simplex. Herpes simplex is a virus that causes painful vesicular lesions on the skin and mucosal surfaces. Shown here are grouped vesicles on erythematous base on the skin. (Courtesy of CDC, Dr. Herrmann, 1964.)

■ Common Rashes

HERPES SIMPLEX

Herpes simplex is a viral infection that involves the skin and mucous membranes. It is transmitted via direct contact between a susceptible person and one who is shedding the herpes simplex virus (HSV). The infection can cause significant systemic symptoms. Orolabial lesions are typically caused by HSV-1 and genital lesions by HSV-2, although either type can be seen in either location (Fig. 4.16).

Signs and Symptoms

There may be a history of recurrent lesions in the same location. The skin lesions consist of multiple vesicles, which cluster and are usually preceded by an area of tender erythema. The vesicles erode, forming ulcerations. The lesions can occur anywhere on the body, although common sites include perioral and peri-genital regions. Herpetic whitlow, a herpetic lesion on the finger, is seen more commonly in dishwashers, health-care workers, or individuals who suck their thumbs. The primary herpes simplex episode can be more severe, with a more painful lesion and greater likelihood of systemic symptoms such as malaise, aches, fever, and lymphadenopathy. Recurrent episodes may be milder in nature. Recurrent herpes simplex in the same area occurs. Sunscreen application at these sites can be very helpful as the sun suppresses the immune system and may cause flare-ups.

Diagnostic Studies

Diagnostic studies are typically not warranted or ordered. Definitive diagnosis can be made by viral culture of the lesion. Serology can differentiate between HSV-1 and HSV-2, and there is a rapid point of care assay for HSV-2.

VARICELLA

The varicella-zoster virus causes chickenpox. Owing to the introduction of the chickenpox vaccine, the incidence of chickenpox/varicella is decreasing (Figs. 4.17 and 4.18).

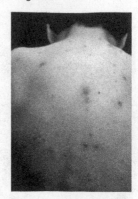

Figure 4.17 Varicella. Hallmark skin eruptions of the acute viral disease known as chickenpox. Typical lesions shown here are generalized papules, vesicles, and crusted lesions in various stages. (Courtesy of CDC, 1995.)

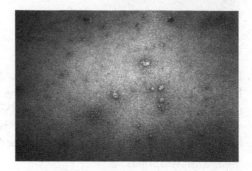

Figure 4.18 Varicella. A number of varicella lesions on the back, cropping in clusters in different developmental stages. (Courtesy of CDC, Dr. John Nobel, Jr.)

Signs and Symptoms

There is often a history of recent exposure, as the incubation period is 14 to 16 days. The onset of the condition often is evident only when the characteristic skin lesions appear, although some patients describe a brief prodromal period of malaise and fever. The prodromal period is more common in adults than in children. The skin lesions appear first randomly scattered on the trunk and then extend to the extremities. Lesions may also appear on the mucosal surfaces. Like other herpes lesions, the lesions progress from an area of redness to form a vesicle; they then become pustular and finally ulcerate. The vesicles look like a dewdrop on a rose petal. New vesicles continue to appear while older lesions ulcerate and crust over, so there is a range of lesion types at a given time. The lesions are intensely pruritic. The systemic symptoms may become severe, and complications include pneumonia, encephalitis, and death.

Diagnostic Studies

Serology studies are helpful in diagnosis.

HERPES ZOSTER (SHINGLES)

Herpes zoster (HZ) is caused by the varicella-zoster virus. The virus resides in the spinal cord area long after the original chickenpox episode is resolved and is released down the dorsal root of the spinal nerve when an individual is immune suppressed (including normal aging) or experiencing stressors (Figs. 4.19, 4.20, and 4.21).

Signs and Symptoms

The skin lesions associated with HZ are usually preceded by a period of regional neuralgia and discomfort, often described as burning and pruritic, as well as a

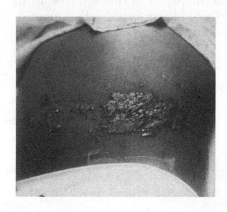

Figure 4.19 Herpes zoster (shingles). Reactivation of the varicella (chickenpox) virus causes inflammation of a few peripheral nerves causing, as shown here, dermatomal distribution of erythematous papules, vesicles, and eroded vesicles in various stages. (Courtesy of CDC, 1995.)

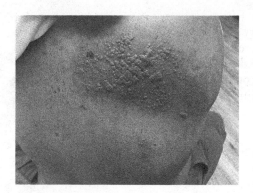

Figure 4.20 Herpes zoster. Dermatomal distribution of inflammation with papules and vesicles. (Copyright Kathleen Hayes.)

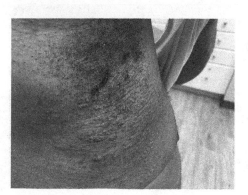

Figure 4.21 Herpes zoster. Dermatomal distribution of inflammation with varied papules and vesicles. (Copyright Kathleen Hayes.)

period of malaise. Skin lesions appear as reddened macules, which later develop as clusters of vesicles and then ulcerate, crusting over. The distribution lies along a dermatome and is almost always unilateral. A bilateral presentation would force a reassessment of the rash. There are many variations of the condition, depending on the affected dermatome. The healing of the lesions is frequently followed by development of postherpetic neuralgia (i.e., long-term nerve pain). There is lymphadenopathy in the region of the skin lesions. In patients who are immunocompromised, the condition may be disseminated. Any facial involvement near the eye necessitates an immediate referral to an ophthalmologist.

Diagnostic Studies

HZ is usually a clinical diagnosis. If any doubt occurs, a HZ culture and serology can be obtained.

CELLULITIS

Cellulitis is an infection of the skin and subcutaneous tissue. The causative organism varies, although staphylococcal and streptococcal infections are common. Superficial cellulitis, called erysipelas, is associated with streptococcal infections (Fig. 4.22).

Signs and Symptoms

The patient often describes a history of a break in the skin from an injury, an insect bite or sting, or a procedure preceding the onset of redness, swelling, and pain at the site. The affected area is tender, swollen, reddened, and warm. There is regional lymphadenopathy. When streptococcal infection is involved, bullae may form on the surface. The lower leg is a common site, usually unilateral.

Diagnostic Studies

A complete blood count and cultures may be warranted.

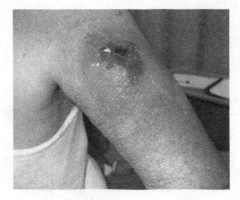

Figure 4.22 Cellulitis. An erythematous and edematous warm area of tenderness caused by a bacterial infection, most commonly *Streptococcus pyogenes* or *Staphylococcus aureus.* (Barankin & Friemann, 2006.)

CONTACT DERMATITIS

Contact dermatitis is an inflammatory response to contact with a chemical, plant, or other agent. The range of potential contactants is immense and includes agents used in grooming; it can also be induced by allergens and irritants (Figs. 4.23 and 4.24).

Signs and Symptoms

The affected area may be mildly or intensely pruritic. The history helps in identifying the offending agent. The dermatitis appears within days following the contact or exposure. The first exposure usually results in a delayed response, whereas reactions to subsequent exposures develop more rapidly, commonly within 1 to 2 days. The distribution and configuration of skin lesions is determined by the exposure. The lesions can range in appearance; they emerge as reddened papules, which form vesicles and later erode and encrust. Any area of skin can be affected. As lesions erupt, the skin is at risk for developing secondary infection.

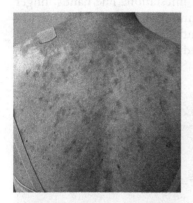

Figure 4.23 Contact dermatitis. In response to skin contact with allergens or irritating substances, erythematous papulovesicular lesions in distribution of the causative agent can occur as seen in this photo. (Reprinted with permission by Margaret Bobonich, DNP, DCNP, FNP-C.)

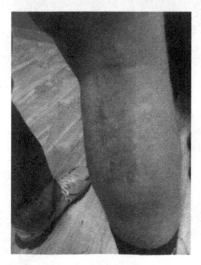

Figure 4.24 Contact dermatitis. Distribution of erythema with papulovesicular lesions in distribution of contactant. (Copyright Kathleen Hayes.)

Diagnostic Studies

None are needed. A patch test may be positive. The most valuable diagnostic approach is a comprehensive history and assessment. If the rash is persistent, serology to measure antibodies to environmental and food sensitivities may be of value.

SCABIES

The mite *Sarcoptes scabiei* is the cause of scabies. Individuals are infected through direct contact. After the mites mate on the skin surface, the females burrow beneath the skin and the infected person develops a delayed sensitivity reaction to the mite, larvae, and fecal material (Figs. 4.25 and 4.26).

Signs and Symptoms

The patient complains of intense pruritus, often worse at night. There is frequently a history of similar symptoms in other family members or contacts. The lesions appear as small red papules, which often form vesicles, erode, and crust. The distribution depends on the area of infestation. The hands, finger webs, wrists, axillae, and pubic areas are commonly involved. The face is a common site on infants, whereas middle-aged individuals have more lesions on the trunk. There can be secondary lesions related to the person's scratching the

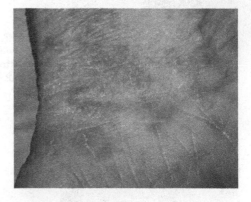

Figure 4.25 Scabies. Skin manifestations of the highly contagious infections of the mite *Sarcoptes scabei* show erythematous papules in a burrows pattern, rarely some vesicles, and excoriations from scratching because of the extreme itching it causes. (Barankin & Friemann, 2006; image courtesy of Loretta Fioroillo, MD.)

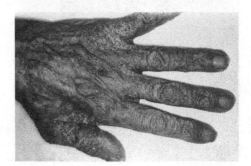

Figure 4.26 Scabies. Patients hand reveals scabies infestation with crusty, erythematous lesions, especially in areas of webbing between fingers. (Courtesy of CDC.)

pruritic primary site. The lesions' configuration is typically linear, as the larvae burrow beneath the skin. Lesions become painful and reddened if secondary infection is present. Norwegian crusted scabies does not exhibit the same symptoms as routine scabies. In these settings, the patients are very contagious and large amounts of the mite are present. The skin can mimic psoriasis in its appearance, and it tends to occur in the older, immobile, and/or immune-compromised patient.

Diagnostic Studies

There is generally no reason to perform diagnostic tests, as the diagnosis is made on the basis of history and physical examination. A scraping from a new lesion placed on a slide with oil and examined under the microscope may reveal mites, eggs, or feces.

DERMATITIS HERPETIFORMIS

Dermatitis herpetiformis is an autoimmune skin disorder associated with celiac disease, but rarely may be seen in associated thyroid disease (Fig. 4.27).

Signs and Symptoms

Pruritus, burning, or stinging at the site often precedes the development of skin lesions. The lesions consist of clustered vesicles on a reddened base. The lesions have a herpetiform configuration, but the distribution is symmetrical. The extensor surfaces of the knees and elbows are often affected, as are the posterior scalp, neck, back, and thighs. The condition is chronic. The oral mucosa is rarely involved, and the palms and soles are not affected. The condition waxes and wanes based on the patient's gluten intake.

Diagnostic Studies

A biopsy will demonstrate characteristic findings.

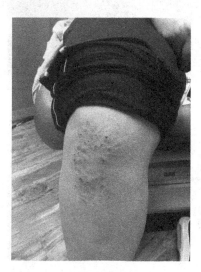

Figure 4.27 Dermatitis herpetiformis. Clustered intact and ruptured vesicles over inflammatory base. (Copyright Kathleen Hayes.)

ERYTHEMA MULTIFORME/STEPHEN-JOHNSON SYNDROME AND TOXIC EPIDERMAL NECROLYSIS SYNDROME

Erythema multiforme is usually a self-limited skin condition that results from exposure to a medication or infection. This condition occurs in varying grades and is commonly classified as erythema multiforme minor, erythema multiforme major, Stevens-Johnson syndrome, and in the most severe case, toxic epidermal necrolysis syndrome.

These are spectral disease states. Both toxic epidermal necrolysis syndrome and Stevens-Johnson syndrome can be fatal and represent dermatological emergencies necessitating hospital admission (occasionally a burn unit). Finding and removing the triggering medication or infectious agent is imperative (Figs. 4.28 and 4.29).

Signs and Symptoms

The patient with erythema multiforme often provides history of having recently taken a drug that caused the disorder or history of another condition such as an autoimmune disorder, malignancy, or infection. The lesions are nonraised, reddened macules or plaques. They may have a "target" appearance, with a deep red outer rim and center, separated by a pale area. The lesions may progress to form vesicles and/or bullae that lie over the reddened base and form crusts as they

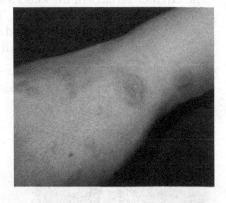

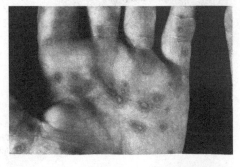

Figure 4.28 Erythema multiforme. The rash shown here often is caused by an immune response to drugs or an infection, such as HSV. It presents with a target lesion with three rings and a vesicular or dusky center. (Barankin & Friemann, 2006.)

Figure 4.29 Erythema multiforme. Patient's palm reveals erythematous, blotchy red rash with round lesions that have begun to coalesce. (Courtesy of CDC, Dr. N. J. Fiumar.)

erode. Although the lesions are generalized, they are usually most prominent over the limbs. The mouth, trunk, and soles of the feet are frequently involved. Any mucosal membrane area may be affected.

Diagnostic Studies

Erythema multiforme may be associated with decreased white blood cell and red blood cell counts, increased erythrocyte sedimentation rate, and increased blood urea nitrogen/creatinine in severe cases. Biopsy of the skin must be performed.

BULLOUS IMPETIGO

Bullous impetigo is usually caused by *Staphylococcus aureus* and is less common than the nonbullous form. Although it can occur at any age, it is most common in children younger than 6 years (Figs. 4.30 and 4.31).

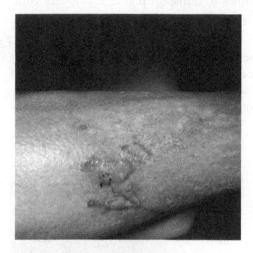

Figure 4.30 Bullous impetigo. Bullous and pustular lesions in varied stages, with reddened base. (Copyright Kathleen Haycraft.)

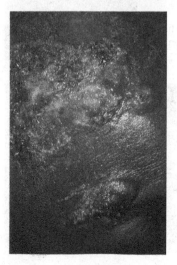

Figure 4.31 Bullous impetigo. Bullous and pustular lesions on forehead. (Courtesy of CDC, Dr. Thomas F. Sellers.)

Signs and Symptoms

The patient or parent may recall being exposed to another person with similar lesions. The bullae progress rapidly, have a thin surface that bursts easily, and subsequently erode. A honey-colored crust is characteristic of impetigo, and smaller lesions may develop near the first. If the crust is removed, a reddened base is visible. Lesions can occur anywhere.

Diagnostic Studies

None are needed. Culture and sensitivity should be performed. Lesions clear with appropriate antimicrobials.

PITYRIASIS ALBA

Pityriasis alba is associated with very dry skin, and inadequate natural moisture results in an inability of the melanosomes to transport pigment. It is very common in children and young adults (Figs. 4.32 and 4.33).

Signs and Symptoms

There are usually no symptoms associated with the lesions, although patients complain of mild pruritus on occasion. There is commonly a family history of atopic diseases, such as asthma and eczema. Occurrence often has a seasonal pattern. The lesions consist of areas of hypopigmented macules or patches, usually

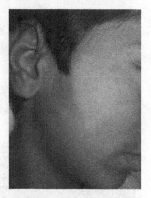

Figure 4.32 Pityriasis alba. Hypopigmented patches with a fine scaly surface that are commonly seen on the face in children. (Barankin & Friemann, 2006.)

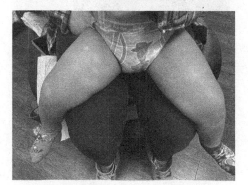

Figure 4.33 Pityriasis alba. Hypopigmented patches distributed along child's lower extremity. (Copyright Kathleen Haycraft.)

covered with a very fine scale. The hypopigmented area is poorly defined and often dry. Over time, the dryness and/or scaling resolves, leaving a smooth area of hypopigmentation. The lesions sometimes arise from an initial area of mild erythema. Common sites include the face and arms. Good skin care and frequent moisturization will improve the appearance.

Diagnostic Studies
None are warranted.

TINEA VERSICOLOR

Tinea versicolor is caused by *Malassezia furfur* (formerly named *Pityrosporum orbiculare*), a yeast-like organism. Tinea versicolor is not contagious (Figs. 4.34 and 4.35).

Signs and Symptoms
Tinea versicolor, also known as *pityriasis versicolor*, consists of scaly patches of hyper- or hypopigmented skin. Although the color can range from paler than the

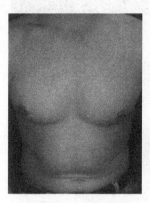

Figure 4.34 Tinea versicolor. Macules and patches varying from hypopigmentation to various colors with a fine scaled surface caused by infection with the fungus *Malassezia furfur*.
(Barankin & Friemann, 2006.)

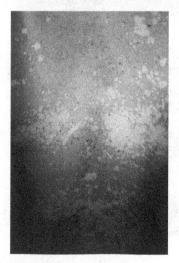

Figure 4.35 Tinea versicolor. A patchy hypopigmented rash of tinea versicolor over upper and lower back.
(CDC, Dr. Gavin Hart.)

surrounding skin to dark brown, an individual's multiple lesions are similar in color. Size of the lesions ranges widely. The margins are irregular and poorly discriminated. This is important to note as it can be confused with vitiligo, which has well-discriminated borders. Itching is often present. It usually occurs in the warm months and in adolescents and young adults.

Diagnostic Studies

Skin scrapings with potassium hydroxide solution reveal hyphae spores under the microscope.

VITILIGO

Vitiligo is a progressive loss of pigmentation due to antibodies attacking the melanocyte. It represents an autoimmune disease and is associated with other autoimmune diseases. Average age of onset is 20 years (Figs. 4.36 and 4.37).

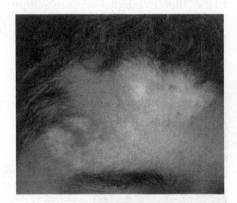

Figure 4.36 Vitiligo. Hypopigmented/white well-defined patches caused by localized loss of melanocytes. (Barankin & Friemann, 2006.)

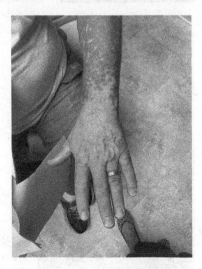

Figure 4.37 Vitiligo. Confluent areas of well-demarcated depigmentation. (Copyright Kathleen Haycraft.)

Signs and Symptoms

The patient often describes a history of the progressive development of small, multiple areas of depigmentation that, over time, become larger and confluent. Lesions frequently start on the fingers and toes. The lesions are well demarcated. There is no overlying scale or vesicle development. Any area of skin can be involved. The hair in the affected area may also lose pigmentation. There is a higher incidence of vitiligo in patients with autoimmune disorders, particularly those affecting the endocrine system, including hypothyroidism, diabetes mellitus, and Addison's disease.

Diagnostic Studies

Biopsy should be performed if diagnosis is in question.

HIDRADENITIS SUPPURATIVA

Hidradenitis suppurativa involves occlusions of hair follicles with associated inflammation and scarring. Sites are commonly under the breast or in the axillae, and under the buttock or groin. The cause or trigger of the occlusion is unknown, but researchers feel it is multifactorial with genetics, immune system, and hormonal balance being cofactors (Fig. 4.38).

Signs and Symptoms

The patient complains of pain at the site of swelling and redness. The lesions range from papules to nodules and are red, warm, and tender. Usually, multiple lesions are present. The lesions are often thought to be secondarily infected; this is not common. The lesions may drain, and/or may form abscesses and, frequently, scar tissue. While they are rarely infected, if lesions rapidly enlarge and drainage color is changed, they may be at risk for MRSA. Lymphadenopathy is usually absent. Without treatment, the lesions can become chronic with prolonged drainage and/or scarring.

Diagnostic Studies

Diagnosis is a clinical one.

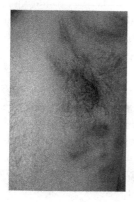

Figure 4.38 Hidradenitis suppurative. Pustules, nodules, abscesses, and/or sinus tracks in the area of hair follicles caused by inflammation of the sweat glands. Often associated with obesity, diabetes, and smoking. (Barankin & Friemann, 2006.)

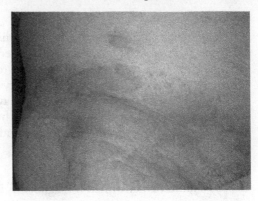

Figure 4.39 Urticaria. An allergic reaction that causes extremely itchy erythematous, edematous papules and/or plaques in varied distributions. (Barankin & Friemann, 2006.)

URTICARIA

Urticaria, commonly called hives, involves a histamine-mediated response that can be either acute or chronic. A wide range of situations are associated with hives, including a variety of infections, allergies to foods and medications, or underlying systemic disease. There are also environmental triggers for urticaria, including heat, water, cold, and exercise (Fig. 4.39).

Signs and Symptoms

The patient may be able to identify a potential trigger based on experience. The complaint may include a recurrence of the pink or red wheals. The lesions are usually very pruritic; they are nonblanching and vary in size. There are often lesions of various stages, as they emerge from pink to red and then gradually fade before disappearing. New lesions appear as others resolve. The lesions are palpable, with a nonpalpable area of peripheral erythema. There may be associated signs of anaphylaxis and/or angioedema. Dermatographism is frequently positive (i.e., pressure on the skin results in elevation and redness). When urticaria occur in the nose, mouth, and airway, it is a much more serious condition called *angioedema* and must be treated urgently.

Diagnostic Studies

Diagnostic studies include punch biopsy, skin tests for allergen identification, serology for allergen identification, complete blood count, and other tests based on assessment and duration of disease state.

ERYTHEMA NODOSUM

Erythema nodosum is believed to be a hypersensitivity reaction to infection, medications, malignancy, or hormones of pregnancy. It is an inflammatory condition of the fat of the lower legs or arms. Erythema nodosum can be acute and isolated or chronic. It is associated with the use of certain medications (e.g., sulfa drugs, oral contraceptives), chronic conditions (e.g., sarcoidosis, Crohn's disease, ulcerative colitis), streptococcal infections, and pregnancy (Figs. 4.40 and 4.41).

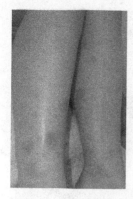

Figure 4.40 Erythema nodosum. Inflammation of the subcutaneous fat (panniculitis) that causes a dull erythematous and tender nodule, frequently on the anterior lower leg. (Barankin & Friemann, 2006.)

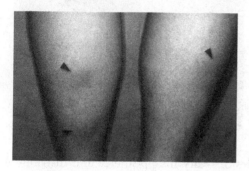

Figure 4.41 Erythema nodosum. Anterior shins reveal number of erythematous areas (see arrows) that appear like bruising but are presentation of erythema nodosum. (Courtesy of CDC and Richard S. Hibbets.)

Signs and Symptoms

The patient may have experienced a period of arthralgia and malaise preceding the development of the skin lesion. The lesion is usually isolated, although multiple sites are possible. The lesion emerges as a firm, tender, reddened nodule, usually along the anterior aspect of the leg, although other sites can be involved. Over a period of up to 2 weeks, the lesion fades in color and the degree of firmness decreases.

Diagnostic Studies

Diagnosis is often clinical. Other appropriate diagnostic studies should be performed if underlying systemic disease or infection is suspected.

SECONDARY SYPHILIS

Secondary syphilis is called the "great imitator" because the associated skin lesions can have a variety of presentations and appearances. The condition is caused by infection with *Treponema pallidum* (Figs. 4.42 and 4.43).

Signs and Symptoms

The patient may provide the history of a more generalized rash developing 2 or more weeks following the primary lesion, which may still be evident. The primary lesion is usually an isolated, single red lesion, which ultimately ulcerates, forming a nontender chancre. There may be a period of malaise preceding the

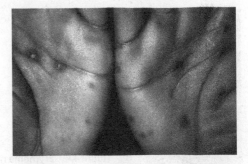

Figure 4.42 Secondary syphilis. A hyperpigmented, papulosquamous rash diagnostic of secondary syphilis on patient's palms. (Courtesy of CDC.)

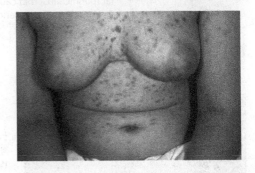

Figure 4.43 Secondary syphilis. Torso reveals macular rash dispersed over trunk and arms, diagnosed as secondary syphilis. (Courtesy of CDC.)

eruption of secondary lesions. These lesions vary in appearance and distribution, but the typical finding is of red maculopapular lesions smaller than 1 cm in diameter. Any portion of skin can be involved, including the scalp, mucous membranes, perineum, and the soles and palms. There is generalized lymphadenopathy. Depending on the involvement of other organs, there may be findings consistent with meningitis, hepatitis, iritis, and arthritis.

Diagnostic Studies
The diagnosis is confirmed by positive serology.

TINEA

Tinea caused by a dermatophyte infection. Depending on the site of the lesion, the condition is referred to differently: tinea capitis (scalp), tinea cruris (groin), tinea faciei (face), tinea pedis (feet), and so on. It is commonly called ringworm. The fungi invade the skin, and the infection is usually limited to the keratin layer. Fungus is the umbrella category for yeast (single cell) and mold (multicellular). (Figs. 4.44, 4.45, and 4.46).

Signs and Symptoms
The patient may recall exposure to another individual with similar lesions or an activity such as gardening or handling animals through which they were exposed to the dermatophyte. The lesion is pruritic. It begins as a small, annular, erythematous, and scaling lesion that develops a central area of clearing as it grows in diameter. The edge may develop vesicles, is typically scaling, and remains palpable and reddened,

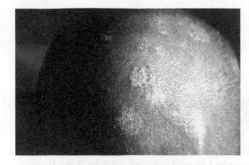

Figure 4.44 Tinea capitus. The patient's scalp displays "ringworm," tinea capitus.
(Courtesy of CDC, Dr. Lucille L. Georg.)

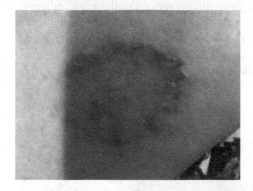

Figure 4.45 Tinea corporis. Annular lesion with vesicular edge and central clearing.
(Copyright Kathleen Haycraft.)

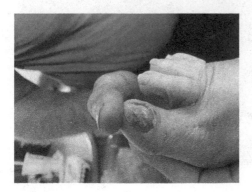

Figure 4.46 Tinea unguium/onychomycosis. Thick, deformed, yellow and brittle toenail.
(Copyright Kathleen Haycraft.)

so that it presents as a ring. The lesion(s) may be localized or diffuse. There is often complaint of intense pruritus over heavily scaled areas and pain at fissures. When blisters occur at sites away from the tinea, it is called an Id reaction (an allergic reaction to the tinea). Tinea can also develop secondary infections, which result in increased pain. The affected area may progress to affect the nails (onychomycosis).

Diagnostic Studies

The diagnosis is typically evident by the appearance of the lesion and the patient's history. However, KOH (potassium hydroxide) skin scraping may reveal hyphae or buds.

PITYRIASIS ROSEA

Pytiriasis rosea is caused by a virus. It is most common in the spring and autumn (Figs. 4.47 and 4.48).

Signs and Symptoms

The patient is usually asymptomatic, although some complain of a prodromal period of malaise preceding the emergence of the rash. The rash is often mildly pruritic. The first sign is typically a "herald patch," which is a 2- to 10-cm annular pink patch that, like tinea, has an area of central clearing with a fine scale. The herald patch is most commonly located on the trunk. The herald patch is followed several days later by a more diffuse set of smaller pink, salmon, or fawn-colored lesions, which, at 0.5 to 1.5 cm, are much smaller than the herald patch. The distribution of the smaller lesions is described as "Christmas tree distribution" because the lesions have a slightly diagonal axis and are distributed along the skin tension lines (see Fig. 4.47). Lesions generally resolve within 12 weeks.

Diagnostic Studies

The diagnosis is a clinical one.

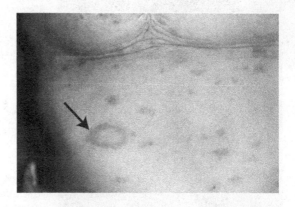

Figure 4.47 Pityriasis rosea. A mild, acute inflammatory condition with a characteristic early rash that is a large macular herald patch and is followed by ovoid, fawn-colored, scaly lesions with a "Christmas tree" pattern, or diagonal, orientation. Occurs most commonly in the spring and fall. (Courtesy of the CDC, 1975.)

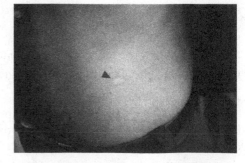

Figure 4.48 Pityriasis rosea. The left flank reveals a 2-week-old herald patch, typically large and scaly. (Courtesy of CDC and Joe Miller.)

ERYTHEMA MIGRANS, LYME DISEASE

Erythema migrans is an early sign of Lyme disease, a tick-borne disease caused by *Borrelia burgdorferi*. It is nicknamed the bull's-eye rash (Figs. 4.49 and 4.50).

Signs and Symptoms

The typical history includes activities in a tick-prone area. A tick bite appears initially as a small red macule. The lesion often expands outwardly with an erythematous border and may include central clearing with the original papule visible, giving it a "target" appearance. The original lesion can expand significantly, reaching 15 to 20 cm in diameter. Regional lymphadenopathy and flu-like symptoms may be present. If untreated, symptomatology may include additional smaller annular lesions, generalized rash, headache, arthritic pain, and cardiovascular symptoms.

Diagnostic Studies

The diagnosis is often evident based on history. Serological antibody testing confirms diagnosis, if uncertain.

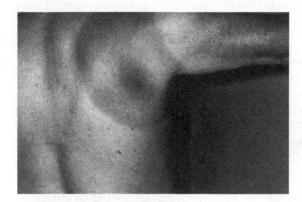

Figure 4.49 Erythema migrans. Named for its resemblance to a target, this early sign of Lyme disease first appears as a macule at the site of a tick bite. An erythematous border expands outwardly. (Courtesy of CDC.)

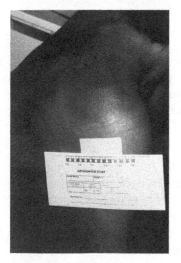

Figure 4.50 Erythema migrans. The posterior shoulder area of patient diagnosed with Lyme disease displays erythema migrans rash. (Courtesy of CDC.)

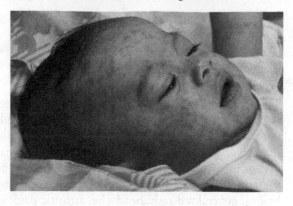

Figure 4.51 Measles. In this highly contagious disease, a generalized macular red rash appears on the neck and face following common viral infection symptoms. Koplik spots are found on the buccal mucosa. (Courtesy of CDC, Rebecca Martin, PhD, 2014.)

MEASLES

Measles is a highly contagious, vaccine-preventable viral condition. While rare in the United States, measles outbreaks have occurred over the past few years. Measles should be considered especially in unvaccinated patients with relevant findings.

Signs and Symptoms

The patient may report exposure 7 to 18 days prior to onset of symptoms. Initially, patients experience symptoms common to viral infections, including aching, cough, sore throat, reddened eyes, and fever. Koplik spots (small white lesions) form on the buccal mucosa, followed by a generalized red macular rash that usually begins on the back of the neck and face, spreading to the trunk. The macules become raised and papular. Complications can develop, including pneumonia and encephalitis (Fig. 4.51).

Diagnostic Studies

Diagnosis is usually based on findings. Serological testing should be employed to identify early outbreaks.

ATOPIC DERMATITIS

Atopic dermatitis, commonly called eczema, is an atopic condition of the skin. It is associated with other atopic diseases, including asthma, conjunctivitis, and eosinophilic disorders. Pathogenesis is unknown but is suspected to be multifactorial with environmental, neuroendocrine, infectious, metabolic, and genetic influences (Figs. 4.52 and 4.53).

Signs and Symptoms

The patient presents with a complaint of recurrent, itchy skin rash. The most common sites involve the flexor surfaces of extremities, neck, and face, although the condition is certainly not limited to these areas. There may be a personal or family history of other atopic conditions. The lesions are erythematous, exudative eruptions that can be intensely pruritic. They often progress to form areas of lichenification due to recurrent scratching, which may become chronic.

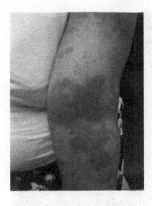

Figure 4.52 Atopic dermatitis. A chronic condition, often seen in families, presents with erythematous, scaly patches and plaques, often along the flexor surfaces. (Reprinted with permission from Margaret Bobonich, CNP, DCNP, FNP-C.)

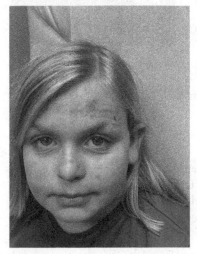

Figure 4.53 Atopic dermatitis. Facial distribution of erythematous lesion with lichenification. (Copyright Kathleen Haycraft.)

The sites are prone to secondary infections. Excessive use of topical steroids can result in hypopigmentation that may be permanent.

Diagnostic Studies

The diagnosis is typically based on history and physical findings.

SEBORRHEIC DERMATITIS

The cause of seborrheic dermatitis is believed to be a combination of oil production and immune response to yeast *Malassezia*. It is an inflammatory skin condition more common in males than females.

Signs and Symptoms

The patient typically presents with complaints of itching and/or burning associated with scaling lesions on the hairy parts of the body, such as scalp, central face, and presternal areas. The lesion consists of a greasy scale lying over an erythematous patch. The problem is chronic. It can become eczematous, allowing for secondary infection. Cradle cap is a form of seborrheic dermatitis seen in children (Fig 4.54).

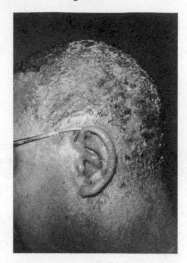

Figure 4.54 Seborrheic dermatitis. Adult patient's head and neck reveal seborrheic dermatitis. (Courtesy of CDC and Susan Lindsley.)

Diagnostic Studies

None are necessary; diagnosis is made based on distribution and appearance of the lesion and the history.

STASIS DERMATITIS

Stasis dermatitis affects the skin in areas with venous insufficiency. It most often affects the lower legs. It is imperative to avoid treating this with recurrent antibiotic therapy as some providers confuse this with recurrent cellulitis (Figs. 4.55 and 4.56).

Signs and Symptoms

There is typically a gradual emergence of patches of erythemic scaling associated with pruritus. Edema is often present. The most frequent site is the medial ankle. Over time, the lesions enlarge and become eczematous so that they weep and form crusting. If the site heals, there is a residual area of discoloration caused by leaking of hemosiderin into the tissues. In advanced cases, the lesions may ulcerate.

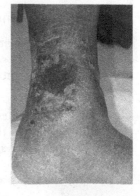

Figure 4.55 Stasis dermatitis. Erythematous, scaly patches on the lower leg, associated with edema, varicosities, and/or hyperpigmentation associated with impaired blood return from the legs. (Barankin & Friemann, 2006.)

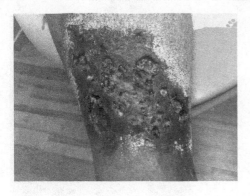

Figure 4.56 Venous stasis ulcer. The patient's leg illustrates advanced venous stasis dermatitis, which is ulcerative. (Copyright Kathleen Haycraft.)

Diagnostic Studies

Deep venous thrombosis may be revealed through Doppler studies. Biopsy reveals characteristic features.

EXANTHEM

An exanthem is a widespread rash caused by drugs, microorganisms, or autoimmune disease. Commonly known diseases such as measles, fifth's disease, Epstein-Barr virus, and strep infections are involved, as are newer diseases such as dengue, West Nile virus, and Chikungunya. In 2020 to 2021, COVID entered the environment, resulting in a wide array of cutaneous rashes. While the range of exanthems is immense, it is important to consider these in differential diagnosis (Fig. 4.57).

Signs and Symptoms

The size and distribution vary depending on the cause; some exanthem distributions are distinct, assisting with diagnosis. Associated signs and symptoms also depend on the cause but may include fever, malaise, and so on. Depending on the cause, many of the symptoms may be prodromal.

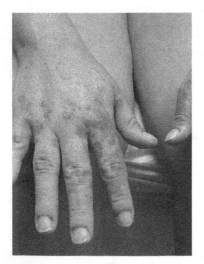

Figure 4.57 Xanthem. Eruption in patient with mild COVID-19. (Copyright Kathleen Haycraft.)

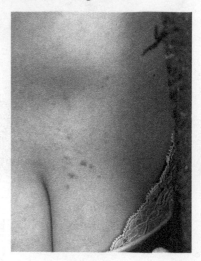

Figure 4.58 Alpha-gal syndrome. Patient with recurrent anaphylaxis, hives, angioedema, and other allergic symptoms. Immunocap panel revealed animal protein allergies. (Copyright Kathleen Haycraft.)

Diagnostic Studies
The need for diagnostic testing will depend on the suspected cause.

ALPHA-GAL SYNDROME

Alpha-gal syndrome involves allergy to red meat, including beef, lamb, pork, and deer, and is also often associated with a tick bite (Lone Star tick), which transmits a sugar called alpha-gal into the system. It is identified by assessment of individuals who have recurrent allergy symptoms, including anaphylaxis and angioedema. The time lag between ingestion or exposure and onset of symptoms may be marked (Fig. 4.58).

Signs and Symptoms
In addition to the development of a rash or hives, other symptoms may include nausea, shortness of breath, and abdominal pain. More severe reactions can be life-threatening.

Diagnostic Studies
ImmunoCAP blood serology is performed to test for allergy to red meats.

POIKILODERMA OF CIVATTE

Poikiloderma of Civatte is associated with sun damage. It involves the area under chin on neck, which is "shielded" from the sun, and patients are often unaware of the pigmentary changes (Fig 4.59).

Signs and Symptoms
The skin changes include atrophy and hypopigmentation or hyperpigmentation.

Diagnostic Studies
None are needed. Typically clinical diagnosis is based on history and presentation.

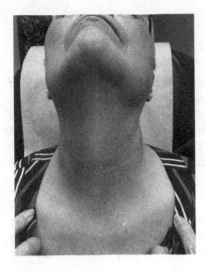

Figure 4.59 Poikiloderma of Civatte. Mottled pigmentation on neck. (Copyright Kathleen Haycraft.)

ERYTHEMA AB IGNE

Erythema ab igne, also known as hot water bottle rash, occurs by extended exposure to heat. The degree of involvement depends on the length of exposure (Fig. 4.60).

Signs and Symptoms

A reticulated red rash develops. Accompanying pruritis or burning may be present. Severe exposure may result in atrophy and hyperpigmentary changes.

Diagnostic Studies

Diagnosis is done by history.

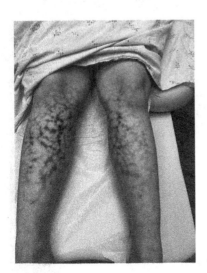

Figure 4.60 Erythema ab igne. Lesions developed in postpartum patient after using space heater located approximately one foot from her leg. (Copyright Kathleen Haycraft.)

■ Chronic Cutaneous Rashes

ACNE

Acne affects most people at some time during their life. The sebaceous unit of the face, back, and chest is influenced by hormones to increase oil production; increased oil production increases an inflammatory bacteria called *Cutibacterium acnes*, resulting in inflammation and dysregulation of the mechanism to remove dead cells. Combined with oil, it creates the "perfect storm" of acne. Severe acne must be treated to avoid serious disfiguring scarring and comorbid disease states (Figs. 4.61 and 4.62).

Signs and Symptoms

The areas most frequently involved include the face, chest, and back. Acne may be mild with comedonal lesions, moderate with papular lesions, or severe with nodular/cystic lesions. The level of pain associated with acne is variable. If acne

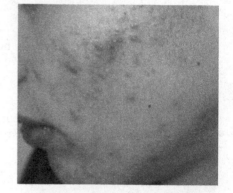

Figure 4.61 Acne. An inflammatory skin condition of the sebaceous follicles exhibiting the inflammatory papules, pustules, and nodules shown here. (Barankin & Friemann, 2006.)

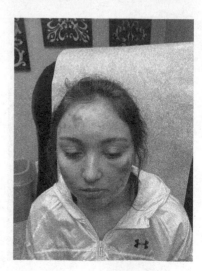

Figure 4.62 Acne. (Copyright Kathleen Haycraft.)

is pruritic, consider a comorbid diagnosis such as atopic disease. If there is fever, leukocytosis, or arthralgia present, prompt dermatology referral needs to occur. Acne is viewed as a chronic condition.

Diagnostic Studies
None are needed.

ROSACEA

Rosacea represents a constellation of increased blood supply to the central face (erythema) with a symbiotic growth of a bacterial and mite complex (inflammation). It is a chronic condition that occurs in both males and females.

Signs and Symptoms
Rosacea occurs on the forehead, cheeks, chin, and periorbital and perioral areas. Initially it is red (telangiectatic rosacea), progresses to papules and pustules (papular/pustular rosacea), and then to thickening of the skin (granulomatous rosacea). Eyes may become dry and gritty at any point of the disease (ocular rosacea). Rhinophyma (more common in men) tends to occur if the disease is not treated in its early phases.

Diagnostic Studies
None are needed.

BACTERIAL FOLLICULITIS

Folliculitis is an inflammation of the hair follicles and is typically associated with staphylococci. Other microorganisms and causes include *Pseudomonas* (associated with hot tubs), *Candida*, tinea barbae, and herpes (Figs. 4.63 and 4.64).

Signs and Symptoms
The patient complains of reddened areas or swelling often associated with a mild pruritic discomfort. Folliculitis lesions often develop as red papules that progress to form pustules. When the lesions erode, crusting occurs. Scarring often develops as the lesions heal. The site of previously healed lesions often has a keloid scar

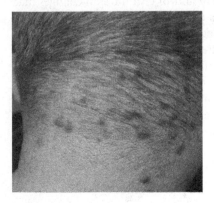

Figure 4.63 Bacterial folliculitis. An inflammatory skin condition of the sebaceous follicles exhibiting the inflammatory papules, pustules, and nodules shown here. (Barankin & Friemann, 2006.)

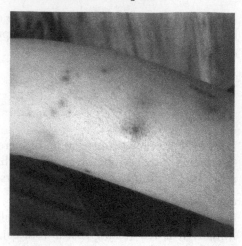

Figure 4.64 Bacterial folliculitis. Reddened papules with central erosion in areas of hair growth. (Copyright Kathleen Haycraft.)

or atrophic scar with no hair growth. Lesions are in the areas with greater hair growth, including the face, scalp, neck, upper trunk, axillae, and inguinal areas. Hot tub folliculitis is intensely itchy and is found in a bathing suit distribution.

Diagnostic Studies

None are generally needed, although a Gram stain and/or culture may be performed.

PSORIASIS

Psoriasis is a chronic autoimmune condition that affects the skin. In addition to severe skin plaques, psoriasis may be associated with disabling psoriatic arthritis and multiple serious comorbid states. The name is derived from the Latin for "itchy plaque." Pain may also be present. Patients may experience worsening of symptoms with stress, infection, trauma, or medications. There is a genetic predisposition (Figs. 4.65 and 4.66).

Signs and Symptoms

The patient often provides a history of recurrent and/or chronic skin changes that most frequently involve the extensor surfaces of extremities and scalp, although other regions are frequently involved. The lesions are often described as itchy, although this is highly variable. There may be associated concurrent arthralgia. The typical psoriasis lesion has a well-demarcated border with a silvery scale overlying an area of obvious erythema. If the scale is removed, the erythematous base reveals minute bleeding points. The shape of most lesions is oval, and several often coalesce to form one larger lesion. Patients frequently exhibit nail pitting and onycholysis.

Diagnostic Studies

Diagnosis may be made on physical findings; however, biopsy will reveal specific histopathologic features.

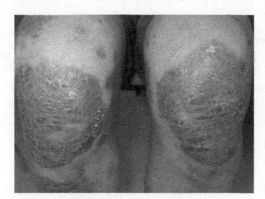

Figure 4.65 Psoriasis. A chronic skin disorder of unknown etiology that causes erythematous and scaly silvery plaques over an erythematous base, frequently found on extensor surfaces. Many variations possible. (Barankin & Friemann, 2006.)

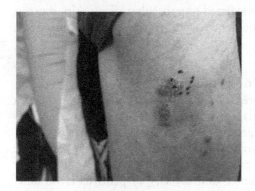

Figure 4.66 Psoriasis. Erythematous based with silver scale. (Copyright Kathleen Haycraft.)

LUPUS ERYTHEMATOSUS

Lupus erythematosus is described in more detail in Chapter 15. However, this chronic connective tissue disorder may manifest as cutaneous symptoms with specific dermatological findings. It is associated with generalized photosensitivity, and patients should avoid ultraviolet radiation. Discoid lupus is a disease that is usually limited to the skin, with less than 5% developing underlying systemic lupus erythematosus (Fig. 4.67).

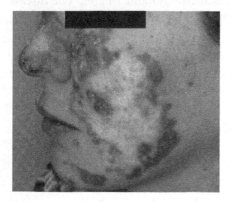

Figure 4.67 Lupus erythematosus. A chronic autoimmune disease of connective tissue that causes a characteristic "butterfly rash" on the face presenting as a fixed erythematous rash that occurs on the cheeks but not in the nasolabial. (Courtesy of the CDC.)

Signs and Symptoms

The patient will have a range of symptoms relevant to the diagnosis, depending on the affected organs. There is often coexisting arthralgia and malaise. The rash is macular and erythematous. It is described as a "butterfly rash" because the distribution resembles a butterfly's wings overlying the forehead and cheeks.

Diagnostic Studies

Biopsy and autoimmune serology testing are valuable.

See Chapter 15.

LICHEN PLANUS

Lichen planus is an autoimmune cell-mediated response that affects skin, mucous membranes, and nails. The highest incidence occurs in the winter months. It is associated with hepatitis C.

Signs and Symptoms

Lichen planus is associated with the "6 Ps": pruritic, planar (flat), purple, polygonal, papules, and plaques. It is important to recognize that in a high Fitzpatrick color, the appearance will vary to a darker purple. The lesions emerge initially on the extremities and then become generalized over a period of days to weeks. They persist for months and may involve the skin overlying all body parts. The lesions are red to purple papules of 1 cm or greater in diameter. They can occur individually or in clusters. The presence and severity of pruritus is variable. The disease may affect the nails.

Diagnostic Studies

If performed, punch biopsy reveals specific histopathologic features. Also screen for hepatitis C.

BULLOUS PEMPHIGOID

Bullous pemphigoid is an autoimmune blistering disease that results from the hemidesmosomes that "glue" the epidermis to the dermis being attacked by antibodies. It is associated with autoantibodies to BP180 and BP230. The disease tends to occur in the older population (Fig. 4.68).

Signs and Symptoms

Tense, firm blisters develop on the flexor surface of the abdomen, arms, and legs. They are usually very pruritic. If mucous membranes are involved, it has a more serious course. It is imperative to refer to a dermatology specialist.

Diagnostic Studies

Always biopsy and perform serological monitoring of BP180 and BP230.

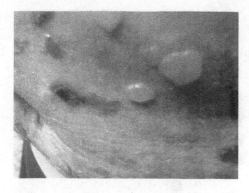

Figure 4.68 Bullous pemphigoid. Tense intact bullae with erupted lesions. (Copyright Kathleen Haycraft.)

PEMPHIGUS VULGARIS

Pemphigus vulgaris is an autoimmune blistering disease in which IgG antibodies attack the "glue" between the epidermal cells. It affects the skin and mucous membranes in middle to older age groups. Diagnosis and early treatment are important as it has a high mortality rate. Dermatology referral is imperative (Fig. 4.69).

Signs and Symptoms

Blisters within the mouth may be the initial symptoms. Pemphigus vulgaris blisters are soft and clear. Oral blisters may make it difficult to eat, and pain associated with ruptured blisters is significant.

Diagnostic Studies

Always biopsy and monitor desmogleins 1 and 3.

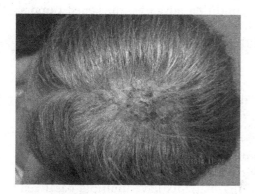

Figure 4.69 Pemphigoid vulgaris. Intact pustular bullae and erosions on scalp. (Copyright Kathleen Haycraft.)

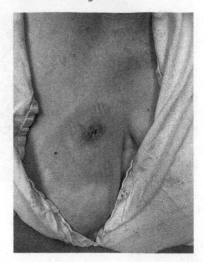

Figure 4.70 Mycosis fungioides. Red-to-violaceous patch over breast. (Copyright Kathleen Haycraft.)

■ Skin Cancer/Cutaneous Carcinoma

MYCOSIS FUNGOIDES

Mycosis fungoides is a cutaneous T-cell lymphoma of the skin that rarely spreads internally. It affects adults older than 50 years (Fig. 4.70).

Signs and Symptoms

Mycosis fungoides evolves with time. The lesions initially appear as flat, scaly patches, ranging from pink to red. Some may be hypopigmented, particularly in darker-skinned individuals. The lesions are often pruritic. The lesions are frequently in the "undergarment" area as they have double sun protection. They generally occur on the abdomen, breast, thighs, and buttocks, and they may be intermittent. With time, the lesions become raised plaques and the color deepens to red or purple. If the condition advances, thickened tumors form. The lesions of mycosis fungoides, as the name implies, are described as looking like mushrooms. This condition can affect other organs, as well (Sezary syndrome).

Diagnostic Studies

It is imperative to refer the patient to a dermatologist for definitive diagnosis.

BASAL CELL CARCINOMA

Basal cell carcinoma is the most common form of cutaneous malignancy and usually involves sun-exposed skin. This malignancy is generally very slow growing. In rare genetic conditions, patients have multiple basal cell cancers. While there is usually a good outcome, it can become quite destructive and invasive if not diagnosed and treated in a timely manner (Figs. 4.71 and 4.72).

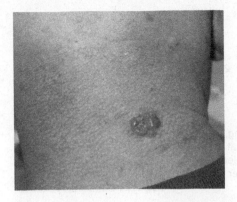

Figure 4.71 Basal cell carcinoma. A pearly, raised border with central induration, often with telangiectasia that define the most common human cancer. The malignancy is associated with sun exposure or other ultraviolet light. (Barankin & Friemann, 2006.)

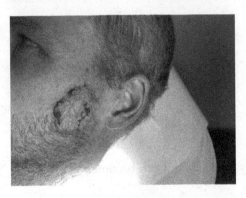

Figure 4.72 Basal cell carcinoma. Advanced lesion with raised, erosive border and central induration on face. (Copyright Kathleen Haycraft.)

Signs and Symptoms

The typical complaint is of a nonhealing sore located on the face, ear, or other sun-exposed area. The patient may complain that the lesion is nonhealing because of repeated trauma. The history often includes previous incidences of basal cell or other skin cancers. The typical lesion has a waxy/pearly appearance with a central indentation, although it may appear as a soft pink or pale papule or patch. Lesions are soft and very prone to bleeding. The surface often reveals telangiectasia. Over time, the central area erodes and becomes crusty. The border of the lesion usually has a "rolled" appearance. However, basal cell carcinoma appears in several variants and can be flat or hyperpigmented, have very indistinct margins, or consist of red papules with telangiectasias.

Diagnostic Studies

The diagnosis is made by shave biopsy.

SQUAMOUS CELL CARCINOMA

Squamous cell carcinoma is second in prevalence only to basal cell carcinoma and involves sun-exposed areas of skin. For patients age 80 years and older, squamous cell cancer is more likely to kill than melanoma. In immune-compromised patients, it has a much higher mortality rate.

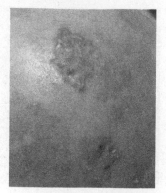

Figure 4.73 Squamous cell carcinoma. Nonhealing, usually slow-growing lesions, often with scaly surface, that appear on skin surfaces exposed to sunlight and ultraviolet light. Second most common form of human cancer after basal cell carcinoma. (Barankin & Friemann, 2006.)

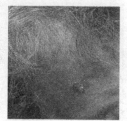

Figure 4.74 Squamous cell carcinoma. Scaly irregular lesion with warty appearance. (Copyright Kathleen Haycraft.)

These carcinomas are more rapidly growing and can become invasive over time (Figs. 4.73 and 4.74).

Signs and Symptoms

The patient complains of a nonhealing lesion that is scaly and usually growing. The lesion is often tender. There is frequently a history of a lesion consistent with actinic keratosis that progressed into the offending lesion. The appearance of squamous cell carcinoma varies from a flat patch to an elevated centrally eroded nodule. The lesion may have a warty appearance, a pink-colored plaque, a nodule, or a papule with eroded surface. The size is usually between 0.5 and 1.5 cm in diameter, although it can be much larger.

Diagnostic Studies

Diagnosis is made by shave biopsy.

MELANOMA

Malignant melanomas are responsible for most skin cancer–related deaths each year. Most arise de novo (70%–80%), with only 20% to 30% occurring at a previous mole (Skin Cancer Foundation, 2021).

Risk factors include individuals with extensive sun exposure; persons with a family history of melanoma, upper third of the back freckling, fair eyes, more than 11 moles on an arm; and persons with a history of atypical moles or many moles on their body. Melanoma is associated with an increased risk of other cancers, such as breast, lymphoma, pancreatic, and others (Figs. 4.75, 4.76, and 4.77.)

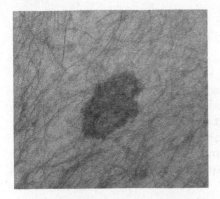

Figure 4.75 Melanoma. A potentially aggressive form of skin cancer of the melanocytes character-ized by asymmetric lesions with irregular borders, variegated coloring, and/or a diameter greater than 6 mm resulting from exposure to sun and ultraviolet light. (Barankin & Friemann, 2006.)

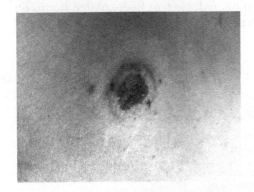

Figure 4.76 Melanoma. Dark, multicolored irregular lesion. (Copyright Kathleen Haycraft.)

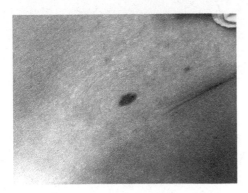

Figure 4.77 Melanoma. Dark, irregular, asymmetric lesion. (Copyright Kathleen Haycraft.)

Signs and Symptoms

There is usually a history of a changing mole or other area of hyperpigmenta-tion. The moles may be dark, pale, consist of multiple colors, or may be simply a white patch with irregular vessels. The lesion is usually greater than 0.6 cm in diameter and has notched or irregular edges, irregular pigmentation, and asym-metry of shape. Like other skin disorders, there are variations in appearance, and there should be a high suspicion for melanoma in any changing pigmented skin lesion or if a mole begins to bleed.

Diagnostic Studies

Diagnosis is made by saucerization shave or excisional biopsy of the lesion.

MERKEL CELL CARCINOMA

Merkel cell carcinoma involves uncontrolled growth of the Merkel cells in the epidermis. Although this is a rare type of skin cancer, its rapid rise in incidence by 95% from 2000 to 2013 is of particular concern (Skin Cancer Foundation, 2021). It occurs in older patients who have significant UV exposure, weakened immune systems, history of other cancers, and fair complexion. Even with treatment, it has the highest mortality rate of skin cancers.

Signs and Symptoms

The Merkel cell cancer can appear as pink, red, blue, or flesh-colored lumps on sun-exposed skin. Lymph nodes may be enlarged at presentations as its potential for spread is high.

Diagnostic Studies

Biopsy is imperative.

REFERENCES

American Academy of Dermatology (2021). *Skin cancer.* https://www.aad.org/media/stats-skin-cancer

Oakley, A. (2012). Fitzpatrick skin phototype. DermNet NZ. https:// https://dermnetnz.org/topics/skin-phototype

Skin Cancer Foundation. (2021). *Skin cancer facts & statistics.* The Skin Cancer Foundation. https://www.skincancer.org/skin-cancer-information/skin-cancer-facts/

Chapter 5

Head, Face, and Neck

Maria Colandrea •

Many conditions can manifest symptoms in the head, face, and neck. Malignancies of the oral cavity, pharynx, larynx, and thyroid are estimated to affect 110,910 Americans in 2021, with approximately 16,820 deaths (Siegel et al., 2021). Other malignancies presenting in the head and neck include cutaneous malignancies, lymphoma, nasopharyngeal cancer, and salivary gland cancer.

Musculoskeletal conditions and infections affecting the head, face, and neck can cause pain. Systemic diseases, affecting the thyroid, kidney, nervous system, heart, skin, and immune systems, may manifest themselves as alterations in the appearance of the head, neck, and face, which may be detectable upon physical examination. This chapter focuses on causes of head, jaw, and facial pain; facial swelling; facial numbness; facial weakness; neck pain; neck mass; and dysphagia. Due to the complexity of the head and neck examination, subsequent content in chapters pertaining to the eye (Chapter 6) and the ear, nose, mouth, and throat (Chapter 7) may also affect the head and neck.

History

■ General Head, Face, and Neck History

The origin of symptoms affecting the head, face, and neck can vary. Obtaining a thorough history will support an accurate diagnosis. Symptom analysis (including symptom onset, timing, duration, associated symptoms, and aggravating and alleviating factors), past medical/surgical history, and social and family history will direct the physical examination and diagnostic testing required to make a diagnosis. A psychosocial and mental health history should be done, especially for any complaints of chronic pain, to determine any relation to stress, anxiety, or other mental health problems. Other, more specific histories should be undertaken according to the chief complaint.

A history of acute trauma or injury to the head may require x-ray, computed tomographic (CT) scan, or magnetic resonance imaging (MRI), depending on the type, location, and extent of the injury. Chronic or acute severe headaches, or new onset headaches in adulthood, may require an MRI and referral to a neurologist. A complaint of syncope or acute, severe vertigo could alert you to the possibility of decreased cerebral blood flow. A complaint of enlarged cervical lymph nodes or neck mass(es), in the absence of infection, can be associated with a malignant process. Symptoms of weight loss, dysphagia, odynophagia, chronic pharyngitis, persistent oral lesions, hoarseness, or voice changes may indicate oropharyngeal or laryngeal cancer. Unilateral nasal obstruction, epistaxis, or cranial nerve (CN) abnormality can indicate a nasal or sinus malignancy. Changes in sense of taste or smell may be symptoms of COVID-19. A complaint of swelling or fullness in the lower anterior neck may be related to thyroid disease. Pain or a decrease in range of motion of the neck can indicate cervical spine arthritis or spinal stenosis. Pain, clicking, or decreased range of motion in the jaw may indicate temporomandibular disorder (TMD).

Past Medical History

The past medical history is an important part of evaluating a patient with symptoms affecting the head, face, and neck. A history of head trauma, chronic diseases, head and neck surgeries, oral health habits, dental disease, autoimmune diseases, medication use, history of radiation exposure, skin cancers, and head and neck cancers should be queried. A history of syncopal episodes, transient ischemic attacks, or cerebrovascular accidents (CVAs) are red flags, and patients with such histories should be referred to a specialist. A history of malignancies of the head, face, or neck raises a high index of suspicion for recurrence. Any past radiation administered to the head and neck may cause long-term side effects, such as mouth sores, dysphagia, xerostomia, dental disease/infections, hoarseness, or hypothyroidism. Past radiation to the neck may increase secondary malignancies to the thyroid and salivary glands.

Family History

A positive family history of cerebrovascular disease, dental disease, thyroid disease, head and neck cancer, cutaneous skin cancers, or migraine creates some increased risk in family members, depending on the age and general health of the patient. Family history of malignancies of any kind should be reviewed. A family history of smoking increases the risk of secondhand smoke exposure in the patient.

Habits

Heavy use of tobacco and alcohol are significant risk factors for malignancies of the head and neck, especially laryngeal cancer. High-risk sexual behavior can increase the patient's risk for human papillomavirus (HPV) infection. Environmental exposures may also cause malignancies, and a thorough occupational and social history should be obtained.

Physical Examination

The physical examination should include visual inspection, palpation, and auscultation of the head, face, and neck. Examination of the head includes visual inspection for symmetry, masses, lesions, skin discolorations and hair

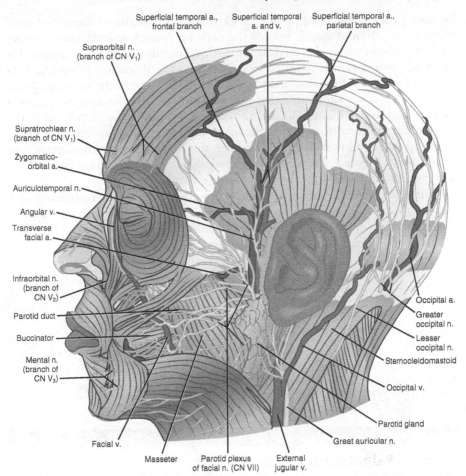

Superficial temporal a.,
frontal branch

Superficial temporal
a. and v.

Superficial temporal a.,
parietal branch

Supraorbital n.
(branch of CN V₁)

Supratrochlear n.
(branch of CN V₁)

Zygomatico-
orbital a.

Auriculotemporal n.

Angular v.

Transverse
facial a.

Infraorbital n.
(branch of
CN V₂)

Parotid duct

Buccinator

Mental n.
(branch of
CN V₃)

Facial v.

Masseter

Parotid plexus
of facial n. (CN VII)

External
jugular v.

Occipital a.

Greater
occipital n.

Lesser
occipital n.

Sternocleidomastoid

Occipital v.

Parotid gland

Great auricular n.

Figure 5.1 Neurovasculature of the head and neck. (From Gilroy, A., MacPherson, B., Schünke, M., Schulte, E., Schumacher, U., Voll, M., Wesker, K. [Eds.]. [4th ed.]. New York: Thieme; 2020. [figure 41.21]. doi:10.1055/b000000417 © 2020. Thieme.)

distribution. Hair should be moved to inspect the scalp for lesions. Palpation of the head will assess for cranial defects, masses, and/or tenderness over the temporal artery (see Figure 5.1 for neurovascular and muscle anatomy of the head and face).

Examination of the face starts with inspection for symmetry, sensation, and motor function (cranial nerves [CNs] V and VII); skin color and lesions; edema; or masses. Palpate the face for tenderness over the sinuses and temporomandibular joints (TMJs). Have the patient open and close the mouth while palpating the TMJ, assessing for crepitus, tenderness, and movement.

The neck should be visually inspected for symmetry, pulsations, lesions, or masses. Visual inspection of the thyroid gland should include having the patient tilt the head back and using a light source pointing downward from the chin, assessing contour of the thyroid gland. Observe movement of the gland by having the patient swallow a sip of water while evaluating contour and symmetry of the thyroid gland. Palpate the neck for masses or tenderness, paying particular attention to the cervical spine, thyroid, salivary glands (submandibular and parotid glands), and cervical lymph nodes. Palpation should be firm enough to detect submucosal masses. Bimanual palpation of the submandibular glands to assess for submandibular stones or masses is performed by placing a gloved hand under the tongue and the other hand under the chin beneath the submandibular gland to compress the submandibular gland between the fingers, assessing for tenderness or masses. Palpate the thyroid for nodules, masses, or hypertrophy. Figure 5.2 depicts thyroid and anterior neck anatomy. See Box 5.1 and Figures 5.3 and 5.4 for thyroid palpation methods.

Auscultate over the carotid arteries and thyroid to detect any turbulent blood flow or bruits, indicating a vascular issue or hyperthyroidism. When auscultating over the neck, ask patients to hold their breath for 5 to 10 seconds to eliminate sound of air movement through the trachea.

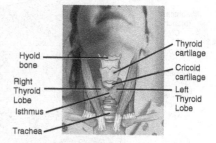

Figure 5.2 Thyroid anatomy. (From Dillon, P. M. [2003]. *Nursing health assessment: A critical thinking, case studies approach.* F. A. Davis, p. 199. Reprinted with permission.)

Labels: Hyoid bone; Right Thyroid Lobe; Isthmus; Trachea; Thyroid cartilage; Cricoid cartilage; Left Thyroid Lobe

---

Box 5.1

Thyroid Palpation Techniques

Posterior approach:
With the patient seated, ask the patient to tilt the neck back slightly, as if looking toward the ceiling. Standing behind the patient, palpate for the thyroid cartilage; placing the fingers just below the thyroid cartilage, ask the patient to swallow. Having water available is helpful for the patient to foster a swallow. As the patient swallows and the isthmus rises, palpate while noting any nodules, firmness, or tenderness. Then displace the trachea to the right using the left hand, while placing the right hand on the right lobe of the thyroid. Ask the patient to swallow, assessing the borders of the right thyroid. Repeat on the left side. See Figure 5.3.

Anterior approach:
With the patient seated, face the patient and locate the thyroid cartilage, palpating the isthmus. Ask the patient to swallow; as the isthmus rises, note any nodules, firmness, or tenderness. Use one hand to retract the sternocleidomastoid muscle and use the other hand to feel the lobe of the thyroid. Have the patient swallow, palpating the thyroid as it rises and falls. Repeat on the other side. See Figure 5.4.

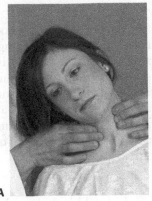
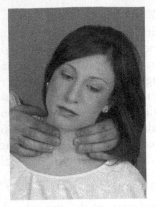

A   **B**

Figure 5.3 Posterior approach to thyroid palpation. (From Dillon, P. M. [2003]. *Nursing health assessment: A critical thinking, case studies approach*. F. A. Davis, p. 235. Reprinted with permission.)

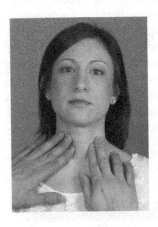

Figure 5.4 Anterior approach to thyroid palpation. (From Dillon, P. M. [2003]. *Nursing health assessment: A critical thinking, case studies approach*. F. A. Davis, p. 235. Reprinted with permission.)

Examination of the mouth, ears, eyes, and nose (covering all the CNs) should also be included in the head and neck exam. See Chapter 6 for the physical examination of the eye and Chapter 7 for the detailed physical examination of the ears, nose, and mouth.

Differential Diagnosis of Chief Complaints

■ Headache
See Chapter 16.

■ Jaw Pain and Facial Pain
Jaw or facial pain can be related to TMD or be referred from another area of the head and neck. Conditions such as ear infections, dental infections, rhinosinusitis, trigeminal neuralgia, giant cell arteritis, and bruxism can cause jaw or facial pain. Other conditions, such as angina, can cause referred pain to the jaw.

History

Determining the location of pain, severity, quality, duration, associated symptoms, and aggravating and alleviating factors will assist in making an accurate diagnosis. Distinguishing the quality and the timing of pain is important, including type of pain and whether the pain is constant or intermittent, occurs at a particular time of day, and so on. Table 5.1 depicts conditions associated with varied qualities of pain. Recent trauma to the face or jaw is a red flag and should alert the provider to a possible facial or mandibular fracture. A history of tobacco use could increase the risk of a neoplasm of the mouth or lips, dental disease, rhinosinusitis, and giant cell arteritis.

Physical Examination

An examination of the entire head and neck should include evaluation of the TMJ, paying attention to range of motion, pain with jaw movement, crepitus, and tenderness to palpation. Examine the ears, assessing for tragal tenderness or pain when pulling on the auricle as seen in otitis externa. Perform an otoscopic examination, assessing the external ear canal and tympanic membrane for infection (see Chapter 7). A complete oral examination should assess dentition for abscesses and caries, as well as the mucosa, tongue, posterior pharynx, and tonsils for lesions. An anterior nasal examination should assess for purulent drainage, turbinate hypertrophy, ulcerations, masses, or polyps. CNs V and VII, which govern jaw clench, facial sensation, and facial movement, should be assessed. If the complaint warrants other system evaluations, such as cardiac or musculoskeletal, those systems should be thoroughly examined.

Table 5.1

Conditions Associated With Varied Pain Qualities

Condition	Pain Quality
Neuropathic	Burning, shock like, or tingling
Trigeminal neuralgia	Paroxysmal, unilateral, sharp pain of the face
Cardiac	More likely to occur with activity; may have associated symptoms such as shortness of breath, chest pain, left arm pain, and palpitations
Dental	Pain to the cheek, ear, or jaw; may have associated swelling in severe dental infections
Giant cell arteritis	Sudden onset of unilateral dull, constant pain in the temple region and may have associated acute vision changes
Acute rhinosinusitis/allergies	Dull ache over the maxillary or frontal sinuses, often associated with nasal congestion, rhinorrhoea, malaise, or recent upper respiratory infection
Salivary stone	Intermittent pain in parotid region

TEMPOROMANDIBULAR DISORDERS

TMD is a group of musculoskeletal and neuromuscular conditions affecting the TMJ and causing chronic orofacial pain. TMD affects 10% to 15% of adults, peaking between the ages of 20 and 40 years (Gauer & Semidey, 2015), and is twice as common in women than in men (Yadav et al., 2018). Contributing factors for TMD include trauma, inflammation, or arthritis to the TMJ, as well as bruxism, cervical spine posture, anxiety, posttraumatic stress disorder, and depression. Stress responses causing an increase in clenching, muscle tension, or bruxism may result in fatigue or spasm of the masticatory muscles, headaches, neck pain, and pain over the TMJ. Other causes include malocclusion, dental disease, and poorly fitting dentures. The pain can be severe and debilitating and can interfere with daily activities, particularly chewing.

Signs and Symptoms

The signs and symptoms range from mild aching to severe, sharp pain in and around the TMJ. Pain is usually associated with movement of the TMJ (e.g., chewing, yawning). There may be pain or tenderness with palpation of the TMJ or surrounding area, including masseter, temporalis, and neck muscles. The pain is often referred to the ear and can cause tinnitus and aural fullness in the setting of a normal ear examination. There may be decreased range of movement or abnormal mandibular movement, jaw locking, clicking, or crepitus with movement. TMD does not cause CN deficits.

Diagnostic Studies

Symptoms and clinical examination findings are most helpful for diagnosing TMD. Panoramic x-rays can be helpful, but CT is superior for evaluating the joint and surrounding structures. MRI is optimal for evaluating the joint and soft tissue.

A referral to a dentist or maxillofacial specialist is recommended. See Figure 5.5 for a TMD management algorithm.

TRIGEMINAL NEURALGIA

Trigeminal neuralgia (TN) is an uncommon cause of chronic facial pain characterized by paroxysmal, recurrent episodes of facial pain occurring along the trigeminal (CN V) route. It is associated with inflammation, degeneration, or pressure on the trigeminal nerve. Prevalence of TN is 0.015%, affecting 4 to 13 out of 100,000 (Jones et al., 2019). It is more commonly seen in adults older than 50 years, affecting women more than men (Jones et al., 2019). Conditions that increase the risk of TN include diabetes, chronic rhinosinusitis, and multiple sclerosis.

Signs and Symptoms

The pain of trigeminal neuralgia is usually unilateral, sharp, stabbing, and paroxysmal. Pain can last from seconds to minutes, but with recurrent paroxysms that may continue for hours. Episodes of neuralgia are recurrent and may be

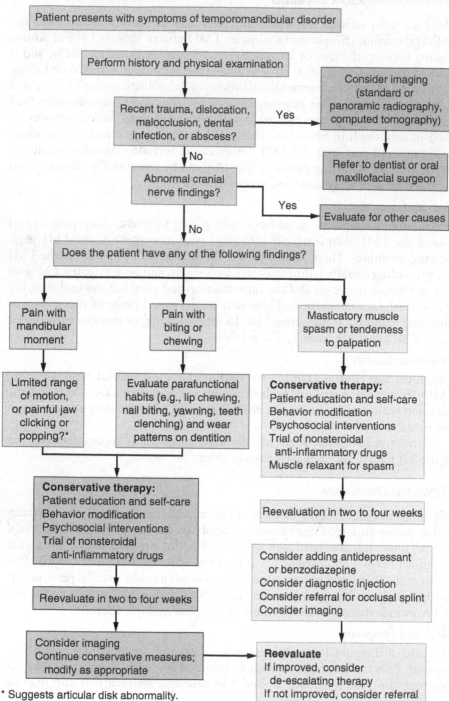

Figure 5.5 Diagnosis and treatment of temporomandibular disorders. (From Gauer, R., Semidy, M. (2015). Diagnosis and treatment of temporomandibular disorders. *American Academy of Family Physicians*, 91(6), 378–386 [figure 2, p. 382]).

triggered by movement such as chewing, brushing teeth, and speaking, as well as exposure to cold temperatures or pressure along CN route. Symptoms may subside for weeks and months without an exacerbation. Because there are three branches to this nerve (ophthalmic, maxillary, and mandibular), the pain radiates from the angle of the jaw to one or more of the three places innervated: the forehead and eye area; the cheek and nose area; or the tongue, lower lip, and jaw area (Fig. 5.6).

Diagnostic Studies

Diagnosis of trigeminal neuralgia is established after three episodes of unilateral pain occurring along one trigeminal nerve route; the pain should not be associated with CN deficits or radiate past the nerve route. The pain must meet two out of the three criteria of severe intensity; sharp, electric, stabbing, or shock-like pain; and paroxysmal episodes lasting 1 to 2 minutes. Neurological deficits in the function of CN V suggest a more serious cause, such as a neoplasm, brainstem lesion, cerebrovascular insult, or multiple sclerosis (MS). Other symptoms that may cause pain similar to TN include Sjögren's syndrome, rheumatoid arthritis, or migraine, although there are generally other defining symptoms with these systemic diseases. MRI with and without contrast is preferred as it provides improved visualization of the trigeminal nerve and soft tissue structures.

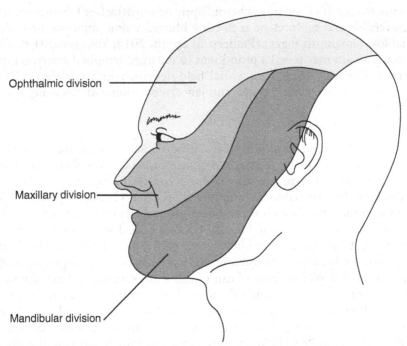

Ophthalmic division

Maxillary division

Mandibular division

Figure 5.6 Branches of the trigeminal nerve (cranial nerve V). (From Swartz, M. H. [1998]. *Textbook of physical diagnosis: History and examination* [3rd ed.]. WB Saunders, p. 509. Reprinted with permission.)

GIANT CELL ARTERITIS

Giant cell arteritis (GCA), also known as temporal arteritis, is caused by inflammation and granulomatous changes to large and medium vessels causing intimal vessel thickness. GCA is considered a medical emergency as it can cause permanent visual loss if left untreated. GCA affects 27 of 100,000 patients older than 50 years, with a lifetime risk of 1% in women and 0.5% in men (Younger, 2019). The disease peaks in the seventh and eighth decades of life (Pradeep & Smith, 2018; Younger, 2019). Risk factors that increase GCA include polyarteritis nodosa, polymyalgia rheumatica (occurs in 40% to 50% of patients with GCA), tobacco use, possessing the HLA-DR4 gene, and being of northern European ancestry (Pradeep & Smith, 2018; Younger, 2019). GCA can cause inflammation of large vessels such as the aorta or affect the cerebral vascular system, which increases the patient's morbidity and mortality risk

Signs and Symptoms

Symptoms are typically insidious but can occur abruptly in some patients. Key symptoms include new onset headaches in the temporal region, with a severity that may disrupt sleep, and scalp tenderness, which can be associated with touch, wearing glasses, or resting the head on a pillow. Pain can be referred to the eye, ear, face, jaw, or neck. Associated symptoms can include fevers, malaise, fatigue, weight loss, and visual loss. Visual loss can occur in 15% to 20% of patients as a result of anterior ischemic optic neuropathy (see Chapter 6), which is irreversible and can present as fleeting blurred vision, diplopia, or transient visual loss (amaurosis fugax) (Pradeep & Smith, 2018; Younger, 2019). Physical examination may reveal a prominent or enlarged temporal artery, temporal artery and/or scalp tenderness, visual field deficits, pupillary defect, CN palsies, absent temporal artery pulse, and jaw claudication with chewing, which is irreversible.

Diagnostic Studies

Diagnosis is based on medical history, clinical evaluation, laboratory data, and diagnostic imaging. The gold standard of diagnosing GCA is obtaining a temporal artery biopsy. Laboratory testing includes complete blood count (CBC), liver enzymes, erythrocyte sedimentation rate (ESR), and C-reactive protein (CRP). Normochromic anemia with thrombocytosis and elevated liver enzymes, ESR, and CRP are most often seen. Normal CRP or ESR does not exclude the diagnosis of GCA. Temporal artery biopsy is the gold standard, particularly when the patient has not been on corticosteroids for less than 2 weeks. Diagnostic imaging such as color Doppler ultrasound can visualize large vessels and blood flow. CT can detect vascular stenosis and dilatation. MRI or magnetic resonance angiography (MRA) can detect intimal vessel wall thickening and edema. Positron emission tomography (PET) can detect increased uptake of fluorodeoxyglucose (FDG), which confirms inflammation. Imaging should not take the place of temporal artery biopsy to confirm diagnosis.

ANGINA

The pain from myocardial ischemia can often be referred to the neck and jaw area, and in rare cases can be the only symptoms indicating a cardiac problem. The provider should retain an index of suspicion for angina being the cause of jaw pain, especially if it is exacerbated with exertion. Proper cardiac history, physical examination, and diagnostic workup will confirm the diagnosis.

Signs and Symptoms

A thorough history of symptoms, comorbid conditions (especially hyperlipidemia and diabetes), social history including tobacco use, and personal and familial cardiac history should lead the examiner in the right direction. Middle-aged patients with a history of cardiovascular disease in themselves or family members should raise the index of suspicion. The red flag complaints that should alert the examiner to the possibility of a cardiac origin are accompanying chest pain, pain with exertion, dyspnea, nausea, or diaphoresis. See Chapter 8.

Diagnostic Studies

The diagnosis of ischemia can be made with an electrocardiogram, if it is obtained while the patient is having pain, or with a graded exercise stress test. If the graded exercise stress test is positive, angiography is warranted. Complete blood count, metabolic panel, lipid panel, and troponin may be helpful in diagnosis. In some patients, chest x-ray may be warranted.

DENTAL PAIN

The most common causes of dental-related jaw pain are the eruption of wisdom teeth and tooth decay or abscess, particularly in the molars. Wisdom teeth generally erupt in the late teens or early 20s, so they should be part of the differential diagnosis in patients of that age. In patients with obviously poor dental hygiene, decay, caries, and abscesses, a dental etiology for the jaw pain should be included in the differential diagnosis at any age. Periodontal disease affects 47% of Americans older than 30 years and 65% older than 65 years and is more common in men than in women (CDC, 2021; Chow, 2019). Periodontal disease can cause jaw pain, caries, cervical adenopathy, swelling of the gingiva, and abscesses. Risk factors include poor dental hygiene, xerostomia, family history, tobacco use, aging, diabetes, and cardiovascular disease. Periodontal pathogens cause inflammation and destruction of dentin.

Signs and Symptoms

Jaw pain can be constant and throbbing with dental carries. On physical examination, discoloration, pits, fissures, or erosions on the tooth surface may be visible. In patients with dental/gingival abscesses, symptoms may include fevers, cervical adenopathy, and pain with eating/chewing. Fluctuant swelling along the diseased tooth/teeth can be visible with or without purulent drainage. In severe cases of mandibular abscesses, cellulitis can cause swelling of the tongue, floor of the mouth, or submandibular space (Ludwig's angina), putting the patient at risk for airway obstruction and sepsis. This is considered a medical emergency and should be referred to the emergency department. In any case, dental caries or abscesses can be quite severe and require analgesics and, if infection is present, antibiotics until a dental referral can be made. With the eruption of wisdom teeth, the pain is milder and generally not constant.

Diagnostic Studies

Diagnosis can be made with a thorough oral examination. Decay and abscesses are quite obvious with an oral examination, whereas other forms of dental disease require in-depth dental evaluation and panoramic x-ray. In any case, dental referral is necessary.

BRUXISM

Bruxism is the clenching or grinding of teeth during sleep. The most common causes are malocclusion or tension and stress.

Signs and Symptoms

Over the long term, bruxism can cause the teeth to wear down, crack, erode, and loosen. Patients are usually not aware of the problem because it occurs during sleep, but they may experience TMD symptoms. Other symptoms include jaw pain, temporalis muscle pain, and headaches. Risk factors include medications, stress, anxiety, sleep apnea, alcohol use, TMD, and family history.

Diagnostic Studies

The diagnosis is usually made via the report of family members witnessing the patient grinding teeth during sleep. Dental examination will also confirm the diagnosis.

SIALADENITIS (PAROTITIS)

There are two types of parotid infection—suppurative (usually caused by *Staphylococcus aureus* [50%–90%], *Streptococcal* species, and *Haemophilus influenza*) and epidemic, more commonly called *mumps* (caused by a paramyxovirus) (Michael & Kiemeney, 2019; Ogle, 2019). In developed countries, mumps is rarely seen because children are immunized against it within the first 2 years of life. Patients with Sjögren's syndrome, diabetes, hypothyroidism, and renal failure are also predisposed to inflammation of the salivary glands (Fig. 5.7)—parotid or submandibular—termed *sialadenitis*.

Signs and Symptoms

In bacterial sialadenitis, the symptoms include fever, chills, acute onset of pain, and unilateral swelling, usually in the preauricular area of the jaw. The gland is firm on palpation, with tenderness and erythema overlying the gland. Purulence from the Stensen's duct may be visible. In chronic or recurrent sialadenitis, symptoms include recurrent episodes of swelling, which usually occur with meals or infections. In mumps, swelling and pain occur on both sides.

Diagnosis

Clinical signs and symptoms most often make the diagnosis of infectious sialadenitis. The examiner should attempt to express pus from the Stensen's duct, which

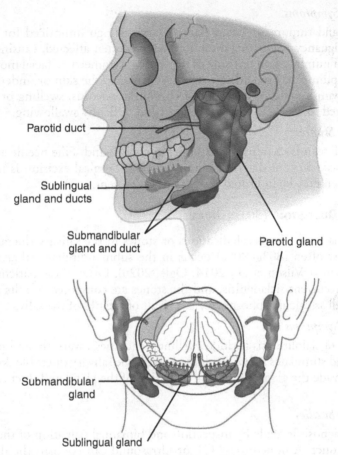

Figure 5.7 Parotid and salivary glands. (From Dillon, P. M. [2003]. *Nursing health assessment: A critical thinking, case studies approach*. F. A. Davis, p. 199. Reprinted with permission.)

can be sent for a culture to confirm the diagnosis and guide antimicrobial therapy. The pus will most often show gram-positive cocci.

SALIVARY GLAND TUMORS

More than 80% of salivary gland tumors are benign, and the majority occur in the parotid gland. The most common benign parotid tumor is pleomorphic adenoma followed by Warthin's tumor. About 16% of salivary gland tumors are malignant; most malignant tumors occur in the submandibular gland and the sublingual and minor salivary glands. Malignant tumors include mucoepidermoid carcinoma and adenoid cystic carcinoma (Ogle, 2020; Carlson & Schlieve, 2019). Face or scalp squamous cell carcinoma can spread to the parotid gland. The only known risk factor is ionizing radiation.

Signs and Symptoms

Salivary gland tumors are often painless and may go unnoticed for months. When malignancy is present, the facial nerve is often affected, causing muscle weakness or numbness on one side of the face or asymmetry of facial movements. Other symptoms may include a mass that is fixed to the skin or underlying tissue, fixed lymph node(s), recurrent or chronic sialadenitis, swelling or ongoing pain localized to the face, neck, or mouth, and difficulty swallowing.

Diagnostic Studies

MRI or CT scan is recommended once a mass is found. Fine needle aspiration (FNA) is necessary for diagnosis and treatment. Surgical excision is necessary, and radiation may be indicated if metastasis is present.

SALIVARY DUCT STONE (SIALOLITHIASIS)

Sialolithiasis results from calcifications or stones in the salivary ductal system. Stones most often (80%–90%) occur in the submandibular rather than the parotid glands (Wilson et al., 2014; Ogle, 2020). Often these patients have a history of recurrent sialadenitis, and the stones are composed of salts and proteins, as well as calcium phosphate, as a result of the pH of the saliva.

Signs and Symptoms

Symptoms of sialolithiasis include swelling, tenderness, warmth, and pain after eating. Food stimulates saliva production; with the salivary ducts blocked, saliva backs up inside the gland. Bimanual palpation of the gland and duct can reveal a stone.

Diagnostic Studies

Clinical diagnosis is made by inspection and bimanual palpation of the salivary gland and duct. A noncontrast CT or ultrasound can confirm the diagnosis. Superficial stones can be expressed by manual manipulation if they are close to the opening of the duct. Stones that are deeper in the gland will require excision. In some cases, sialendoscopy, a miniature endoscopy procedure to retrieve and flush out stones and protein buildup, can be performed to avoid surgery (Fig. 5.8).

TRAUMA

A history of trauma to the jaw alerts the examiner to the need for x-ray or CT imaging to evaluate the presence of a fracture or dislocation of the mandible. Fistfighting and boxing are the most common causes, as well as other sources of trauma, such as motor vehicle accidents or sports injuries.

Signs and Symptoms

Bruising may be present, as well as lacerations to the face, chin, or jaw. Pain over a TMJ, abnormal movement, and difficulty with opening and closing of the jaw are the hallmark symptoms.

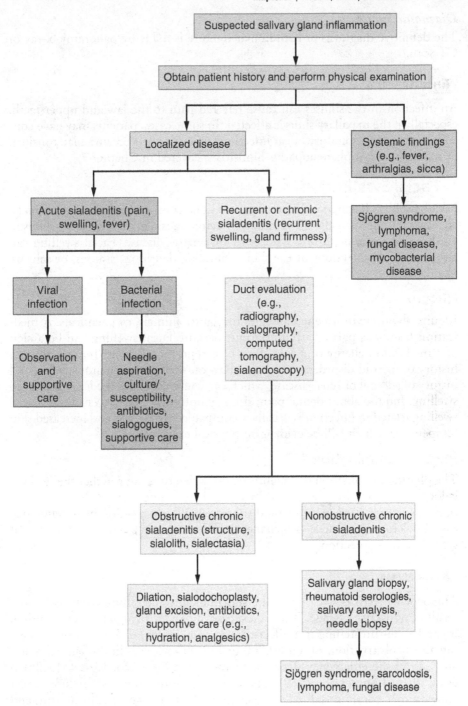

Figure 5.8 Evaluation of salivary gland disorders. (From Wilson, K. F., Meier, J. D., & Ward, P. D. [2014]. Salivary gland disorders. *American Family Physician, 89*(11), 882–888 [figure 1, p. 884]).

Diagnostic Studies

The definitive diagnosis of mandibular fracture is made by panoramic x-ray or CT scan.

RHINOSINUSITIS

An infection in the sinuses can cause referred pain to the jaw and upper teeth, especially if the maxillary sinus is affected. In some cases, patients may have concomitant upper respiratory or ear infections that can cause preauricular, tonsillar, or mandibular lymphadenopathy. Sinusitis is covered in Chapter 7.

■ Facial Swelling

Facial swelling has many different causes. The most common cause of facial edema is related to an allergic reaction. Systemic causes include hypothyroidism, Cushing's disease, nephrotic syndrome, or hepatic disease. Facial swelling can also stem from infections of the skin (cellulitis), dentition, sinuses, or salivary glands.

History

Inquire about environmental allergies to plants, animals, or chemicals. A medication history is particularly important because facial swelling can be a sign of a medication allergy or a side effect of certain medications. Inquire about a history of thyroid disorders, which can be a cause of myxedematous facies, and history of adrenal or renal disease, which can cause generalized edema and facial swelling. Inquire about dental pain, sinus symptoms, or any recent fever. Facial swelling related to infection is usually accompanied by redness and increased skin temperature, which will be evident on physical examination.

Physical Examination

The physical examination is straightforward in determining whether the swelling is localized, which may be caused by a problem or infection in the underlying tissues, or generalized, which would suggest an allergic reaction or systemic disease. Look for any redness, skin changes, tenderness, and lymphadenopathy that would indicate infection.

ANGIOEDEMA

Angioedema (AE) is swelling of the subcutaneous and submucosal tissue as a result of vasoactive cascade. While most cases of AE are benign and self-limiting, it can be life-threatening if it affects the tongue, larynx, or upper airway, causing airway obstruction. About 80,000 to 112,000 patients in the United States are seen in the emergency department each year for angioedema (Moellman et al, 2014; Long et al., 2019). The causes are numerous and include insect stings; atopic conditions; food allergies (typically nuts, eggs, shellfish, fruit, and sulfites); drug allergies; allergy desensitization injections; a reaction to blood products; a response to exercise, cold, or pressure; heredity; and vasculitis.

Angiotensin-converting enzyme inhibitors and NSAIDs are common causes of angioedema.

Signs and Symptoms

The most commonly affected sites include the eyelids, lips, tongue, and larynx. Patients may have urticaria, which presents as wheals and is usually seen around the mouth, nose, eyes, mucous membranes, and hands and feet. AE resulting in anaphylaxis is accompanied by systemic reactions; therefore, abnormal vital signs, such as hypotension, dyspnea associated with stridor, bronchospasm, and wheezing should be immediately identified and referred to the emergency department. Angioedema is usually self-limiting and lasts 1 to 7 days, but it can be a chronic, recurring condition, depending on the cause.

Diagnostic Studies

The diagnosis is based on clinical symptoms and physical examination. Allergy testing may be helpful in ruling out causes such as food, environmental, or drug allergies.

CELLULITIS

Cellulitis is defined as an acute inflammation of cellular or connective tissue, usually confined to the skin and subcutaneous tissue, but it may extend to deeper tissues (see Chapter 4). Group A β-hemolytic streptococcus is the most common organism responsible for superficial cellulitis. It can occur from a wound or bite or as a complication of infections of the eyes, ears, mouth, or nose. Patients who are at greater risk include those with diabetes, especially with uncontrolled blood glucose, and immunocompromised patients.

Signs and Symptoms

The symptoms include redness, warmth, edema, leukocyte infiltration, tenderness, and regional lymphadenopathy. The skin may have a thick, orange-peel appearance, and the borders are usually indistinct. If there is purulent drainage or an abscess, incision and drainage or aspiration is necessary. If systemic symptoms such as fever, tachycardia, hypotension, or rapid progression of erythema, are present, an emergency department visit and treatment with parenteral antimicrobial therapy is warranted. Otherwise, response to oral antimicrobials should be followed.

Diagnostic Studies

The diagnosis can be made solely by history and physical examination. A CBC can help monitor trends in white blood cell counts. Wound or tissue cultures will identify the causative organism and direct antimicrobial therapy. Cellulitis in the head and face should be treated promptly and can usually be accomplished with outpatient antimicrobials.

CUSHING'S DISEASE

See Chapter 17.

LONG-TERM USE OF STEROIDS

A cushingoid look can occur in patients who take long-term steroids for chronic diseases, including respiratory, hematological, and autoimmune.

Signs and Symptoms
The typical symptoms are those of Cushing's disease, with a rounded "moon face" appearance and truncal obesity.

Diagnostic Studies
In the case of steroid use, the diagnosis is made by history.

MYXEDEMA

Myxedema is related to hypothyroidism. See page 143 in this chapter.

NEPHROTIC SYNDROME

See Chapter 17.

■ Facial Numbness and Weakness

Numbness, tingling, or hypersensitivity in the face should be taken seriously because the causative conditions can be grave neurological diseases, such as MS or CVA. Bell's palsy is the most common cause of facial neuropathy; rarely, infectious and inflammatory diseases such as HIV, Lyme disease, and sarcoidosis may present with facial numbness.

■ History

Obtain history pertaining to onset and location of numbness/weakness, past medical and surgical history, associated symptoms, precipitating factors, and so on. Inquire about the presence of other neurological symptoms, such as weakness, unsteadiness, hemiparesis, disequilibrium, severe headache, acute/severe vertigo, and diplopia or other visual changes, which are possible indications of either CVA or MS. Inquire about masses or skin cancers of the head and neck. Bell's palsy, a frequent cause of facial weakness or paralysis, occurs at any age, often as a sequela of a viral illness. MS occurs more in the young adult population, whereas CVA occurs more in the older population, especially in those with hypertension or diabetes. A thorough family history may disclose a predisposition to CVA, hypertension, diabetes, and other neurological diseases. Twin studies show a genetic susceptibility for MS.

■ Physical Examination

The physical examination should include a complete head and neck examination focusing on the CNs. Assess facial sensation on each side of the face (CN V) as well as movement by having the patient perform various facial expressions (CN VII). A complete mental status examination and neurological examination can help rule out a CVA. Diagnostic imaging with MRI will rule out brain tumor, parotid lesion, CVA, or MS.

BELL'S PALSY

Bell's palsy is a rapid onset, unilateral weakness or paralysis of the face. It most commonly occurs between the ages of 15 and 45 years (Baugh et al., 2013). The degree of weakness or paralysis is variable among patients. The etiology is uncertain, but the paralysis is thought to be due to an inflammation of CN VII secondary to a viral infection, a large percentage being herpes simplex virus. Other risk factors include diabetes, immunocompromised status, or pregnancy. The condition is usually self-limiting, but care should be taken if there is incomplete closure of the eye, which could result in eye injury.

Signs and Symptoms

The onset of Bell's palsy is sudden (less than 72 hours), and the symptoms are unilateral. The affected side of the face droops with asymmetrical facial movement; patients may complain of pain in or around the ear, excessive lacrimation and salivation, inability to close the eye, and/or altered sense of taste. The facial weakness may be partial or complete paralysis. No tactile sensory loss is demonstrable. The affected eye must be kept moist with lubricating drops/ointments and patched to avoid excessive dryness and injury. Figure 5.9 depicts one approach to the diagnosis of Bell's palsy.

Diagnostic Studies

The diagnosis is made by physical examination. There are no recommended diagnostic tests for initial diagnosis, but an electromyogram can be helpful to determine the extent of the nerve damage. Recovery from partial paralysis occurs in 2 to 6 months; complete recovery from total paralysis varies from 20% to 90%. High-dose corticosteroids should be prescribed as a 10-day course. Antivirals are optional and should only be prescribed concomitantly with corticosteroids and within 72 hours of symptom onset.

MULTIPLE SCLEROSIS

Multiple sclerosis (MS) is a progressive autoimmune disease of the central nervous system attacking the white matter of the brain. It typically affects young adults and has a variety of neurological symptoms affecting the motor, sensory, mental, and central and autonomic nervous systems. See Chapter 17.

Signs and Symptoms

The onset of MS is insidious and may go undiagnosed for months or years. Symptoms are intermittent with relapses and remissions. Unilateral facial paresthesia or pain occasionally is seen early in the disease process; eye symptoms are most common early in the disease and include optic neuritis, abnormal ocular movements, and nystagmus.

Diagnostic Studies

History helps guide diagnosis, especially one that describes remissions and exacerbations of the symptoms, which can raise an index of suspicion for MS. MRI with and without contrast, lumbar puncture, and evoked potentials are all part of the diagnostic workup.

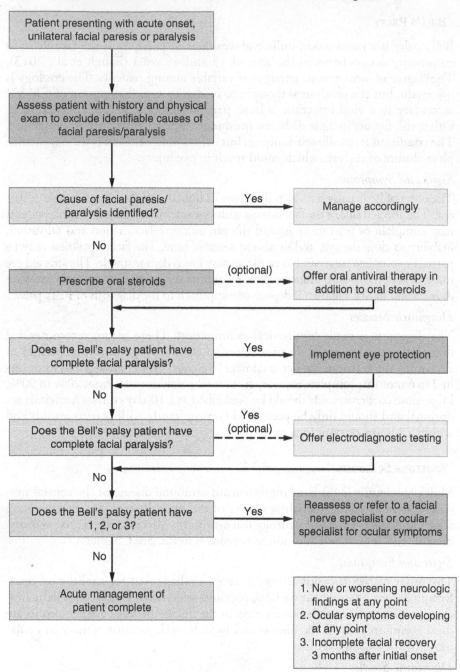

Figure 5.9 Evaluation of Bell's palsy. (From Baugh, R. F., Basura, G. J., Ishii, L. E., Schwartz, S. R., Drumheller, C. M., Burkholder, R., Deckard, N. A., Dawson, C., Driscoll, C., Gillespie, M. B., Gurgel, R. K., Halperin, J., Khalid, A. N., Kumar, K. A., Micco, A., Munsell, D., Rosenbaum, S., Vaughan, W. [2013]. Clinical practice guideline: Bell's palsy. *Otolaryngol Head Neck Surgery, 149*(3 Suppl), S1–27. https://doi.org/10.1177/0194599813505967 [figure 1, p. S22]).

CEREBROVASCULAR ACCIDENT

Although it would be unusual for facial numbness to be the presenting complaint for stroke, it can certainly cause facial weakness or paralysis and should be considered in the differential diagnosis. Age, comorbidities, and past medical and family history are very helpful in raising the index of suspicion for CVA. A thorough physical examination, focusing on the neurological system, and diagnostic imaging are definitive. See Chapter 16.

■ Scalp and Face Pruritus

History

It would be unusual for pruritus in the head and neck to indicate anything except a skin condition/disease or infestation. If the patient is a school-age child, pediculosis is an obvious consideration, and the child's friends and school administrators should be questioned about recent outbreaks. Inquire about history of skin conditions such as eczema, psoriasis, and seborrheic dermatitis, which can all cause pruritis of the scalp and face. Ask about personal or family history of skin cancer, sun exposure, and blistering sunburns, since skin cancers can occur in the scalp of both men and women, although they are more common in men due to thinning hair and, consequently, increased sun exposure.

Physical Examination

The physical examination includes careful inspection of the head and scalp for nits or actual lice. Nits are fixed to the hair shaft and are grayish white in appearance. Unlike the flakiness of seborrhea, nits cannot be easily dislodged. The skin of the head and face should be inspected for lesions, color changes, new or changing moles, crusting, scaling, ulceration, or bleeding, which might be indicative of cancer. Patches of scaling, crusting areas with surrounding erythema can be indicative of eczema or psoriasis. Further discussion of various dermatological problems causing pruritus can be found in Chapter 4 for adult and Chapter 19 for pediatric patients.

■ Neck Fullness, Mass, or Pain

History

Gather a thorough history of present illness, as well as past medical and surgical history; personal and family history for cancer and thyroid disease; medication use; injuries to the neck; and arthritis. Ask about history of neck strain, cervical spondylosis, spinal stenosis, cervical radiculopathy, arthritis, injury, or TMD, as well as frequent infections, allergies, and chronic problems affecting the ears, nose, and throat. Obtain a social history including tobacco use, illicit drug use, alcohol use, and secondhand smoke exposure. Ask about living arrangements, as living in close quarters, such as classrooms and college dormitories, can predispose patients to a variety of infections and perhaps secondhand smoke. Inquire about high-risk sexual behaviors.

Symptoms vary depending on the underlying cause. In thyroid disease, patients may describe a feeling of having something in their throat. The complaint is more likely to be one of fullness rather than of pain or dysphagia. The history should inquire about signs and symptoms of hyper- or hypothyroidism, such as weight loss or gain, nervousness or fatigue, diarrhea or constipation, intolerance to heat or cold, insomnia or lethargy, menstrual irregularities, and skin or hair changes. Laboratory studies and thyroid scanning can diagnose most problems.

Lymphadenopathy has numerous causes but can generally be placed into two categories: infection or malignancy. Lymphadenopathy may be a normal finding in children; however, cervical lymphadenopathy, in the absence of infectious symptoms, is an indication of malignancy in an adult. Infection often presents with fever, pharyngitis, rhinorrhea, otalgia, cough, and malaise. A recent history of an upper respiratory infection is common.

Symptoms of head and neck malignancies are more likely to be associated with a unilateral mass, unilateral otalgia, dysphagia, odynophagia, chronic pharyngitis, hemoptysis, hoarseness, and/or weight loss. Lymphoma symptoms include fatigue, weakness, anorexia, weight loss, fever, night sweats, bleeding, and easy bruising. A history of tobacco and/or alcohol use or abuse may be present in neoplasms of the head and neck, especially laryngeal and oral cancers. As oropharyngeal cancers are often related to HPV, high-risk sexual behaviors or known exposure to HPV should be questioned.

Physical Examination

Complete head and neck examination is essential when a patient presents with a neck mass. Pay special attention to the scalp, ears, and cheeks for skin lesions or dryness. Examine the mouth, nose, ears, and oral and nasal cavities for lesions or infection. Conduct a complete CN examination focusing on CNs V and VII. The physical examination includes inspection and palpation of the thyroid for enlargement, asymmetry, or nodules. Look for periorbital edema, which may be present in hypothyroidism. Check the vital signs for hyper- or hypotension, tachycardia or bradycardia, and fever or subnormal temperature. Notice any tremor. Check the deep tendon reflexes, noting hyper- or hyporeflexia. Abnormalities in any of these areas would indicate the need for further thyroid studies, including thyroid-stimulating hormone (TSH), free T_4, and possibly a thyroid ultrasound or radionuclide scan.

A complete examination of the mouth, throat, nose, ears, and eyes should be performed, particularly if risk factors or symptoms of head and neck malignancy are present. Assessing lesions, masses, ulcerations, or tonsil asymmetry can require referral to a specialist for biopsy. Palpate for lymphadenopathy in other areas of the body, which might be present in malignancies such as in lymphoma. If mononucleosis is suspected, palpate for splenomegaly.

A CBC might be warranted to check for leukocytosis or leukopenia. A positive "mono spot" would definitively diagnose mononucleosis. A chest x-ray may be necessary to look for mediastinal lymphadenopathy, indicating Hodgkin's disease or other malignancy. Depending on sexual practices, a *Neisseria gonorrhoeae* or *Chlamydia trachomatis* culture of the throat or blood studies for rapid plasma reagin or HIV may be necessary.

GOITER

Goiter, an enlargement of the thyroid gland, may be associated with hypothyroidism or hyperthyroidism, but patients with goiter also may be euthyroid, a condition termed *nontoxic goiter*. In underdeveloped countries, iodine deficiency is the number-one cause of goiter, which is especially prevalent in the U.S. immigrant population or in visitors to the country and may be associated with autoimmune Hashimoto's thyroiditis and Grave's disease.

SIMPLE NONTOXIC GOITER (EUTHYROID GOITER)

Simple nontoxic goiter is the most common type of thyroid enlargement. While iodine deficiency is rare in the United States, it may be seen in patients from other countries. Some patients are susceptible to goiter due to congenital defects in thyroid enzyme activity. Medications such as amiodarone and lithium may also cause euthyroid goiter. Simple nontoxic goiter is frequently noted at puberty, during pregnancy, and at menopause. The cause at these times is usually unclear.

Signs and Symptoms

Patients are generally asymptomatic except for an enlarged thyroid. The thyroid may be diffusely enlarged or nodular and not associated with hyperthyroidism, hypothyroidism, inflammation, or cancer.

Diagnostic Studies

Diagnosis is through physical examination and laboratory testing to determine thyroid function to rule out hypo- or hyperthyroidism or malignancy. TSH and free T4, thyroid ultrasound, or thyroid radioactive iodine uptake scan are recommended. Compensatory small elevations in TSH may occur, preventing hypothyroidism, but the TSH stimulation results in goiter formation. Thyroid antibodies should be measured if the patient has signs or symptoms of hypothyroidism to rule out Hashimoto thyroiditis. Treatment is directed at the cause, but partial surgical removal may be required for very large symptomatic goiters that cause shortness of breath or dysphagia.

THYROID NODULES/MULTINODULAR GOITER

Although rare in the United States, iodine deficiency is one of the most common causes of nodular goiter. Thyroid nodules are extremely common, and most are benign (Burman & Wartofsky, 2015; Detweiler et al., 2019; Haugen, et al., 2016). The causes are multifactorial, but thyroid nodules are known to increase with age, with women having a higher prevalence of thyroid nodules than men. In general, the development of multinodular goiter is due to a mix of genetic and environmental factors. There are two forms of multinodular goiter: nontoxic and toxic. In nontoxic goiter, normal amounts of thyroid hormone are produced. Toxic goiter is associated with higher production of thyroid hormones, leading to a suppressed TSH and hyperthyroidism. (See "Hyperthyroidism," Chapter 17.)

Signs and Symptoms

Most thyroid nodules are asymptomatic, although if large enough they may be palpable and visualized, and in rare instances, the cause of difficulty swallowing or shortness of breath. Some thyroid nodules may cause oversecretion of thyroxine, mimicking hyperthyroidism with symptoms of unexplained weight loss, sweating, tremor, nervousness, and palpitations/tachycardia.

Diagnostics

Several diagnostics can and should be used to determine if the nodule is cystic or solid, nontoxic or toxic, benign or malignant.

- TSH and free T_4.
- Thyroid ultrasound differentiates between cysts and solid nodules and number of nodules, which can help determine if a thyroid scan and/or FNA should be performed. The ultrasound may also be used as a guide if FNA is performed.
- Thyroid scan involves use of an isotope of radioactive iodine injected in an arm vein. Nodules that produce excess thyroid hormone, "hot nodules," show an increased uptake of the isotope; "cold nodules" are nonfunctioning and appear as holes in the scan. Hot nodules are typically noncancerous; cold nodules may be benign or malignant, thus warranting a FNA to differentiate benign from malignant cold nodules (Figure 5.10).

THYROID CANCER

Patients are often asymptomatic with thyroid cancer, and it is commonly found by the patient or practitioner as a nontender nodule. About 8% to 15% of thyroid nodules are malignant (Burman & Wartofsky, 2015; Detweiler et al., 2019; Haugen et al., 2016). Predisposing factors include young age; female sex; family history; and a history of radiation exposure to the head, neck, or chest. There are four main types: papillary, follicular, medullary, and anaplastic; the papillary type accounts for 85% of all thyroid cancers and has the best clinical outcomes. The other types are less differentiated, more difficult to treat, and have less favorable outcomes.

Signs and Symptoms

Clinical signs are usually absent, except for a painless enlargement of the thyroid gland. A history of rapid enlargement and a hard, fixed mass should raise the index of suspicion for carcinoma. The presence of enlarged anterior cervical lymph nodes is also a suspicious finding for thyroid metastasis. Thyroid function tests are usually normal.

Diagnostic Studies

Ultrasound of the neck is the first-line evaluation to determine size, location, and characteristics of the thyroid lesion. Radiographic evidence of a solid hypoechoic nodule or solid hypoechoic component with cystic characteristics indicates high

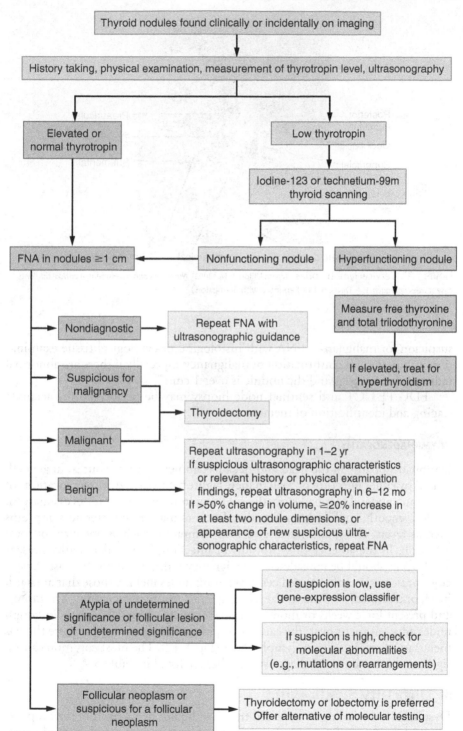

Figure 5.10 Assessing thyroid nodules. (Burman, K., Wartofsky, L. [2015]. Thyroid nodules. *New England Journal of Medicine, 375*:24, 2347–2356 [figure 1]).

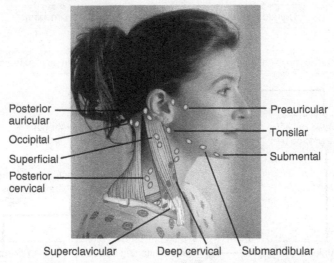

Posterior auricular
Occipital
Superficial
Posterior cervical
Preauricular
Tonsilar
Submental
Superclavicular   Deep cervical   Submandibular

Figure 5.11 Cervical lymph nodes. (From Dillon, P. M. [2003]. *Nursing health assessment: A critical thinking, case studies approach*. F. A. Davis, p. 199. Reprinted with permission.)

suspicion for malignancy. FNA with histological or cytological tissue examination is indicated for confirmation of malignancy, especially if there are abnormal radiographic findings and the nodule is over 1 cm.

FDG PET-CT and sentinel node biopsy may be performed for accurate staging and identification of metastases.

LYMPHADENOPATHY

Lymphadenopathy in the head and neck has numerous causes but is, in general, caused by either infection or malignancy. Figure 5.11 illustrates exact locations of the lymph nodes. Lymphadenopathy resulting from infection produces enlarged, tender, smooth, mobile lymph nodes. Patients may have systemic symptoms such as fevers, chills, and malaise or local symptoms such as abscesses or local infection. In the absence of symptoms of infection, lymphadenopathy present for 2 weeks should be considered a malignancy unless proven otherwise. Suspicious presentations of enlarged cervical lymph nodes include those that are hard, fixed, or ulcerated; >1.5 cm in size; accompanied by other concerning symptoms; and present for 2 weeks or more. Lymphadenopathy generally occurs in lymph nodes adjacent to, or near, the cause, except in some malignancies where there is metastatic disease to distant lymph nodes (Fig. 5.12). The most common causes, signs, and symptoms and diagnostic studies are listed in Table 5.2.

■ Difficulty Swallowing

Dysphagia is the feeling of impaired transit of liquids or solids from the oropharynx to the stomach. Dysphagia symptoms can be caused by a multitude of issues, such as oropharynx, pharynx, or esophageal transport disorders; lesions of the pharynx, hypopharynx, and esophagus; or neuromuscular disorders that cause

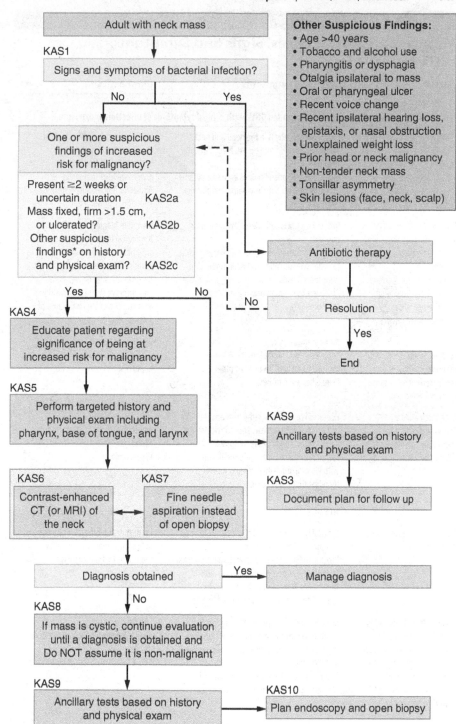

Figure 5.12 Algorithm for assessing neck mass. (From Pynnonen, M. et al. [2017]. Clinical practice guideline: Evaluation of the neck mass in adults. *Otolaryngology–Head and Neck Surgery, 157*(2), S1–S30. https://doi /10.1177/0194599817722550 [figure 1, p. S9]).

Table 5.2

Lymphadenopathy: Causes, Signs and Symptoms, and Diagnostic Studies

Causes	Signs and Symptoms	Diagnostics
Viral/Bacterial **Workup of the below symptoms is recommended ONLY with clinical symptoms of infection or exposure.**		
Pharyngitis/tonsillitis *Viral most common* *Bacterial causes include* *Group A streptococcus*	Lymphadenopathy is in the head and neck. Symptoms include sore throat, fever, difficulty swallowing. Physical examination findings include erythema of tonsils with exudate, erythematous posterior pharynx	Throat culture, specifically strep, viral if herpes viral simplex is suspected and/or *Neisseria gonorrhoeae* or *Chlamydia trachomatis* if sexually transmitted infection is suspected
Mononucleosis caused by the Epstein-Barr Virus (EBV) • *transmitted by intimate contact* • *Chronic EBV can increase risk of B cell lymphoma, T cell lymphoma, Hodgkin's lymphoma*	Diffuse cervical lymphadenopathy is usually dramatic. Symptoms include fever, severe pharyngitis, tonsillar swelling and exudate, fatigue, URI symptoms, headache. Physical examination findings include rash, splenomegaly.	Complete blood count (CBC) and serological testing for heterophil antibodies ("mono spot"), Epstein-Barr virus antibody titer. Treatment is supportive; steroids may improve symptoms; caution against contact sports because of splenomegaly.
HIV *Consider in individuals with exposure to HIV or with clinical symptoms or acute or chronic infections.*	Initial stages Cervical lymphadenopathy Symptoms include flu-like symptoms, headache, fever, rashes.	Serological screening testing HIV antibody (ELISA) Rapid tests
Cat scratch disease *Transmitted by scratch or bite from a cat infected with* Bartonella henselae	Regional lymphadenopathy near an injury but can present with cervical, supraclavicular and submandibular lymphadenopathy. Symptoms may include abdominal pain with visceral organ involvement, ocular manifestations, and fever. Physical findings may include signs of bite or scratch.	CBC Serological testing (EIA or IFA IgG titers) Wound culture
Dental caries/dental abscesses	Cervical lymphadenopathy Symptoms include fever, pain. Physical findings of caries, gum changes, swelling Ludwig's angina is swelling and cellulitis of the tongue, floor of mouth, or submandibular space. Can cause airway obstruction or sepsis.	Prompt dental referral is necessary. In Ludwig's angina, emergency room visit to drain abscess.
Mycobacterium tuberculosis (TB) of the head and neck (extrapulmonary). Cases are seen in patients emigrating from or in contact with others from countries with high TB rates.	Chronic cervical lymphadenopathy (scrofula) Symptoms may include malaise, weight loss, night sweats, cough, rhinorrhea, pharyngitis, and dysphagia. Head and face physical findings may include ulcerations or indurations of mucosa.	Clinical diagnosis Serological testing for lymphotropic disease. CBC, CT neck/MRI, FNA of neck mass

Table 5.2

Lymphadenopathy: Causes, Signs, and Symptoms, and Diagnostic Studies—cont'd

Causes	Signs and Symptoms	Diagnostics
Malignancies		
Cervical lymphadenopathy should be considered malignancy in the absence of infectious symptoms.		
Metastatic head and neck carcinoma (e.g., oral cancer, oropharyngeal cancer, hypopharyngeal cancer, laryngeal cancer, nasopharyngeal cancer, salivary gland cancer, thyroid cancer, metastatic skin cancer of the head and neck)	Stand-alone symptoms suspicious for head and neck cancer include: • Neck mass present for more than 2 weeks • Absence of infectious symptoms • Firm, fixed neck mass • Size of neck mass over 1.5 cm • Ulceration of skin over the neck mass	CT neck with and without contrast or MRI FNA is necessary for diagnosis, and referral to an otolaryngology provider for thorough examination including laryngoscopy, nasal endoscopy, direct laryngoscopy under anesthesia.
Leukemia: Malignant neoplasm of the blood-forming cells in the bone marrow. Besides being acute or chronic, leukemias are classified according to cell type: lymphoblastic or myeloid.	Generalized lymphadenopathy Symptoms include fatigue, weakness, anorexia, weight loss, fever, night sweats, bleeding, and easy bruising.	Diagnosis is made through hematological studies and bone marrow biopsy. Prompt referral to a hematologist and/or oncologist is necessary.
Lymphomas: This group of neoplasms arises from the lymphatic system and lymphoid tissues. The most common types are Hodgkin's lymphoma, which occurs more often in younger patients, and non-Hodgkin's lymphoma, which occurs more in the older population. Burkitt's lymphoma and mycosis fungoides are rare types.	Cervical and mediastinal lymphadenopathy often occurring in clusters and often preceding systemic symptoms. Systems include fever, night sweats, weight loss, fatigue. Physical examination findings include extranodal tumors/lesions of the head and neck.	CT or MRI imaging Diagnosis is made through hematological studies and bone marrow biopsy. If lymphoma is suspected, prompt referral to a hematologist and/or oncologist is warranted.

functional limitations. It is important to differentiate between pre-esophageal dysphagia, which occurs mostly in patients with neuromuscular disorders, and esophageal disorders, which can include obstructive or motor disorders. Neuromuscular disorders include CVA, myasthenia gravis, muscular dystrophy, dermatomyositis, and poliomyelitis. The obstructive disorders include cancer, peptic stricture secondary to gastroesophageal reflux disease (GERD), and esophageal rings. The obstructive esophageal disorders are often limited to solid food. Motor disorders can affect both solid and liquid intake and are caused by impaired esophageal peristalsis, which occurs with such conditions as diabetes, achalasia, and scleroderma.

History

The history is particularly important in these patients because physical examination is of little value in diagnosing dysphagia. It is important to clarify if the dysphagia is acute or chronic. Inquire if there is difficulty swallowing only with liquids or with both solids and liquids. The most important question is whether the patient is coughing or choking on food or liquids, as this could be concerning for aspiration. Ask about associated symptoms such as pharyngitis, odynophagia, weight loss, globus, or hemoptysis. Identifying where the difficulty in transit is felt by the patient is important in determining whether the cause is pre-esophageal or postesophageal. In oropharyngeal dysphagia, patients may have difficulty getting the food or liquid to the back of the throat to swallow. In esophageal dysphagia, patients may feel like foods are getting stuck after swallow is initiated. Ask if the dysphagia occurs constantly or intermittently and what makes it worse or better. Identifying a history of cancer, CVA, neuromuscular or autoimmune diseases, or GERD is important, as these conditions affect swallowing. Inquire whether there have been frequent bouts of pneumonia or a chronic cough, which might alert you to aspiration as a cause. Inquire as to all medications. The bisphosphonates, a drug class used for treating osteoporosis, can cause esophagitis if not taken with a full glass of water. Ask about habits, such as smoking and alcohol intake, because cancers of the head and neck are more common in individuals with a history of tobacco and/or alcohol use or abuse.

Physical Examination

Physical examination is not helpful other than as an observation of patient discomfort when swallowing or a regurgitation or cough following attempted swallowing. Definitive diagnosis will require swallow studies and/or endoscopy or laryngoscopy to determine the exact cause of the problem.

ACHALASIA

The term *achalasia* refers to an esophageal motility disorder. Achalasia is rare, affecting 20,000 to 40,000 patients in the United States, with a peak incidence between the ages of 30 and 60 years (Vaezi et al., 2020). Symptoms occur with both liquids and solid foods. In addition, GERD, strictures, and neoplasms are more common in older patients, which also contribute to aspiration prevalence in this population.

Signs and Symptoms

With achalasia, the patient will complain of progressive dysphagia to solids and liquids. Symptoms include GERD, chest pain, regurgitation, weight loss, and discomfort or fullness in the throat. In the older patient who is nonverbal, aspiration may be the first sign.

Diagnostic Studies

The diagnosis of achalasia is made with barium swallow studies, esophageal manometry, and endoscopy. Having the patient take small amounts of food, eat a soft diet, and sit while eating are helpful preventive measures.

ESOPHAGITIS

Esophagitis is a general term referring to an inflammation of the esophagus that can occur with GERD, *Helicobacter pylori* (*H. pylori*) infection, gastroesophageal junction incompetence, esophageal strictures, certain medicines (especially when not taken with enough fluid), ingestion of caustic substances, neoplasms, chemotherapy, or radiation.

Signs and Symptoms
The patient with esophagitis describes burning and pain in the esophagus with or without dysphagia. Patients may also experience globus, hypersalivation, and/or regurgitation. The symptoms may occur more with eating or drinking, especially spicy or citrus foods, chewing gum, or mints, and at night when the patient is recumbent.

Diagnostic Studies
The diagnosis of esophagitis is made with endoscopy, pH manometry, and biopsy for *H. pylori*. Removal of the causative agent, if possible, helps toward healing. Medicines such as H_2 blockers and proton pump inhibitors may be necessary as well as diet modification, weight loss, and not eating before lying down.

BARRETT'S ESOPHAGUS

This condition is caused by the mucosal lining of the esophagus changing from normal columnar epithelium to stratified squamous epithelium as a result of chronic GERD and is characterized by inflammation of the lower esophagus with possible ulceration. Barrett's esophagus is associated with an increased frequency of esophageal squamous cell carcinoma (Clermont & Falk, 2018).

Signs and Symptoms
As with esophagitis, patients may describe globus, dysphagia, or a burning sensation in the throat.

Diagnostic Studies
The diagnosis is made by endoscopy with a biopsy of the mucosal tissue. Due to the increased risk for squamous cell carcinoma in these patients, regular follow-up is necessary.

SCHATZKI'S RING

Schatzki's ring is a mucosal narrowing of the distal esophagus at the squamocolumnar junction. It is thought to be congenital but may not manifest until later in life.

Signs and Symptoms
Dysphagia is the presenting symptom in patients with Schatzki's ring, especially with ingestion of solid foods.

Diagnostic Studies
The diagnosis is made by endoscopy, and the treatment includes stretching of the stricture to alleviate the symptoms. Recurrence is common, and repeat dilations or resection may be necessary.

SCLERODERMA

Scleroderma is a chronic disease of unknown etiology characterized by a progressive systemic fibrosis of the skin, joints, and internal organs, especially the esophagus, gastrointestinal tract, heart, lung, and kidney. It affects women three times more often than men and generally occurs in the third to fifth decade of life.

Signs and Symptoms

There is a wide range in the severity of the symptoms and the prognosis. It may affect only the skin and manifest as generalized thickening, which is the most common type of scleroderma, or it may be systemic, involving the vital organs and resulting in death. The initial symptoms usually involve gastrointestinal complaints, such as dysphagia or reflux; shortness of breath due to pulmonary fibrosis or pulmonary hypertension; polyarthralgia; or Raynaud's disease, causing a thickening and stiffening of the skin on the hands and feet. The symptoms may worsen with time and involve numerous systems: skin, musculoskeletal, gastrointestinal tract, cardiorespiratory, and kidneys. It may take several years for these manifestations to occur, and the constellation of symptoms is often called CREST (**c**alcinosis, **R**aynaud's, **e**sophageal dysfunction, **s**clerodactyly, and **t**elangiectasias) syndrome.

Diagnostic Studies

A positive antinuclear antibody is present in more than 90% of patients. An anticentromere antibody is present in a high portion of patients who progress to CREST syndrome.

NEUROMUSCULAR DISEASES

Several neuromuscular disorders can cause pre-esophageal dysphagia, including myasthenia gravis, muscular dystrophy, dermatomyositis, and poliomyelitis.

Signs and Symptoms

Dysphagia is one of the common presenting symptoms in these neuromuscular diseases. Other symptoms vary according to the underlying disease but include proximal limb weakness, general muscle fatigability, ocular muscle weakness, quadriparesis, polyarthralgia, skin eruptions, muscle spasms, and loss of deep tendon reflexes, to name only a few. Aspiration can be a risk in these patients.

Diagnostic Studies

Diagnosis depends on the underlying disease, which is beyond the scope of this text. These patients need to be immediately referred to a neurologist for diagnosis and follow-up.

REFERENCES

Baugh, R. F., Basura, G. J., Ishii, L. E., Schwartz, S. R., Drumheller, C. M., Burkholder, R., Deckard, N. A., Dawson, C., Driscoll, C., Gillespie, M. B., Gurgel, R. K., Halperin, J., Khalid, A. N., Kumar, K. A., Micco, A., Munsell, D., Rosenbaum, S., & Vaughan, W. (2013). Clinical practice guideline: Bell's palsy. *Otolaryngology–Head and Neck Surgery, 149*(3 Suppl), S1–27. https//doi.org/10.1177/0194599813505967

Burman, K., & Wartofsky, L. (2015). Thyroid nodules. *New England Journal of Medicine, 375*:24, 2347–2356.

Carlson, E. R., & Schlieve, T. (2019). Salivary gland malignancies. *Oral and Maxillofacial Surgery Clinics of North America, 31*(1), 125–144. https://doi.org/10.1016/j.coms.2018.08.007

Centers for Disease Control. (2021). Disparities in Oral Health. Retrieved June 3, 2021, from https://www.cdc.gov/oralhealth/oral_health_disparities/index.htm

Chow, A. (2019). Epidemiology, pathogenesis, and clinical manifestations of odontogenic infections. In UptoDate. Durand, M., Bogorodskaya, M. (Eds). Retrieved July 8, 2021, from https://www.uptodate.com/contents/epidemiology-pathogenesis-and-clinical-manifestations-of-odontogenic-infection https://www.uptodate.com/contents/epidemiology-pathogenesis-and-clinical-manifestations-of-odontogenic-infections?search=epidemiology-pathogenesis-and-clinical-manifestations-of-odontogenic-infection&source=search_result&selectedTitle=1~26&usage_type=default&display_rank=1

Clermont, M., & Falk, G. W. (2018). Clinical guidelines update on the diagnosis and management of Barrett's esophagus. *Digestive Diseases and Sciences, 63*(8), 2122–2128. https://doi.org/10.1007/s10620-018-5070-z

Detweiler, K., Elfenbein, D. M., & Mayers, D. (2019). Evaluation of thyroid nodules. *Surgical Clinics of North America, 99*(4), 571–586. https://doi.org//10.1016/j.suc.2019.04.001

Gauer, R., & Semidey, M. (2015). Diagnosis and treatment of temporomandibular disorders. *American Academy of Family Physicians, 91*(6), 378–386.

Haugen, B., Alexander, E., Bible, K., Doherty, G., Mandel, S., Nikiforov, Y., Pacini, F., Randolph, G., Sawka, A., Schlumberger, M., Schuff, K., Sherman, S., Sosa, J., Steward, D., Tuttle, R., & Wartofsky, L. (2016). 2015 American Thyroid Association management guidelines for adult patients with thyroid nodules and differentiated thyroid cancer: The American Thyroid Association Guidelines Task Force on Thyroid Nodules and Differentiated Thyroid Cancer. *Thyroid, 26*(1), 1–133 https://doi.org/10.1089/thy.2015.0020

Jones, M., Urits, I., Ehrhardt, K., Cefalu, J., Kendrick, J., Park, D., Cornett, E., Kaye, A., & Viswanath, O. (2019). A comprehensive review of trigeminal neuralgia. *Current Pain and Headache Reports, 23*(74), 1–7.

Long, B. J., Koyfman, A., & Gottlieb, M. (2019) Evaluation and management of angioedema in the emergency department. *Western Journal of Emergency Medicine, 20*(4), 587–600. https://doi.org/10.5811/westjem.2019.5.42650

Michael, R., & Kiemeny, M. (2019). Infections of the neck. *Emergency Medicine Clinics of North America, 37*(1), 95–107.

Moellman, J. J., Bernstein, J. A., Lindsell, C., Banerji, A., Busse, P. J., Camargo, C. A. Jr., Collins, S. P., Craig, T. J., Lumry, W. R., Nowak, R., Pines, J. M., Raja, A. S., Riedl, M., Ward, M. J., Zuraw, B. L., Diercks, D., Hiestand, B., Campbell, R. L., Schneider, S., & Sinert, R. (2014). A consensus parameter for the evaluation and management of angioedema in the emergency department. *Academic Emergency Medicine, 21*(4), 469–484. https://doi.org/10.1111/acem.12341

Ogle, O. E. (2020). Salivary gland diseases. *Dental Clinics of North America, 64*(1), 87–104. https//doi.org/10.1016/j.cden.2019.08.007

Pradeep, S., & Smith, J. (20) Giant cell arteritis: Practical pearls and updates. *Current Pain and Headache Reports, 22*(2), 1–8. https//doi.org/10.1007/s11916-018-0655-y

Pynnonen, M., Gillespie, M., Roman, B., Rosenfeld, R., Tunkel, D., Bontempo, L., Brook, I., Chick, D., Colandrea, M., Finestone, S., Fowler, J., Griffith, C., Henson, Z., Levine, C., Mehta, V., Salama, A., Scharpf, J., Shatzkes, D., Stern, W., Youngerman, J., & Corrigan, M. (2017). Clinical practice guideline: Evaluation of the neck mass in adults. *Otolaryngology–Head and Neck Surgery, 157*(2), S1–S30. https//doi.org/10.1177/0194599817722550

Siegel, R. L., Miller, K. D., Fuchs, H., & Jemal, A. (2021). Cancer statistics, 2021. *CA: A Cancer Journal for Clinicians, 71*, 7–33. https://doi.org/10.3322/caac.21654

Vaezi, M. F., Pandolfino, J. E., Yadlapati, R. H., Greer, K. B., & Kavitt, R. T. (2020). ACG clinical guidelines: Diagnosis and management of achalasia. *American Journal of Gastroenterology, 115*(9), 1393–1411. https://doi.org//10.14309/ajg.0000000000000731

Wilson, K. F., Meier, J. D., & Ward, P. D. (2014). Salivary gland disorders. *American Family Physician, 89*(11):882–888.

Yadav, S., Yang, Y., Dutra, E., Robinson, J., & Wadhwa, S. (2018) Temporomandibular joint disorders in the elderly and aging population. *Journal of the American Geriatric Society, 66*(6), 1213–1217.

Younger, D. (2019). Giant cell arteritis. *Neurologic Clinics, 37*(2):335–344. https://doi.org/10.1016/j.ncl.2019.01.008

Chapter 6

The Eye

- James Blackwell
- Mary Jo Goolsby

E ye disorders are common in all age groups, although the nature of the problems varies across the life span. Eyes are visual system organs that are similar to cameras, focusing light on a membrane that is then converted into electric signals and relayed to the brain for interpretation. Of all eye disorders, those resulting in visual impairment are the source of greatest disability. The incidence of vision loss is rising, despite the fact that much blindness can be prevented. The prevalence of eye disease increases with age. In the United States, approximately 1.3 million people are legally blind, 2.9 million have low vision, and 4.2 million have some visual impairment (AAO, n.d.).

The most common forms of visual impairment are refractive errors; more than 150 million Americans reportedly use corrective lenses for refractive errors. Cataracts are extremely common; more than 24.4 million adults over 40 have cataracts, and this number doubles to about 50% for those 75 and older. Less prevalent but still common causes of visual impairment include advanced macular degeneration associated with age (2.1 million among Americans age 50 or older), diabetic retinopathy (over 7.7 million among Americans age 40 or older), and glaucoma (2.7 million among Americans age 40 and older). Dry eye syndrome affects 3.2 million, including 1.68 million men age 50 and older (AAO, n.d.).

Figure 6.1 illustrates basic eye anatomy. Table 6.1 provides a summary of characteristics that help differentiate among the causes of visual change.

History

■ General Eye History

When a patient has concerns about the eyes or vision, it is necessary to obtain a thorough analysis of symptoms and a general history related to the eyes. The history of the present illness can help determine a general category of vision loss/ eye problem and is key to communicating problems to an ophthalmologist or optometrist, who have the expertise and equipment to perform a comprehensive

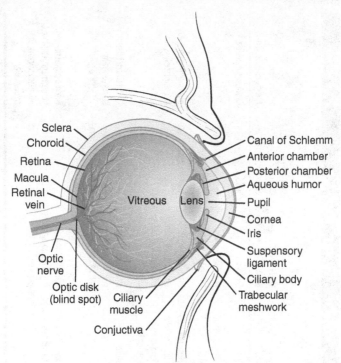

Figure 6.1 Basic eye anatomy. (Courtesy of National Eye Institute, National Institutes of Health.)

ophthalmic examination. A good mnemonic for an eye history is to ask "RSVP" questions. If all of these questions elicit a positive response, then an urgent ophthalmology consult is required.

R: Redness
S: Sensitivity to light (unable to keep the eyes open)
V: Vision loss
P: Pain

The timing of the ophthalmic problem should be established, as well as whether it was a sudden or gradual onset. The vision loss should be established as either unilateral or bilateral, since a bilateral vision loss is indicative of a visual pathway disorder. The presence and quality of pain, along with the presence or absence of redness, should be noted. Any associated symptoms such as nausea and vomiting, rhinorrhea, tearing, balance or depth perception issues, and history of trauma should be noted.

▪ Past Medical History

Past medical history should specifically include a focus on vascular disease entities such as diabetes mellitus, coronary artery disease, hypertension, hypercoagulability disorders, and stroke; glasses or contact lens use; and previous eye

Table 6.1

Differentiating Among Causes of Vision Changes

	Cataracts	Chronic Open-Angle Glaucoma	Acute Closed-Angle Glaucoma	Amaurosis Fugax	Retinal Detachment	Ischemic Ocular Neuropathy	Macular Degeneration
Onset	Gradual	Gradual	Sudden	Sudden	Sudden	Sudden	Gradual to sudden
Associated symptoms			Head/eye pain, nausea, eye redness	Neurological deficits possible	Possible signs of trauma	Head, jaw, temple pain or soreness	
Severity of vision change	Ranges from cloudy, hazy, to vision loss	Gradual darkening may range to complete vision loss	Blurring, halos; can range to total vision loss	Complete but transient loss initially; may lead to complete vision loss	Flash of light, darkened areas; may progress to complete loss	Affected portion lost	Blurring may progress to complete loss
Portion of vision affected	Unilateral or bilateral	Unilateral or bilateral; peripheral vision lost first	Unilateral	Unilateral	Unilateral, often specific fields affected; can be complete loss	Unilateral; may affect only a portion but progress to complete loss	Unilateral or bilateral; starts centrally
Inspection	Clouding; loss of red reflex	Cup/disc ratio change; late afferent effect possible	Red eye, ciliary flush, fixed pupil, corneal edema	Pale retina with red fovea, embolus	Wrinkling and graying of retina, afferent pupil defect		Altered pigmentation; hemorrhage, exudates, microaneurysms, or neovascular

examinations and surgeries. Include previous eye disorders such as glaucoma, strabismus, amblyopia, cataracts, retinopathy, and macular degeneration. Determine whether the patient uses corrective lenses (either glasses or contact lenses) and, if so, how they are worn and whether they successfully correct the vision. Soft contact lens users are at a higher risk of pseudomonal keratitis, corneal abrasions, and recurrent conjunctivitis. In the older population, ask about keratoconjunctivitis sicca (dry eye related to lack of tear production), the severity of symptoms, and current treatment, if any.

All medications, including over-the-counter medicines, herbal supplements, and vitamins, should be identified in order to investigate possible medication side effects. For example, angle-closure glaucoma may be associated with anticholinergics and topiramate, yellow vision may be associated with digoxin use, and blue vision may be associated with sildenafil use. Box 6.1 includes a list of commonly prescribed drugs that affect the eyes or vision. Finally, knowing what medications the patient routinely takes may suggest the need for a more detailed medical history if it is found that the patient is taking drugs for disorders that were not disclosed earlier.

■ Family History

Identify the family history of eye disorders, including those conditions mentioned in the preceding paragraphs. Determine whether immediate relatives have refractive errors requiring correction.

■ Social History

Social history should include occupational and recreational activities that may predispose the individual to eye injuries, such as being a welder or participating in possible contact sports such as handball or basketball, and the use of protective

---

Box 6.1

Examples of Drugs With Oculotoxic Effects

- Amiodarone
- Amphetamines
- Anticholinergic agents
- Antihistamines
- Bisphosphonates
- Chloramphenicol
- Chloroquine
- Contraceptives (oral)
- Corticosteroids
- Digitalis
- Ethambutol
- Gold salts
- Hydroxychloroquine
- Isotretinoin
- Isoniazid
- Phenothiazines
- Phosphodiesterase inhibitors
- Quinine
- Retinoids
- Rifampin
- Selective serotonin reuptake inhibitors
- Sympathomimetics
- Tamoxifen
- Topiramate

eye wear. If the patient wears contact lenses, determine how long the lenses are worn, how often they are changed, and how they are cleansed and stored between wearings.

Physical Examination

■ Order of the Examination

Inspection is the primary technique used in the eye examination. The general appearance of the eyes should be noted. This includes the position and spacing of the eyes, the eye color, sclera and conjunctiva appearance, presence of discharge or tearing, pupillary size, symmetry and reactivity, eye movement, and eyelid and periorbital appearance, paying particular attention to any asymmetry. When a mass or lesion is discovered, palpation of the area is indicated. If the patient has complained of discharge, palpation of the punctum, lids overlying the meibomian glands, and the region of the medial canthus may express the discharge. The globe also can be palpated gently to determine tone. If the patient has experienced a sudden onset of eye pain, it is important not to dilate the eyes before determining whether acute angle glaucoma is present because dilating the eye may increase the intraocular pressure. Gently palpate surrounding bony structures and tissue with a history of trauma.

■ Visual Acuity

Visual acuity should be measured in a well-lighted area with and without corrective lenses, if lenses are worn. Testing the visual acuity assesses central vision and should be performed one eye at a time and then with both eyes simultaneously. Visual acuity can be measured by using a standardized chart that employs either symbols or letters, typically with the patient standing 20 feet from the chart. Snellen or Sloan eye charts use letters and should not be used with patients who cannot read. For children or adults who cannot read or do not know the letters of the alphabet, a LEA chart or "tumbling E" chart can be used. The LEA uses four simple objects (circle, square, pentagon/house, and apple). The "E" chart displays the capital letter E facing different directions. The examiner may also have the patient count fingers, identify gross hand motion, or detect light if the patient is unable to adequately see the chart. Near vision may be tested by using a handheld chart, such as a Rosenbaum chart, typically held 14 inches from the eyes. Color vision can be grossly tested by using the color strips (green and red) on the Snellen chart or by asking the patient to identify the colors of other objects. Ishihara or Hardy-Rand-Rittler plates can be used for a more thorough assessment of color vision. Peripheral vision is tested separately.

■ Visual Field Assessment/Peripheral Vision

Visual field assessment is conducted by having the person face the examiner and focus on a particular part of the examiner's face, such as the nose. The examiner either wiggles their fingers or holds up a certain number of fingers with their arms fully extended and asks the patient to indicate when the fingers come into the patient's visual field, which should match the examiner's visual field. Assess each of the four visual field quadrants (superior, inferior, lateral, and medial). Carefully identify the location of any visual defects. Alternatively, peripheral field perimetry can be measured more objectively using equipment designed specifically for this purpose.

■ Alignment

Ocular alignment is evaluated by observing eye motion, performing the cover/uncover test, and assessing the light reflex. For motion, observe the eyes as the patient follows an object as it is moved smoothly through the six cardinal positions, approximately 12 inches in front of the face. Alignment is tested by comparing the corneal light reflex while holding a light source in front of the patient as they stare straight ahead. A symmetric reflection in the center of each pupil is indicative of normal eye alignment. Ocular alignment and strabismus may be assessed with the cover-uncover test. As the patient looks at a near object, one eye is then covered for 5 seconds and then uncovered as the covered eye is observed. The opposite eye is then tested in the same fashion. The test is then repeated for both eyes while fixating on a far object. A normal test is when neither eye moves out of alignment or "drifts."

■ Accessory Structures

Inspect the eyebrows and lashes for symmetry and orientation. Inspect lids for symmetry and placement; palpate the lids for masses or tenderness. Observe for areas of discoloration, masses, and xanthomas.

■ External Eye Structures

Inspect the conjunctiva, cornea, and sclera, noting the condition of the surface, clarity, color, and vascularity. Differentiation between "muddy" and icteric sclera can be done by observing the sclera under the lower eyelids. Red eyes may be caused by conjunctivitis or subconjunctival hemorrhages. Epithelial hyperplasia is a yellow-white lesion of the bulbar conjunctiva that may be uncomfortable, whereas a pterygium is a painless lesion that may grow over the cornea. Figures 6.2, 6.3, and 6.4 depict examples of abnormalities. Box 6.2 reviews the procedure for performing a fluorescein stain to assess for potential corneal lesions.

■ Pupils

Observe the shape and symmetry of the pupils, including the response to light and accommodation. While testing for light response, have the patient focus on a distant point in order to avoid confusing light and accommodation responses. The pupils provide important indications of the cause for vision change. Examples of abnormal findings and causes are noted in Table 6.2. The cornea is also assessed during the pupil examination. Box 6.3 describes assessment of the pupils.

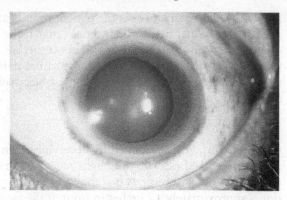

Figure 6.2 Arcus senilis. White or gray ring at corneal margin seen in older adults and caused by fat deposits in the cornea or hyaline degeneration. (Reprinted with permission from Dr. Julia Haller, Ophthalmologist in Chief. Permission granted by Michael D. Allen, Esquire, at Wills Eye Institute.)

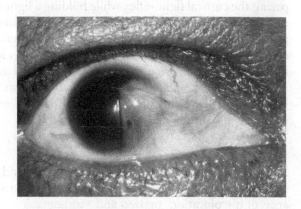

Figure 6.3 Pterygium. Wedge-shaped and raised conjunctival growth, usually extending from nasal side. May be related to chronic irritation. (Reprinted with permission from Dr. Julia Haller, Ophthalmologist in Chief. Permission granted by Michael D. Allen, Esquire, at Wills Eye Institute.)

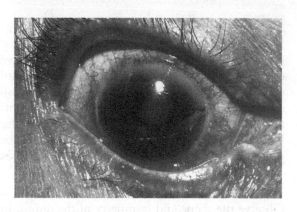

Figure 6.4 Ciliary flush. A condition where conjunctival vessels are most dilated around the corneal edge. (Reprinted with permission from Dr. Julia Haller, Ophthalmologist in Chief. Permission granted by Michael D. Allen, Esquire, at Wills Eye Institute.)

■ Anterior Chamber and Lens

Determine the approximate depth and clarity of the anterior chamber using oblique lighting. The anterior chamber should be clear and free of opacities, debris, or blood. Hyphema refers to blood in the anterior chamber; hypopyon is a condition in which white blood cells and exudate (sterile pus) collect in the

Box 6.2   SPECIAL PROCEDURE

Fluorescein Stain Technique to Assess Corneal Integrity

After determining that the patient has no relevant allergies, inspect the cornea and sclera without staining, if tolerated. A topical ocular anesthetic improves tolerance of further examination. Approximately 1 minute after installation of topical anesthetic, moisten the tip of a fluorescein stain strip with sterile saline. Holding the lids open with thumb and index finger, apply the stain by touching the moistened strip to the lower conjunctiva. Ask the patient either to blink or to move their eye up and down and side-to-side with their eyelid closed to disperse the stain. If both eyes are being stained, use a separate strip for each eye to avoid cross-contamination.

Once the stain has been distributed by blinking, inspect the cornea and conjunctiva beneath the upper and lower lids using a cobalt blue light source, held obliquely to the structure being examined. The stain should be uniformly distributed; areas of stain uptake, indicating abrasion to the cornea, will fluoresce bright green. Any visible and superficial foreign body should be removed if possible.

Following inspection, flush the stain with sterile saline solution.

anterior chamber. Also with the oblique lighting, assess the clarity of the lens. During the funduscopic examination, the clarity of the lens is also identified when the red reflex is noted. A good rule of thumb is to remember "If the cornea or anterior chamber is not clear, ophthalmology needs to be here."

■ Cranial Nerves

The eye examination includes an assessment of cranial nerves (CNs) II, III, IV, and VI, which is accomplished during assessment of visual acuity, peripheral acuity, extraocular movements, accessory structures, and pupils. CN II is assessed by visual acuity and visual fields. CN III, IV and VI are assessed by ocular

Table 6.2

Pupil Abnormalities

Horner's syndrome	Miosis is present unilaterally. Pupillary responses are intact. Associated with ptosis and appearance that eye is "sunken" on affected side, with lack of sweating on opposite side. Caused by sympathetic lesion.
Benign anisocoria	Some asymmetry of the pupil size is considered normal if the difference is less than 0.5 mm.
Argyll-Robertson pupil	The pupil is small and may have an abnormal shape. Although the pupil does not respond to light, it exhibits a brisk response to accommodation (near vision). Usually bilateral involvement. Associated with neurosyphilis.
Tonic pupil	No response to light (direct or consensual). Accommodation usually also affected. Most common in female patients. Unilateral. Caused by denervation of the ciliary muscle and sphincter.

Box 6.3   SPECIAL PROCEDURE

Pupil Testing

The assessment of pupil shape, size, and reactivity provides much data. It is important to always assess direct and consensual pupillary response. If these are abnormal, you should then also assess for accommodation. By using the "swinging penlight" test in assessing the response to light, afferent defects—in which the consensual response is more pronounced than the direct response—are more easily detected. This method is performed by holding the light source in front of the patient and directing it toward one eye. At this point, observe both pupils, noting the direct response of the eye receiving the direct light and the consensual response in the opposite eye. Leave your attention on the opposite eye, continuing to note the consensual response as you briskly swing the light source in the direction of this eye. Note whether the pupil response is a slight constriction, slightly more pronounced with direct light, which is normal, or the pupil slightly relaxes so that the response is slightly less pronounced with direct light, which is an abnormal, Marcus-Gunn effect. Then observe the opposite eye, swinging the light back to that eye as you note any change between the indirect and direct responses. In some optic nerve disorders, such as ischemic optic neuropathy and optic neuritis, as well as other conditions that affect the pathway anterior to the optic chiasm, this afferent defect may be the only objective finding.

movements and pupil. Ocular movements are assessed by having the individual follow the examiner's finger or other object in an "H-shape" fashion. Pupils are assessed for size, shape, and response using the PERRLA acronym (i.e., are pupils equal, round, and reactive to light and accommodation). (See Box 6.3.) The optic nerve is finally directly observed during the funduscopic examination.

■ Funduscopic Examination

Ophthalmoscopic examination requires constant practice as it is a diminishable skill. It is best done in a darkened room and should include the visualization of the red reflex, anterior chamber, iris and lens, and retina and optic disc (Box 6.4). The retina is examined, visualizing the optic disc, blood vessels, and the macula, located laterally to the optic disc. The optic disc may be found by following the retinal blood vessels as they converge into the optic disc. The posterior chamber should be clear and free of opacities, debris, or blood. Blood in the posterior chamber indicates a vitreous hemorrhage. The iris and lens should be observed for the presence of cataracts, which may be congenital or acquired. It is important to recognize that there are limitations in the portion of the eye that is seen through an undilated pupil as performed in the typical primary care setting. Table 6.3 lists several abnormalities, with the related significance for each. Also refer to Figures 6.5 through 6.10, which illustrate the normal fundus and selected abnormal findings.

Box 6.4 SPECIAL PROCEDURE

Funduscopic Examination

Successful use of the ophthalmoscope is challenging. Practice and patience are required to locate, identify, and assess retinal structures. The ophthalmoscope provides the ability to directly visualize both the external and internal structures of the eye, including the blood vessels. It is important that the examiner be familiar with adjusting the intensity of the light source, varying the apertures, and adjusting the diopters to best see the target structures. As the dial on the ophthalmoscope is moved counterclockwise, the diopters shift from positive to negative. Because the more negative diopters direct the focus posteriorly, by moving from the positive to negative diopters, your focus will shift from the anterior eye to the posterior eye, retina, and optic disc. Adjustment of the ophthalmoscope while inspecting the eye takes considerable practice and coordination. As the retinal vessels branch out as they leave the optic disc, one way to locate the optic disc is to follow the branches as they converge or toward the trunk of the vessels. Since only a portion of the retina is visible at any time, repositioning or directing of the ophthalmoscope is necessary to visualize different areas of the background. The newer panoptic ophthalmoscope provides a magnified view and is easier to manipulate than traditional equipment and is increasing in usage. However, the traditional ophthalmoscope is most commonly found in most practice settings.

Table 6.3

Retinal and Background Abnormalities

Finding	Significance
Flame hemorrhages (superficial)	Linear hemorrhages, often associated with extreme elevation of blood pressure.
Preretinal hemorrhages	Superficial hemorrhage, often characterized by a rounded inferior margin and a linear upper visible margin. Associated with both diabetic and hypertensive retinopathy and retinal tears.
Microaneurysms	Tiny rounded dilations of retinal arteries, frequently associated with hypertension.
Neovascularization	Proliferation of new, fragile vessels on the surface of retina, which have increased likelihood of bleeding. Associated with diabetes.
Dot/blot hemorrhages (deep)	Deeper, rounded and irregularly shaped hemorrhages associated with diabetes.
Cotton wool exudate	Yellow to white "fluffy" areas of ischemia. Associated with both diabetic and hypertensive retinopathy.
Hard exudate	Very discrete yellow to white lesions, often distributed in a circular pattern. Associated with leakage of fluids into retinal tissue. Associated with both diabetic and hypertensive retinopathy.

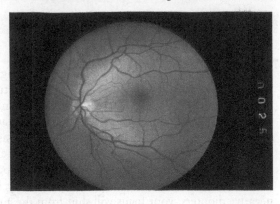

Figure 6.5 Normal fundus. Well-defined disc, paired arteries and veins; bright red arteries; AV ratio 2:3; no nicking, exudates, hemorrhages. (Reprinted with permission from Dr. Julia Haller, Ophthalmologist in Chief. Permission granted by Michael D. Allen, Esquire, at Wills Eye Institute.)

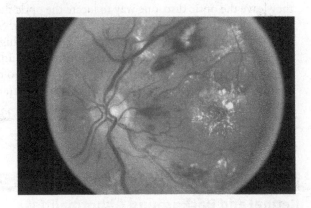

Figure 6.6 Diabetic retinopathy. Soft and hard exudates; soft and hard hemorrhages. (Reprinted with permission from Dr. Julia Haller, Ophthalmologist in Chief. Permission granted by Michael D. Allen, Esquire, at Wills Eye Institute.)

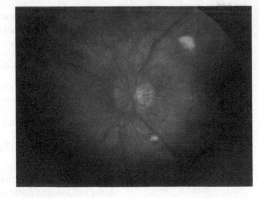

Figure 6.7 Diabetic proliferative retinopathy. Extensive microvascular changes, with exudates and other background changes that occur in advanced stage diabetes when abnormal new blood vessels and scar tissue form on the surface of the retina. (Courtesy of National Eye Institute, National Institutes of Health.)

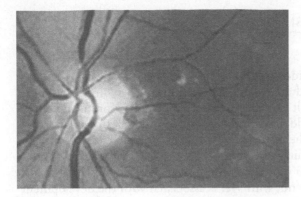

Figure 6.8 Hypertensive changes. Narrowing arteries, increased light reflex, crossing changes, and exudates commonly seen with long-term hypertension. (Reprinted with permission from Dr. Julia Haller, Ophthalmologist in Chief. Permission granted by Michael D. Allen, Esquire, at Wills Eye Institute.)

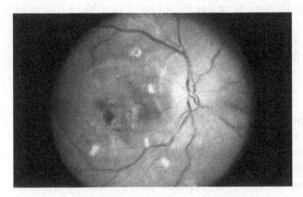

Figure 6.9 Malignant hypertension. Blurred disc margins, papilledema, narrowed arteries, crossing changes, and exudates are seen in malignant hypertension. (Reprinted with permission from Dr. Julia Haller, Ophthalmologist in Chief. Permission granted by Michael D. Allen, Esquire, at Wills Eye Institute.)

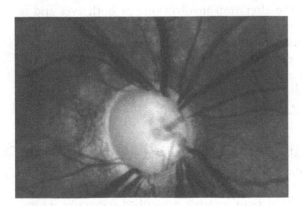

Figure 6.10 Glaucomatous optic nerve. Increased cup and disc ratio is a common finding when visualizing the optic nerve in a patient with glaucoma. (Reprinted with permission from Dr. Julia Haller, Ophthalmologist in Chief. Permission granted by Michael D. Allen, Esquire, at Wills Eye Institute.)

Differential Diagnosis of Chief Complaints

■ Visual Disturbances

Visual disturbances cover a wide range of complaints, including blurred vision, loss of vision, blind spots, and altered color perception. When altered vision is the patient's chief complaint, it is crucial to be alert for indications of potential irreversible loss of vision. Sudden loss of vision is considered an ocular emergency, regardless of whether the disturbance is partial or complete and whether or not it is accompanied by pain.

Altered vision can refer to decreased visual acuity with intact visual fields. This is a common complaint and, with age, is associated with the development of cataracts. It can also be associated with relatively benign refractive errors or with hyperglycemia and diabetes, macular degeneration, or glaucoma. In contrast, the loss of vision—whether limited to a specific visual field or area, one eye, or both eyes—typically indicates a very significant health problem that may result in permanent visual loss and disability. Acute profound painless vision loss (especially less than 20/200) that has occurred within 24 to 48 hours requires an urgent ophthalmology consult.

History

When patients complain of altered vision, it is important to obtain a history of any other eye symptoms or disease and to explore the altered vision. Determine when the patient first noticed the altered vision, how, if at all, it has progressed since onset, and whether it has been transient or persistent. Ask whether the visual disturbance has affected the patient's ability to perform any normal activities and whether the patient has been exposed to chemicals or trauma. Always determine what the patient means if the patient complains of decreased or blurred vision; discriminate between decreased visual acuity and episodes of actual vision loss as well as perceived glare or haze, distortion, flashing, or quivering of image. Ask whether the alteration involves one or both eyes and is limited to central, peripheral, near, or distant vision. Figures 6.11 through 6.14 illustrate examples of normal and select types of altered vision. Establish the date and results of the patient's last visual examination and whether corrective lenses are prescribed and used. Find out whether there is history of systemic diseases, such as diabetes, and what medications the patient has recently taken. The family history of eye disease and other chronic diseases is important.

Physical Examination

The physical examination for altered vision starts with a determination of visual acuity. Both far and near vision are tested in each eye alone and then in combination. Adaptations must be made for patients with very low vision. If applicable, vision should be tested with the patient wearing prescribed corrective lenses. Although it is tempting to go directly from testing visual acuity to the funduscopic examination, the assessment should next include inspection of the external

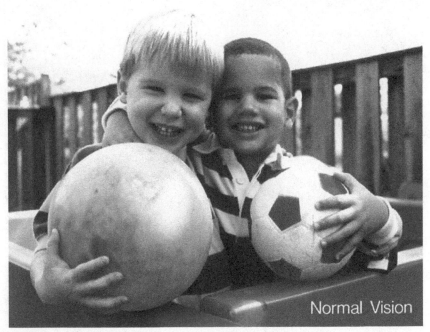

Figure 6.11 Normal vision. (Courtesy of National Eye Institute, National Institutes of Health.)

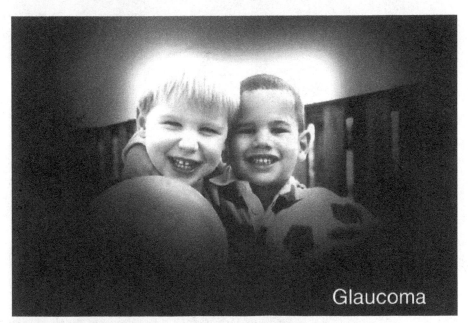

Figure 6.12 Glaucoma scene. (Courtesy of National Eye Institute, National Institutes of Health.)

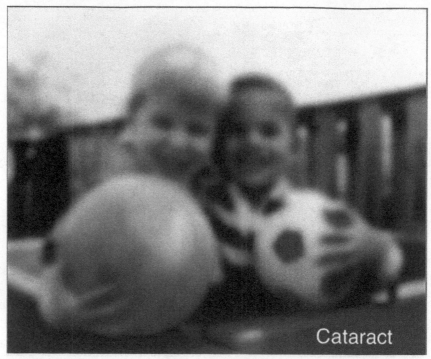

Figure 6.13 Cataract scene. (Courtesy of National Eye Institute, National Institutes of Health.)

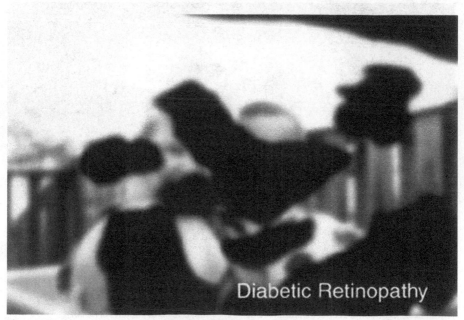

Figure 6.14 Diabetic retinopathy scene. (Courtesy of National Eye Institute, National Institutes of Health.)

RED FLAG	**Warnings for Visual Disturbances**

- *Eye pain; photophobia*
- *Eye redness*
- *Sudden onset*
- *Headache, weakness, slurred speech*
- *Scalp or temple tenderness*
- *Flashes*
- *Nausea and vomiting*
- *History of trauma*

structures, eye movement, peripheral vision/visual fields, and pupil reactions. Assess the appearance of the cornea and anterior chamber as well as the quality of the red reflex. A funduscopic examination should be performed, with rare exceptions, such as when vision change is accompanied by severe eye pain and photophobia, as occurs with acute closed-angle glaucoma. Funduscopic examination also may be difficult with lens cloudiness, as occurs with advanced cataracts.

The decision to examine other systems should be determined in the context of the patient's history and general survey. For instance, if eye movement or pupil reaction is asymmetrical, a neurological examination is warranted. With a history of diabetes, blood glucose and other signs of diabetes control should be determined. As necessary, the physical examination should include careful assessment of the cardiovascular and neurological systems.

In many situations, definitive diagnostic studies such as dilation of the eye, intraocular pressure measurement, and magnification are not performed at a general practice site but by a specialist to whom the patient is referred. The history taking and physical examination must be adequate to identify the need for prompt referral to another specialist—for instance, a neurologist. Although it is beyond the scope of this chapter to address the full range of disorders that could result in visual disturbance, many of the characteristic disorders are identified here.

CATARACTS

Cataracts are opacities of the optic lens and most typically occur as a disease of aging. However, cataracts can be caused or accelerated by conditions such as exposure to ultraviolet light and to certain drugs (e.g., corticosteroids) as well as systemic diseases (e.g., diabetes).

Signs and Symptoms

Patients with cataracts generally describe progressive and painless decreased visual acuity. The altered vision includes general blurring, dimming, and haziness of vision as well as the development of halos and glares in response to bright lights or when driving in the dark. The opacities may be visible as gray or whitening areas over the pupil. The opacity makes ophthalmologic examination difficult, obscuring the visualization of the posterior chamber and retinal structures.

Diagnostic Studies

Early cataracts are best detected through ophthalmic examination of the dilated eye, using magnification.

CHRONIC OPEN-ANGLE GLAUCOMA

Glaucoma is characterized by increased intraocular pressure, which results in neuropathy of the optic nerve. This most common form of glaucoma results in a gradual and progressive altered vision. The incidence of chronic glaucoma is highest among black patients, patients with diabetes, and those older than 35 years, particularly if they have a positive family history. Use of corticosteroids is an associated secondary cause of chronic open-angle glaucoma.

Signs and Symptoms

Patients with chronic open-angle glaucoma generally have no complaints until the disease progresses to the point where they perceive the decreased vision. The visual disturbance then progresses from blurring to complete vision loss if not recognized and treated. The patient may have required frequent corrective prescription changes up until definitive diagnosis. The vision loss begins peripherally; central vision is preserved until late in the disorder. The physical examination identifies an increased cup-to-disc ratio and elevated intraocular pressure.

Diagnostic Studies

A normal tonometric value is under 21, although the value can vary or fluctuate. Tonometry must be considered in combination with retinal signs of glaucoma and visual fields. Ophthalmologists perform additional tests, including gonioscopy, which assesses the drainage angle to determine whether it is open or closed.

ACUTE CLOSED-ANGLE GLAUCOMA

This less common form of glaucoma results in acute visual disturbance. The increased intraocular pressure may be transient and triggered by conditions that cause pupillary dilatation, such as darkened rooms. As the intraocular pressure acutely increases, the patient typically experiences significant symptoms, which may resolve before the patient arrives for evaluation. It is very important that the examiner *not* dilate the eyes when a patient presents with a history of unilateral eye pain and visual disturbance because the dilation may further exacerbate the increased intraocular pressure.

Signs and Symptoms

During episodes of acute closed-angle glaucoma, patients usually experience severe, unilateral eye pain. Corneal edema is reflected by a dulling of the corneal light reflex or a gray or white color of the cornea. Sudden onset of corneal edema in acute open-angle glaucoma is typically associated with nausea and vomiting and reports of colored halos around lights, along with severely elevated intraocular pressure, usually in the 40 to 80 mmHg range. Hardness may be noted on palpation of the affected eye if formal tonometry is not available. The eye may be tearing, red, and painful. The pupil may be fixed in a mid-dilated position.

Diagnostic Studies

Whenever acute closed-angle glaucoma is suspected, the patient must be immediately referred to an ophthalmologist, who can complete tonometry and, if intraocular pressure is elevated, determine diagnosis in order to provide prompt definitive treatment and to preserve vision.

AMAUROSIS FUGAX

Amaurosis fugax is a monocular, transient loss of vision. It stems from transient ischemia of the retina and presents an important warning sign for impending stroke. Depending on the circumstances reported, the patient should be immediately referred to either a cardiovascular or neurological specialist. Four broad causes of amaurosis fugax are emboli, retinal vascular insufficiency, arterial spasms, and idiopathy.

Signs and Symptoms

An episode of vision loss that accompanies amaurosis fugax may last from only seconds to minutes. The patient often describes the episode as if a shade had been pulled over one eye in a descending fashion and then, a short time later, the shade was raised and vision restored. Unlike acute glaucoma, there is no associated pain during the episode. Depending on the duration of the episode, the funduscopic examination may reveal the retina as whitened with a bright red fovea. If the occlusion is of the carotid, the patient may report or exhibit transient sensorimotor deficits consistent with a transient ischemic attack. The funduscopic examination may reveal emboli, altered vessels, microaneurysms, and blot hemorrhages. Carotid bruits may be present.

Diagnostic Studies

Depending on the setting, noninvasive carotid studies such as Doppler ultrasound or magnetic resonance angiography (MRA) may be obtained before the patient is seen by the specialist. If valvular embolus has caused the disorder, the embolus may be visible.

RETINAL DETACHMENT

Retinal detachments may occur spontaneously but may also be caused by trauma or by the traction caused by diabetic retinal disease and other causes of preretinal fibrosis. Regardless of the cause, patients suspected of having a retinal detachment should be immediately referred to an ophthalmologist.

Signs and Symptoms

The patient usually provides a history of a contributing condition or trauma followed by a sudden visual disturbance, such as flashing light, floaters or black dots, or scotoma. The visual defect may advance or progress as the retinal detachment enlarges, but central vision will be retained unless the macula is involved. Some patients may report a visual disruption or field defect that they describe as a shadow or "a curtain being pulled down." Retinal detachment is not painful, nor does it result in a red eye. Depending on the size of the defect, the patient may exhibit an afferent pupil defect in which the pupil of the affected eye dilates rather than constricts when exposed to direct light. The affected retina appears wrinkled and gray. Patient should be referred immediately for an ophthalmology assessment and possible urgent surgical repair.

ISCHEMIC OCULAR NEUROPATHY

The visual disturbances of ischemic ocular neuropathy stem from chronic ischemia, and the resulting vision loss is irreversible. However, unilateral loss of vision in patients older than 65 years may be caused by giant cell (temporal) arteritis; in this case, the patient is at risk for losing vision in the opposite eye. Other risk factors include use of drugs, such as amiodarone or phosphodiesterase inhibitors, and various conditions, including diabetes and atherosclerosis.

Signs and Symptoms
The visual loss is unilateral and may be limited to either the upper or the lower visual field. There is no associated pain of the eye. However, patients with temporal arteritis will have previously experienced pain of the head, temple, or face and more generalized symptoms of polymyalgia rheumatica, including joint pain, malaise, weakness, fatigue, and even weight loss.

Diagnostic Studies
With giant cell arteritis, the erythrocyte sedimentation rate (ESR) and C-reactive protein are often elevated. A temporal artery biopsy is diagnostic, although treatment must not be withheld pending the biopsy.

MACULAR DEGENERATION

Most commonly, macular degeneration is associated with aging and results either from atrophy of the macula or exudation and hemorrhage of the vessels in the macular region.

Signs and Symptoms
Visual alterations associated with macular degeneration are typically unilateral, vary from gradual to sudden in onset, and can range from blurring to complete blindness. The retina may show altered pigmentation, hemorrhage, or hard and soft exudates. In diabetics, neovascularization and microaneurysms may be visible.

Diagnostic Studies
An ophthalmologist will further evaluate the patient's central vision and perform fluorescein angiography. A commonly used test, the Amsler grid, assesses the patient's ability to accurately see a set of grids.

TRAUMA

Blunt trauma to the eye or orbit can be associated with altered vision. Depending on the type of trauma, the history should provide details of the event and the physical examination may allow detection of other signs of trauma.

Signs and Symptoms

An orbital fracture should be suspected if there is periocular ecchymosis, pain with lateral or vertical gaze, diplopia (which is usually caused by ocular muscle entrapment), disconjugate gaze while looking vertically or horizontally, decreased sensation in the infraorbital area, and tenderness, bony step-off, or crepitus in the zygomatic arch or maxillary sinus areas. The globe may be sunken or bulging. Ophthalmological changes will depend on degree and type of trauma and injury. Patient should be urgently referred to an ophthalmologist for definitive evaluation and treatment.

Diagnostic Studies

Evaluation will include radiological imaging, usually with computed tomography (CT). Other tests include eye motility diplopia fields assessment.

■ Reddened Eye

Eye redness can be caused by a wide range of disorders, from conjunctivitis to acute closed-angle glaucoma. Eye redness may herald a disorder that has no associated visual impairment or other disorders associated with complete loss of vision. Although most causes of eye redness are self-limiting, it is essential to perform a complete assessment when this is the presenting complaint.

History

When a patient complains of a reddened eye, first determine whether the patient has experienced eye trauma or any associated vision disturbance. Obtain a history of the redness and its progression, then ask about other symptoms, such as eye itching, pain, swelling, discharge, or photophobia. Ask about exposures to chemical agents. If the patient wears contact lenses, determine the type and how the lenses are cared for, as well how long the lenses are worn. Ask about systemic symptoms such as general malaise, skin rashes, and cold or allergy symptoms. Ascertain whether the patient has had previous episodes of eye disorders or systemic problems, such as atopic or rheumatic disorders. Identify any drugs or other products that have been used around or on the eyes. For example, old mascara has been shown to be full of bacteria. Determine whether there is a family history of eye conditions, such as glaucoma, iritis, or allergic conjunctivitis, as well as relevant systemic disorders. Autoimmune disorders and HIV are associated with certain eye diseases that may cause redness. Determine the patient's tetanus status if the patient has had eye trauma and/or corneal abrasion.

Physical Examination

The physical examination must begin by determining the patient's corrected visual acuity, then observing the general characteristics of the redness, and

RED FLAG	**Warnings for Eye Redness**

- *Pain (not discomfort or irritation)*
- *Decreased vision*
- *Profuse discharge*
- *Corneal defect grossly visible*

finishing with a rapid assessment to rule out signs of trauma. Note whether there is any photophobia and adjust the light to the patient's comfort if possible. Assess the outer and appendage structures, looking for swelling, redness, discharge, or lesions. Next, focus on the eye itself, observing the cornea and conjunctiva for redness and noting the degree, pattern, and location of the redness. Identify any shadowing by passing oblique lighting over the anterior chamber. Assess the palpebral and tarsal conjunctiva beneath the lids; observe for foreign bodies or lesions. Assess the size, shape, and responsiveness of the pupils. If tolerated, perform a funduscopic examination. Depending on the history and examination of the eyes, it may be necessary to extend the assessment to the skin, ears, nose, throat, and joints to assess for infections, allergy, or rheumatic disorders.

Diagnostic studies are generally not warranted for eye redness. However, it may prove necessary to obtain a culture from the conjunctiva or to determine the intraocular pressure through tonometry. If foreign body or corneal abrasion is suspected, the examination should include fluorescein staining and examination of the eye with a Wood's lamp. If a foreign body is suspected, a slit lamp examination is necessary, and referral to an ophthalmologist is warranted.

CONJUNCTIVITIS

Conjunctivitis, which is a catch-all term for any inflammation of the conjunctiva, may be caused by infections, allergies, irritants, crying, or systemic problems. The conjunctiva is usually transparent, but may appear pink or red when it is inflamed and is different from the fine blood vessel dilation, usually called "injected" (i.e., "bloodshot"). Conjunctivitis is a clinical diagnosis, usually made from the history and physical examination and does not generally require any testing, although a rapid test is available to diagnose adenoviral conjunctivitis. Infectious conjunctivitis may be classified as viral or bacterial. Both are highly contagious.

Signs and Symptoms

The primary symptom of conjunctivitis, eye redness, is fairly consistent among the various causes. The degree of accompanying eye symptoms, such as discomfort, itching, and discharge, as well as extraorbital symptoms, helps to define the problem. Examination of the eyes also provides important information to

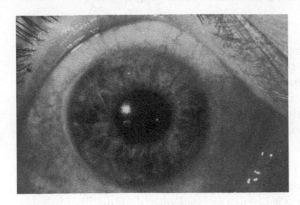

Figure 6.15 Conjunctivitis. Inflammation of the conjunctiva that is most commonly caused by viral, gonococcal, and chlamydia organisms. Presentation is generalized vessel injection with dilation greatest peripherally. (Reprinted with permission from Dr. Julia Haller, Ophthalmologist in Chief. Permission granted by Michael D. Allen, Esquire, at Wills Eye Institute.)

identify the cause. Eye discharge should be noted as coming from one or both eyes. Purulent discharge is consistent with a bacterial infection, although chemical irritant may also cause discharge. Figure 6.15 depicts one presentation of conjunctivitis. Tearing alone is not specific to conjunctivitis, as it can result from allergies, foreign bodies, viral infections, blocked tear duct, or glaucoma. The presence of photophobia suggests a cause other than conjunctivitis. Table 6.4 differentiates among the signs and symptoms of viral, bacterial, and allergic conjunctivitis.

Diagnostic Studies

On occasion, diagnostic tests are helpful in assessing conjunctivitis. Studies can include viral and bacterial cultures of the conjunctiva or tests for atopy. For findings consistent with bacterial conjunctivitis that do not respond to treatment, consider and test for gonococcal and chlamydia infection.

Table 6.4

Differentiating Conjunctivitis

Finding	Allergic Conjunctivitis	Bacterial Conjunctivitis	Viral Conjunctivitis
Pain/discomfort	Itchy sensation	Burning or gritty sensation	Foreign body or gritty sensation
Discharge	Watery, thin, clear Usually bilateral	Mucopurulent, viscous Often unilateral May collect at lid margins	Mucoid to watery Often starts in one eye, may involve other
Preauricular nodes	Nonpalpable/normal	Usually nonpalpable; palpable in hyperacute cases	Palpable
Accompanying symptoms	Allergy symptoms often present; history of allergies, recurrent episodes	May have URI symptoms	May have URI symptoms

URI: upper respiratory infection.

CORNEAL ABRASION

The cornea can become scratched or abraded by a variety of situations, including trauma and foreign bodies. A common foreign body involved in corneal abrasions is a contact lens. It is important to identify how the abrasion occurred in order to determine the risk of complications, including infection and ulceration (Fig. 6.16). For instance, the abrasion is more likely to be contaminated and at risk for infection if caused by contact lenses or an animal scratch than if caused by a grain of sand.

Signs and Symptoms

The patient usually reports eye pain, "scratchiness," and a reluctance to open the eye. A foreign body sensation is often associated with blinking. Photophobia and significant tearing are common with abrasions. The symptoms generally have a sudden onset after some exposure and can be severe. Patients typically have normal visual acuity and a normal pupillary response. Decreased vision with blurring is likely to occur in the affected eye. The redness may be either diffuse or in a ciliary flush pattern. Foreign bodies are not always evident upon gross examination, which should include an upper eyelid eversion to detect any foreign body located in this area. Fluorescein staining and a cobalt blue light or Wood's lamp (see Box 6.2) identifies an obvious break in the corneal surface with uptake of the stain, which will appear as green areas around the regions of the affected conjunctival epithelium. Examination of the fundus is normal. Unless the patient has delayed assessment, there should be no discharge or enlargement of the preauricular nodes, indicating infection.

Diagnostic Studies

Diagnostic study is not indicated unless signs of infection are evident. With appropriate treatment, abrasions generally resolve in 24 hours. Patients should be rechecked to ensure that the abrasion is resolving as anticipated. If not, the patient should be referred to an ophthalmologist as ulceration is common.

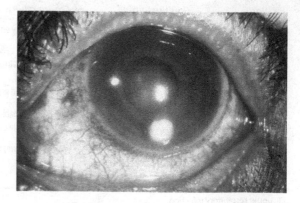

Figure 6.16 Corneal ulceration. Well-circumscribed ulcer following fluorescein staining. Not always visible to the naked eye. (Reprinted with permission from Dr. Julia Haller, Ophthalmologist in Chief. Permission granted by Michael D. Allen, Esquire, at Wills Eye Institute.)

FOREIGN BODY

Foreign bodies can be retained in or on the cornea. Examples include pieces of metal, glass, or even hair. Persons with occupations such as construction or operating heavy equipment are at higher risk and should wear eye protection.

Signs and Symptoms

The patient usually complains of a foreign body sensation and eye pain. The history may include accidental injury without eye protection. Visual acuity may be normal or diminished. The foreign body may be visible on the cornea or under eyelids. If the foreign body is metallic, an area of rust discoloration may be visible. Eye redness is often prominent.

Diagnostic Studies

Diagnosis is usually confirmed by visualization and removal of the object. Fluorescein staining may be helpful in locating the object. If unable to identify the object, referral for specialty assessment and imaging, as needed, should be done. Embedded objects require urgent referral to ophthalmologist.

SUBCONJUNCTIVAL HEMORRHAGE

While subconjunctival hemorrhages may appear worrisome to laypersons, they are usually benign and self-limiting, although they may be caused by injury or inflammation (Fig. 6.17). Subconjunctival hemorrhages occur when tiny blood vessels break underneath the clear surface of the conjunctivae, resulting in a bright red patch within the white of the eye. The cause may be unknown, although they may result after intense sneezing or coughing; heavy lifting, straining, or vomiting; or as a side effect of blood thinners. Typically, no treatment is required for this harmless condition, which usually resolves within 2 weeks. However, other conditions such as corneal abrasions or perforations should be ruled out as a cause or associated condition for the red eye.

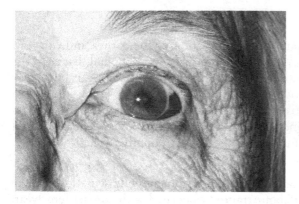

Figure 6.17 Subconjunctival hemorrhage. Hemorrhage beneath the conjunctiva usually caused by injury. (Reprinted with permission from Dr. Julia Haller, Ophthalmologist in Chief. Permission granted by Michael D. Allen, Esquire, at Wills Eye Institute.)

Signs and Symptoms

Subconjunctival hemorrhage is not associated with vision loss, photophobia, or pain. The onset of the redness is sudden and typically limited to one eye; it may be localized to one region of the affected eye. With the exception of the deep redness, other findings are within normal limits.

UVEITIS

Uveitis involves inflammation of the uveal tract, which includes the iris, ciliary body, and choroid. As the uveal tract includes the iris, this condition includes iritis as well. The inflammation may be caused either by infection or as part of a reaction associated with a systemic disorder. For instance, an increased incidence of uveitis is associated with autoimmune disorders, such as Crohn's disease, ankylosing spondylitis, and HIV infection. It is important to identify any systemic source of the problem and to refer the patient for a thorough ophthalmic examination.

Signs and Symptoms

Vision changes associated with uveitis stem from altered responsiveness of the pupil and lens. If the inflammation is in the anterior structure of the eye, the patient may report a red eye with painful light sensitivity; if the inflammation is in the intermediate or posterior structure, the patient may complain of floaters and the eye may appear normal, but with a diminished red reflex. There may be a ciliary flush and a constricted pupil. Precipitates may be visible on the posterior surface of the cornea, and hypopyon may be present. If an autoimmune disorder is involved, the patient may complain of other systemic symptoms, such as joint pain and altered bowel habits and abdominal pain.

Diagnostic Studies

The ophthalmologist will perform diagnostics related to the eye disorder, but if the uveitis is recurrent and/or has a suspected systemic cause, further diagnostic studies should be considered, including ESR, autoimmune panel, and HIV testing.

KERATITIS

Disorders in this category result in inflammation of the cornea and can lead to blindness in the affected eye. Keratitis can be caused by viral, bacterial, or fungal infections and trauma, including chemical exposures, foreign bodies, or corneal abrasions. It can be triggered by eye dryness or denervation; it may also be secondary to conjunctivitis. Keratitis is noteworthy because it can lead to ulcerations, opacities, and blindness of the affected eye; thus, patients suspected of this disorder should be immediately referred to an ophthalmologist.

Signs and Symptoms

Patients with keratitis may complain only of a foreign body sensation or may complain of severe pain. Ask about trauma associated with contact lens wear.

Although vision may not be initially affected, it can be altered as the condition advances. The eye is usually tearing, red, and painful or irritated. Gray infiltrate may be visible on examination, and there may be a ciliary flush. Fluorescein stain demonstrates diffuse epithelial cell loss or a dulling of the corneal light reflex.

If ulcerative keratitis is involved, perforations may be evident on staining. A hypopyon ulcer may develop, with pus collecting in the anterior chamber.

Diagnostic Studies

On referral, the ophthalmologist will perform a variety of studies to identify the causative agent of the situation, including bacterial, fungal, and viral cultures and slit lamp examination.

SCLERITIS AND EPISCLERITIS

Scleritis and episcleritis are inflammatory problems involving the sclera and episclera, respectively. Most cases of scleritis are associated with chronic autoimmune disorders, such as rheumatoid arthritis, systemic lupus erythematosus, and sarcoidosis. In contrast, episcleritis is self-limiting and not associated with chronic disorders. They are best differentiated by the degree of involvement. Although they do not typically affect the vision, both conditions are often chronic and warrant referral to an ophthalmologist. With time, scleritis can evolve to cause cataracts and glaucoma (Fig. 6.18).

Signs and Symptoms

Visual acuity can be altered with advanced scleritis. While episcleritis is generally painless, scleritis may cause extreme pain, including deep eye discomfort. Although photophobia is not common with either disorder, it is more likely to occur with scleritis. Neither disorder is associated with altered pupils, and the redness may be localized or diffuse. However, the redness associated with scleritis may be intense—almost purple—and is darker than is typically seen with episcleritis. The discoloration lies immediately below the conjunctiva, and the sclera may develop inflammatory nodules and engorged vessels. Episcleritis,

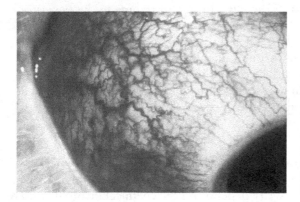

Figure 6.18 Episcleritis. Inflammation of the conjunctival layer of the sclera characterized by localized, sectoral conjunctival vessels dilated peripherally. (Reprinted with permission from Dr. Julia Haller, Ophthalmologist in Chief. Permission granted by Michael D. Allen, Esquire, at Wills Eye Institute.)

in contrast, is more localized but can also be associated with localized engorged vessels and nodular changes.

Diagnostic Studies

Episcleritis requires no specific diagnostic studies. However, if scleritis is suspected or the diagnosis is uncertain, the patient should be referred to an ophthalmologist for definitive diagnosis and treatment. Laboratory studies include complete blood count, ESR, and antinuclear antibody; in addition, rheumatoid factor should be considered.

■ Eye Pain

Eye pain can be caused by urgent problems that threaten vision, such as acute closed-angle glaucoma, various traumatic injuries, and infectious agents. There is a lot of overlap among the disorders that cause eye pain and those that cause eye redness; thus, the history and physical examination are similar for both complaints.

History

When the chief complaint includes eye pain, first establish whether there is a history of chemical exposure or burn, trauma, or vision loss. In the case of chemical burn, further assessment must be delayed until the eye has been thoroughly irrigated. Once chemical exposure and trauma has been excluded, explore the onset and characteristics of the pain. For instance, determine whether the pain had sudden onset or developed gradually. Ask about the type of pain—for instance, whether it is sharp, dull, throbbing, or aching, and whether it is superficial or deep, focused or diffuse, periorbital or ocular. Identify any associated symptoms, including malaise, vision change, discharge, photophobia, and redness.

■ Physical Examination

If tolerated, test visual acuity before proceeding with further examination. Carefully inspect the accessory and external eye structures. Note any lacerations, lesions, discolorations, swelling, redness, and discharge. Assess the size, shape, and responsiveness of the pupils. If there is a history of trauma to the eye, carefully assess the corneal surface. Grossly inspect for signs of perforation, such as bleeding or "leakage" from the globe, altered shape, and obvious entry points. If perforation can be excluded by history and examination, fluorescein stain should be applied so that the corneal surface can be inspected using a Wood's lamp. Assess the cornea for clarity, and note the anterior chamber depth. If tolerated, a funduscopic examination should be performed.

CHEMICAL BURNS

Ocular chemical burns result from contact with either acidic or alkaline substances and require emergency evaluation and treatment to prevent permanent damage and vision loss. Injury severity depends on the chemical involved, with alkaline substances being more damaging than acidic ones, the duration of the exposure, and the depth of the chemical penetration.

Signs and Symptoms

Patients with chemical burns usually present with decreased vision, eye pain, an inability to open the eyelids (blepharospasm), conjunctival redness, and photophobia. Inspect the face and periorbital region for blisters, redness, and other signs of a burn. There may be significant redness, tearing, pain, and swelling of the eye and accessory structures. It is essential that the offending chemical be identified quickly, if possible, and that the appropriate decontamination measures be instituted immediately. It may be impossible to clearly assess visual acuity, owing to photophobia, pain, and tearing, which can blur vision.

Chemical ophthalmic burns represent an emergency situation. The patient should be referred immediately to an ophthalmologist to determine the severity of injury and to implement necessary treatment and follow-up. Chemical burns are treated with continuous irrigation with either water or saline until a neutral eye pH is obtained, which may take 30 to 60 minutes; irrigation should be initiated, depending on time of transfer.

HERPES ZOSTER

Herpes zoster, or shingles, involves a reactivation of latent varicella zoster infection, which occurs as a painful, unilateral vesicular eruption following a dermatome. Risk factors for herpes zoster include being older than 50 years, being immunocompromised, or having an autoimmune disease or certain comorbidities such as cancer or chronic lung or kidney disease. When herpes zoster involves the ophthalmic portion of the fifth CN, it can be a potentially sight-threatening condition. There is a high correlation with eye involvement with vesicular lesion on the side or tip of the nose.

Signs and Symptoms

The development of herpes zoster skin and mucous membrane lesions is usually preceded by a period of several days during which the patient experiences malaise and neuralgia along the affected nerve root. The pain is severe and often accompanied by systemic symptoms, including fever and fatigue. Photophobia may be present. Other associated symptoms may include headache, unilateral pain or a decreased sensation affecting the involved eye and forehead, and eye redness, whether conjunctivitis, uveitis, or keratitis. Accessory structures may be inflamed and swollen. Vision may be altered in the affected eye. Inspection of the cornea following fluorescein stain may reveal punctate or dendritic ulcerations.

Diagnostic Studies

Whenever eye involvement of herpes zoster is suspected, the patient should be referred to an ophthalmologist. Although the actual diagnosis may be evident, referral allows specialized examination—including slit lamp to assess the degree of involvement—and the timely initiation of appropriate and individualized treatment to minimize complications. Viral cultures may be obtained.

DRY EYE SYNDROME

Dry eye syndrome (keratoconjunctivitis sicca) is a multifactorial condition resulting in inadequate tear production or quality. It is more commonly idiopathic, occurring more often with increased age and female sex (especially with hormonal changes). Other causes include autoimmune diseases, such as diabetes mellitus, Parkinson disease, Sjögren syndrome, and systemic lupus erythematosus; systemic medications, such as antihistamines, anticholinergics, and selective serotonin receptor antagonists; ocular medications that contain preservatives; contact lens wear; nutritional deficiencies; and low-humidity environments.

Signs and Symptoms

Common complaints include dryness, conjunctival redness, and chronic discomfort ranging from itching, grittiness or burning, or foreign body sensation, to more severe pain. There may be paradoxical excessive tearing, blurry vision, and photosensitivity may be present. Symptoms may wax and wane dependent on weather or other environmental factors, such as windy or cold weather, low humidity, and time of day.

Diagnostic Studies

While the diagnosis is usually based on clinical presentation, a Schirmer test can be conducted to measure tear production.

TRAUMA

Trauma should always be considered with the presentation of eye pain. (See p. 173.)

FOREIGN BODY

Foreign body is discussed under "Reddened Eye," p. 177.

ACUTE CLOSED-ANGLE GLAUCOMA

Acute closed-angle glaucoma is described under "Visual Disturbances," p. 170.

CORNEAL ABRASION AND EROSION

Corneal abrasions are discussed under "Reddened Eye," p. 176.

CONJUNCTIVITIS

Conjunctivitis is discussed under "Reddened Eye," pp. 174–175.

UVEITIS, IRITIS, AND SCLERITIS

Each of these inflammatory disorders affecting the eye is covered in the section on "Reddened Eye," pp. 178–179.

■ Eye Discharge

Eye discharge is most commonly associated with infectious disorders but can also be associated with other inflammatory conditions or systemic diseases affecting the eye. The most common causes of eye discharge are the various forms of conjunctivitis.

History

Ask about the onset of the discharge and whether the discharge is persistent or instead occurs in certain settings. Note associated eye symptoms, such as pain, altered vision, photophobia, or swelling. Ask about extraocular symptoms, such as sneezing, itching, fever, and malaise. Determine the history of atopic disorders and exposure to infectious diseases.

Physical Examination

Test visual acuity, and then perform a general inspection, observing for the quantity and location of any discharge and noting the consistency and color. Although not generally necessary, a culture of the discharge may be warranted. To obtain a culture, retract the lower lid and place a conjunctival swab in the palpebral space.

DACRYOCYSTITIS/CONGENITAL NASOLACRIMAL DUCT OBSTRUCTION

Dacryocystitis is an infection of the lacrimal sac and is most common in infants, secondary to congenital stenosis of the lacrimal duct. In adults, it can be caused by hypertrophic rhinitis, polyps, or trauma. Older adults lose the elasticity of the drainage system so that the duct is not flushed by tears, and dacryocystitis may result.

Signs and Symptoms

If the duct is occluded, constant tearing may occur. The lacrimal sac may be edematous, red, and tender. Pressure over the sac produces purulent discharge. The surrounding area can become inflamed, tender, and swollen. Associated conjunctivitis or blepharitis may be present.

Diagnostic Studies

Diagnostic studies are generally not warranted.

ERYTHEMA MULTIFORME/STEVENS-JOHNSON SYNDROME

Erythema multiforme involves inflammation of the mucous membranes and skin. It is often related to an infection or can be due to almost any medication. Often, no specific cause is identified. The most severe form is called Stevens-Johnson syndrome. Because the condition can be fatal, it is important to immediately recognize and treat.

Signs and Symptoms

The patient appears acutely ill and has systemic symptoms, including malaise, fever, and arthralgias so that the eye findings are not isolated. In Stevens-Johnson syndrome, conjunctivitis with copious amounts of purulent discharge may occur.

The eyes become painful. Conjunctival bullae and ulcerations may develop. Patients develop erythematous lesions and bullae over the skin and hemorrhagic lesions of the mucous membranes.

Diagnostic Studies

The diagnosis is often made by identifying the classic skin lesions, which consist of red-centered bullae surrounded by white areas. In addition to the eye tissue, the palms, soles, anus, vagina, nose, and mouth are commonly affected.

CONJUNCTIVITIS

See the section on "Reddened Eye," p. 174, for differentiation of allergic, bacterial, and viral conjunctivitis.

■ Ptosis

Ptosis, or drooping of an eyelid, can be related to simple aging, with natural loss of elasticity and lid drooping, or it can result from a variety of other causes. The causes of ptosis are often categorized as congenital and acquired. Causes occurring after birth include trauma, conditions adding mass to the eyelid, and conditions that affect the nerves or muscles controlling the lid's position. In 75% of the cases, the first manifestation of myasthenia gravis is ptosis.

History

It is important to determine how and when the ptosis developed, including whether the onset was sudden or gradual. Identify any associated altered vision and whether the patient believes the vision has been obscured by the drooping eyelid. Ask about all other medical disorders and medications. Determine whether the patient has a history of hypertension, peripheral vascular disease or other risk factors for stroke, or a history of myasthenia gravis. Ask about any recent trauma to the head or eye region.

Physical Examination

Assess visual acuity. Closely inspect the lids, noting the degree of ptosis and location of the lid margin relative to other eye structures, such as the iris or pupil. Measure the palpebral fissure, comparing one eye with the other. While inspecting the lids and determining the degree of asymmetry, ensure that there is not merely an illusion of ptosis caused by a contralateral retraction of the opposite lid, as seen in conditions causing exophthalmos. Palpate the lids for masses or swelling; observe for redness and discoloration. Assess CN III and muscle function by testing extraocular movements. Perform a general assessment of the face and CNs. Assess the pupils for symmetry, shape, and reaction to light.

HORNER'S SYNDROME

Horner's syndrome is caused by decreased sympathetic innervation to the structures of the eye. Horner's syndrome can be caused by a variety of lesions, including trauma, tumors, and ischemia.

Signs and Symptoms

The symptoms vary but usually include unilateral ptosis, reduced sweating of the face, and miosis. The ptosis is typically incomplete, and although there is no true enophthalmos, the eye appears to have receded. The pupil reaction to light and accommodation remains intact.

Diagnostic Studies

A complete history and physical examination should be performed to identify likely etiologies. Based on findings, referral and/or imaging studies should be ordered.

MECHANICAL PTOSIS

Lacrimal gland tumor is an example of a mechanical cause of ptosis, adding bulk to the upper lid. The degree of ptosis depends on the size of the tumor. Other causes of mechanical ptosis include chalazion and hordeolum.

Signs and Symptoms

Pain is often associated with a lacrimal gland tumor and with chalazion and hordeolum. When inflammation is involved, the abnormal lid may be reddened and tender. If a lacrimal gland tumor is involved, there may be some degree of exophthalmos and deviation of the eye, depending on tumor size.

AGING

Senile involutional ptosis is a common cause of ptosis, particularly in patients with advanced age.

Signs and Symptoms

The lids and other accessory structures will have a thin, inelastic appearance. No masses, inflammation, or systemic signs will be evident.

MYASTHENIA GRAVIS

Myasthenia gravis causes skeletal muscle weakness owing to a dysfunction of the acetylcholine receptors; this dysfunction results in reduced muscle innervation. It is a common cause of ptosis. Ptosis is the most common initial sign of myasthenia gravis, which often occurs at an earlier age in women than in men.

Signs and Symptoms

In myasthenia gravis, patients often have intermittent diplopia in addition to the ptosis. The ptosis is often intermittent. The patient may attempt to compensate by raising the opposite lid. The ptosis of myasthenia gravis can be accentuated by having the patient maintain an upward gaze or forcibly blink for an extended time. Alternatively, the icepack test, where a bag of crushed ice is placed over the closed affected lid for 1 minute, may reveal a subsequent temporary decrease in the ptosis. The pupils are within normal limits and not affected by the disorder.

Diagnostic Studies

Myasthenia gravis is definitively diagnosed by the Tensilon test, which involves administration of edrophonium chloride to counteract acetylcholine. If myasthenia gravis is present, any mild weakness will rapidly become exaggerated for a brief period of time following the Tensilon test. Alternatively, serology studies, such as acetylcholine receptor antibodies, may be ordered.

OCULOMOTOR NERVE DEFICIT

The oculomotor nerve, CN III, stimulates most of the extraocular muscles, so this disorder was chosen as an exemplar of CN disorders. Deficits can be caused by a wide range of problems, including diabetes and tumors.

Signs and Symptoms

The affected eye may have a "down-and-out" deviation, and the pupil is dilated. The ptosis is significant: The lid occludes the pupil, and the patient cannot see from the affected eye. Facial muscle movement and strength are affected, as is sensation. The exact findings depend on which CNs are affected; CNs III, V, and VII may be involved.

Diagnostic Studies

Recent onset of third nerve palsy should trigger immediate neurology consultation for thorough assessment, which is likely to include a CT scan, magnetic resonance imaging (MRI), or MRA.

BOTULISM

Botulism is caused by toxins from the bacillus *Clostridium botulinum*, which can be either food borne or a wound contaminant. Following ingestion of the botulism toxin, the incubation period ranges from hours to several days. The incubation period following wound contamination may be as long as 2 weeks.

Signs and Symptoms

The earliest symptoms involve the CNs; neurological involvement then follows a descending pattern. Symptoms are generally symmetrical. Ptosis is an early symptom and may be preceded by diplopia. When wound contamination is the source of the condition, symptoms are limited to the neurological system. However, when ingested, systemic symptoms such as nausea, vomiting, and diarrhea occur. Immediate referral to a neurologist or emergency department should be made because botulism can be life-threatening.

▪ Double Vision

Double vision, or diplopia, usually occurs when the extraocular muscles do not work in a coordinated manner and the patient sees one object as two. There are a variety of causes for diplopia, including both neurological and muscular disorders. Only in rare circumstances is monocular diplopia a problem, as this typically stems from eye deformities or retinal abnormalities.

History

For the complaint of double vision, it is important to fully analyze the symptom, determining how severe the visual disturbance is, when it occurs, and so on. Determine whether there is a recent history of head injury. Ask about any associated symptoms, such as other weaknesses, headache, or pain. Explore whether the diplopia most commonly occurs in certain circumstances, including particular times of day. Ask about substance use and abuse, including alcohol intake. Identify any history of systemic disorders, including neuromuscular, endocrine, and neurological diseases.

Physical Examination

The physical examination should start with visual acuity testing. Determine whether the diplopia occurs only when the patient uses both eyes or is limited to only one eye. Carefully assess the placement and symmetry of the eyes, performing a cover/uncover test and observing for the corneal light reflex. Note any lack of conjugate movement as the patient follows an object through the six cardinal fields of gaze.

PROPTOSIS AND EXOPHTHALMOS

Proptosis is the general term for anterior displacement of the eye; *exophthalmos* specifically describes proptosis related to endocrinopathy, usually thyroid disease. In thyroid disorders, the eye muscles thicken and thereby move the eyes forward so that their ability to move conjugately is affected and the lids may fail to close completely. Movement in all directions may be affected, although most commonly the patient finds it difficult to look upward. In addition to diplopia, patients may experience dry eyes, ulcerations, and diminished vision. Less common causes of proptosis include infections and tumors affecting the structures of or near the eye.

Signs and Symptoms

The patient may complain of signs of thyroid disease, primarily those of hyperthyroidism, such as nervousness, anxiety, weight loss, and so on. The thyroid may be nodular or enlarged, the heart rate elevated, and a fine tremor may be present. A fever may accompany the proptosis, regardless of whether the cause is from thyroid disease or infection. There may also be complaints of visual disturbances in addition to the diplopia, a dry or gritty sensation, and eye tenderness.

Diagnostic Studies

The initial tests are to assess thyroid function, with complete blood count and other studies obtained subsequently, as needed. A Hertel exophthalmometer can be used to measure the degree of anterior displacement.

OCULOMOTOR NERVE DISORDERS

Lesions of CNs III, IV, and VI may result in diplopia, either vertical or horizontal. The third, fourth, or sixth CN palsies are usually benign, self-limited, and resolve in weeks to months. They commonly occur in patients who have hypertension or diabetes. However, a mass-occupying lesion should be excluded.

Signs and Symptoms

If CN III is affected, accompanying ptosis usually occurs; the lid obscures the vision in the affected eye, and the patient's main complaint may not be double vision. If CN IV is involved, the diplopia will be vertical, whereas CN VI palsy results in horizontal diplopia. Depending on the cause, the patient may exhibit signs or complaints consistent with herpes zoster, other infections, or neurological involvement.

Diagnostic Studies

The patient who experiences new onset of diplopia related to nerve disorder should be promptly referred to an ophthalmologist for further evaluation and determination of subsequent assessment needs.

MYASTHENIA GRAVIS

See p. 185.

BOTULISM

See p. 186.

■ Eyelid Problems

Eyelid (blepharal) problems stem from a range of ailments affecting the accessory eyelid structures. Common problems include irritation of the lid margin and other eyelid lesions, masses, growths, and nodules. The eyelids are subject to some unique problems (e.g., blepharitis, hordeolum, chalazion) as well as many conditions affecting the skin in general (e.g., allergic rashes, herpes zoster, skin cancers). Because the eyelids cover and protect the cornea and help to distribute tears, associated problems can have significant implications.

Drooping eyelid is discussed under "Ptosis," pp. 184–186.

History

For any problems related to the eyelids, determine details regarding onset and progression of the condition, such as when it developed, any contributing factors, whether it has remained constant or is intermittent, and any related visual changes. Identify any associated symptoms, such as pain or itching, discharge, vision change, or blurring. Ask about other medical disorders and medications. Determine whether the patient has been exposed to topical or aerosol irritants or to infections. Ask about any similar skin lesions on other regions of the body.

Physical Examination

The physical examination primarily consists of inspection of skin and mucous membranes of the lids, with palpation of any noted areas of tenderness, swelling, or nodules. Use a bright light to enhance visualization as the upper and lower lids are inspected. Observe the lids opening and closing, comparing bilaterally. Note and document any areas of inflammation, erythema, swelling or thickening, and rash or vesicles of the lids, as well as signs of corneal irritation. Focus on any lesions, maintaining suspicion of potential malignancy.

BLEPHARITIS

Blepharitis involves chronic inflammation of the lid margin structures. It is often associated with meibomian gland dysfunction in the case of seborrheic blepharitis. Seborrheic blepharitis involves greasy scaling of the eyelid margin, which may obstruct the meibomian glands. However, the causes are multifactorial, including infections and demodex mites involving lash follicles.

Signs and Symptoms

The patient may complain of burning and itching of the eyelid, often worse in the morning. The lid margins are usually reddened with crusting and telangiectasias; crusting or debris may cling to the base of eyelashes. The obstruction of meibomian glands associated with debris may cause chalazion. Patient may also exhibit seborrheic crusting or peeling of the scalp or eyebrows.

Diagnostic Studies

The diagnosis is usually made based on clinical presentation. If unresponsive to treatment or chronic, lesions should be cultured. Malignancy should be ruled out for chronic lesions.

PERIORBITAL (PRESEPTAL) CELLULITIS AND ORBITAL CELLULITIS

Periorbital and orbital cellulitis are two distinct infections. While periorbital cellulitis is an infection of the eyelid and surrounding skin anterior to the orbital septum, orbital cellulitis involves infection posterior to the orbital septum and is an emergency situation. They may be initially confused, as both cause eyelid swelling, redness, pain, and warmth. Periorbital cellulitis usually stems from, for example, an infected injury, hordeolum, or insect bite of the eyelid and skin surrounding the eyes. Orbital cellulitis begins posterior to the orbital septum, usually stemming from spread of ethmoid or frontal sinusitis. Orbital cellulitis carries a risk of vision loss, meningitis, and cerebral abscess.

Signs and Symptoms

Periorbital cellulitis symptoms include lid tenderness or pain, redness, swelling, and warmth. The lid may be swollen shut, making examination of the eye and visual acuity difficult. A fever may be present. If the eye can be examined, visual acuity is unaffected, ocular movement is maintained, and there is an absence of proptosis (bulging eye).

Orbital cellulitis also involves swelling, redness, pain, and warmth of the eyelid. However, eye examination reveals hyperemia of the conjunctiva, decreased ocular movement, proptosis, and altered visual acuity. Accompanying symptoms include headache and lethargy when meningitis is present.

Diagnostic Studies

Periorbital cellulitis is a clinical diagnosis. However, the patient should be urgently referred if orbital cellulitis cannot be ruled out. Imaging (CT or MRI) is used to diagnose or exclude orbital cellulitis.

HORDEOLUM (STYE) AND CHALAZION

Hordeola and chalazia are frequently confused and involve the glands and tissue surrounding lash follicles. Both often result in an inflamed nodule, which may be tender. The causes are different. Chalazion is caused by meibomian gland plugging with sterile material accumulating. However, a secondary infection may develop.

Hordeolum (stye) may be internal (under the lid) or external. Hordeolum is caused by infectious thickening matter involving a meibomian gland (internal) or Zeiss or Moll gland (external). While chalazion is often nontender with only mild inflammation, a hordeolum can be quite tender and inflamed, evolving to a painful edema, abscess, or nodule.

Signs and Symptoms

Both hordeolum and chalazion often present initially as diffuse swelling and mild inflammation of the lid. The chalazion will form a nontender or mildly tender nodule. The hordeolum will progress, causing induration, inflammation, and significant pain. On inspection, the hordeolum often will reveal a pustule near the base of an eyelash. Both lesions usually spontaneously drain with the application of warm compresses.

Diagnostic Studies

Diagnosis is made on clinical findings. However, if a hordeolum or chalazion fails to respond to treatment, the diagnosis should be reconsidered and malignant growth ruled out.

EYELID MALIGNANCY

The eyelid is a common site for skin cancer and is subject to the full range of skin malignancies. The most common eyelid malignancy is basal cell carcinoma. While this is unlikely to metastasize, it may expand, invading deeper tissue and structures. Melanoma and squamous cell carcinoma are rarer than basal cell but do occur on the eyelids.

Signs and Symptoms

Eyelid cancer often presents as a chronic lesion and is sometimes mistaken for a nonmalignant problem. The lesion may present as an ulceration or nonhealing sore, swelling, pearly or red nodule, colored mass, or chronic infection.

Diagnostic Studies

Any eyelid lesion that grows, ulcerates, or does not heal should be biopsied or subjected to another diagnostic procedure.

ENTROPION

Entropion involves inward turning of the lid margin and lashes toward the surface of the eye. Entropion most commonly involves the lower lid. Incidence increases with age; the most common form is involutional entropion, which occurs with age-related changes in facial and periorbital fatty tissue and collagen. Cicatricial entropion is associated with tissue scarring from autoimmune, inflammatory, traumatic, and other factors.

Signs and Symptoms

The lashes and lid margin rubbing against the eye often cause blurred vision, a foreign body sensation, redness, and tearing.

Diagnostic Studies

The diagnosis is clinical. The patient should be referred to determine whether surgical repair is indicated.

ECTROPION

Ectropion involves the turning of the lid margin and lashes outward, away from the eye. Typically, lower lids are involved. The causes are similar to those of entropion, with involutional ectropion due to age-related changes being most common. Scarring of tissue can cause cicatricial ectropion.

Signs and Symptoms

Besides the abnormal appearance and position of the eyelid, complaints include decreased lubrication of the eye, with a foreign body sense, redness, and tearing.

Diagnostic Studies

The diagnosis is clinical. Patient should be referred to determine whether surgical repair is indicated.

REFERENCE

American Academy of Ophthalmology (AAO). (n.d.). *Eye health statistics.* Retrieved March 23, 2022 from https://www.aao.org/newsroom/eye-health-statistics#refractiveerrors

Chapter 7
Ear, Nose, Mouth, and Throat

• Maria Colandrea

Complaints affecting the ears, nose, sinuses, mouth, and throat make up a significant component of primary care visits. The common cold is the leading cause of upper respiratory tract symptoms in children and in adults who care for young children. Viruses such as rhinovirus, influenza, parainfluenza, respiratory syncytial virus, and adenovirus are common in day-care settings and are known to cause symptoms such as cough, otalgia, ear infections, headaches, rhinosinusitis, pharyngitis, fevers, and malaise. These symptoms are self-limiting and likely resolve within 7 to 10 days; however, a small percentage of cases (<5%) can progress to a superimposed bacterial infection (Allan & Arroll, 2014). Nonviral causes such as allergic and non-allergic rhinitis can also cause upper respiratory complaints such as rhinorrhea, postnasal drip, pharyngitis, pruritis of the throat, palate, eyes, and rhinosinusitis. Upper respiratory complaints related to the ear, nose, mouth, and throat affect all ages and are responsible for lost days of work and school. It is essential to recognize and rapidly treat conditions that can affect breathing and nourishment. Other common complaints in the outpatient setting include ear pain owing to infection or trauma, foreign body (seen mostly in the pediatric population), and hearing loss from age, loud noise exposure, or cerumen impaction aggravated by hearing aid wear. Figures 7.1, 7.2, and 7.3 identify the major landmarks of the upper respiratory system.

History

■ General History

A general history of the ear, nose, mouth, and throat should include current or recent exposure to sick contacts with respiratory infections such as flu or colds. Inquire if children are in day-care settings or if adults have young children in those settings. Ask about onset, acuity, and duration of symptoms, as well as associated symptoms. Duration, acuity and type of symptoms can help the provider determine if they are related to a virus, allergy, or bacterial infection. A personal history of recent flu, upper respiratory infection, frequent sinus

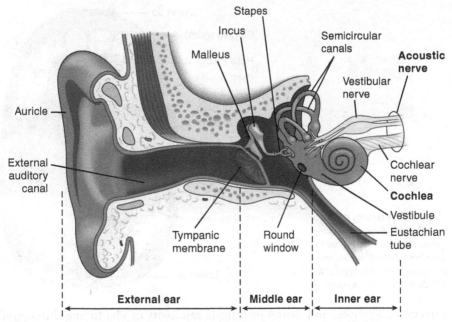

Figure 7.1 Anatomy of the ear. (From Dillon, P. M. [2003]). *Nursing health assessment: A critical thinking, case studies approach*. Philadelphia, PA: F. A. Davis. Reprinted with permission.)

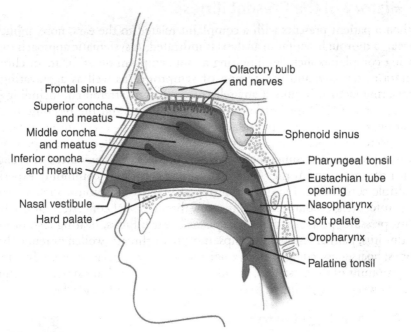

Figure 7.2 Anatomy of the nose. (From Dillon, P. M. [2003]). *Nursing health assessment: A critical thinking, case studies approach*. Philadelphia, PA: F. A. Davis. Reprinted with permission.)

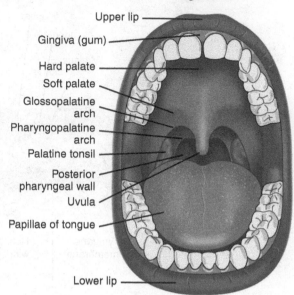

Upper lip

Gingiva (gum)

Hard palate

Soft palate

Glossopalatine arch

Pharyngopalatine arch

Palatine tonsil

Posterior pharyngeal wall

Uvula

Papillae of tongue

Lower lip

Figure 7.3 Anatomy of the mouth and oropharynx. (From Dillon, P. M. [2003]). *Nursing health assessment: A critical thinking, case studies approach.* Philadelphia, PA: F. A. Davis. Reprinted with permission.)

infections, allergies, and dental infections can assist in identifying differential diagnoses. A history of exposure to mononucleosis or strep and a history of smoking are also important.

■ History of the Present Illness

When a patient presents with a complaint related to the ears, nose, mouth, or throat, a thorough symptom analysis is indicated. A systematic approach to evaluating complaints includes inquiring about symptom onset (acute or chronic), duration, severity, and progression of symptoms, as well as aggravating and alleviating factors. Inquire if any self-treatment was attempted, including over-the-counter (OTC) medications or home remedies and the response to those treatments. Inquire if symptoms are cyclical (occurring every spring or fall) or if they occur with specific exposures to triggers such as pollen, dust, or pets. When pain is present, determine the exact location as well as any areas of radiation. With ear, nose, and throat (ENT) conditions, patients commonly experience multiple complaints. Inquire about any associated symptoms, such as pain or discomfort (e.g., mouth, nose, sinus, ear, throat); nasal congestion or discharge; sinus pressure; postnasal drainage; epistaxis; ear fullness, hearing loss, otorrhea, or tinnitus; pain or lesions of the lips, mouth, or throat; swollen or tender lymph nodes; hoarseness, cough, or sneezing; and itchy eyes, palate or nose. In addition to symptoms of the ears, nose, mouth, and throat, ask about systemic symptoms such as weight loss, fatigue, fever, myalgia, malaise, and headache.

■ Past Medical History

Determine history and frequency of upper respiratory infections, such as strep throat/tonsillitis, rhinosinusitis, and otitis media (OM). It is important to know how many times the patient was treated with antibiotics within the last 6 to

12 months for the same or similar symptom(s). Establish whether the patient has ever had surgery or other procedures performed on the ears, nose, mouth, or throat; include cosmetic/aesthetic procedures as well as therapeutic ones. Identify any other major medical conditions such as seasonal allergies, diabetes, autoimmune disease, immunosuppressive disorders, recent viral infections/exposures, head and neck cancer, or inflammatory disorders. Ask about history of rhinitis or other atopic conditions, such as asthma, allergic conjunctivitis, and dermatitis. Determine whether the patient has a prior history of skin or other malignancies. Obtain a history of all current and recent medications as well as immunizations and vaccinations. Prior diagnostic studies such as hearing tests (audiogram), vestibular testing, laboratory testing, cultures, diagnostic imaging, along with the results, should be obtained and reviewed if possible. The use of hearing aids should be noted.

■ Family History

Obtain a family history of hearing disorders and conditions, such as autoimmune diseases, hearing loss, otological diseases, Meniere's disease, allergies, head and neck malignancies, and asthma. Determine whether others in the family are ill with similar symptoms.

■ Habits

Exposure to recreational and occupational noise is important when assessing hearing complaints. Assess whether the patient works in an area that requires hearing protection and the type of protection used. Ask about activities that involve barometric pressure changes, such as scuba diving and flying, which may affect ear equilibrium. Determine whether the patient's activities involve exposure to toxins, trauma, or chemicals and any medications used (both prescribed and OTC). For exposures to environmental sounds and toxins, ask about use of protection. Ask about the use of smoked and smokeless tobacco, alcohol, and recreational drugs. Assess high-risk sexual behavior and use of barrier contraceptives. Establish the patient's living conditions, including the method of cooling and heating the home and any exposure to pets or environmental allergens. Determine how often the patient sees a dentist and identify any dental conditions.

■ Review of Systems

Based on the initial history, complete a review of other systems. If balance is a complaint, inquire about cardiovascular symptoms, vision, peripheral neuropathy, stroke, and neurological history.

Physical Examination

■ Order of the Examination

Note the patient's vital signs and complete a general survey. Develop a systematic approach to examining the ear, nose, mouth, and throat. These components are often incorporated into the examination of the head, face, and neck, described in Chapter 5.

Examination of the Ears

The ear examination begins with inspection of the external ear. Note the placement and symmetry of the ears. Inspect the external ears, noting the condition of the skin and the integrity of the structures. Assess any skin changes as described in Chapter 4. Identify any deformities, lesions, areas of enlargement, or other abnormalities. Observe for inflammation, signs of a foreign body, trauma, and drainage. Assess any piercings for healing, signs of tearing, or infection. Palpate the external ear, noting any areas of tenderness or deformities. In suspected otitis externa, patient will present with tenderness when pushing on the tragus or pulling on the pinna. Palpate the preauricular and postauricular lymph nodes for size, tenderness, consistency, and mobility.

The otoscope is then used to examine the canal and middle ear. If symptoms are unilateral, assess the asymptomatic ear before proceeding to the area of complaint. Use the largest ear speculum that is comfortable. Inspect the canal and associated structures for patency, erythema, tenderness, masses, ulcerations, exudate, deformity, and drainage. Note the integrity of the tympanic membrane (TM) and the quality of the light reflex. Observe the visibility and placement of the bony landmarks posterior to the TM. Evaluate the TM for inflammation, perforations, retraction, or bulging. In children, observe for the presence of pressure-equalizing tubes. Assess for bubbles or purulence behind the eardrum. Purulence will indicate an OM. Air-fluid level, bubbles, and yellow-orange hue behind the TM will indicate a serous OM. A pneumatic otoscope may be used to evaluate TM motility. Figure 7.4 depicts a normal TM. Table 7.1 lists some abnormalities detected on the ear examination. See also the Red Flag box for presentations related to the ear.

Hearing can be grossly assessed using the whisper test, watch ticking, and tuning forks (see next subsection). If screening indicates a deficit or if the patient complains of hearing loss, an accurate assessment of hearing requires a pure-tone hearing assessment known as an audiogram, which is conducted by a licensed audiologist.

Special Maneuvers

Weber Test and Rinne Test

The Weber test is performed with a tuning fork (512 Hz). The test measures the patient's ability to hear sound bilaterally. The tuning fork is tapped gently, lightly vibrating the tuning fork. The base of the tuning fork is placed on the midline

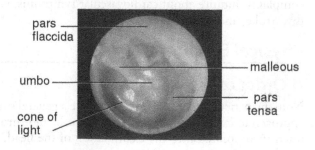

Figure 7.4 Normal tympanic membrane. (From Dillon, P. M. [2007]). *Nursing health assessment: A critical thinking, case studies approach*, 2nd ed. Fig. 12-19, p. 376. Philadelphia, PA: F. A. Davis. Reprinted with permission.)

pars flaccida

umbo

cone of light

malleous

pars tensa

Table 7.1	

Abnormalities of Inspection: Ear

Finding	Significance
Diffuse erythema and edema of the auricle or ear canal associated with severe pain	Malignant otitis externa/mastoiditis
Erythema and edema of ear canal with or without otorrhea	Otitis externa
Bloody discharge	External ear canal wound, malignancy, skull fracture, traumatic perforation of tympanic membrane
Yellow or brown matter that occludes the tympanic membrane	Cerumen impaction
Purulent discharge	Infection or foreign body
Bulging tympanic membrane with purulence noted behind tympanic membrane	Otitis media
White plaques on the tympanic membrane	Scarring from chronic infections or pressure-equalizing tubes
Bubbles with yellow/orange hue behind tympanic membrane	Serous otitis media
Keratinizing squamous epithelial tissue eroding the tympanic membrane or superior ear canal	Cholesteatoma
Gray, white, black or brown debris with fungal spores	Fungal otitis externa
Red tympanic membrane	Acute otitis externa, fever, crying

RED FLAG ◄ **Warnings for the Ear**

- *Sudden hearing loss is a medical emergency. Patient must be urgently referred to an audiologist for a stat audiogram and an otolaryngologist for prompt treatment with corticosteroids. Diagnostic imaging, such as magnetic resonance imaging (MRI), is needed to rule out acoustic schwannoma.*

- *Erythema, an edematous auricle that is very painful (pain is out of proportion to ear examination, especially pain worse at night) in the setting of a patient with diabetes or immunosuppression, could be a malignant otitis externa or mastoiditis. Urgent referral to an otolaryngologist or emergency room is indicated. Diagnostic computed tomography (CT) imaging is indicated.*

- *Auricular lesions that are irregular, ulcerated, discolored and with rapid growth pose a significant risk of cancer and should be biopsied or referred to a specialist for biopsy.*

- *Clear fluid draining from the ear, especially after a head injury, may be associated with cerebral spinal fluid and must be referred for prompt diagnostic imaging (CT or MRI).*

of the patient's scalp or on the upper front teeth (must not have false teeth/dentures). The patient should hear the vibration equally in both ears, which indicates no conductive or sensorineural hearing loss.

The Rinne test uses a tuning fork to assess and compare the patient's ability to hear both through bone and air conduction. The lightly vibrating tuning fork (512 Hz) is placed on the patient's mastoid bone (bone conduction). When the patient indicates the tuning fork is no longer heard, the examiner positions the tines of the fork 1 to 2 cm in front of the ear canal (air conduction) until the patient signals that the sound is no longer heard in that manner. The amount of time the patient hears the vibration in both positions is noted, and the maneuver is repeated on the opposite side. Air conduction should be twice as long as bone conduction, and the results should be similar for both ears.

The Weber and Rinne tests are useful only if performed and interpreted together. Interpretation also must be integrated with overall hearing assessment, and abnormal findings should be followed by audiogram.

- Normal: Air conduction louder than bone conduction both ears, no lateralization
- Conductive hearing loss: In affected ear, bone conduction greater than air conduction, lateralization to the affected ear
- Sensorineural hearing loss: In affected ear, air conduction greater than bone conduction, lateralization to "good" ear

Hearing Tests

A licensed audiologist using a soundproof booth should conduct pure-tone audiometry with speech discrimination. Before the audiogram is performed, ears should be examined for any cerumen buildup or acute infections. Patients with symptoms of an acute ear infection should not be tested.

Tympanocentesis

Tympanocentesis, which involves aspiration of middle ear fluid by a specialist, should be considered in patients with recurrent OM to identify the causative organisms.

Pneumatic Otoscopy

Pneumatic otoscopy should be used to confirm the diagnosis of serous otitis externa or OM (acute or chronic). Pneumatic otoscopy evaluates the mobility of the TM. Immobility indicates fluid within the middle ear.

Examination of the Nose and Sinuses

The examination of the sinuses begins with inspection of the face, noting any swelling or edema. Palpate over the frontal and maxillary sinuses, noting any tenderness.

Observe the external nose for placement and any obvious deformity or discharge. Observe the patient's respiratory pattern, noting whether the patient is mouth breathing or has adequate airflow through the nose. Identify any flaring of the nostrils or nasal obstruction. Palpate the external nose, noting any deformities, masses, or tenderness. If the patient is experiencing significant nasal symptoms, the internal examination of the nose is best accomplished after asking the patient to blow the nose. Using a speculum and light, inspect the anterior nasal cavity by tilting the patient's head back. The examiner's nondominant hand and thumb can be used to stabilize the nose and forehead with slight pressure of the thumb upward on the nose tip as a nasal speculum is gently inserted to observe the nasal mucosa and turbinates. Assess for discharge, noting the color, amount, and consistency. Thick, purulent discharge is associated with infection, and clear, profuse discharge is often associated with allergies or viral illness.

Assess the nasal mucosa for integrity, color, moistness, edema, lesions, or ulcerations. Assess the nasal septum for deviations, perforations, or sources of bleeding. The turbinates should be assessed for color and size. Pale, boggy turbinates suggest allergies; erythematous, swollen turbinates are often seen with infection or non-allergic rhinitis. Table 7.2 lists several abnormalities that can be identified during examination of the nose. See the Red Flag box for concerning presentations for the nose.

Olfactory sensation is typically a component of the cranial nerve (CN) examination. However, depending on the patient's complaints, it may be part of the limited ENT examination.

Table 7.2

Abnormalities of Inspection: Nose

Finding	Significance
External nasal redness, papules, hyperplasia	Rosacea
Transverse nasal crease (allergic salute) Pale, boggy turbinates Turbinate hypertrophy Clear, watery rhinorrhea Pruritis of the nose, eyes, and palate	Allergies
Erythematous turbinates Turbinate hypertrophy Nasal discharge (clear or colored)	Non-allergic rhinitis Rhinosinusitis
Soft tissue mass	Nasal polyps Papilloma Malignancy
Telangiectasias	Alcohol abuse Rendu-Osler-Weber disease
Asymmetric nasal dorsum/crooked nose	Deviated septum (may be acquired or congenital)
Septal perforation	Cocaine use or resulting from surgical complication

> | RED FLAG ◀ | **Warnings for the Nose and Sinuses** |
>
> - *Epistaxis that is acute, severe, chronic, unilateral, and persistent is concerning.*
>
> - *Frequent sinus infections that require antibiotic management (three to four infections in 1 year) warrants further investigation.*
>
> - *Acute rhinosinusitis associated with severe headaches, sinus pain, facial numbness, neurological changes, periorbital edema, ophthalmoplegia, proptosis, visual changes, or frontal swelling can indicate a serious complication needing urgent referral.*
>
> - *Unilateral nasal obstruction with unilateral epistaxis or sinus drainage can indicate an obstruction caused by a mass or malignancy.*
>
> - *Skin lesion on the nose that is irregular, ulcerated, discolored, and with rapid growth poses a significant risk of cancer and should be biopsied or referred to a specialist for biopsy.*
>
> - *Clear, copious, salty tasting rhinorrhea that is worse when bending forward can indicate a cerebral spinal fluid leak.*

Examination of the Mouth and Throat

The examination of the mouth and throat should begin with an inspection of all the structures that can be readily observed, followed by an examination that requires touching and moving the structures in order to thoroughly examine the oral cavity. The examination should end with palpation of the structures, paying particular attention to observed abnormalities. Gloves should always be worn during palpation. Ask the patient to remove any dental appliances, and then systematically examine the mouth and the pharynx. The use of a tongue depressor facilitates examination of the inner cheeks/buccal mucosa, floor and roof of the mouth, gums, posterior mouth, and tongue.

Inspect the size, shape, and symmetry of the lips. Obvious lesions, asymmetry, or abnormalities should be noted and their characteristics recorded. To inspect the oral cavity and the pharynx, use a good light source.

First, note the general condition of the internal structures of the mouth, including the tongue, buccal mucosa, hard and soft palates, gums, and teeth. Observe any abnormalities, such as lesions, ulcers, masses, exudate, discolorations, inflammation, and missing or decayed teeth. Identify any tongue or lip piercings, which may cause microscopic enamel cracks to teeth as a result of constant abrasion. Using a tongue depressor to displace the lips and cheeks, inspect areas of the buccal mucosa that are not otherwise visible, including the sites of the Stensen's duct and retromolar trigone. As the patient lifts the tongue to touch the palate, sticks it out, and moves it side to side, observe the lateral and ventral surfaces of the tongue, the sublingual mucosa, floor of mouth, Wharton's duct, and the frenulum. Assess the movement of the tongue and soft palate, looking for decreased or asymmetric movements or tongue fasciculations. As the oral cavity is inspected, the general integrity of the mucosal coverings and structures should be continually noted.

Inspect the oropharynx, tonsils, and uvula, taking care not to trigger an unwanted gag reflex. Observe the posterior pharynx to identify any inflammation, petechiae, ulcerations, discolorations, edema, swelling, tonsil asymmetry, lesions, and exudate or postnasal drainage. Observe the movement of the soft palate and uvula as the patient says "Ah." Make sure the uvula is midline and not deviated. Identify whether the tonsils are present and, if present, their size, symmetry, and color and the presence of exudate or masses/ulcerations. Smell the breath for acetone, ammonia, or foul breath (fetor oris). See Table 7.3.

Finally, accessible structures should be palpated, including the tissue between the cheeks and buccal mucosa, the floor of the mouth, bilateral tonsils, and the tongue. To palpate the floor of the mouth, use both hands, with one hand under the tongue palpating the floor of mouth and the other hand placed externally over the submandibular region directly below the floor of mouth. Apply upward pressure so that any masses will be displaced upward and toward the palpating hand. Use a similar technique to apply external, lateral pressure when palpating the buccal mucosa so that masses are not pushed away by the examining hand. Bilateral tonsils should be palpated using fingers and sweeping from the superior pole of the tonsil to the inferior pole, if a lesion is suspected. Note any areas of tenderness and masses. Masses should be assessed for consistency, firmness, dimensions, mobility, tenderness, and shape.

Table 7.3

Abnormalities of Inspection: Mouth

Finding	Significance
Hard, bony growths on the hard palate and anterior floor of mouth	Palatine or mandibular tori
Vesicular lesions on lips with crusting	Herpes simplex virus
White, patchy plaque on tongue or oral mucosa that can be removed with tongue depressor	Oral candidiasis
Painful ulcers with yellow or white centers with surrounding erythema that resolve	Aphthous ulcers
Fissuring of the oral lip commissures	Angular cheilosis
Papule white or pink in color that looks like a verrucous (wart) lesion	Papilloma
Painful, swelling in the gingival tissue with or without purulent drainage	Dental abscess
White, hyperkeratotic patch of mucosa	Leukoplakia or lichen planus

RED FLAG ◀	**Warnings for the Mouth and Throat**

- *Persistent, rapidly growing, painless mouth lesions or lesions concerning for malignancy require urgent referral for biopsy.*

- *Sore throat associated with severe pain, odynophagia, drooling, or stridor indicates potential epiglottitis or peritonsillar abscess.*

- *Sore throat lasting more than 1 week, associated with tonsil erythema, edema, or exudates and skin rashes without viral respiratory symptoms can suggest group A streptococcal (GAS) pharyngitis or tonsillitis.*

- *Asymmetric tonsils with or without masses should be referred to an otolaryngologist, as this can indicate tonsil malignancy.*

- *Prolonged symptoms of pharyngitis associated with odynophagia, dysphagia, unilateral otalgia, hoarseness, and trismus can be an indication that patient may have a head and neck malignancy. Referral to an otolaryngology specialist for evaluation is indicated.*

Differential Diagnosis of Chief Complaints: Ear

■ Ear Pain (Otalgia)

Ear pain can be primary or referred and is one of the most common complaints seen in primary care. It is most often seen in children and is usually associated with bacterial or viral upper respiratory infections. Complaints of ear pain in the summer are often associated with otitis externa (OE), otherwise known as swimmer's ear. Complaints of primary ear pain in older adults are often related to OE or cerumen impaction, especially in hearing aid users, or herpes zoster oticus (Ramsay Hunt syndrome). Referred ear pain can be related to temporal mandibular disorder, sinus infections, dental infection/abscess, or head and neck malignancy.

History

The history should include information related to the location of the pain (unilateral or bilateral); quality, quantity, and severity; onset; timing; and duration. The presence of sinus and nasal congestion is relevant because OM is typically secondary to a cold or sinus infection. Other historical information includes air travel, deep-sea diving, ear trauma, chronic ear infections, otological surgeries, allergies, dental disease, associated hearing loss/tinnitus, jaw pain or tenderness, pharyngitis, odynophagia, weight loss, trismus, or neck pain. In adults, possible underlying conditions, such as diabetes mellitus, and chronic inflammatory conditions, such as psoriasis, could be contributing factors exacerbating ear infections. A child's history should include exposure to secondhand smoke, day care, and swimming. A compromised immune status should be considered in those patients who have atypical OM or who do not respond to therapy.

Physical Examination

The physical examination should include inspection of the external auditory structures, palpation and manipulation of the tragus and auricle, and otoscopic inspection of the canal and TM. Attention should be paid to detecting inflammation and exudate in the canal and the condition of the TM, noting color, light reflex, translucency, and perforation. The examination should also include screening for hearing acuity. In a patient who presents with a complaint of otalgia with a normal ear examination, it is essential to assess other areas for referred pain, such as the temporomandibular joint (TMJ), oral cavity, posterior pharynx, neck, and cervical lymph nodes.

Diagnostic Studies

Diagnosis is based on findings from the physical examination. A culture and sensitivity (C&S) test should be considered if there is a purulent discharge. If a complete blood count (CBC) is done, there may be an associated leukocytosis and elevated erythrocyte sedimentation rate.

ACUTE OTITIS MEDIA

Acute OM (AOM) involves infection of the fluid in the middle ear space. AOM is one of the most common diagnoses affecting children, peaking between 6 months and 15 months of age (Gaddy et al., 2019). In children, the eustachian tube (ET) is shorter and the angle is less acute. Microorganisms of the nasopharynx easily enter the ET, predisposing children to AOM. The three bacterial organisms most often associated with AOM are *Streptococcus pneumoniae*, *Haemophilus influenzae*, and *Moraxella catarrhalis*. Frequently, viral organisms (rhinovirus, adenovirus, coronavirus, influenza, and respiratory syncytial virus) coexist with one of the preceding bacterial causes (Fig. 7.5). Adults who are immunocompromised may develop AOM; however, this is uncommon. If an adult presents with recurrent episodes of AOM, referral

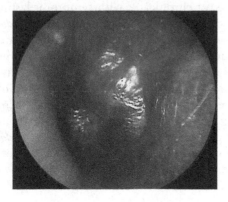

Figure 7.5 Acute otitis media.

to an otolaryngology specialist should be made to evaluate masses that can obstruct the ET.

Signs and Symptoms

The patient often complains of unilateral ear pain, which may radiate to the neck or jaw. There is commonly a current or recent history of symptoms consistent with an upper respiratory infection, including nasal congestion, sinus pressure/fullness, or sore throat. General hearing acuity will be diminished on the affected side, with bone conduction enhanced on that side. The external ear has a normal appearance unless there is drainage from the perforated TM. The TM is typically dull, may be inflamed, and bulges so that the posterior landmarks are obscured. The light reflex is distorted or obscured. If myringitis (inflammation of the TM) is present, the TM is reddened. Purulent or yellow fluid may be evident posterior to the TM, with diminished TM mobility. The examination is associated with increased pain. There are often other findings of upper respiratory infection. With ET dysfunction, OM with effusion (OME), also known as serous OM, may result. This condition is discussed under "Decreased Hearing or Hearing Loss" later in this chapter.

Diagnostic Studies

Pneumatic otoscopy should be performed to confirm middle ear effusion. Tympanometry can also be performed to confirm middle ear effusion. A tuning fork examination should also be performed to assess and confirm conductive hearing loss. In recurrent AOM, tympanocentesis or insertion of pressure-equalizing tubes can be performed by an otolaryngology specialist to alleviate discomfort and obtain a culture when the anticipated response to therapy is not achieved. In adults with recurrent AOM (more than two episodes in 1 year) or AOM that persists over 6 weeks, nasolaryngoscopy should be performed by an otolaryngology specialist to rule out mechanical obstruction of the ET (Gaddy et al., 2019).

OTITIS EXTERNA

OE is an inflammation of the lining of the ear canal. It can occur acutely, with symptoms lasting less than 6 weeks, or chronically, with symptoms lasting over 6 weeks. In acute OE, the most common causative bacteria are *Pseudomonas aeruginosa* and *Staphylococcus aureus*. In chronic OE, fungal organisms are commonly the causative pathogen. Acute OE is frequently associated with swimming and warm and humid climates, as well as mechanical trauma, which may occur through attempts to clean the ear with cotton-tipped swabs or other objects. Immunocompromised patients are at increased risk for developing necrotizing OE (malignant OE). Necrotizing OE extends to the temporal bone and is a medical emergency that requires prompt treatment and referral. *Pseudomonas aeruginosa* is the cause in 90% of necrotizing OE. Patients with diabetes, HIV, or any other immunosuppressive disorder must be closely monitored when diagnosed with OE to ensure they do not progress to necrotizing OE (Fig. 7.6).

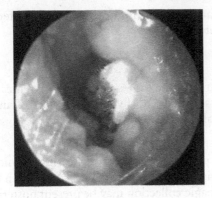

Figure 7.6 Otitis externa.

Signs and Symptoms

In acute OE, there is often pain, which is exacerbated when the auricle or tragus is touched or moved, making the examination difficult. On otoscopy, there is inflammation and edema of the canal. Drainage or exudate may be present, ranging in consistency from purulent to blood tinged or serous, and may have a foul order. Depending on the amount of swelling and exudate, the distal portion of the canal and TM may not be visible.

In necrotizing OE, severe pain is the most common complaint, associated with severe headache. Pain is worse at night, which causes a disruption in sleep and is often out of proportion to the physical examination. On examination, there may be significant edema and granulation tissue within the external ear canal that may progress to the outside of the auricle. Patients may have pain in the TMJ and cervical lymphadenopathy. The facial nerve should be assessed in these patients to ensure there are no deficits.

In chronic OE, the most common symptom is significant pruritis. Depending on the amount of exudate, patients may also complain of decreased hearing acuity and aural fullness. Pain is not a common finding in chronic OE. On otoscopy, there may be whitish-gray, brown, or black discharge with fungal spores. Patients may also present with dry, eczematic inflammation within the ear canal.

Diagnostic Studies

For uncomplicated acute OE, there is no indication for diagnostic studies. Otorrhea can be cultured and a sensitivity test performed to provide culture-directed therapy, especially if initial treatment has failed. Antibiotic otic drops are usually curative; however, before prescribing otic drops, the provider must ensure the TM is intact and not perforated. Patients should be closely monitored for resolution of symptoms, especially if they are at high risk for developing necrotizing OE.

For chronic OE with suspected fungal pathogen, antifungals are indicated. If the patient does not experience resolution of symptoms, referral to an otolaryngology specialist is indicated. In patients with suspected necrotizing OE, MRI or CT scan is indicated to evaluate and confirm diagnosis. Imaging will reveal erosion of bone within the ear canal. Close monitoring and stat referral to an otolaryngology specialist is indicated.

BAROTRAUMA

Barotrauma is injury to the structures of the ear resulting from extremes of atmospheric pressures, such as those associated with flying or deep-sea diving. Onset typically occurs within 24 hours of the exposure.

Signs and Symptoms

Complaints include ear pressure, pain, altered acuity of hearing, tinnitus, sinus pain/pressure, and headache. Vertigo may be present. The TM is often inflamed and may be perforated. A hemorrhagic collection may be present posterior to the TM. Benign positional vertigo and/or sinus tenderness may be evident.

Diagnostic Studies

No specific diagnostics are warranted unless the patient also has symptoms of decompression sickness.

TRAUMA

Direct trauma as a cause of ear pain is most seen in children, who frequently insert foreign objects into their ears. However, it may occur in adults as the result of overzealous ear cleaning or with hearing aid use. Indirect trauma can be associated with blunt blows to the head, jaw, or ear.

Signs and Symptoms

The signs and symptoms depend on the type of trauma and the structures injured. In direct trauma, the pain is consistent with OE or perforated TM. In blunt trauma, the signs and symptoms are consistent with the history of the injury. The actual findings may be from a source of referred pain (e.g., a fractured jaw) or from resultant perforation of the TM. The history of the traumatic event is important.

Diagnostic Studies

For mild traumatic injuries, no diagnostic studies are warranted. However, in the case of trauma to the head, diagnostics should be accomplished as recommended in Chapter 16.

MASTOIDITIS

Mastoiditis refers to inflammation of the middle ear mucosa lining of the mastoid bone. Mastoiditis results from a complication of AOM. The most common pathogens of acute mastoiditis are *Streptococcus pneumonia* and *Streptococcus pyogenes*. The pneumococcal conjugate vaccine (PCV13) has decreased the incidence of mastoiditis within the United States.

Signs and Symptoms

In mastoiditis following an AOM, symptoms include radiating ear pain, malaise, lethargy, and fever. The hearing on the affected side is usually significantly diminished. As the condition progresses, there is swelling, erythema, and tenderness over the mastoid bone. The swelling can be so advanced as to displace the auricle. Complications can be extracranial, including facial paralysis resulting from facial nerve compression, hearing loss, osteomyelitis, or abscess of the mastoid bone. Intracranial complications include infection of the cerebrospinal fluid (CSF), causing meningitis or brain abscess.

Diagnostic Studies

The patient should be referred promptly to an otolaryngology specialist for definitive diagnosis and treatment. On referral, diagnostics will likely include a CBC, a culture of fluid, and a CT scan to determine the degree of involvement.

FOREIGN BODY

Any foreign body in the ear canal, such as beads, cotton, insects, or toys, can cause ear pain. The presence of a foreign body is most common in young children. However, in adults using hearing aids or cotton-tipped swabs, hearing aid domes or cotton from the swab can become lodged inside the ear canal.

Signs and Symptoms

Pain is often the presenting complaint and may be associated with unilateral, purulent discharge from the canal. Other symptoms include altered hearing acuity and aural fullness. Physical findings often include tenderness on manipulation of the ear and with the examination, as well as visualization of the foreign body. Depending on the amount of trauma caused by the offending object, the canal may be inflamed or edematous and have exudate consistent with a resultant OE.

Diagnostic Studies

Diagnostic studies are typically not warranted. The offending object can usually be flushed out and retrieved with alligator forceps. In the case of an insect in the ear canal, it is important to suffocate the insect before removal. Inserting warm oil (mineral, olive, vegetable, or baby oil) inside the ear canal will suffocate the insect and prevent the insect from trying to burrow inside the ear. This will make the extraction less traumatic and painful for the patient.

REFERRED PAIN

A variety of conditions can result in pain that is referred to the ear. These include TMJ pain, dental pain/infections, head and neck cancers, neck mass/pain, tonsillitis, temporal arteritis, and trigeminal neuralgia. The variety of conditions is beyond the scope of the discussion for ear pain but can be found in other chapters, particularly Chapters 5 and 16.

■ Ear Discharge (Otorrhea)

Discharge emanating from the ear often indicates a condition warranting urgent diagnosis and treatment. Purulent discharge is most often related to an infectious process. Clear liquid can indicate a CSF leak, which can be caused by head trauma, congenital malformations, or spontaneous CSF leaks. Bloody discharge associated with recent head trauma may indicate a skull fracture. Bloody discharge can also be caused by malignancy of the ear canal.

History

Immediate proximal causes for ear discharge, such as AOM with perforation, OE, mastoiditis, chronic ear infections, or a foreign body, should be investigated. Inquire about serious conditions such as head trauma if an immediate proximal cause is ruled out. Ask how long the discharge has been present and about its consistency, color, and odor. Ask about other medical conditions such as diabetes or immunosuppression. Explore the possibility of direct or indirect trauma as well as secondary or complicated infections. Obtain a history of previous episodes of ear discharge, ear infections, or other conditions. A thorough review of systems is warranted, particularly as related to other components of the upper respiratory and neurological systems.

Physical Examination

Examination usually includes the head, ears, nose, and throat. Begin by assessing the patient's general health and mental status. If there is no history of head trauma and the patient's general neurological status is intact, proceed to examination of the ears. Observe both external ears, comparing for symmetry of appearance. Identify areas of inflammation, swelling, deformity, or distortion of landmarks and signs of trauma. Note the color, odor, and consistency of any visible discharge. Palpate the structures of the external ear, noting any tenderness or palpable abnormalities. Observe the distal portion of the canal for swelling, erythema, discharge, or obvious foreign body. Complete the otoscopic examination, noticing the condition of the canal walls, TM, and visible portion of the middle ear structures.

Diagnostic Studies

Diagnosis is usually based on history and physical examination. Some specific diagnoses and other conditions that can be associated with discharge are discussed in the preceding sections.

ACUTE OTITIS MEDIA WITH PERFORATION

Particularly in children, spontaneous rupture of the TM may occur owing to the pressure in the middle ear, resulting in a white or purulent discharge from the ear. In addition to the typical findings of AOM, there may be a visible perforation. See the preceding section on AOM and Figure 7.7.

CEREBROSPINAL FLUID LEAKAGE

Otorrhea caused by a CSF leak can be associated with head trauma, surgery, tumors of the skull base, congenital abnormalities, or chronic intracranial hypertension, or it may be idiopathic. Patients would complain of clear, watery otorrhea that increases with the Valsalva maneuver. If the history and/or physical

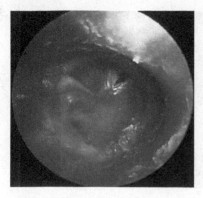

Figure 7.7 Acute otitis media with perforation.

examination suggest the potential for leakage of CSF, the drainage can be tested for beta-2 transferrin, which distinguishes CSF from other watery discharge from the nose or ear after a traumatic injury to the brain or spine. Providing the patient is stable, an emergency referral is warranted for definitive diagnosis because CSF leakage indicates a heightened potential for the development of meningitis. Further diagnostic studies, including imaging, will be completed following referral.

CHOLESTEATOMA

A cholesteatoma is an abnormal growth of epithelial tissue causing a cyst in the middle ear (Fig. 7.8). The tissue can grow to invade surrounding bone and/ or extend into the inner ear. Cholesteatomas can present as white squamous debris or yellow/white masses behind the TM. Patients with ET dysfunction and retracted TMs are at highest risk for developing a cholesteatoma.

Signs and Symptoms
The patient often complains of chronic ear infections and otorrhea. An associated sense of aural fullness and/or decreased hearing may be experienced in the affected ear. Over time, pain and dizziness can develop. The examination will reveal otorrhea and/or epithelial tissue in the canal with canal erosion. The drainage is often mucopurulent. If infection is present, inflammatory changes may be evident, as seen with AOM. The cholesteatoma may also present behind the TM. Because of the risk of permanent hearing loss from the erosion of the ear bones and risk of meningitis from erosion of the skull base, the patient should be referred to an otolaryngology specialist for definitive diagnosis and surgical intervention.

Diagnostic Studies
No studies are indicated in a primary care setting.

OTITIS EXTERNA

See p. 209.

MASTOIDITIS

See p. 206.

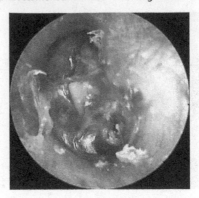

Figure 7.8 Cholesteatoma.

FOREIGN BODY

See p. 207.

■ Decreased Hearing or Hearing Loss

Hearing loss is defined as a decrease in hearing threshold of 25 dB or more in one or both ears and can be classified as mild, moderate, severe, or profound. Hearing loss rates double for every 10 years of life after age 50 years (Gorman & Lin, 2016). Hearing loss affects 2 out of every 1,000 children and about 15% of adults older than 18 years (NIDCD, 2021). As patients age, the prevalence of hearing loss increases. The rate of disabling hearing loss is 25% between the ages of 65 and 74 years and 50% over age 75 years (Gorman & Lin, 2016). Hearing loss affects men at a higher rate than women.

Hearing loss is identified as conductive or sensorineural. In conductive hearing loss, there is a disruption in the conduction of sound waves funneled into the ear canal, which prevents the TM and ossicles from vibrating and opening the oval window. This prevents sound from getting into the cochlea. In sensorineural hearing loss, there is a dysfunction of hair cells within the cochlea or damage in conduction of sound through the vestibulocochlear nerve (CN VIII). The most common cause of sensorineural hearing loss is associated with aging (presbycusis), with onset noticed in the sixth decade. This is followed by repetitive exposure to loud noise, which may occur with both occupational and recreational activities. In children, sensorineural hearing deficits are often associated with congenital cytomegalovirus and genetic causes. In adults, the most common cause of conductive hearing loss is mechanical obstruction of the ear canal by cerumen or a foreign body. In children, the most common cause of conductive hearing loss is OME. The list of conditions and factors that can result in an altered sense of hearing is extensive (Table 7.4). It includes a variety of infectious diseases, autoimmune disorders, chronic systemic diseases (e.g., diabetes, thyroid disease, vascular and neurological conditions), medications, and many more.

Table 7.4	

Common Causes of Hearing Loss

Causes of Conductive Hearing Loss From Most to Least Common	Causes of Sensorineural Hearing Loss From Most to Least Common
Cerumen	Presbycusis
Otitis media with effusion (most common in children)	Noise exposure
Acute otitis media	Hereditary
Tympanic membrane perforation	Ototoxicity (drug induced)
Otosclerosis	Sudden idiopathic hearing loss
Otitis externa	Autoimmune hearing loss
Ear canal mass/middle ear mass (glomus tumor, osteomas)	Meniere's disease
Tympanosclerosis	Vestibular schwannoma
Cholesteatoma	Infections (meningitis, syphilis, mumps, viral labyrinthitis)
	Stroke
	Congenital malformation of the ossicles
	Temporal bone fractures

History

It is essential to explore the onset and progression of the hearing loss, determining whether the onset was progressive (over time) or acute, and regardless of the onset, how it has progressed since first noticed. Inquire if one or both ears are affected and if the hearing is diminished, fluctuating, or completely absent. Investigate the severity with questions regarding the impact of the hearing loss on the patient's ability to communicate. Identify associated symptoms, including tinnitus (ringing in the ear[s]), pain, fullness, vertigo, otalgia, fevers, otorrhea, headaches, disequilibrium, or acoustic trauma. Have the patient identify all prescribed, OTC, and recreational substances used before and since onset as possible causative agents. Medications with ototoxic effects include aminoglycoside antibiotics; platinum-based antineoplastics and methotrexate; loop diuretics; salicylates and anti-inflammatories; and quinine-based medications such as quinine, chloroquine, hydroxychloroquine, and mefloquine. A history of noise exposure is important, including occupational and recreational exposure. Prolonged noise levels of 85 dB and higher put the patient at higher risk for sensorineural hearing loss (CDC, 2018b)

Explore the patient's general state of health from the period just before and since the altered sense of hearing was noticed, asking about other conditions and infections, including upper respiratory infections, family history of hearing loss, otological surgeries, or head and neck cancers; Meniere's disease; OE and OM. Identify the history of systemic disorders, such as diabetes, head and neck malignancies, hypertension, strokes, and vascular disorders. Ask about recent barotrauma as well as other trauma to the head or ear. In pediatric patients, ask if the patient has speech or learning difficulties, behavior issues, history of cleft palate, history of birth weight less than 3.3 pounds, and if the patient's mother had perinatal viral infections.

Physical Examination

A complete examination of the ears should be performed, along with assessment of the other upper respiratory structures. As indicated by the patient's age and presenting history, general appearance, and ear findings, consider expanding the examination to include neurological, cardiovascular, and other systems. It is reasonable to grossly test hearing with the whisper test, a ticking watch, or fingers being rubbed together. The type of loss (sensorineural or conductive) may be grossly evaluated using tuning fork techniques. Evidence supports that these hearing tests have good specificity but poor sensitivity (Box 7.1). Based on the results of these gross screenings, an audiogram should be obtained.

Diagnostic Studies

An audiogram is required to quantitatively assess hearing acuity. This should be performed by a licensed audiologist to include pure-tone audiometry with speech discrimination, as well as impedance testing. Other diagnostic procedures depend on the suspected cause of hearing loss. Pneumatic otoscopy and/or tympanogram should be performed if OM is suspected.

CERUMEN IMPACTION

Cerumen is produced by glands within the outer two-thirds of the external ear canal to keep the pH of the ear acidic, preventing infections. The ear canal is supposed to be self-cleaning; however, in some patients, cerumen impaction can occur, causing symptoms of hearing loss, tinnitus, aural fullness, otalgia, otorrhea, and infections. Cerumen impaction affects 1 in 10 children and 1 in 20 adults. Cerumen impaction causes about 12 million people to seek medical care yearly (Schwartz et al., 2017). Risk factors include use of hearing aids, use of cotton-tipped swabs, narrow ear canals, and increased hair within the ear canal. Cerumen impaction is a common cause of altered hearing, particularly in older patients.

Box 7.1

Accuracy of Gross Hearing Tests

In a study by Boatman et al. (2007), each of the following tests was performed on 107 adults, 50 to 88 years of age, and compared to audiogram results. The sensitivity and specificity are based on patients with hearing loss >25 dB/>40 dB.

Test	Sensitivity (Hearing Loss: >25 dB/>40 dB)	Specificity
Finger rub	0.27/0.35	0.98/0.97
Whispered speech	0.40/0.46	0.83/0.78
Watch tick	0.44/0.60	1.0/0.99
Rinne (256 Hz)	N/A	1.0/1.0
Weber (256 Hz)	0.30/0.26	0.74/0.74

Signs and Symptoms

The patient typically complains of progressive decreased hearing acuity, although in some patients, onset may be sudden. The cerumen may cause discomfort and/or itching in the canal. In older patients, there is often a history of previous cerumen impactions, especially with those who wear hearing aids. Hearing loss is conductive (a Weber test would lateralize to affected ear). The examination reveals the mass of cerumen within the canal. On occasion, the cerumen causes excoriation of the canal walls. Patient will have immediate relief of subjective hearing loss once cerumen impaction is removed.

Diagnostic Studies

No studies are indicated.

PRESBYCUSIS

Presbycusis is an age-related cause of sensorineural hearing loss and involves diminished hair cell function within the cochlea as well as a decrease in the vestibulocochlear nerve's (CN VIII) transmission of sound vibrations, affecting high-frequency hearing. Although the changes associated with presbycusis often start in early adulthood, the decreased hearing acuity is usually not noticed until the individual is older than 65 years. In addition to age-related changes, onset can be associated with exposure to environmental noise and influenced by genetic predisposition. Other risk factors include family history of hearing loss, diabetes, cardiovascular disease, and tobacco use. Hearing loss can be associated with depression, isolation, and decreased quality of life. When presbycusis is suspected, the patient should be referred to an audiologist for definitive diagnosis and assessment for the use of hearing aid(s).

Signs and Symptoms

Symptoms of presbycusis occur gradually and progressively over many years. It usually affects the ears symmetrically and has associated symptoms of tinnitus and aural fullness. Some patients complain of disequilibrium or vertigo. Commonly, patients report that family members complain about the television being too loud or about being frequently asked to repeat words. The physical examination of the ear is normal.

Diagnostic Studies

Audiogram identifies the degree of hearing loss, usually affecting the higher frequencies, making the diagnosis of presbycusis.

OTOSCLEROSIS

Otosclerosis is caused by calcifications to the bony structures of the middle ear, specifically the stapes. This results in the gradual onset of low-frequency conductive hearing loss, as the bones lose their vibratory ability. Otosclerosis affects white people and women at a higher rate, with an average age of onset of 30 years (Batson & Rizzolo, 2017). Genetic history is a strong predictor with about 60% having a family history of otosclerosis (Batson & Rizzolo, 2017).

Signs and Symptoms

The patient typically complains of painless, progressive changes in lower frequency hearing. Symptoms are usually bilateral but can present as unilateral early in the disease. It is often associated with tinnitus and aural fullness. The physical examination is normal. A tuning fork examination will reveal conductive hearing loss.

Diagnostic Studies

Audiometry quantifies the deficit, which usually involves the lower frequencies, showing a Carhart notch at 2,000 Hz. A referral to an otolaryngology specialist, specifically an otologist, is warranted, as surgical intervention (stapedectomy) is often successful. The specialist may order CT imaging to confirm the diagnosis.

OTITIS MEDIA WITH EFFUSION

OME, or serous OM, results from the dysfunction of one or both ETs and may follow or contribute to the development of AOM. OME affects five out of six children (90%) before school age (NIDCD, 2021; Rosenfeld et al., 2014). The presence of residual middle ear fluid can cause significant conductive hearing loss. In adults, this is an uncommon finding. It may result from AOM, ET dysfunction, or blockage of the ET from a nasopharyngeal mass (Fig. 7.9).

Signs and Symptoms

Parents and/or teachers often relate that the child does not listen well, has delayed language, or has behavior issues. Symptoms include a sense of ear fullness and a need to "pop" the ear(s). Hearing acuity is decreased on the affected side. The external ear and canal are normal in appearance. The TM may be bulging, with a yellowish hue from the fluid collected posteriorly in the middle ear chamber. There may be visible bubbles behind the TM. The TM mobility is diminished or absent on pneumatic otoscopy.

Diagnostic Studies

A tympanogram reveals decreased compliance of the TM.

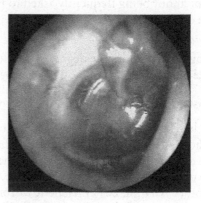

Figure 7.9 Otitis media with effusion.

INFECTIOUS DISEASE

A variety of infectious conditions can affect hearing acuity. These include the conditions that are usually responsible for AOM and OE (described earlier in this chapter), as well as herpes simplex, herpes zoster, syphilis, meningitis, mononucleosis, mumps, rubella, and rubeola. Infections are responsible for both conductive and sensorineural hearing loss.

Signs and Symptoms

Complaints and findings are consistent with the specific infection and may include malaise, fever, myalgia, headache, and pain. Physical examination should reveal findings consistent with AOM or OE if either is present. In addition to physical ear findings, there may be generalized signs of upper respiratory infection, skin rash or lesions, lymphadenopathy, and other changes. Tuning fork tests may reveal either conductive hearing loss (associated with bacterial or viral AOM) or sensorineural loss (common with syphilis, meningitis, or herpes zoster). It is possible that the signs of a causative infection may have resolved by the time the patient presents with hearing loss; thus, the history will be important in identifying this as a possible etiology.

Diagnostic Studies

The selection of diagnostic studies will be guided by the history of exposure, symptomatology, and risk factors, as well as the physical findings.

SUDDEN SENSORINEURAL HEARING LOSS

Sudden sensorineural hearing loss (SSNHL) is the acute, rapid, unilateral (within 72 hours) loss of hearing. SSNHL affects 66,000 patients annually (Chandrasekhar et al., 2019). It is considered a medical emergency and should prompt the primary care provider to expedite evaluation and management to prevent permanent hearing loss. SSNHL may occur after an upper respiratory viral infection, although most of the time it is idiopathic. Nonidiopathic causes of SSNHL include stroke, autoimmune disease, Meniere's disease, multiple sclerosis, meningitis, or acoustic neuroma.

Signs and Symptoms

Patients complain of painless, sudden hearing loss, which may be accompanied by tinnitus, aural fullness, and/or vertigo. Identify precipitating events such as head trauma, upper respiratory infections, or viral infections. Also ask if the patient has associated otalgia, otorrhea, chronic ear infections, or ear surgeries; this may help to distinguish if the hearing loss is conductive or sensorineural in nature. In SSNHL, the ear examination will be normal. A neurological examination, assessing CNs for deficits, is important to rule out a nonidiopathic cause of SSNHL such as vestibular schwannoma. On the Weber examination, a tuning fork will reveal a lateralization away from the affected ear, indicating a sensorineural hearing loss.

Diagnostic Studies

Urgent referral to an audiologist and an otolaryngology specialist is indicated. Diagnosis is made by confirmed hearing loss >30 dB at three consecutive frequencies. Laboratory testing is not routinely indicated unless there is suspicion of a viral or autoimmune etiology. Once referral to an otolaryngology specialist is made, treatment with high-dose steroids, either orally or intratympanic, with a repeat audiogram is the recommended treatment. MRI of the brain, assessing the internal auditory canal and ruling out vestibular schwannoma, should be performed.

VESTIBULAR SCHWANNOMAS

Vestibular schwannomas ([VSs] acoustic neuromas) are rare, benign tumors affecting the vestibulocochlear nerve (CN VIII). The overall incidence of VS is 1.09 per 100,000 per year and increases with age between 65 to 74 years to 2.93 per 100,000 per year (Goldbrunner et al., 2020). The onset of symptoms usually occurs after age 30. Therapeutic interventions include surgery and radiation.

Signs and Symptoms

Symptoms depend on the size of the tumor. Most patients present with asymmetric hearing loss and tinnitus.

Some patients will present with SSNHL and/or vertigo and unsteadiness. As the tumor advances, symptoms may include headache, facial paresis, ataxia, nausea/vomiting, and lethargy. On physical examination, the ear structures appear normal.

Diagnostic Studies

An audiogram is essential to determine the severity of hearing loss in the affected ear. MRI is the gold standard in diagnosing VS. The patient should be referred for definitive diagnosis and treatment.

MENIERE'S DISEASE

Meniere's disease is described in Chapter 16.

MEDICATIONS

A variety of medications can potentially cause a symmetric hearing loss. The most common are antibiotics (aminoglycosides); quinine derivatives; antineoplastics (platinum-based and methotrexate); loop diuretics; and NSAIDs, both salicylate-based and others. When hearing loss is identified, a list of all agents taken by the patient may identify a potentially ototoxic drug. Medication-related ototoxicity can be permanent or reversible, depending on the agent.

CHOLESTEATOMA

See p. 209.

■ Tinnitus

Tinnitus (ringing in the ears) is the perception of sound without an external cause. Tinnitus affects over 50 million people within the United States and is the number one service connection issue for veterans (Tunkel et al., 2014). Tinnitus affects men and white people at a higher rate. Risk factors include hearing loss, loud noise exposure, anxiety, obesity, hypertension, insomnia, psychiatric conditions, and stress. Primary tinnitus is associated with sensorineural hearing loss or may be idiopathic in 10% of cases. Secondary tinnitus is associated with an underlying cause. Pulsatile tinnitus is described as a heartbeat or pulse in the ear and can indicate cardiovascular cause of symptoms. Tinnitus refers to a wide range of sounds mimicking whistles, crickets, ringing, buzzing, ticking, and the like. It is typically persistent and bilateral. Tinnitus is most often associated with hearing loss.

History

Ask the patient to describe the quality of the tinnitus, if it is pulsatile or not, onset, duration, and affected ear(s). Identify if the patient has associated hearing loss, vertigo, otalgia, otorrhea, or facial weakness. If the patient complains of pulsatile tinnitus, ask about cardiovascular or vascular disease. Obtain a list of current medications and the amount and frequency of dosing. Ask about recent exposure to loud noise or chemical agents through activities, including work, hobbies, and recreation. A history should be obtained for other ear disorders and symptoms, including labyrinthitis, Meniere's disease, or progressive hearing loss. Inquire about sleep patterns, depression, anxiety, alcohol use, and ear surgeries.

Physical Examination

A thorough ENT and neurological examination should be performed. In the absence of a structural abnormality or infection, the physical examination should be normal. There may be a decrease in gross hearing acuity and in performance during a tuning fork examination because tinnitus is associated with the causes of hearing loss. In complaints of pulsatile tinnitus, a full head and neck examination is warranted, as well as a cardiovascular examination, auscultating the carotid artery for bruits.

Diagnostic Studies

Diagnostic studies are related to the specific suspected etiology associated with the tinnitus but should include audiometry. The major causes of tinnitus are listed in Box 7.2.

■ Aural Fullness

The etiology of aural fullness is multidimensional. Fullness can be related to fluid in the middle ear as a result of OM, hearing loss, changes in barometric pressure, or ET dysfunction. The most common causes vary by age: Children

Box 7.2

Causes of Tinnitus

Otological	Hearing loss
	Meniere's disease
	Vestibular schwannoma
	Eustachian tube dysfunction
	Cerumen impaction
	Otosclerosis
	Cochlear abnormalities
Neurological	Multiple sclerosis
	Head injury
Metabolic	Thyroid disorder
	Hyperlipidemia
	Vitamin B_{12} deficiency
Psychogenic	Depression
	Anxiety
	Fibromyalgia
Pulsatile Tinnitus	Vascular neoplasm
	Vascular anomality
	Vascular malformation within the ear or head and neck
Substances	Ototoxic medications
	Alcohol
Other	Temporal mandibular joint syndrome
	Arthritis of the neck
	Myoclonus
	Intercranial hypertension

are more likely to experience ear fullness associated with OME and ET dysfunction; older adults are more likely to have cerumen impaction and/or hearing loss.

History

Complete a symptom analysis, especially noting the timing of the symptom. Ask whether the onset was gradual or sudden. Determine whether the fullness is affected by the patient's position. Identify any other concurrent or recent ENT symptoms or respiratory conditions.

Physical Examination

Examine the external ear structures. Manipulate the external ear to identify any tenderness before inserting the otoscope speculum. Examine the canal for masses or swelling. Observe the TM to detect any dullness, decreased

Box 7.3	
Causes of Aural Fullness	
Otological	Hearing loss
	Meniere's disease
	Eustachian tube dysfunction
	Cerumen impaction
	Otosclerosis
	Ear infections (otitis media, otitis externa)
	Otitis media with effusion
	Mass
Systemic	Allergies
Substances	Ototoxic medications
Other	Temporal Mandibular Disorder

light reflex, bulging, retraction, or inflammation, which may indicate fluid or infection.

Diagnostic Studies

Pneumatic otoscopy will assist in determining the presence of fluid in the middle ear. An audiogram can be helpful in determining if there is a hearing loss associated with aural fullness. The common causes of complaints of ear fullness are listed in Box 7.3.

Differential Diagnosis of Chief Complaints: Nose

■ Epistaxis (Nose Bleeds)

Epistaxis is a common symptom affecting about 60% of the U.S. population, with a peak incidence affecting children younger than 10 years and adults between the ages of 70 and 79 years (Tunkel et al., 2020). Three out of four children have at least one episode of epistaxis in their lifetime, usually caused by digital trauma, nasal dryness/crusting, nasal inflammation, or foreign bodies (Tunkel et al., 2020). The most common site of nose bleeds (90%) is the anterior nasal septum, known as Kiesselbach's plexus. These bleeds are typically easy to control with direct pressure and are self-limiting (Chaaban et al., 2017). In about 10% of patients, bleeding occurs from the posterior septum, known as Woodruff's plexus; this site most often affects older adults. Posterior nose bleeds are more difficult to manage and often result in hospitalizations (Tunkel et al., 2020). Bleeding from the nose typically occurs spontaneously, is bright red, and is often profuse but can usually be controlled within a few minutes after applying pressure and cold. See Box 7.4 for causes of epistaxis.

Box 7.4

Causes of Epistaxis

Causes	Causes and Associated Symptoms
Trauma	Digital manipulation Trauma/injury to nose Forceful nasal blowing
Nasopharyngeal carcinoma	Unilateral bleeding Unilateral nasal obstruction Chronic sinusitis Facial numbness/paresis Unilateral otalgia or ear infections Cervical neck mass Weight loss
Medication-induced epistaxis	Intranasal corticosteroids Cocaine Oral anticoagulants Aspirin NSAIDs
Nasal structural deformities	Deviated septum Perforated septum
Juvenile nasopharyngeal angiofibroma	Early symptoms: epistaxis, nasal obstruction, chronic sinus infections and rhinorrhea Late-stage symptoms: Headaches, facial numbness, swelling of cheeks, droopy eyelids, protruding eyes, watery eyes, blindness or double vision, and hearing loss
Chronic allergies/sinus infections	Chronic sinus infections Purulent drainage Rhinorrhea Nasal polyposis
Chronic medical illness or bleeding disorders (high association with posterior epistaxis)	Chronic illnesses: Hypertension, cirrhosis, renal disease, cancer (especially Hodgkin's disease) Bleeding disorders: Hemophilia, von Willebrand disease, hereditary hemorrhagic telangiectasia

Worrisome symptoms include unilateral recurrent, persistent epistaxis with nasal obstruction, chronic unilateral sinus infections, or facial weakness/paresis, which could indicate a nasal carcinoma or juvenile nasopharyngeal angiofibroma. Nasal compression of the lower two-thirds of the nose for 5 minutes or more usually stops anterior epistaxis. Intranasal medication such as oxymetazoline can also be used to vasoconstrict the blood vessels. In profuse or prolonged epistaxis, nasal packing, and occasionally artery ligation, may be necessary to control the bleeding. Any unexplained, recurrent epistaxis warrants investigation and possible referral to an otolaryngology specialist.

History

Inquire about onset, duration, laterality (unilateral or bilateral nares), and frequency of epistaxis. Ask if the bleeding comes out of the front of the nose or drains down the back of the throat and what the patient does to stop the bleeding. Inquire about associated symptoms such as unilateral nasal obstruction, facial paresis, headaches, unilateral otalgia, weight loss, or neck mass. Ask about medications the patient is taking that could be contributing, such as anticoagulants, aspirin, or NSAIDs, and the presence of other medical problems, such as hematologic, liver, or vascular disease. Social history such as intranasal cocaine use, occupational and chemical exposures, and tobacco use need to be explored. A complaint of recent trauma is a straightforward cause of epistaxis. Ask about frequent sinus infections and the use of nasal sprays, obtained by prescription or OTC; steroid or antihistamine nasal sprays can cause dryness, irritation, and bleeding. Chronic epistaxis warrants referral to an otolaryngology specialist to determine a structural or vascular cause.

Physical Examination

The physical examination should start with an inspection of the external nose for alignment, airflow, and the presence of any skin lesions. Using a speculum and light, visualize the nasal mucosa for redness, purulent discharge, lesions, ulcerations, masses, and signs of bleeding. Assess CN for facial paresis.

Diagnostic Studies

An x-ray can detect gross facial fractures, but a CT scan is diagnostic for sinus disease, fracture, tumor, and polyps. MRI is more sensitive in identifying neural invasion. C&S of nasal discharge can be taken for resistant infections. CBC with differential, platelet count, and coagulation studies might be needed to rule out hematologic or vascular causes. A liver profile might be needed to identify a hepatic cause of the epistaxis.

TRAUMA

Bleeding accompanied by edema and asymmetry of the nose indicates a possible fracture. Ice and pressure on the sides of the nose with the head tilted forward usually controls the bleeding, at least temporarily. Use of oxymetazoline nasal spray can also help to vasoconstrict the blood vessels. If bleeding does not stop, packing or cautery may be necessary.

Signs and Symptoms

There is a history of a blow to the nose. If the cause of apparent trauma is not reported by the patient, be alert for and inquire about any signs of abuse. Edema occurs rapidly after a blow to the nose and is obvious on visual inspection. There may be abrasions or lacerations present, and asymmetry is seen with fracture.

Diagnostic Studies

A CT scan should be done to look for a fracture. If the CT is positive for a fracture, the patient should be referred to the otolaryngologist and/or a plastic surgeon.

MEDICATIONS

Anticoagulant medications such as warfarin (Coumadin), heparin, or any of the newer direct factor Xa and thrombin inhibitors are the most common medications to cause epistaxis. Other drugs that might cause bleeding include aspirin, NSAIDs, nasal sprays, and ginkgo biloba.

Signs and Symptoms

A thorough medication history identifies prescription, OTC, or herbal preparations associated with epistaxis. In addition to the nasal bleeding, an over-anticoagulated patient may have bruising over the body from everyday minor contusions, particularly on the limbs. Bleeding from the gums also is commonly seen with over-anticoagulation.

Diagnostic Studies

If the patient is taking anticoagulants, a prothrombin time with international normalization ratio or a factor Xa level should be done, depending on the drug class.

HEMATOLOGIC DISORDERS

Hematologic disorders likely to cause increased bleeding include thrombocytopenia, leukemia, aplastic anemia, and hereditary coagulopathies (hemophilia, von Willebrand disease, hereditary hemorrhagic telangiectasia). Multiple hematologic disorders can be seen with liver disease, including anemia, thrombocytopenia, leukopenia, leukocytosis, and impaired synthesis of clotting factors causing increased prothrombin time.

Signs and Symptoms

A history of hematologic disorders will quickly point toward the cause of the bleeding. There may be a history of bruising, fatigue, shortness of breath, fever, or frequent infections. The patient may have a personal or family history of liver disease and/or alcohol use or abuse. Risk factors for hepatitis may be present.

Except for the epistaxis, the physical examination may be unremarkable. Fever, bruising, or petechiae may indicate leukemia, thrombocytopenia, or coagulopathies. A rapid heart rate and/or heart murmur as well as cyanosis around the lips or nails may be present with long-standing anemia. Capillary refill may be altered. Hepatomegaly or ascites may be present in liver disease.

Diagnostic Studies

If hematologic disorders are suspected, a CBC, platelet count, liver profile, and coagulation studies should be done. A bone marrow aspiration may need to be performed by the hematologist or oncologist to confirm the diagnosis.

INTRANASAL DRUG USE

Cocaine use runs the gamut of socioeconomic class, age, and gender. It is important not to stereotype individuals as being or not being at risk for cocaine use.

Signs and Symptoms

A history of any kind of illegal drug use or alcohol abuse should alert the practitioner to the possibility of cocaine use. Typical symptoms associated with cocaine use are tachycardia, tachypnea, elevated blood pressure, arrhythmias, dilated pupils, nervousness, euphoria, hallucinations, and friability of the nasal mucosa leading to epistaxis. An overdose may lead to tremors, seizures, delirium, respiratory failure, and cardiovascular collapse. On examination, patients may present with an anterior perforation of the nasal septum.

Diagnostic Studies

A drug screen should be performed for suspected cocaine use. An electrocardiogram, blood pressure monitoring, and pulse oximetry may be necessary until the heart and respiratory rates and blood pressure return to a normal range.

MUCOSAL DRYNESS, IRRITATION, AND INFECTION

Dry climates, especially during the winter months, may cause nasal mucosal irritation and bleeding, which is usually scanty. OTC nasal sprays and corticosteroid or antihistamine nasal sprays may dry the mucosal lining of the nose and cause bleeding. Intranasal steroids can thin the lining of the septum, causing epistaxis. Patients should be educated on proper use of intranasal steroids before prescribing them. Infection, particularly recurrent or chronic infection, can lead to sinus and mucosal inflammation and irritation resulting in bleeding, which is usually scanty unless the infection is severe enough to erode the mucosal surface.

Signs and Symptoms

A history of a dry environment or recent sinus infections, fever, sinus pressure or pain, and purulent nasal discharge may be present. Bleeding may be aggravated by blowing the nose. Dry crusting found in the nares, along with areas of irritation, may indicate the etiology of the bleeding. Infections cause the nasal mucosa to look beefy red; some areas may be raw and bleeding. Infection is usually accompanied by fever and purulent discharge.

Diagnostic Studies

Diagnostic studies are usually not warranted. CT scan of the sinuses may be necessary with a history of recurrent and/or chronic sinus infections.

VASCULAR DISORDERS

The most serious vascular etiology of epistaxis is Rendu-Osler-Weber disease, also known as hereditary hemorrhagic telangiectasia, an autosomal dominant disease caused by vascular malformation. It affects both men and women. It can cause severe, recurrent epistaxis resulting from arteriovenous aneurysms in the mucous membranes. A less common vascular cause is hypertension, particularly uncontrolled or episodic hypertension. Juvenile nasopharyngeal angiofibroma is a rare, benign, invasive vascular tumor affecting male adolescents. It is highly aggressive and needs to be surgically managed.

Signs and Symptoms

A thorough family history is essential to uncover Rendu-Osler-Weber disease. The patient may give a history of recurrent, profuse nosebleeds. The patient may give a family or personal history of elevated blood pressure. The patient may either admit to nonadherence with the prescribed regimen or be unaware of the hypertension. Symptoms may include headache, lightheadedness, and pounding or swishing sounds in the ears. Hypertension is easily uncovered with blood pressure measurement. In Rendu-Osler-Weber disease, small telangiectatic lesions on the face, lips, oral mucosa, nasal mucosa, fingertips, and toes are characteristic, and the nosebleeds are profuse. Similar lesions occur internally in the mucosa of the gastrointestinal (GI) tract, which can cause major GI bleeding.

Diagnostic Studies

Diagnosis is usually made by history and physical examination. In Rendu-Osler-Weber disease, laboratory studies are normal except in iron-deficiency anemia, which may be severe. Genetic testing is necessary for definitive diagnosis. For hypertension, blood chemistries and renal studies, including 24-hour urine for catecholamines, should be done to rule out kidney or adrenal disease.

MALIGNANT NASAL AND SINUS TUMORS

Nasopharyngeal cancers are rare, causing less than 1% of all cancers. It is more common in the Asian population, affecting males at a higher rate than females (Chen et al., 2019). The most common cancers seen in this area are squamous cell carcinomas. Less common types in this area include adenocarcinoma, melanoma, sarcoma, and lymphoma. Risk factors include Epstein-Barr virus, which can cause a rare form of non-Hodgkin's lymphoma that affects nasal passages and paranasal sinuses; family history; tobacco use; and alcohol use.

Neoplasms can be found in the nasopharynx or paranasal sinuses, causing unilateral nasal obstruction, OM, and sinus infections. Patients are often asymptomatic until late in the course.

Signs and Symptoms

Patients often complain of persistent unilateral nasal congestion/obstruction, epistaxis, or ear fullness. Patients may also present with recurrent unilateral sinus or ear infections and/or pain that has failed symptomatic and antibiotic treatment. The red flag is the symptom of recurrent unilateral complaints. In advanced disease, there may be facial paresis if there is perineural invasion of the facial nerve or obvious swelling of the cheek or around the eye.

Diagnostic Studies

An MRI or CT scan is needed to define the extent of the tumor. Biopsy is necessary to confirm the diagnosis and the type of neoplasm.

■ Congestion and Drainage

Nasal congestion with associated drainage is one of the common complaints seen in the family practice setting. It is common in the winter months with the concomitant increase in upper respiratory infections. Complaints of congestion and drainage in the fall and spring may be due to allergies, and a thorough history and physical examination will assist in differentiating infection from allergy. Nasal congestion and drainage may be associated with non-allergic rhinitis or hormonal causes such as pregnancy.

History

As with any history, start with the onset of the symptoms, to include frequency, persistence, and progression. Ask about the presence of fever and about the color and consistency of the mucous drainage. Persistent fever and thick, yellow-green mucus indicate bacterial infection. Inquire about allergies to pollen and animals and the presence of environmental exposures to chemicals or noxious fumes. Explore related symptoms, such as sore throat, ear pain, headache, or cough. Ask about facial and/or sinus pain, which might indicate sinus involvement. Pruritis of the nose, palate, throat, and eyes differentiates allergic from non-allergic rhinitis. Some patients complain that their upper teeth hurt, which may indicate dental disease or sinus infection because the maxillary sinuses are located just above the upper teeth. Include questions regarding exposure to family members or coworkers with similar symptoms and whether they are being treated. A history of honey-colored sinus drainage following head trauma is a red flag because it may indicate a skull fracture.

Physical Examination

Vital signs are a good place to start looking for fever, which would indicate infection. Inspect the nasal mucosa with the nasal speculum as you look for septal deviation or lesions, redness, irritation, friability, and discharge. Nasal discharge should be assessed for its amount and color and any associated symptoms. Clear, profuse discharge is allergic in nature; yellow-green purulent discharge indicates infection. Palpate the sinuses for tenderness. Examine the pharynx, ears, lungs, and lymph system in the head and neck.

COMMON COLD

Differentiating a viral cold from a bacterial infection of the sinuses is one of the more challenging diagnostic exercises for any practitioner. The similarity of symptoms between viral and bacterial illnesses, accompanied by the patient expectation that antibiotics will cure all things, can make management difficult.

Signs and Symptoms

If the patient experienced malaise and fever initially but feels well aside from the congestion, then the cause is likely viral in nature. The viral illness will usually run its course in 5 to 7 days. When a viral cold is present, the physical examination is usually unimpressive in that it does not reveal any of the following: fever, TM dullness or redness, sinus pain/tenderness, or chest congestion.

Diagnostic Studies

No diagnostic imaging is recommended as diagnosis can usually be made with a history and physical.

RHINOSINUSITIS

Rhinosinusitis is an inflammation of the sinonasal mucosa caused by a viral or bacterial infection. Rhinosinusitis affects about 29 million people in the United States each year, costing approximately $11 billion (CDC, 2021a). Rhinosinusitis can be acute, with symptoms for less than 4 weeks; chronic, with persistent symptoms for more than 12 weeks; or recurrent, with four or more episodes of acute rhinosinusitis (ARS) per year with interim symptom resolution. ARS is further classified as acute viral rhinosinusitis (AVRS) and acute bacterial rhinosinusitis (ABRS). AVRS is most often caused by rhinovirus, but coronavirus, influenza A and B, parainfluenza, RSV, adenovirus, and enterovirus are also causative pathogens. Only 0.5% to 2% of AVRS progress to ABRS (Rosenfeld et al., 2015). Risk factors for ARS include smoking, air travel, exposure to changes in atmospheric pressure, asthma and allergies, dental disease, immunodeficiency, and anatomic blockages (deviated septum, nasal polyps, nasal mass). Pathogens most commonly responsible for ABRS are *Streptococcus pneumonia* (20%–43%), *Haemophilus influenza* (22%–33%), *Moraxella catarrhalis* (2%–10%), *Staphylococcus aureus* (3%–10%), and *Streptococcus pyogenes* (7%) (Rosenfeld et al., 2015; Patel & Hwang, 2018). Complications of ABRS can result in infection outside the paranasal sinuses and nasal cavity extending to the orbit and intercranial regions. Orbital complications are commonly seen in children and are a result of infection of the ethmoid, maxillary, or frontal sinuses. Worrisome symptoms include periorbital edema/erythema, displaced globe, double vision, ophthalmo-plegia, reduced visual acuity, severe headache, frontal swelling, signs of sepsis, or other neurological signs.

Chronic rhinosinusitis (CRS) symptoms can persist over 12 weeks and present with nasal obstruction and/or nasal discharge, facial pressure/pain, and reduction or loss of smell. CRS can be a result of allergic rhinitis (AR) with nasal polyposis, chronic allergies, fungal infections, autoimmune or inflamma-tory conditions such as Wegner's granulomatosis (rare autoimmune vascular disease affecting the sinuses, lungs, and kidneys), sarcoidosis, Samter's triad (characterized by asthma, nasal polyps, and ASA/NSAID intolerance), dental infections, and anatomic obstructions such as deviated septum or concha bullosa. Risk factors associated with CRS include smoking, asthma, chronic obstructive pulmonary disease, and immunosuppression (HIV, diabetes, neutropenia).

Signs and Symptoms

Symptoms of ARS are classified as having two or more symptoms: nasal obstruc-tion and/or nasal discharge, facial pain/pressure or both, and reduction and/or loss of smell. Viral symptoms are usually self-limiting and last 10 days or less. ABRS should be considered if patient presents with three or more symptoms: fevers, double worsening (symptoms improve but suddenly get worse), purulent drainage, unilateral symptoms, or severe sinus pain. Symptoms of ABRS persist over 10 days or can worsen over 5 days of initial onset. Therefore, it is important to elicit duration of symptoms from the patient. Patients may present with fever, frontal headache, severe sinus congestion, sinus and ear pain and/or pressure, difficulty breathing, sore throat, purulent nasal discharge, and malaise. Bacterial infection often worsens with time, which can help the provider make the diagno-sis of ABRS. The examination may reveal inflamed nasal mucosa; thick, purulent discharge; sinus tenderness; an accompanying dull or inflamed TM; pharyngeal erythema; and perhaps cervical lymphadenopathy. In CRS, nasal polyps or devi-ated septum may be identified.

Diagnostic Studies

In ARS, diagnostic studies are not recommended. Recurrent rhinosinusitis or persistent sinusitis after a course of antibiotics should be further investigated with a CT scan of the sinuses. A CBC may confirm a bacterial cause, and a C&S of the nasal discharge may identify the organism responsible for chronic infections. Patients with persistent, recurrent, or chronic sinusitis symptoms should be referred to an otolaryngology specialist for nasal endoscopy to rule out nasal polyposis, anatomic obstructions, nasal masses, and so on. Referral to an otolaryngology specialist also must be initiated in symptoms of periorbital edema, double vision, ophthalmoplegia, severe headache, frontal swelling, and/or neurological deficits.

See Figures 7.10 and 7.11 for algorithms for ARS and CRS.

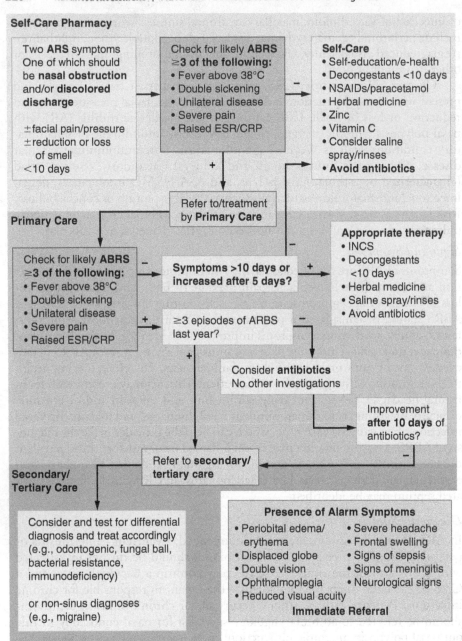

Figure 7.10 Acute rhinosinusitis algorithm. (From Fokkens, W. J., Lund, V. J., Hopkins, C., Hellings, P. W., Kern, R., Reitsma, S., et al. European Position Paper on Rhinosinusitis and Nasal Polyps 2020 Rhinology. 2020 (Suppl. 29), 1–464. Fig 1.4.1, page 9.)

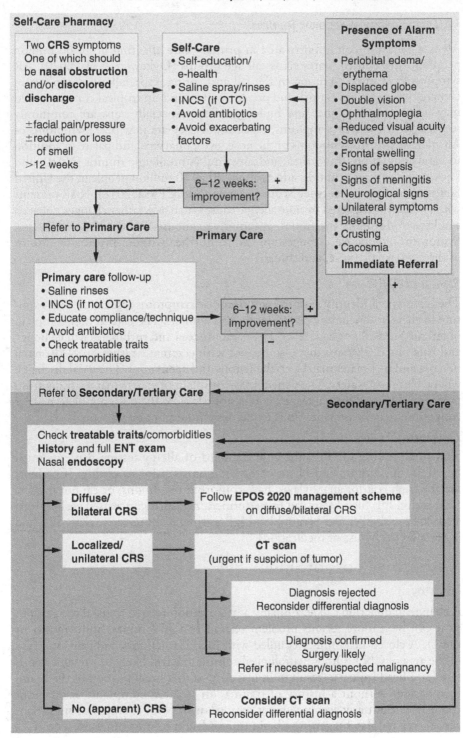

Figure 7.11 Chronic rhinosinusitis algorithm. (From Fokkens, W. J., Lund, V. J., Hopkins, C., Hellings, P. W., Kern, R., Reitsma, S., et al. European Position Paper on Rhinosinusitis and Nasal Polyps 2020 Rhinology. 2020 (Suppl. 29), 1–464. Fig 1.6.1, page 13.)

ALLERGIC AND NON-ALLERGIC RHINITIS

AR is a common condition treated in primary care affecting up to 60 million people in the United States across all age groups (Dykewicz et al., 2020). AR symptoms are more common in the fall and spring, especially in damp, warm climates where foliage is thick and present year-round. In tropical climates, mold may be present in homes and buildings. Pets, especially cats, are commonly responsible for allergy symptoms, especially if they are new pets. Symptoms of AR include pruritis symptoms of the nose, eyes, pharynx, and palate in addition to nasal congestion, rhinorrhea, and sneezing. Non-allergic rhinitis (NAR), also known as vasomotor rhinitis, affects about 20 to 30 million people in the United States, affecting women twice as often as men (Sur & Plesa, 2018). NAR presents with symptoms triggered by non-allergic causes such as weather changes, tobacco smoke, strong odors (perfumes, automotive exhausts), and hormonal causes. Symptoms include nasal congestion and rhinorrhea without pruritis symptoms of the eyes, palate, nose, and throat.

Signs and Symptoms

The history will identify seasonal symptoms or symptoms associated with exposure to allergens, including plants, foods, and animals. The patient may complain of fatigue but will not have fever. The nasal mucosa and turbinates will be boggy and pale in AR. Patients may also present with eczematic rashes. In NAR, nasal mucosa and turbinates may be erythematous and edematous. The nasal discharge will be clear and watery. The patient may complain of sore throat resulting from postnasal drip, and there may be a cobblestone look to the posterior pharynx. Ear congestion may be present. Sinus tenderness should not be present.

Diagnostic Studies

Skin prick testing (SPT) is the gold standard of allergy testing. Patients must be off antihistamines and H_2 receptor antagonists prior to testing. If patients are at a high risk for anaphylaxis, have comorbid conditions, or cannot tolerate SPT, serum IgE blood tests can be performed, measuring increased eosinophilia associated with allergies. Serum blood IgE testing is less sensitive than SPT and is not affected by use of medications.

■ Anosmia (Loss of Smell)

History

A change in olfaction can accompany any condition related to nasal congestion, or it can be a more serious problem related to CN I injury from trauma or tumor. A closed head injury coupled with loss of smell may indicate an injury in the area of CN I. Other neurological complaints will likely be present, as it is rare for a head injury to result in injury only to this small portion of the brain. In a patient without a history of trauma, an isolated complaint of olfactory changes without any accompanying symptoms of cold, allergies, or sinus congestion is a red flag suggesting a brain tumor. Brain tumors can cause a decrease in olfaction or, in some cases, olfactory hallucinations. Headache along with olfactory changes increases the index of suspicion for a tumor etiology. More recently, COVID-19 has emerged as a cause of anosmia, and it can persist for months.

Diagnostic Studies

A CT scan or MRI of the head is necessary to determine the presence of a tumor. A thorough neurological examination should be performed to detect other neurological abnormalities. See Chapter 16 for a more in-depth discussion.

Differential Diagnosis of Chief Complaints: Mouth

■ Mouth Sores (Painful and Painless)

Many conditions manifest with lesions on the lips and/or oral mucosa. Most are self-limiting conditions, such as aphthous ulcers; others, such as Behçet's syndrome and oral cancers, can result in significant morbidity if not recognized and treated promptly. Oral lesions associated with pain can be very distressing to patients. Labial lesions (those on the lips) cause distress because they are obvious and difficult to conceal. Painful lesions, both on the lips and in the mouth, can significantly impair a patient's ability to take food and fluids by mouth. A diagnosis of herpes simplex can be very upsetting to a patient because of the associations between herpes simplex and genital findings as well as the complexity and chronicity of the condition. A nonpainful lesion on the lips can be a malignancy, more common in those with significant sun exposure.

History

When a patient presents with a mouth sore, it is helpful to determine early in the history whether the lesion is painful, as certain conditions are more likely than others to cause painful lesions. It is important to obtain a thorough analysis of the symptoms, including when the lesion was first noticed, whether the lesion was preceded by other symptoms, and whether there is a history of similar symptoms in the past. Identify any associated symptoms, including fever, malaise, joint pain, shortness of breath, nausea, vomiting, diarrhea, photosensitivity, and so on. Identify any chronic or coexisting conditions as well as any prescribed or OTC medications taken.

Physical Examination

The physical examination should include measurement of vital signs, particularly noting the presence of fever. A thorough assessment of the specific lesion should be performed, noting the type of lesion involved (e.g., ulcer, vesicle, papule) as well as the dimensions, coloring, shape, distribution, and other details. The surrounding tissue should be closely inspected, noting edema, erythema, or pallor.

A thorough examination of the entire oral mucosa is necessary, with careful palpation of all accessible areas to note indurations, thickenings, nodules, or other palpable changes. Cervical lymph nodes should be palpated. Depending on the patient's presenting history and findings, examination may include other systems.

Diagnostic Studies

For most mouth sores, diagnostic studies are not indicated. However, lesions can be cultured to provide definitive diagnosis of candida, herpes simplex, or other infectious causes. In recurrent or persistent lesions, biopsies may be indicated to diagnose or rule out malignancy or systemic cause.

APHTHOUS ULCERS

The cause of aphthous ulcers (canker sores) is unclear. Several theories exist, including genetics, infection, stress, vitamin deficiencies, and food sensitivities. Recurrent aphthous ulcers occur in 20% of the population, more commonly in children (France & Villa, 2020). Systemic disease, such as inflammatory bowel disease, should be suspected in patients who present with anemia and GI conditions (Fig. 7.12).

Signs and Symptoms

The ulcers are painful and usually small (less than 1 cm), shallow, and surrounded by erythema and mild edema. The base of the ulcer is pale yellow or gray. Often only one ulcer is present, although patients may have multiple ulcers. On occasion, patients experience larger ulcers, which take longer to heal and are associated with increased pain. The patient often has had previous ulcers, which healed in approximately 1 week.

Diagnostic Studies

None are warranted. Occasionally, the ulcers can be cultured to rule out herpes simplex virus (HSV). Biopsies are usually not indicated unless systemic disease or malignancy is suspected. If anemia is present, folic acid and iron blood tests are recommended.

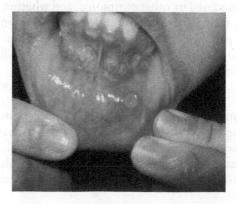

Figure 7.12 Aphthous ulcer.

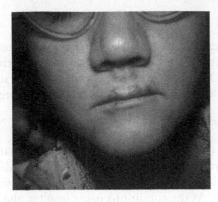

Figure 7.13 Herpes simplex.

HERPES SIMPLEX

Orolabial ulcers are often caused by HSV type 1. In 20% to 30% of patients, lesions present as painful ulcerations lasting 7 to 10 days (France & Villa, 2020). HSV is contagious and usually spreads through sexual or intimate contact. It can also be spread through sharing drinks and utensils and can be passed from mother to infant during childbirth (Fig. 7.13).

Signs and Symptoms
The patient often complains of a history of intermittent mouth sores, with onset in youth. The ulcers are typically preceded by a prodromal phase of tenderness, followed by edema at the site where an individual or cluster of vesicles forms and progresses to ulceration. The prodromal phase may also include malaise and fever. The vesicles have an erythematous base, and the ulcerated lesion often becomes crusted.

Diagnostic Studies
None are usually warranted. The vesicles can be cultured for definitive diagnosis; a Tzanck smear can be performed in the office for rapid diagnosis.

HERPES ZOSTER

Herpes zoster is described in Chapter 4. Compared with other painful mouth lesions, herpes zoster typically occurs in older individuals. Because the virus affects a dermatome, there are usually extra-oral findings and complaints.

CHEMICAL AND THERMAL BURNS

As with any of the integument, the oral mucosa is at risk for chemical and thermal burns. The history is extremely important to identify whether the patient has been exposed to chemical agents or to a thermal source that resulted in the painful lesion. The distribution of the lesion(s) should be consistent with the history of exposure.

HAND-FOOT-AND-MOUTH DISEASE

Hand-foot-and-mouth disease is caused by coxsackievirus 16 and enterovirus 17. It is common in children younger than 5 years, with symptoms lasting 7 to 10 days (France & Villa, 2020). Outbreaks are most common in the summer and fall months. In rare serotypes, the condition is occasionally associated with meningitis.

Signs and Symptoms

Painful skin and oral lesions are often preceded by a period of malaise and fever. The patient often presents once the lesions appear on the lips and/or oral mucosa. The lesions erupt as vesicles, which later ulcerate. Multiple lesions are located on the lips and oral mucosa. As the condition's name implies, the lesions often appear on the hands and feet as well as in the mouth. They may also be evident on the genitalia and buttocks.

Diagnostic Studies

Diagnostic studies are not usually warranted. The patient's hydration status should be monitored if the lesions impair ability to take food and/or fluids by mouth.

CANDIDIASIS

Candidiasis is caused by a species of the fungal genus *Candida* (Fig. 7.14). Risk factors for candidiasis include an impaired immune system, use of inhaled steroids, antibiotic therapy, malignancy, and recent surgery or trauma. Candidiasis affects a variety of systems and tissues, including the oral mucosa.

Signs and Symptoms

Candida infections of the oral mucosa take several forms. Thrush, or pseudo-membranous candida, results in white patches or plaques overlying a very red base. The plaques can be scraped off with a tongue blade. Erythematous candida results in erythematous lesions and, on occasion, ulcerative lesions. Angular stomatitis results in lesions at the corners or angles of the mouth. The amount of associated pain is variable.

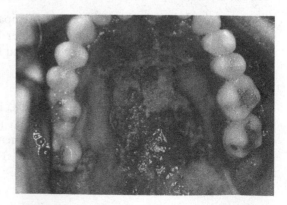

Figure 7.14 Candidiasis.

Diagnostic Studies

Studies are not usually necessary because the diagnosis is based on the findings. Fungal cultures can be used to isolate specific organisms.

BEHÇET'S SYNDROME

Behçet's disease is considered a syndrome because it involves a variety of problems, including oral lesions. Other characteristic findings include uveitis, arthralgia, genital lesions, and non-genital skin lesions. The condition affects males more often than females and is more common in young adults. Although rare, Behçet's syndrome can lead to significant morbidity, and the patient should be referred to a specialist for definitive diagnosis and treatment if the condition is suspected. The cause of Behçet's syndrome is unknown. It may be an autoimmune disorder, but it is likely that genetic and environmental factors also play a role. Several genes have been found to be associated with the disease. Some researchers believe a virus or bacterium may trigger Behçet's disease in people who have certain genes that make them susceptible.

Signs and Symptoms

The patient complains of recurrent episodes of oral lesions that are consistent with aphthous ulcers. The number of lesions ranges from one to several; the size of the ulcers varies from less than to greater than 1 cm. Like aphthous ulcers, the lesions are well defined, with a pale yellow or gray base surrounded by erythema. Most patients also develop lesions on the genitals or other skin. Eye findings are varied and include conjunctivitis, keratitis, uveitis, and others. The condition can, over time, lead to decreased visual acuity and blindness. Several other miscellaneous findings and/or complaints may include the GI, musculoskeletal, neurological, and cardiovascular systems.

Diagnostic Studies

There is no definitive laboratory test specific to Behçet's syndrome. Patients may have anemia, leukocytosis, elevated sedimentation rate, or elevated C-reactive protein. Rheumatoid factor and/or antinuclear antibody tests are negative.

ORAL LICHEN PLANUS

Lichen planus (LP) affects 1% to 2% of the population, affecting women between ages 30 and 60 years most often (Maymone et al., 2019). The exact cause of LP is not known. The condition causes inflammatory changes in the mouth, with the development of mucosal changes that are primarily white in color. Although the relationship between LP and oral cancers is not clear, there is a slight increased risk of malignancy (1.1%) in patients with LP, especially erosive LP (Maymone et al., 2019) (Fig. 7.15).

Signs and Symptoms

LP most often presents with white, lacy lines called Wickham striae. The most common sites include the buccal mucosa, gingiva, and tongue. LP forms include

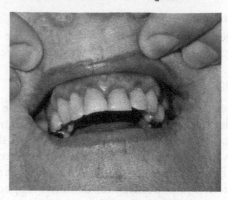

Figure 7.15 Oral lichen planus.

papular, plaque, erythematous or atrophic, erosive, or bullous (Maymone et al., 2019). Although pain is not always an early symptom, many patients complain of discomfort at the affected sites, especially when eating spicy foods. The more inflammatory and erosive lesions are usually painful. Episodes of LP are often recurrent. Some patients develop extra-oral pruritic skin lesions of the extremities, genitalia, and/or scalp, as well as nail changes.

Diagnostic Studies

Diagnostic studies are often not required. However, biopsies can be performed to rule out malignancy and to provide definitive diagnosis.

ERYTHEMA MULTIFORME

Erythema multiforme is described in detail in Chapter 4. Oral lesions are common manifestations of erythema multiforme, ranging from shallow, crusted lesions of the lips to deeper ulcerations of the lips and oral mucosa. Depending on the severity, lesions may have a necrotic appearance.

INFECTIOUS CAUSES OF ORAL LESIONS

In addition to the infections noted previously, many others have painful oral mucosal manifestations. These include gonorrhea, syphilis, HIV, and chickenpox.

NONINFECTIOUS SYSTEMIC CONDITIONS

A wide range of systemic conditions, including Crohn's disease, ulcerative colitis, anemia, and sarcoidosis, are associated with oral lesions. It is important to explore the other potential symptoms when the patient presents with unexplained oral lesions.

LEUKOPLAKIA

Leukoplakia is a common premalignant lesion of the oral mucosa presenting as white, hyperkeratotic, nonscrapable lesions. Leukoplakia is more common in men older than 40 years and has a malignant transformation rate from 0.1% to 36% (Maymone et al., 2019). The cause of most episodes of leukoplakia is not determined. Risk factors for the development of leukoplakia include chronic/recurrent trauma to the affected site, a use of smokeless and smoked tobacco, human papilloma virus (HPV), betel quid, and use of alcohol.

Signs and Symptoms

The lesions are painless, so the patient will usually have noticed the lesion after looking in the mouth. Most lesions present as a flat, white, superficial plaque on mucosal lining of the oral cavity. Some lesions become "warty" and raised, and thus a patient can feel the lesion's presence. However, most are flat and smooth. Unlike thrush, these lesions cannot be rubbed or scraped away.

Diagnostic Studies

The diagnosis is usually based on the history and physical examination. However, biopsy should be considered to rule out dysplasia. The patient should be clinically evaluated on a routine basis to make sure the area does not change in size or other features.

ERYTHROPLAKIA

Erythroplakia presents as an erythematous lesion most commonly affecting the buccal mucosa, palate, ventral tongue, and floor of mouth. Erythroplakia has a 50% risk of malignant transformation (Maymone et al., 2019). Risk factors include tobacco and alcohol use and HPV-16 and -18. These lesions often coexist with leukoplakia in the form of "speckled leukoplakia," where leukoplakia lesions are superimposed on larger erythemal lesions.

Signs and Symptoms

These lesions are painless, so the patient may not notice the lesion unless the patient has inspected the oral mucosa for some reason. The lesions are usually flat or depressed below the mucosal surface and often have a velvety texture. Some erythroplakia lesions are "pebbly," with raised areas. The red lesions vary in size and are often very well demarcated. On palpation, they may be firm or soft.

Diagnostic Studies

Biopsies are obtained on referral to a specialist for definitive diagnosis. Complete excision of the lesion is indicated for severe dysplasia. Monitoring for recurrence is recommended.

MALIGNANCY

The annual incidence of oral cancer is 5% to 15% per 100,000, affecting males at a greater rate than females (3:1) (Maymone et al., 2019). The most common form of oral cancer is squamous cell cancer. More than 50% of oral cavity cancers originate in the tongue or floor of mouth. The risk factors associated with cancer of the oral cavity include tobacco use, alcohol use, betel quid, poor oral health, sun exposure (lip carcinoma), systemic disease, and premalignant lesions. As tobacco use has decreased in the United States, there is a growing incidence of oropharyngeal cancer, especially among younger, white, nonsmoking males, as a result of an increasing incidence of HPV infections. Approximately 70% of oropharyngeal cancer is related to HPV variants 16 and 18. Risk factors include high-risk sexual behaviors and other sexually transmitted infections (Maymone et al., 2019).

Oral mucosal melanoma is uncommon (1%), affecting white males at a higher incidence. The hard palate and maxillary gingiva are the most common sites for oral malignant melanoma. Because many oral cancers are not diagnosed until they are quite advanced, there is a high risk of metastasis, resulting in a poor prognosis.

Signs and Symptoms

Cancers of the oral cavity can present as white patches (leukoplakia) or reddened patches (erythroplakia), progressing to areas of induration/thickening, ulceration, or necrotic lesions. In small, early cancers, patients may be asymptomatic; however, as the lesion grows, pain can be a common symptom. Pain can be referred to the ear and throat. Patients may also complain of odynophagia, dysphagia, globus sensation, hemoptysis, bleeding from lesion, chronic OM, trismus, decreased movement of the tongue, and/or weight loss.

Lesions of malignant melanoma are painless, irregular lesions that have varied pigmentation, including brown, blue, and black. On palpation, lesions that appear flat and smooth may be nodular, indurated, or fixed to adjacent tissue on palpation. The cervical lymph nodes may be enlarged and could be the only presenting symptom.

Diagnostic Studies

Oral malignancy is diagnosed by biopsy. Diagnostic imaging (CT with contrast or MRI) is used to evaluate size, invasion, and metastasis to lymph nodes.

KAPOSI'S SARCOMA

Kaposi's sarcoma is a vascular tumor often associated with HIV. It is believed that a herpes virus is implicated in the development of this condition.

Signs and Symptoms

Like the other oral malignancies described in the preceding subsections, the lesions of Kaposi's sarcoma are usually painless. The lesions most commonly occur on the palate, which is not easily seen by the patient, although it can occur on any of the oral mucosa. Initially flat, the lesions often become nodular with time. The coloring of the lesions is consistent with a vascular tumor and range from deep reddish brown to purple. The patient may provide a history of HIV.

Diagnostic Studies

Diagnosis is made by biopsy.

DENTURE OR ORTHODONTIC DERMATITIS

Individuals wearing dentures and orthodontic devices are at risk for developing oral lesions, which may be related to an allergic reaction to a component of the device or to chronic rubbing and irritation from the device.

Signs and Symptoms

These lesions may result in mild discomfort or be painless. The history and physical findings should be consistent with use of the appliance that has caused the irritation.

Diagnostic Studies

No diagnostic studies are indicated.

■ Mouth Pain Without Obvious Lesions

On occasion, patients present with mouth pain yet have no visible lesions. In this case, the history should be directed to a careful analysis of the pain from the time it was first noticed. A thorough review of systems and a history of present illness and medications taken are necessary. Ask the patient about recent trauma, systemic diseases, or previous episodes of similar pain.

A careful examination of the mouth should be conducted. Most patients experiencing mouth pain without the clinical signs to guide diagnosis should be referred to a dentist or otolaryngology specialist for assessment.

DENTAL PAIN

See Chapter 5.

HERPES

Both herpes simplex and herpes zoster affect the oral mucosa. The appearance of skin lesions is often preceded by a prodromal phase that may include tingling and pain.

Signs and Symptoms

The patient with herpes simplex may report a history of recurrent painful mouth sores, often preceded by discomfort, before an eruption of herpetic lesions. A patient who is developing herpes zoster may describe pain distributed along a specific dermatome. There may be some palpable induration and lymphadenopathy, particularly with herpes simplex infections. Mouth pain may be the presenting complaint in a patient who is experiencing postherpetic neuralgia after the visible signs of herpes zoster have resolved.

Diagnostic Studies

There are no diagnostic studies warranted if either early herpes simplex or early herpes zoster is suspected. Follow-up should be arranged to confirm diagnosis.

See Chapter 5.

BURNING MOUTH SYNDROME

Burning mouth syndrome is characterized by burning pain of the oral structures with absence of clinical signs. It is more common in women than in men. The onset is typically sudden and is sometimes variable through the day. The cause is uncertain, although there are several theories under consideration, including diabetes, nutritional deficit, dry mouth, and emotional disorders (depression, anxiety, and stress).

Signs and Symptoms

The patient complains of significant burning pain that may affect the ability to sleep or to focus on normal daily activities. Many patients also complain of altered taste. There are no visible clinical signs or abnormalities.

Diagnostic Studies

The condition is a diagnosis of exclusion. The patient should be referred for specialist assessment.

Differential Diagnosis of Chief Complaints: Throat

■ Pharyngitis

Pharyngitis (sore throat) is a very frequent complaint in primary care settings. Most episodes of sore throat are associated with self-limited viral upper respiratory infections. Bacterial infections such as group A Streptococcus, gonorrhea, and syphilis can also be the cause. Gastroesophageal reflux disease can also cause pharyngitis. Prolonged pharyngitis can be associated with head and neck cancers.

History

The history should begin with a thorough analysis of the throat pain, including onset, duration, description (scratchy sore throat to excruciating throat pain), dysphagia, odynophagia, and weight loss. In addition to determining the characteristics of the pain, identifying all associated symptoms and past medical history is helpful in narrowing the differential diagnosis. It is important to identify any other recent illnesses as well as recent exposures to others who are ill. Determine whether the patient is experiencing any respiratory difficulty.

Physical Examination

The physical examination for sore throat should include comprehensive assessment of the upper and lower respiratory systems, including ears, nose, mouth, throat, and lungs. The neck assessment should include, at a minimum, assessment of the cervical lymph nodes. A more thorough neck assessment is indicated if thyroiditis is suspected.

Diagnostic Studies

Strep screens, throat cultures, and mononucleosis screens are common diagnostic studies used to narrow the differential diagnosis of sore throat. A CBC with differential count is helpful in determining the cause of sore throat.

INFECTIOUS PHARYNGITIS

Most cases of pharyngitis are viral in origin, and any number of the respiratory viruses can cause inflammation of the throat. Most viral pharyngitis cases are self-limited. Herpes infections can also affect the pharynx. GAS pharyngitis is a bacterial infection of the pharynx, commonly called strep throat. Complications of GAS pharyngitis, although rare, include rheumatic heart disease and glomerulonephritis, and the condition requires prompt diagnosis and definitive treatment. Most patients with GAS pharyngitis are children and teenagers. Other bacterial causes of pharyngitis include mycoplasma pneumonia, gonorrhea, syphilis, and diphtheria.

Signs and Symptoms

Complaints typically include malaise, headache, rhinitis, and/or cough in addition to the throat pain, which can range from mild, scratchy discomfort to severe pain. The onset can be sudden, as with influenza, or it may develop over many hours. Fever and chills may be present. In all cases of pharyngitis, the pharynx is reddened, and tender lymphadenopathy is often present. The findings associated with varied causes of non-GAS pharyngitis are summarized in Table 7.5.

The classic symptom of GAS is a severe sore throat with sudden onset. The patient often also complains of nausea, vomiting, fever, headache, and malaise. Unlike other forms of pharyngitis, the patient does not usually experience

Table 7.5

Differential Diagnosis of Infectious Pharyngitis

Cause	Onset	Associated Symptoms	Pharyngeal Signs	Anterior Lymphadenopathy
Respiratory viruses	Variable	Headache, fever, chills, malaise, rhinitis, conjunctivitis, cough, nausea, diarrhea	Inflamed pharynx	Present
Rhinitis/sinusitis	Evolves over few days	Rhinorrhea, thick nasal discharge, headache, fever	Inflamed pharynx from post-nasal drip	Usually present
Herpes pharyngitis	Evolves with prodromal phase	Malaise, fever	Inflamed with ulcerative lesions	Present
Herpangina or hand-foot-and-mouth disease	Evolves over few days	Malaise; lesions in mouth, on hands, feet, buttocks, and/or genitalia	Inflamed with ulcerative lesions	Present

(cont. on page 242)

Table 7.5

Differential Diagnosis of Infectious Pharyngitis—cont'd

Cause	Onset	Associated Symptoms	Pharyngeal Signs	Anterior Lymphadenopathy
Diphtheria	Evolves over 1 to 2 days	Headache, rhinitis, fever/chills, dysphagia, difficulty breathing	Inflamed pharynx with thick, gray membrane	Present
Group A streptococcal pharyngitis	Sudden onset	Malaise, nausea, vomiting, diarrhea, headache, sandpaper rash Absence of rhinitis, cough, conjunctivitis	Inflamed uvula, pharynx, tonsils; white-gray tonsillar exudate	Present
Mycoplasma pneumonia	Variable	Cough, dyspnea, pharyngitis, fever, headache	Wheezing Pneumonia diagnosed on CXR	Varies
Early HIV	Variable	Malaise, fatigue, fever, headache, pharyngitis, night sweats, weight loss	Ulcers or exudate of the posterior pharynx	Present
Oral neisseria gonorrhea			Dysphagia, pharyngeal lesions, cervical lymphadenopathy	
Syphilis			Chancres, on lips, tip of tongue, gums and/or posterior pharynx	
Noninfectious causes	Variable			Absent
GERD		Cough		
Allergic Rhinitis		Clear nasal discharge Postnasal drip	Cobble-stoning, boggy nasal mucosa	
Tobacco use		Hoarse voice		
Dysphonia		Hoarse voice		

rhinitis or cough. The patient often appears quite ill and lethargic. The findings of GAS include very inflamed pharynx, uvula, and tonsils. The tonsils are enlarged, usually with a white or gray-white exudate. There is tender cervical lymphadenopathy. Although some patients with viral pharyngitis may have an exanthem, GAS can present with a fine scarlatina rash, often described as "sandpaper" rash owing to the tiny, punctate pink-red lesions.

The modified Centor criteria score provides a commonly used decision tool for possible GAS. The formula assigns points for fever, tonsillar exudates, tender cervical lymphadenopathy, and absence of cough. A point is added if the patient is age 3 to 14 years and deducted if the patient is 45 years or older. Patients with no more than two points are presumed to not have GAS so that further testing is not advised (Harris et al., 2016).

Diagnostic Studies

With GAS pharyngitis, a throat culture and/or rapid strep assay is positive. If sexually transmitted infection is suspected, a throat culture is needed to rule out gonorrhea, chlamydia trachomatis, and syphilis (especially in HIV patients).

MONONUCLEOSIS

Mononucleosis is common among teenagers and young adults, usually caused by the Epstein-Barr virus, although it can result from other viruses. Even though complications are rare, they can lead to significant morbidity or death. The potential list of complications is broad and includes hepatitis, splenic rupture, myocarditis, meningitis/encephalitis, and hemolytic anemia.

Signs and Symptoms

The patient often complains of an onset over several days or more than a week. The sore throat may be preceded by prodromal symptoms that include malaise, fevers, fatigue, generalized aches, and headache. Throat pain is usually severe and is associated with lymphadenopathy of the posterior cervical nodes in addition to generalized lymphadenopathy. The pharynx is inflamed, and the tonsils are usually involved, with inflammation and exudate that ranges from white to yellow or green. The pharynx is often similar in appearance to GAS. Petechiae over the palate are often identified. A maculopapular generalized rash frequently occurs. Other skin changes may include jaundice. Splenomegaly is common, and hepatomegaly may also be present.

Diagnostic Studies

The white blood cell count is increased, with an increased ratio of lymphocytes. A rapid Monospot test is often positive in the clinical setting. Liver function tests are often elevated. Depending on the degree of findings suggesting one of the previously listed potential complications, consultation of or referral to the appropriate specialist should be completed. If no referral is warranted, close follow-up in the primary care setting is essential.

TONSILLITIS

Tonsillitis involves infection of the tonsils, most commonly as a result of a viral infection; however, GAS can be a bacterial cause and be associated with more serious complications (Fig. 7.16 and Fig. 7.17). Most cases of tonsillitis are diagnosed in school-aged children and adolescents. Patients can develop chronic tonsillitis and/or have frequent recurrences of the condition.

Signs and Symptoms

The patient complains of severe throat pain and difficulty swallowing. A fever is present, and the patient appears ill. The patient is usually mouth breathing, has a deepened voice, and may have difficulty articulating and moving the mouth because of the swelling and pain. Pain may be referred to the ears. The tonsils are edematous and have exudate that varies in color. If Epstein-Barr virus is present,

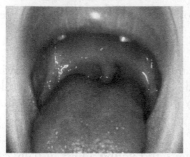
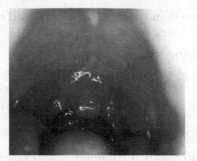

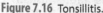

Figure 7.16 Tonsillitis.   **Figure 7.17** Tonsillitis.

palatal petechiae may be visible. If herpes virus is present, tonsillar ulcerations are visible. Lymphadenopathy is present, and the patient limits neck motion owing to pain. The history may reveal previous episodes.

Diagnostic Studies

Definitive diagnosis is made by throat culture, rapid strep, and/or a Monospot test.

PERITONSILLAR ABSCESS

Peritonsillar abscesses (PTA) may occur at any age, although most cases peak in young adults ages 15 to 19 years. The incidence in the United States for ages 5 to 59 years is 30 per 100,000 (Gupta & McDowell, 2021). Many cases evolve as a complication of tonsillitis, but others develop as PTA without a history of tonsillitis. The condition involves infection of the peritonsillar space. There are many pathogens that cause PTA; however, GAS and *Fusobacterium necrophorum* are responsible for more than 50% of infections (Klug et al., 2020). Complications of PTA include airway obstruction, poststreptococcal sequelae (rheumatic fever, glomerulonephritis), and extension of infection to the deep neck, mediastinum, and/or lung secondary. Identifying and treating PTA is essential to preventing complications.

Signs and Symptoms

The patient describes the onset of sore throat, fever, and malaise over several days. Symptoms progress to a severe sore throat, localized to one side, with associated symptoms of odynophagia, dysphagia, and ipsilateral otalgia. The severe odynophagia causes the patient to drool because it hurts to swallow saliva. It becomes increasingly difficult for the patient to move the neck and speak. The patient's voice is a muffled or "hot potato" voice. The patient's breath is fetid. Respiratory distress is possible and should be identified early to avoid life-threatening airway obstruction. Pharyngeal examination can be difficult, as the patient may have trismus, an inability to open the jaw because of the swelling. On examination of the pharynx, there is swelling and erythema of the anterior tonsil pillar and soft palate. The tonsil is often displaced with deviation of the uvula away from the infected tonsil. There may be signs consistent with dehydration, including dry skin and tachycardia.

Diagnostic Studies

The patient should be referred to the emergency department or otolaryngology specialist, who may aspirate the abscess to obtain a culture or obtain a culture at the time of therapeutic incision and drainage. The white blood cell count is elevated. An ultrasound or CT scan is used to confirm diagnosis.

EPIGLOTTITIS

Epiglottitis is an inflammation of the epiglottis and supraglottic structures caused by a bacterial infection. Before the immunization of *Haemophilus influenza* vaccine (HIB), children between the ages of 2 and 6 years were commonly affected. There has been a shift toward the adult population developing epiglottis; however, it can occur at any age. Although rare, it can cause significant respiratory obstruction resulting in death. Causes most commonly include bacterial infections such as GAS and *H. influenza.*

Signs and Symptoms

The patient presents with rapidly developing sore throat, fever, cough, and difficulty swallowing. The patient's voice is a muffled, "hot potato" voice, and there is drooling. Stridor and/or varying signs of respiratory distress may be evident. The patient often leans forward and breathes with the mouth open while sitting to maximize airway opening (tripod position). The patient has a very ill appearance, and gentle palpation over the larynx causes significant pain. Cervical adenopathy is present. Inspection of the posterior pharynx should not be attempted until the patient is in a location with access to intubation and/ or emergency tracheotomy.

Diagnostic Studies

The patient should be closely monitored for complete airway obstruction, but urgent referral for emergency care via an ambulance is indicated prior to performing any diagnostic evaluation, because the potential exists for sudden loss of airway.

THYROIDITIS

Painful subacute thyroiditis involves inflammation of the thyroid gland. It is a self-limiting condition and includes a hyperthyroid phase, followed by a period of hypothyroidism, before the patient regains a euthyroid state. More women than men are affected. A variant, postpartum thyroiditis occurs within 6 months of giving birth and is generally painless. Although the etiology of painful subacute thyroiditis is not clear, it may have a viral trigger.

Signs and Symptoms

Patients commonly complain of pain in the throat and/or neck, with radiation to an ear. Onset is described as relatively sudden, and associated symptoms include fever, malaise, and achiness. The throat pain may be associated with dysphagia. The patient may not complain of symptoms of hyperthyroidism or hypothyroidism during those phases; however, the severity of metabolic symptoms is quite variable. On physical examination, the thyroid region is very tender and enlarged.

Diagnostic Studies

Depending on the phase during which diagnosis is made, thyroid studies may be increased or decreased. The sedimentation rate is usually elevated. If radioactive iodine uptake is performed, uptake will be low. Thyroid antibodies may be elevated in painful thyroiditis.

Chronic Sore Throat

Most sore throat complaints involve acute conditions. Figure 7.18 depicts an algorithmic approach to chronic sore throat (i.e., sore throat existing for over 12 weeks in spite of conventional treatment).

■ Hoarseness (Dysphonia)

Hoarseness affects 1 in 13 adults in the United States, affecting women at a higher rate (Lenell et al., 2020). While the causes of hoarseness can be self-limiting, typically secondary to a viral upper respiratory infection, prolonged hoarseness can be caused by other etiologies that warrant further work up. Risk factors for voice disorders include increased age and occupation (teachers, drill sergeants, ministers) because of voice overuse.

Voice overuse or stress is a common cause of hoarseness. It can occur at any age and may be a recurrent problem for patients who use their voice extensively in lecturing, singing, or speaking in loud environments. The patient provides a history consistent with voice overuse or abuse. The hoarseness may tend to occur toward the end of the day or with prolonged speaking and improve the next morning after some period of rest. The hoarseness may be associated with a sensation of muscle tension and/or discomfort in the neck.

Other causes of hoarseness result from vocal trauma, smoking, emotional or psychological conditions, vocal cord paresis, vocal cord mass (benign and/or malignant), vocal cord leukoplakia, tumor of the lung or mediastinum, neurological conditions (Parkinson's disease, stroke), and endocrine and rheumatologic conditions (Wegner's granulomatosis, sarcoid) (see Table 7.6 for causes of hoarseness).

History

When a patient presents with hoarseness or voice alteration, it is important to obtain an explanation of how the voice has changed—in tone, volume, and so on. Quality of voice is also important, identifying if the patient has a breathy or gravelly voice or loses the breath with speaking. Determine whether the onset was sudden or gradual and whether the change has been constant or intermittent. Also determine the patient's typical pattern of voice use and whether any unusual use (e.g., singing, lecturing, shouting) occurred before the onset of hoarseness. The presence of associated symptoms, such as sore throat, unilateral otalgia, weight loss, dysphagia, odynophagia, neck mass, neck pain, postnasal drainage, heartburn, and/or cough, is important. Identify the use of alcohol and

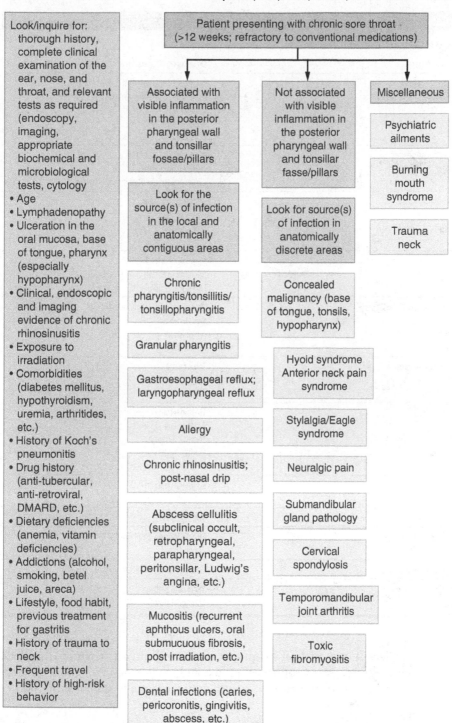

Figure 7.18 Chronic sore throat algorithm. (From Kundu, S., Dutta, M., Adhikary, B., & Ghosh, B. [2019]). Encountering chronic sore throat: How challenging is it for the otolaryngologist? *Indian Journal of Otolaryngology and Head and Neck Surgery*, 71(Suppl. 1), 176–181. Figure 1.)

Table 7.6

Causes of Hoarseness

Systems	Diseases/Conditions
Neoplastic	Laryngeal squamous cell carcinoma Recurrent respiratory papillomatosis Chondroma Lymphoma Leukoplakia
Neurological	• Spasmodic dysphonia • Vocal cord paresis • Essential tremor/Parkinson's disease
Endocrine	Hypothyroidism Diabetes Menopause Hormone therapy
Infectious	Upper viral infection Bacterial infection Laryngeal candidiasis
Autoimmune	Granulomatosis (Wegner's disease) Sarcoidosis Amyloidosis Rheumatoid arthritis
Inflammatory	Tobacco use Polypoid corditis Allergy
Surgical	Thyroidectomy or parathyroidectomy Anterior spinal surgery Thoracic surgery Cardiac surgery Neurosurgery and skull base surgery
Traumatic	Laryngeal fracture Intubation injury
Behavioral	Voice overuse
Musculoskeletal	Muscle tension dysphonia Cervicalgia
Gastrointestinal	Gastroesophageal reflux disease
Congenital	Vocal cord web Laryngeal cleft

tobacco. Identify the medical history of such conditions as thyroid disorders, pulmonary disease, gastroesophageal reflux, and malignancy. Ask about surgical history (recent surgery/intubation) as well as any trauma to the neck or chest.

Physical Examination

The physical examination specific to a complaint of hoarseness should include the ears, nose, throat, neck, lungs, and CNs (particularly CN IX and CN X).

Diagnostic Studies

For persistent hoarseness, referral to an otolaryngology specialist is warranted for direct laryngoscopy. Laryngoscopy is a diagnostic procedure using a flexible scope with a camera to view the upper airway. The larynx is assessed for movement and function of the vocal cords, masses, polyps, and/or edema of the vocal cords. See Table 7.6 for causes of hoarseness and associated findings.

REFERENCES

Allan, G. M., & Arroll, B. (2014) Prevention and treatment of the common cold: Making sense of the evidence. *Canadian Medical Association Journal, 186*(3),190–199. https://doi.org/10.1503/cmaj.121442

Batson, L., & Rizzolo, D. (2017). Otosclerosis: An update on diagnosis and treatment. *Journal of the American Academy of Physician Assistants, 30*(2), 17–22.

Boatman, D. F., Miglioretti, D. L., Eberwein, C., Alidoost, M., & Reich, S. G. (2007). How accurate are bedside hearing tests? *Neurology, 68*(16), 1311–1314.

Centers for Disease Control. (2018a). Summary Health Statistics: National Health Interview Survey, Table A-2. Selected respiratory diseases among adults aged 18 and over, by selected characteristics: United States, 2018. Retrieved August 11, 2021, from https://ftp.cdc.gov › SHS › 2018_SHS_Table_A-2.pdf

Centers for Disease Control and Prevention. (2018b). The National Institute for Occupational Safety and Health (NIOSH) Noise and Hearing Loss Prevention: Risk Factors. Retrieved August 9, 2021, from https://www.cdc.gov/niosh/topics/noise/default.html

Centers for Disease Control and Prevention. Chronic Sinusitis. (2021). Retrieved August 11, 2021, from https://www.cdc.gov/nchs/fastats/sinuses.htm

Chaaban, M., Zhang, D., Resto, V., & Goodwin, J. (2017). Demographic, Seasonal, and Geographic Differences in Emergency Department Visits for Epistaxis. *Otolaryngology-Head and Neck Surgery, 56*(1), 81–86.

Chandrasekhar, S., Tsai Do, B., Schwartz, S., Bontempo, L., Faucett, E., Finestone, S., Hollingsworth, D., Kelley, D., Kmucha, S., Moonis, G., Poling, G., Roberts, J., Stachler, R., Zeitler, D., Corrigan, M., Nnacheta, L., & Satterfield, L. (2019). Clinical practice guideline: Sudden hearing loss (Update). *Otolaryngology Head and Neck Surgery, 161*(1 Suppl), S1–S45, doi.org/10.1177/0194599819859885

Chen, Y-P., Chan, A., Le, Q-T., Blanchard, P., Sun, Y., & Ma, J. (2019). Nasopharyngeal Carcinoma. *Lancet, 394*(10192), 64–80. doi: 10.1016/S0140-6736(19)30956-0

Dykewicz, M., Wallace, D. V., Amrol, D., Baroody, F., Bernstein, J., Craig, T., Dinakar, C., Ellis, A., Finegold, I., Golden, D. B. K., Greenhawt, M., Hagan, J., Horner, C., Khan, D. A., Lang, D., Larenas-Linnemann, D., Lieberman, J., Meltzer, E., Shaker, M., Shaw, J., . . . Wang, J. (2020). Rhinitis 2020: A practice parameter update. *Journal of Allergy Clinical Immunology, 146*(4), 721–767.

Fokkens, W., Lund, V., Hopkins, C., Hellings, P., Kern, R., Reitsma, S., Toppila-Salmi, S., Bernal-Sprekelsen, M., & Mullol, J. (2020). Executive summary of EPOS 2020 including integrated care pathways. *Rhinology, 58*(2), 82–111.

France, K., & Villa, A. (2020). Acute oral lesions. *Dermatologic Clinics,* 38, 441–450.

Gaddey, H. L., Wright, M. T., & Nelson, T. N. (2019). Otitis media: Rapid evidence review. *American Family Physician, 100*(6), 350–356.

Goldbrunner, R., Weller, M., Regis, J., Lund-Johansen, M., Stavrinou, P., Reuss, D., Evans, D., Lefranc, F., Sallabanda, K., Falini, A., Axon, P., Sterkers, O., Fariselli, L., Wick, W., & Tonn, J-C. (2020). EANO guideline on the diagnosis and treatment of vestibular schwannoma. *Neuro-Oncology, 22*(1), 31–45.

Goman, A., & Lin, F. (2016). Prevalence of hearing loss by severity in the United States. *American Journal of Public Health, 106*(10),1820–1822.

Gupta, G., & McDowell, R. (2021). Peritonsillar abscess. *NCBI StatPearls.* https://www.ncbi.nlm.nih.gov/books/NBK519520/

Harris, A., Hicks, L., & Qaseem, A. (2016). Appropriate antibiotic use for acute respiratory tract infection in adults: Advice for high-value care from the American College of Physicians and the Centers for Disease Control and Prevention. *Annals of Internal Medicine, 164*(6), 425–434.

Klug, T., Greve, T., & Hentze, M. (2020). Complications of peritonsillar abscess. *Annals of Clinical Microbiology and Antimicrobials, 19*(32), 1–17.

Kundu, S., Dutta, M., Adhikary, B., & Ghosh, B. (2017). Encountering chronic sore throat: How challenging is it for otolaryngologists? *Indian Journal Otolaryngology Head and Neck Surgery, 71*(Suppl 1), S176–S181.

Maymone, M., Greer, R., Kesecker, J., Sahitya, P., Burdine, L., Cheng, A-D., Maymone, A., & Vashi, N. (2019). Premalignant and malignant oral mucosal lesions: Clinical and pathological findings. *Journal of the American Academy of Dermatology,* 81, 59–71.

National Institute on Deafness and Other Communication Disorders. (2021). Quick statistics about hearing. Retrieved August 16, 2021, from https://www.nidcd.nih.gov/health/statistics/quick-statistics-hearing

Patel, Z,, & Hwang, P. (2018). Acute Bacterial Rhinosinusitis. National Institutes of Health. Infections of the Ears, Nose, Throat and Sinuses. May 4, 133-143. doi: 10.1007/978-3-319-74835-1_11.

Rosenfeld, R., Schwartz, S., Cannon, C., Roland, P., Simon, G., Kumar, K., Huang, W., Haskell, H., & Robertson, P. (2014). Clinical practice guideline: acute otitis externa. *Otolaryngology Head and Neck Surgery, 150*(IS), S1–S24. https//doi.org/10.1177/0194599813517083

Rosenfeld, R., Piccirillo, J., Chandrasekhar, S., Brook, I., Kumar, K., Kramper, M., Orlandi, R., Palmer, J., Patel, Z., Peters, A., Walsh, S., & Corrigan, M. (2015). Clinical Practice Guideline (Update): Adult sinusitis. *Otolaryngology-Head and Neck Surgery, 152*(2), S1–S39.

Schwartz, S., Magit, A., Rosenfeld, R., Ballachanda, B., Hackell, J., Krouse, H., Lawlor, C., Lin, K., Parham, K., Stutz, D., Walsh, S., Woodson, E., Yanagisawa, K., & Cunningham, E. (2017). Clinical practice guideline (update): Earwax (cerumen impaction). *Otolaryngology Head and Neck Surgery, 156*(1S), S1–S29.

Sur, D., & Plesa, M. (2018). Chronic nonallergic rhinitis. *American Family Physician, 98*(3), 171–176.

Tunkel, D., Bauer, C., Sun, G., Rosenfeld, R., Chandrasekhar, S., Cunningham, E., Archer, S., Blakley, B., Carter, J., Granieri, E., Henry, J., Hollingsworth, D., Khan, F., Mitchell, S., Monfared, A., Newman, C., Omole, F., Phillips, C., Robinson, S., Taw, M., . . . Whamond, E. (2014). Clinical practice guideline: Tinnitus. *Otolaryngology Head and Neck Surgery, 15*(2S), S1–S40.

Tunkel, D., Anne, S., Payne, S., Ishman, S., Rosenfeld, R., Abramson, P., Alikhaani, J., Benoit, M., Bercovitz, R., Brown, M., Chernobilsky, B., Feldstein, D., Hackell, J., Holbrook, E., Holdsworth, S., Lin, K., Lind, M., Poetker, D., Riley, C., Schneider, J., . . . Monjur, T. (2020). Clinical Guideline: Nosebleed (Epistaxis). *Otolaryngol Head Neck Surg, 162*(1_suppl), S1–S38. doi: 10.1177/0194599819890327.

Chapter 8

Cardiac and Peripheral Vascular Systems

Laurie Grubbs ·

Leslie L. Davis ·

CARDIAC SYSTEM

Cardiovascular disease (CVD) is the leader in all-cause morbidity and mortality regardless of age or sex. It includes heart failure (HF), cerebrovascular disease, peripheral vascular disease (PVD), hypertension (HTN), valvular heart disease, and coronary artery disease (CAD), which accounts for about 50% of all CVD. Men are affected more than women by CVD, especially before the age of 50, but after age 50, the incidence rate for women increases and eventually surpasses the incidence of cases for men. CVD often goes undetected, especially among women. Early detection and intervention can save many lives, and advanced practice registered nurses can have a significant impact in terms of prevention, early detection, and treatment.

Anatomy and Physiology

Figure 8.1 illustrates the anatomy and electrical pathway of the heart.

■ The Conduction System

The conduction pathway of the heart begins in the sinoatrial (SA) node and travels through the atria to the atrioventricular (AV) node, the bundle of His, the bundle branches, the Purkinje fibers, and finally to the ventricular muscle. When the electrical impulse travels normally through this pathway, it is considered a normal sinus rhythm, with a rate of 60 to 100 beats per minute (bpm), but it may be lower in older patients, in athletes, or in patients taking medications that lower heart rate (such as digoxin, beta blockers, calcium channel blockers, or other antiarrhythmic agents).

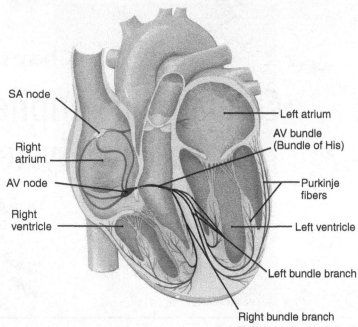

Figure 8.1 Anatomy of the heart. (From Scanlon, V. C., & Sanders, T. [2015]. *Essentials of anatomy and physiology* [7th ed.]. Philadelphia, PA: F. A. Davis. Reprinted with permission.)

■ The Cardiac Cycle

The cardiac cycle is diagrammed in Figure 8.2. Blood is returned to the right atrium via the superior and inferior vena cavae and to the left atrium via the pulmonary veins. As the blood fills the atria during early diastole, the pressure rises until it exceeds the relaxed pressure in the ventricles, at which time the mitral and tricuspid valves open and blood flows from the atria to the ventricles. At the end of diastole, atrial contraction produces a slight rise in pressure termed the *atrial kick*. As ventricular contraction begins, the rise in pressure in the ventricles exceeds that of the atria, causing the mitral and tricuspid valves to close. This closure produces the first heart sound (S_1). As ventricular pressure rises, it exceeds the pressure in the aorta and pulmonary artery, forcing the aortic and pulmonic valves to open. As the blood is ejected from the ventricles, the pressure declines until it is below that of the aorta and pulmonary artery, causing the aortic and pulmonic valves to close and producing the second heart sound (S_2). As the ventricles relax, the pressure falls below the atrial pressure, the mitral and tricuspid valves open, and the cycle begins again.

■ Heart Sounds

S_1 is the closing of the mitral valve (in the following diagram, M_1), and with the tricuspid (T_1) valve, together they are known as the *AV valves*.

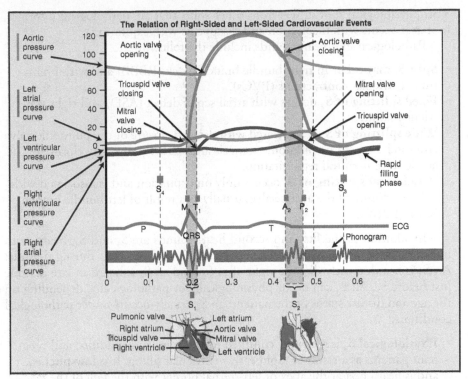

Figure 8.2 The cardiac cycle and mechanisms of heart sounds. (From Dillon, P. M. [2016]. *Nursing health assessment: A critical thinking, case studies approach*. Philadelphia, PA: F. A. Davis. Reprinted with permission.)

S_2 is the closing of the aortic (A_2) and pulmonic (P_2) valves; together they are known as the *semilunar valves*.

S_1 represents the beginning of systole; S_2 represents the beginning of diastole.

S_1 systole	S_2 diastole	S_1 systole	S_2 diastole
$M_1 T_1$	$A_2 P_2$	$M_1 T_1$	$A_2 P_2$

Normally, the S_1 and S_2 occur as single sounds each. In some conditions, these sounds may be split and occur as two sounds. In healthy young adults, a physiological split of S_2 may be detected in the second and third left interspaces during inspiration as a result of changes in the amount of blood returned to the right and left sides of the heart. During inspiration, there is an increased filling time and therefore increased stroke volume of the right ventricle, which can delay closure of the pulmonic valve, causing the second heart sound to be split.

This physiological split differs from other splits that are pathological in origin, in that it occurs with inspiration and disappears with expiration.

Pathological split heart sounds include the following:

- **Split S₁** may occur in right bundle branch block (RBBB) and with premature ventricular contractions (PVCs).
- **Fixed splitting of S₂** occurs with atrial septal defect (ASD) and right ventricular failure.
- **Wide splitting of S₂** is associated with delayed closure of the pulmonic valve and can be caused by pulmonic stenosis and RBBB or by early closure of the aortic valve in mitral regurgitation.
- **Paradoxical splitting of S₂** occurs only on expiration and is associated with delayed closure of the aortic valve, usually as a result of left bundle branch block (LBBB).

In addition to the first and second heart sounds are S₃ and S₄, heard both in normal and pathological conditions. Both S₃ and S₄ occur during diastole: An S₃ is heard in early diastole right after S₂, and an S₄ is heard in late diastole just before S₁. An S₃ can occur physiologically or pathologically, depending on the age and disease status of the patient; an S₄ usually occurs under pathological conditions:

- **Physiological S₃** is generally confined to children, young adults, and pregnant patients as a result of rapid early ventricular filling. It is low-pitched and is heard best at the apex or left sternal border with the bell of the stethoscope.
- **Pathological S₃**, also called a *ventricular gallop*, is heard in adults and is associated with decreased myocardial contractility, HF, and volume overload conditions, as can occur with mitral or tricuspid regurgitation. The sound is the same as a physiological S₃ and is heard just after S₂ with the patient supine or in the left lateral recumbent position. The sound is very soft and can be difficult to hear.
- **S₄**, also called an *atrial gallop*, occasionally occurs in a normal adult or well-trained athlete but is usually due to increased resistance to filling of the ventricle. Possible causes of a left-sided S₄ include HTN, CVD, cardiomyopathy, and aortic stenosis. Possible causes of a right-sided S₄ include pulmonic stenosis and pulmonary HTN. S₄ is heard just before S₁ with the patient supine or in the left lateral recumbent position. The sound can be as loud as S₁ and S₂. S₄ is not heard in patients with atrial fibrillation due to no distinct atrial kick.

Other heart sounds may occur in pathological conditions and include opening snaps and pericardial friction rubs.

- **Opening snap** is caused by the opening of a stenotic mitral or tricuspid valve and is heard early in diastole along the lower left sternal border. It is high-pitched and heard best with the diaphragm of the stethoscope.

- **Friction rubs** occur frequently after a myocardial infarction (MI) or with pericarditis. The sound is a high-pitched grating, scratching sound—resulting from inflammation of the pericardial sac—that issues from the parietal and visceral surfaces of the inflamed pericardium as they rub together.

History

■ General History for the Cardiac and Peripheral Vascular System

In many instances, the history may be more telling than the physical examination. It is important to take a thorough history for signs and symptoms of heart disease. Investigate complaints of chest pain, pressure, or heaviness; left arm, jaw, or neck pain or numbness; dyspnea at rest or with exertion; cough; paroxysmal dyspnea; hemoptysis; syncope; palpitations; fatigue; or edema. Complaints indicating PVD, such as claudication, skin changes especially in the lower extremities, dependent edema, or pain, also should be investigated. Determine the date of the last chest x-ray and electrocardiogram (EKG). Inquire about comorbid conditions or other factors that may increase the patient's risk for heart disease and PVD (Box 8.1). A detailed risk estimator, published in 2013 by the American College of Cardiology/American Heart Association (ACC/AHA), may be used to calculate patients' 10-year risk of heart disease and stroke. The atherosclerotic cardiovascular disease (ASCVD) 10-year risk estimator, designed for primary prevention, is used for patients with no prior history of MI or stroke. The 10-year ASCVD risk estimate provides information for clinicians and patients to guide shared decision-making regarding use of preventive therapies to reduce CVD risk (for example, blood pressure, lipid, and diabetes management). Based on the 2019 ACC/AHA primary prevention of CVD guideline, clinicians should routinely assess traditional cardiovascular risk factors and calculate the 10-year ASCVD risk in asymptomatic adults age 40 to 75 years who

Box 8.1	
Risk Factors for Heart and Peripheral Vascular Disease	
Hypertension	Stress
Smoking	Age: >45 years for men and >55 years for women
Diabetes	Sex: men and postmenopausal women
Obesity	Positive family history
Dyslipidemia	Sedentary lifestyle

are free from ASCVD. For adults age 20 to 39 years, assessment of ASCVD risk factors should occur at least every 4 to 6 years. For adults older than 75 years, the ACC/AHA recommends that clinicians and patients discuss the potential benefits of preventive therapies in the context of comorbidities and life expectancy (ACC, 2019).

■ Past Medical History

History of heart disease includes any previous diagnoses of congenital heart disease, murmurs, palpitations, arrhythmias, abnormal EKGs, acute coronary syndrome (ACS; includes unstable angina with or without MI), angiography, angioplasty, stent placement, or coronary artery bypass grafting.

■ Family History

Family history is particularly important for cardiac assessment because CVD, HTN, dyslipidemia, and other vascular diseases often have a familial association that is not easily ameliorated by lifestyle changes. If there are deaths in the family related to CVD, determine the age and exact cause of death, because having immediate family members who have had CVD at a young age (men younger than 55 and women younger than 65) carries an increased risk of CVD. Ask about sudden death, which might indicate a family history of life-threatening arrhythmias or congenital heart conditions (such as prolonged QT syndrome or Marfan's syndrome). This is especially important to ask during pre-sports physicals because sudden death in athletes is often related to congenital or familial heart disease. In addition, familial dyslipidemia, an autosomal dominant genetic disorder, often leads to CAD and MI at a young age. Family history of obesity and type 2 diabetes are also secondary risk factors for heart disease because the familial tendency for these is strong. Ask about smoking in the house, as second-hand smoke is a risk factor for respiratory and cardiac disease.

■ Habits

The social history should include habits or lifestyle behaviors that increase the risk for heart disease, such as smoking, physical inactivity, high-fat diet, drug or alcohol abuse, and increased stress. Lifestyle changes may be necessary to decrease CVD risk. For example, smoking cessation for people who smoke cigarettes can reduce their risk of developing heart disease by 50% to 70%.

Physical Examination

■ General Assessment

General signs of heart or circulatory disease include diaphoresis, pallor, cyanosis, edema, restlessness, and confusion. Vital signs should be thoroughly assessed. Changes in classification of blood pressure (BP) from the most recent ACC/AHA guidelines for prevention, detection, evaluation, and management of high BP in adults indicate that systolic BP readings at or above 120 mm Hg and/or diastolic BP readings at or above 80 mm Hg should be further evaluated along with implementing lifestyle modification counseling (Whelton et al. [2018]). Heart rates above 90 bpm may be seen in noncardiac conditions, such as fever, anxiety, pain, medication, thyroid disease, dehydration, anemia, or pulmonary disease, but if other clinical signs or symptoms are present, a 12-lead EKG is warranted. Heart rates below 50 bpm can be seen in young trained athletes, but otherwise, there should be a high index of suspicion for other causes, such as heart block, and a 12-lead EKG is recommended. Diminished or accentuated peripheral pulses, pulsus paradoxus (decreased pulse amplitude at the end of inspiration, associated with pericarditis), pulsus alternans (alternating weak and strong pulsation, associated with left ventricular failure), and a bisferious pulse (having two systolic peaks, associated with aortic regurgitation or hypertrophic cardiomyopathy [HCM]) are indicative of valvular heart disease or tamponade. Jugular venous distension and hepatojugular reflux suggest an increase in right ventricular pressure. Wheezes, rhonchi, crackles, or significant increase in respiratory rate should alert the examiner to the possibility of pulmonary disease or HF.

■ Inspection

A general inspection of the patient is necessary, noting particularly short or tall stature, which may be associated with Turner's or Marfan's syndromes—both linked to congenital heart defects. Inspect the skin for changes in temperature or color and for ulcerations or sores that will not heal. Pallor, coolness, ulcerations, or hyperpigmentation of the extremities suggests arterial or venous insufficiency. Cyanosis of the nailbeds or, in more severe cases, circumoral cyanosis, suggests hypoxia. A red, ruddy complexion can be seen in HTN and in alcohol abuse. Inspect the skin around the eyes for xanthelasma seen in dyslipidemia. Inspect the configuration of the chest, noting thoracic scoliosis or pectus excavatum that may be associated with restrictive lung or cardiac disease. Check the respiratory rate and effort, looking for dyspnea. Palpate the point of maximal impulse (PMI) and the precordium for heaves or lifts, seen in ventricular hypertrophy. The apical impulse is easily observed in the pediatric client but is not always visible in the adult. An accentuated or displaced apical impulse may indicate ventricular hypertrophy. Inspect the neck for the jugular venous distension seen in right-sided HF.

■ Auscultation

Auscultation is generally the most useful part of the cardiac examination. First, identify the rate and rhythm of the heart. Identify S_1 (heard louder at the apex) and S_2 (heard louder at the base). S_1 is synchronous with the carotid pulse, and it is helpful to palpate the carotid pulse while listening for S_1 and S_2 to be certain you are differentiating the two sounds correctly. Determine if these are heard as single sounds or if there are splits. A physiological split of the second heart sound is common and varies with respiration, in that S_2 splits on inspiration and is heard as a single sound on expiration. This is due to changes in intrathoracic pressure during inspiration that cause increased filling time of the right ventricle and therefore increased stroke volume and a slightly later closing of the pulmonary valve (P_2). Note any fixed splitting of the first and second heart sounds, which can occur in a variety of pathological conditions, including RBBB, LBBB, PVC, right ventricular failure, ASD, pulmonic stenosis, and mitral regurgitation. Next, identify any extra sounds, such as an opening snap heard early in diastole in mitral or tricuspid stenosis, an early systolic ejection click heard in aortic or pulmonic stenosis, the midsystolic ejection click of mitral valve prolapse (MVP), a ventricular gallop (S_3) heard just after S_2, an atrial gallop (S_4) heard just before S_1, or a systolic or diastolic murmur. Auscultating the carotid arteries for bruits and amplitude is an important part of the cardiovascular examination. Audible bruits should be further evaluated with a carotid duplex scan to assess the amount, if any, of carotid artery stenosis or occlusion. Occlusion of the carotid artery should alert the examiner to the increased risk of stroke, and prompt referral should be made to the surgeon.

■ Palpation

It is important to palpate the precordium because palpation of a sustained apical or ventricular impulse can give information about heart size. A lift or heave caused by right ventricular hypertrophy can be palpated along the left sternal border, and a left ventricular lift or heave can be palpated at the apex. Thrills associated with grade IV, V, and VI murmurs are palpated over the precordium and are vibratory in nature. Palpate the carotid, femoral, and dorsalis pedis arterial pulses for amplitude and regularity. To assess for hepatojugular reflux, perform deep palpation of the liver by applying steady firm pressure to the right-upper quadrant of the abdomen for 10 seconds while the patient takes a deep inspiration. A positive test in a patient lying with the head of the bed elevated at 30 to 45 degrees is noted if the neck veins are distended 3 cm or more, which is typically seen in conditions of volume overload such as HF or in rare conditions such as constrictive pericarditis, cardiac tamponade, and inferior vena cava obstruction.

■ Percussion

Percussion of the heart borders is not often performed owing to its low sensitivity; however, it may be useful in some conditions—such as in pericardial effusion with or without cardiac tamponade—and especially in emergency situations when x-ray is not readily available. In addition, when the heart is either located or displaced to the right of the sternum, as in dextrocardia or tension pneumothorax of the left chest, percussion can be helpful. In patients with known HF, it is helpful to percuss the upper and lower borders of the liver to assess for hepatomegaly due to volume overload.

Cardiovascular Laboratory Tests

Table 8.1 presents normal values for common laboratory tests used in assessment of the cardiovascular system, along with the significance of each test.

Table 8.1

Cardiovascular Laboratory Tests

Laboratory Test	Normal Value	Significance
Lactate dehydrogenase (LDH)	45–90 U/L	An enzyme released when organ or tissue is destroyed, particularly myocardial tissue. Can also be elevated in hemolytic states, hyperthyroidism, kidney disease, gastric malignancy, and megaloblastic anemia.
Troponin I (cTnI)	<0.35 ng/mL	This index is useful in the diagnosis of acute myocardial injury. After 4 hours, it is equally as sensitive as CK-MB for up to 48 hours. Troponin I remains elevated longer than CK-MB and is more cardiac specific.
Troponin T (cTnT)	<0.2 mg/L	The sensitivity of cTnT for detecting acute MI is 100% from 10 hours to 7 days after onset. The sensitivity begins to decrease after 7 days.
Potassium (K+)	3.5–5 mEq/L	Most importantly, elevated K+ levels can cause ventricular fibrillation. Other changes in the EKG include widened P waves, peaked T waves, widened QRS complex, depressed ST-segment, and heart block. Decreased K+ can cause inverted T waves, U waves, and depressed ST-segment. Variations in K+ levels place patients at risk for digitalis toxicity.
Sodium (Na+)	135–145 mEq/L	Na+ is important for fluid balance, particularly when dehydration may be an issue or in HF, where Na+ less than 130 indicates a poor prognosis.
Calcium (Ca+)	8.5–10.6 mg/dL	The hypercalcemic effects on the heart include shortening of the QT interval and atrioventricular block. The effect of hypocalcemia is prolongation of the ST-segment.
Glucose	70–100 mg/dL	Changes in blood glucose can have indirect effects on the heart. Diabetes significantly increases the risk for MI and dyslipidemia.
Creatinine	0.6–1.2 mg/dL	Chronic kidney disease may elevate blood pressure, which, over time, will increase the risk for ASCVD. Creatinine level is also important when prescribing certain medications for HTN and HF, particularly ACE inhibitors and diuretics. A loop diuretic should replace thiazide diuretic if creatinine is greater than 1.5.
Cholesterol	Total, <200 mg/dL LDL, <130 mg/dL HDL, >40 mg/dL	Increased total cholesterol and LDL-C and decreased HDL-C increase the risk for ASCVD. Cause may be inherited or acquired, secondary to obesity, thyroid disease, or high-fat diet.
Triglycerides	<150 mg/dL	Elevated levels increase the risk for ASCVD.
Thyroid-stimulating hormone	0.4–4.2 mIU/L	In older patients, hypothyroidism may contribute to the development of HF. Hyperthyroidism may present as atrial fibrillation or other arrhythmias in patients older than 50 years.
Hemoglobin (Hgb)	11.5–15 g/dL	Anemia may be a cause or a result of many forms of heart disease.
Hematocrit (Hct)	34%–44%	Anemia may be a cause or a result of many forms of heart disease.
Oxygen saturation	95%–97%	Pulse oximetry can be helpful in patients with severe myocardial damage and HF to evaluate clinical status.
D-dimer	A level of 500 ng/mL or higher is elevated.	Part of the diagnostic testing to rule in/out a DVT.

ASCVD = arteriosclerotic cardiovascular disease; CK-MB = creatine kinase-myocardial band; EKG = electrocardiogram; HF = heart failure; HDL-C = high-density lipoprotein cholesterol; LDL-C = low-density lipoprotein cholesterol; MI = myocardial infarction.

Differential Diagnosis of Chief Complaints

■ Palpitations or Arrhythmia

The Conduction System

The conduction pathway of the heart begins in the SA node and travels through the atria to the AV node, the bundle of His, the bundle branches, the Purkinje fibers, and finally to the ventricular muscle. When the electrical impulse travels normally through this pathway, it is considered a normal sinus rhythm, with a rate of 60 to 100 bpm, but it may be lower in older patients, in athletes, or in patients taking medications that lower heart rate (such as digoxin, beta blockers, or calcium channel blockers).

The EKG

Following are the elements of the EKG (Fig. 8.3). Each small block on the EKG represents 0.04 seconds, and each large block represents 0.20 seconds.

- *P wave*—Represents depolarization of the atria. The absence of P waves may indicate atrial arrhythmias, junction rhythm, or an idioventricular rhythm.
- *P-R interval*—0.12 to 0.20 seconds, measured from the beginning of the P wave to the beginning of the QRS. Prolongation of the P-R interval indicates a conduction delay producing first-, second-, or third-degree heart block. A shortened P-R interval is seen in Wolff-Parkinson-White and Lown-Ganong-Levine syndromes.
- *QRS complex*—0.08 to 0.12 seconds. The QRS complex represents depolarization of the ventricles. A wide QRS complex is seen in conduction delays in the ventricles, such as bundle branch blocks and complete heart block, and in ventricular ectopic beats, such as PVCs. The amplitude of the R wave is decreased in MI, owing to altered depolarization or decreased myocardial contractility, and in pericardial effusion.
- *T wave*—Represents repolarization of the ventricles. Repolarization of the atria is not represented on the EKG tracing because it takes place within the QRS complex. Configuration of the T wave should be upright. Myocardial ischemia, injury, and necrosis may cause inversion of the T wave due to altered repolarization. Hyperventilation and laboratory abnormalities may also cause inverted T waves.
- *QT interval*—Should not be more than 0.50 seconds. Prolongation may result in syncope and sudden death due to the R-on-T phenomenon causing ventricular tachycardia. A corrected QT interval (noted on a 12-lead EKG) adjusts for the patient's heart rate and is more accurate than a noncorrected value.
- *ST-segment*—Should not be more than 0.5 mm below or 1.0 mm above the isoelectric line in most leads. Variations in the ST-segment in two or more leads of the 12-lead EKG that are above or below the isoelectric line may represent acute ischemia (such as ACS or MI). ST-segment variations occur in the leads that reflect the area of injury or infarct.

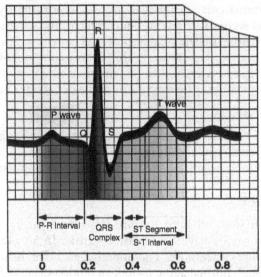

Figure 8.3 The electrocardiogram. (From Scanlon, V. C., & Sanders, T. [2015]. *Essentials of anatomy and physiology* [7th ed.]. Philadelphia, PA: F. A. Davis. Reprinted with permission.)

- *Q wave*—May represent death (infarction) of the muscle and is due to the absence of depolarization in dead tissue. A pathological Q wave measures greater than 0.04 seconds and is greater than one-third the height of the QRS complex.

History

Occasional palpitations occur physiologically in the majority of the population and in some people as a result of other, noncardiac conditions, such as anxiety, exercise, hyperthyroidism, and anemia. They can also occur with valvular heart disease, increased or decreased stroke volume, and during arrhythmias. The patient may complain of palpitations or skipped beats, or an arrhythmia may be seen on an EKG. Patients are often aware if their heart rate is slower or faster than normal or if it is irregular. With some arrhythmias, patients may complain only of fatigue, shortness of breath, weakness, or syncopal episodes. These are common symptoms in patients who have atrial fibrillation, and, if the ventricular response is slow, the patient may be unaware of the arrhythmia. Ask the patient about the frequency and duration of the palpitations and the presence of associated symptoms, such as loss of consciousness, syncope, lightheadedness, chest pain or pressure, shortness of breath, nausea, or vomiting.

Ask about history of heart disease, heart attack (i.e., MI), or valvular heart disease. In young women, MVP is a common cause of palpitations, which are generally benign in nature but unsettling to the patient. Ask patients how long they have had the symptoms and whether they are constant or intermittent.

Paroxysmal supraventricular tachycardia occurs intermittently and lasts anywhere from several seconds to several hours. Determine whether there is chest pain, because myocardial ischemia predisposes the patient to ventricular arrhythmias. Age and other risk factors are an important component of the history. Occasionally, young, otherwise healthy patients may have frequent PVCs that are benign in nature but warrant investigation to rule out serious causes.

Physical Examination

Although the EKG remains the major diagnostic tool, a thorough cardiac examination, including vital signs and carotid and jugular venous pulsation, as well as an examination of the extremities and peripheral vascular system, are necessary.

BRADYARRHYTHMIAS

A pulse rate lower than 60 bpm is considered bradycardia, although many trained athletes normally have a sinus bradycardia. In an older or untrained individual, it is more concerning. The underlying cardiac history is of utmost importance. Although normal aging includes a modest delay in SA and AV node conduction, thus increasing the likelihood of bradycardia, sinus node pathology and heart blocks should be suspected in older patients or in patients with underlying heart disease. A thorough medication history is also imperative because many medications, including many for the heart, can cause bradycardia or heart block. Electrolyte imbalance, particularly potassium (K^+), should be excluded. See Table 8.2 for common causes of bradyarrhythmias.

Table 8.2	
Common Causes of Bradyarrhythmias	
Cause	Description
Sick sinus syndrome	This term describes sinus arrest, sinoatrial block, and persistent sinus bradycardia of unknown origin. Often caused or exacerbated by drugs, particularly digitalis, calcium channel blockers, beta blockers, and antiarrhythmics.
First-degree heart block	This rhythm is characterized by a lengthening of the P-R interval greater than 0.20 seconds.
Second-degree heart block: • Mobitz type I or Wenckebach • Mobitz type II	In Mobitz type I, the P-R interval progressively lengthens until a QRS complex is completely dropped, and the pattern is repeated. In Mobitz type II, there is a regular P-R interval, and a QRS is absent on a regular interval.
Third-degree (complete) heart block	There is a complete dissociation between the atrial and ventricular rhythms. None of the electrical activity originating in the sinoatrial or atrioventricular node is being conducted through the ventricles. The atria continue beating at the normal rate, while the ventricles are beating at rate of 30–40 bpm.
Interventricular conduction defect/bundle branch block	Electrical impulse is slowed or blocked in one of the branches of the bundle of His. The right and left ventricles will not beat in complete synchronization, causing a widened and slightly delayed QRS.

Signs and Symptoms

Fatigue and shortness of breath are common symptoms of bradyarrhythmias. In older patients, weakness, confusion, dizziness, and syncope may occur as cerebral perfusion is decreased due to decreased cardiac output. HF may ensue in older patients or in patients who already have some degree of cardiac compromise.

Diagnostic Studies

- *EKG*—A 12-lead EKG is the first step in diagnosing arrhythmias. However, if the problem is intermittent, it may not show on a single EKG.
- *Holter monitor*—This device gives a continuous EKG reading for 24 hours or more and is useful in identifying paroxysmal arrhythmias.
- *Electrolytes*—An electrolyte panel, particularly to obtain potassium, calcium, and magnesium levels, is necessary because problems with potassium balance can cause arrhythmias. Medications such as loop and thiazide diuretics may lead to hypokalemia. Other potassium-sparing diuretics, angiotensin-converting enzyme (ACE) inhibitors, or angiotensin receptor blockers may lead to hyperkalemia.
- *Thyroid functions*—A low level of thyroid-stimulating hormone (TSH) or an elevated level of triiodothyronine (T_3) and thyroxine (T_4) may indicate thyroid disease as a cause for the arrhythmia.
- *Cardiac enzyme studies*—Elevations in troponin levels suggest myocardial ischemia/injury as a cause of the arrhythmia.
- *Medication levels*—It may be necessary to measure blood levels of medications such as digoxin, theophylline, and some antidepressants that can cause arrhythmias. Other medications may affect cardiac rhythms, and patients' medication lists should be carefully reviewed.

TACHYARRHYTHMIAS

A pulse rate over 100 bpm is considered tachycardia and should be investigated. Tachycardia can result from many noncardiac conditions, including hyperthyroidism, respiratory disease, infection (or sepsis), anemia and blood loss, illegal drugs, prescription medications, heat exhaustion, dehydration (or fluid volume deficit), strong emotions, and exercise. The underlying cardiac history is also important to rule out a cardiac origin. See Table 8.3 for common causes of tachyarrhythmias.

Signs and Symptoms

The symptoms vary greatly depending on the cause of the arrhythmia, the ventricular rate, and the cardiac output. Those with mild to moderate increases in ventricular rate may be asymptomatic. With higher rates, patients will complain of weakness, dizziness, syncope, and shortness of breath, and they may lose consciousness.

Diagnostic Studies

See "Diagnostic Studies" under "Bradyarrhythmias."

Table 8.3

Common Causes of Tachyarrhythmias

Cause	Description
Sinus tachycardia	When the heart rate is greater than 100 bpm but the impulse is via the normal sinus pathway, it is a sinus tachycardia. This is due to outside influences, such as fever, pain, anemia, volume depletion as in shock, or volume overload as in HF, thyrotoxicosis, drugs, fear or other emotions, and exercise.
Supraventricular tachycardia (SVT)	The heart rate ranges from 140 to 240 bpm, and SVT may last a few seconds to several hours. The usual mechanism is reentry, which is initiated by a premature atrial or ventricular beat involving dual pathways within the atrioventricular node. Most do not involve structural heart disease. SVT may be a result of digitalis toxicity. Patients may complain of dizziness, shortness of breath, or mild chest pain, or they may be asymptomatic except for the sense of a racing heart rate.
Ventricular tachycardia	The usual ventricular rate is 160–240 bpm and results in syncope owing to decreased stroke volume. The usual mechanism is reentry, which is initiated by a premature atrial or ventricular beat. Causes include MI, cardiomyopathy, myocarditis, and, occasionally, MVP.
Atrial fibrillation	Atrial fibrillation may or may not result in tachycardia. Although the atria are not beating regularly, there may be a controlled ventricular response. In many cases, there is a rapid ventricular response resulting in tachycardia.
Atrial flutter	In atrial flutter, the atrial rate is often over 250 bpm, but there is a variable ventricular response. In 2:1 or 3:1 flutter, the ventricular response may be close to normal, and the patient may have few or no symptoms.

■ Chest Pain/Chest Pressure

RED FLAG ◄ Red Flags for Chest Pain/Chest Pressure
• *Sudden onset of chest pain/pressure*   • *Severe, "crushing" chest pain/pressure*   • *Pain/pressure lasting more than 15 minutes*   • *Pain/pressure that worsens with exertion/physical activity*   • *Pain/pressure that occurs early in the morning or awakens the patient*   • *Pain/pressure accompanied by shortness of breath, diaphoresis, nausea, and/or vomiting*   • *Pain/pressure radiating to the left arm, neck, or jaw*   • *Pain/pressure accompanied by change in vital signs—tachycardia, bradycardia, hypotension*

The coronary arteries supply blood to the heart muscle. A narrowing in one of the coronary arteries results in decreased blood supply, and, when the lesion becomes significant, myocardial ischemia and chest pain or other ischemic symptoms occur. Typically, symptoms occur once there is approximately 70% or more blockage, but an MI can occur in some patients at 50% blockage. Blockage in the right coronary artery results in damage to the posterior/inferior area of the heart. The left coronary artery branches off to the left anterior descending artery and the left circumflex artery. A highly stenotic left coronary artery or proximal left anterior descending artery can cause significant and often fatal heart damage. Blockage in the left anterior descending artery results in damage to the anterior portion of the heart. Blockage in the circumflex branch artery results in damage to the posterior and lateral areas.

While the history and physical examination may not be definitive, they are a very important part of the overall assessment of ACS in determining the etiology of the symptoms.

History

Any complaint of chest pain or other symptoms suggestive of ischemia should be thoroughly investigated in all patients. Initially, determine whether the patient is having active cardiac symptoms during the evaluation, which would require emergent transport to the closest emergency department via emergency medical services for a full cardiac workup. Although it may be a low likelihood in seemingly young, healthy patients, a cardiac origin for the chest pain/pressure should always be kept on the list of differential diagnoses for all adults. Start by asking the patient about current medicines and comorbidities. Ask whether this is the first episode of chest pain/pressure (or other ischemic symptoms) or whether the symptoms have been recurrent. Ask how long the symptoms have been going on, whether symptoms are constant or intermittent, and whether symptoms radiate to either arm, back, neck, or jaw. Ask how long the symptoms last when they occur, and ask for a description of the quality of the symptoms and the level of symptom intensity (on a scale of 0 to 10, with 0 representing no symptoms and 10 being the worst one could imagine). Inquire about associated symptoms, such as shortness of breath, sweating, dizziness, syncope, nausea, vomiting, palpitations, or cough. Determine if the symptoms have a trigger or if they are associated with certain activities, such as exercise, sexual intercourse, eating, sleeping, stress, or strong emotions. Be sure to inquire about sports or exercise activities that could have resulted in injury to the intercostal muscles, ribs, or chest wall. Ask about alleviating or aggravating factors and whether the patient is taking any kind of medicine for the symptoms (prescription or over-the-counter medications, home remedies, or alternative treatments).

Suspicion of a cardiac origin of the symptoms warrants prompt evaluation by a cardiology specialist or a referral to the emergency department. Typical characteristics that indicate ACS include crushing, substernal chest pain/pressure with radiation to the neck or left arm, an association with exertion or stress with relief on rest, a duration of several minutes or more, and associated symptoms of nausea, diaphoresis, weakness, or shortness of breath. Less common classic symptoms, which may come on gradually and be intermittent, occur more often in women, older patients, and patients with diabetes and include jaw pain, fatigue, weakness, indigestion, and upper back pain.

Physical Examination

Assess the patient's pain level and associated signs, such as changes in color (paleness or cyanosis) and the presence of dyspnea, diaphoresis, nausea, or vomiting. Listen to the heart and note rate and rhythm (R&R), any murmurs, arrhythmias, bradycardia, or tachycardia. Auscultate the lungs for crackles or decreased breath sounds that might signal a pulmonary origin for the chest pain. If a pulmonary origin is suspected, percuss the lungs for areas of dullness and assess for voice sounds. For patients with obvious dyspnea, a pulse oximetry reading provides useful information. Palpate the chest wall for tenderness. An EKG and chest x-ray can assist in differentiating a cardiac from a pulmonary etiology. However, if the patient is actively having symptoms and you suspect ACS, emergency medical services should be notified for immediate transport to the closest emergency department for a full cardiac workup.

With angina and MI, acute ischemic changes may be seen on the 12-lead EKG. Each lead reflects an area of the heart, and the EKG can determine the location of the ischemia. The lateral wall of the heart is reflected in leads I, aVL, V_5, and V_6. The inferior wall is reflected in leads II, III, and aVF. The anterior wall is reflected in leads V_1, V_2, V_3, and V_4. The posterior wall is reflected in leads V_1, V_2, and V_3. With ischemia, EKG changes need to occur in two contiguous leads. Reciprocal EKG changes can be seen in the area of the heart opposite the injured area.

Diagnostic Studies

- *CK-MB*—Many facilities have stopped using CK-MB testing, relying primarily on troponin testing. The levels can also be elevated following trauma or with progressive muscular dystrophy.
- *Troponin*—An inhibitory protein found in muscle fibers, troponin is elevated within 4 hours of an MI and stays elevated for 7 to 10 days. It is more sensitive and specific than creatine kinase for cardiac muscle but may be falsely elevated in patients with kidney dysfunction. Many institutions are starting to use high-sensitivity troponin testing, which more accurately conveys diagnosis and prognosis for patients with myocardial ischemia and MI.
- *12-lead EKG*—The practitioner should look for signs of acute ischemia, such as ST-segment elevation or depression, arrhythmias, and conduction delays. EKG is minimally helpful in diagnosing pericarditis, except in the case of cardiac tamponade or constrictive pericarditis, where decreased amplitude may be seen. Keep in mind that the majority of patients with ACS will have a normal EKG, typically ruling in for myocardial ischemia by troponin values.

- *Graded exercise test*—The stress test can assist in diagnosing CAD and angina and establishing safe exercise levels. The addition of the radioactive substance thallium helps determine the extent of coronary artery blockage and blood flow both at rest and with exercise.
- *Imaging*—Studies such as computed tomography (CT) scan, electron beam computed tomography (EBCT) scan, positron emission tomography (PET) scan, magnetic resonance imaging (MRI), and single photon emission computed tomography (SPECT) scan can assist in diagnosing CAD, aortic aneurysms, cardiac masses, myocardial disease, and pericardial disease.
- *Arterial blood gases*—These measures evaluate oxygenation and acid–base balance and can assist in ruling out pulmonary disease.
- *Chest x-ray*—Pneumonia, pulmonary masses or other pulmonary disease, heart size, and aortic aneurysms can be identified on x-rays.
- *Echocardiography*—The most widely used technique is 3D transesophageal echocardiography, which gives a detailed analysis of anatomical cardiac pathology, particularly type and severity of valvular heart disease, cardiomyopathy, and HF. Transthoracic echocardiography, an older, noninvasive technique, is used for simple assessments of overall cardiac health, including aneurysms, pericardial effusion, and other structural abnormalities in the chest.
- *Cardiac catheterization*—If symptoms are highly suggestive of ischemia, cardiac catheterization can assess the need for revascularization (coronary angioplasty/stenting or coronary artery bypass grafting). Urgent reperfusion with angioplasty or coronary artery stenting must be performed promptly, ideally within 90 minutes of the onset of MI symptoms, in order to minimize the amount of cardiac muscle damage.
- *Endoscopy*—Once a cardiac origin is ruled out, endoscopy can rule out a gastric cause for the pain.
- *Amylase/lipase*—Once a cardiac origin is ruled out, blood laboratory tests for gastrointestinal causes should be initiated. Amylase/lipase measures will assist in the diagnosis of pancreatitis and cholecystitis.
- *Complete blood count (CBC), erythrocyte sedimentation rate, and chemistry panel*—These tests should be done if pericarditis is suspected.

ANGINA AND MYOCARDIAL INFARCTION

With a complaint of chest pain or pressure, the most life-threatening diagnosis should be ruled out first. A thorough history identifying the quality and quantity of the pain, alleviating and aggravating factors, and associated symptoms assists in raising or lowering your index of suspicion for a myocardial origin of the symptoms. Age, sex, weight, vital signs, family history, and medical history also assist in diagnosis.

Signs and Symptoms
Signs and symptoms that are suspicious for acute myocardial ischemia include substernal chest pain or discomfort that may radiate into the neck or left arm, diaphoresis, nausea, shortness of breath, and perhaps weakness. Chest discomfort

that increases with exertion and resolves with rest or sublingual nitroglycerin is highly suggestive of myocardial ischemia. Chest discomfort that occurs in the early morning or wakes a patient at night may also be cardiac in origin. Chest discomfort or pain at rest is worrisome because it may signify ACS (unstable angina with or without acute MI). Less classic symptoms such as jaw pain, fatigue, indigestion, and upper back pain are more common in women, older patients, and patients with diabetes.

PERICARDITIS

Pericarditis, inflammation of the pericardium, is usually not a solo disease process but is seen in conjunction with other diseases or conditions. Pericarditis may occur as a complication of MI (Dressler's syndrome) or coronary artery bypass grafting. It is also more commonly seen in patients with connective tissue disorders such as rheumatoid arthritis, systemic lupus erythematosus, scleroderma, and sarcoidosis. Bacterial, viral, or fungal infections, including HIV, are risk factors for pericarditis. Pericarditis can occur with kidney failure or metastatic neoplasias or as a reaction to medication, particularly phenytoin, hydralazine, and procainamide. Rarely, it is idiopathic and the cause unknown, although a common viral infection is suspected. Cardiac tamponade can occur as a serious complication, and it is an emergency requiring immediate pericardiocentesis. Constrictive pericarditis can occur over time due to scarring of the pericardial sac.

Signs and Symptoms
Unlike the symptoms associated with ACS, the pain accompanying pericarditis is sharp and stabbing; it may worsen with inspiration or when lying flat or leaning forward. Associated symptoms may include shortness of breath, fever, chills, and malaise.

THORACIC/ABDOMINAL AORTIC ANEURYSM

Thoracic aneurysms account for less than 10% of aortic aneurysms, are rarely symptomatic, and are usually found in routine examinations for other reasons. The history should include any chest trauma; hereditary connective tissue disorder, especially Marfan's or Ehlers-Danlos syndromes; congenital cardiac anomalies, such as coarctation, patent ductus arteriosus, or bicuspid aortic valve; and severe, long-standing HTN. Control of HTN is imperative to prevent progression of the aneurysm.

Signs and Symptoms
Symptoms are often described as tearing or ripping in the chest, back, or abdomen and substernal or thoracic back pain. There also may be symptoms related to pressure on the trachea or esophagus, such as dyspnea, cough, hoarseness, and dysphagia. Superior vena cava syndrome may accompany thoracic aneurysm. The systolic murmur of aortic regurgitation may be heard in aneurysms of the ascending aorta. The risk of rupture depends on the diameter of the aneurysm.

The long-term prognosis is generally poor. Surgical intervention is also risky, with a high rate of morbidity and mortality.

GASTROESOPHAGEAL REFLUX DISEASE AND PEPTIC ULCER DISEASE

It is often difficult to differentiate the symptoms of gastroesophageal reflux disease (GERD) or peptic ulcer disease (PUD) from cardiac symptoms. A thorough history and diagnostic tests are necessary. Patients with a history of GERD or PUD should still be worked up for a cardiac etiology, particularly if the characteristics of the symptoms or the history have changed to raise the index of suspicion for cardiac disease.

Signs and Symptoms

The pain of GERD and PUD can be severe and anxiety provoking. Symptoms are typically substernal and may be accompanied by nausea and diaphoresis if severe enough. Unlike cardiac symptoms, GERD tends to be worse at night when the patient is lying down, which is helpful in differentiating it from cardiac symptoms. Pain relieved by sublingual nitroglycerin or a "GI cocktail" (mixture of Mylanta, viscous lidocaine, and Donnatal) cannot rule in or rule out a cardiac origin because GERD, PUD, esophageal spasm, and angina often respond to either or both treatments. (See also Chapter 11.)

CHOLECYSTITIS

The history and location of the pain are good indicators for differentiating cholecystitis from angina. Cholecystitis is more common in young to middle-aged women and is seen more in those with a positive family history.

Signs and Symptoms

The pain of cholecystitis is generally colicky in nature and localized to the right upper quadrant. It is often accompanied by nausea and vomiting, and Murphy's sign is positive. Often there is fever and an elevated white blood cell count. Attacks are intermittent and are usually related to large or high-fat meals. See Chapter 11.

PANCREATITIS

Alcohol abuse accounts for more than 80% of pancreatitis, making the history most helpful. Other causes include dyslipidemia, drugs, toxins, infection, structural abnormalities, surgery, vascular disease, trauma, hyperparathyroidism and hypercalcemia, kidney transplantation, and hereditary pancreatitis.

Signs and Symptoms

The pain of pancreatitis is severe, steady, and "boring"—radiating from the epigastric region through to the back. It is often accompanied by nausea and vomiting, tachycardia, hypotension, and diaphoresis. These symptoms are also seen in MI; however, the exquisite abdominal tenderness present in pancreatitis assists in differentiating it from cardiac pain. See Chapter 11.

CHEST WALL PAIN AND COSTOCHONDRITIS

Chest wall pain can often be differentiated from cardiac pain through history. A history of injury, heavy lifting, contact sports, excessive coughing, or late-stage pregnancy (which stretches the intercostal muscles) leads the examiner to consider chest wall pain. This often occurs in a younger population with no cardiac risk factors.

Signs and Symptoms

One of the most helpful differentiating symptoms is that the pain is increased with movement, cough, or in some cases, respiration. The pain tends to be less severe than with other causes and, generally, no accompanying symptoms occur.

PULMONARY DISEASE

Several pulmonary conditions can cause chest pain, most commonly pulmonary embolism (PE), pneumonia, pleurisy, and tumor. The symptoms vary widely, depending on the underlying disease. See Chapter 9.

Signs and Symptoms

Except in the case of PE, in which the pain can be sudden and severe, the pain accompanying pulmonary disease is often more insidious in onset, localized to the area of disease, less acute in nature, and less severe than the pain of myocardial ischemia. Shortness of breath is almost always an accompanying symptom, and in some cases, cough is present. See Chapter 9.

■ Patient History of Heart Murmur

Heart murmurs fall into two general categories: systolic and diastolic. Systolic murmurs are further categorized into pathological, functional, and innocent murmurs. Diastolic murmurs are generally not considered to be functional or innocent. The following are the broad categories of the causes of murmurs with parenthetical examples:

- Flow across a partial obstruction (valvular stenosis)
- Flow across a valvular irregularity (bicuspid aortic valve)
- Increased flow through normal structures (anemia, pregnancy)
- Flow into a dilated chamber (aneurysm)
- Backward or regurgitant flow across an incompetent valve (valvular incompetence)
- Shunting of blood out of a high-pressure chamber through an abnormal passage (atrial or ventricular septal defect)

History

One of the first questions to ask patients when a murmur is heard on examination is whether they have ever been told that they have a murmur and if any diagnostic testing has been done, particularly an echocardiogram. Inquire about palpitations, weakness or syncope, cough, exercise intolerance, endocarditis, and respiratory problems. A medical history is important for congenital anomalies or rheumatic fever.

Physical Examination

A thorough cardiac examination is performed with the patient sitting, leaning forward, lying, and in the left lateral recumbent position. Some murmurs are heard better in different positions. Listen over the carotids for radiation of an aortic or pulmonic murmur; in the left midaxillary line for radiation of a mitral murmur; and in the epigastric area for a bruit, indicating an aneurysm. Assess the peripheral vascular system for bruits, pulses, and edema. Auscultate the lungs for crackles, which might indicate respiratory involvement.

Grading of murmurs is based on a scale of I through VI. Grading murmurs is an experiential process, but the following characteristics can be used as a guide (Box 8.2):

Box 8.2

Grading of Murmurs

- Grade I—very faint, not heard in all positions
- Grade II—soft but easily heard
- Grade III—moderately loud
- Grade IV—loud, may be associated with a thrill
- Grade V—very loud, may be heard with the stethoscope barely on the chest, associated with a thrill
- Grade VI—may be heard with the stethoscope off the chest, associated with a thrill

---

Murmurs should be described according to grade (intensity), location, radiation, pitch (high, medium, low), quality (blowing, rumbling, harsh, musical), and where they occur in the cardiac cycle.

SYSTOLIC MURMURS

Systolic murmurs occur between S_1 and S_2 and are broken down into ejection murmurs and regurgitant murmurs. Ejection murmurs are the most common type of systolic murmurs and are associated with forward flow through the semilunar valves. They have a crescendo–decrescendo pattern. Because systolic ejection murmurs are often physiological, especially in children and pregnant patients, they are further classified as pathological, functional, or physiological/innocent. Pathological murmurs result from obstruction to forward flow through the semilunar valves (aortic stenosis, pulmonic stenosis, and HCM) or backward flow through the AV valves (mitral regurgitation, tricuspid regurgitation).

AORTIC STENOSIS

Aortic stenosis is heard best in the second right intercostal space with the client leaning forward. The murmur is harsh, loud, and often associated with a thrill. It may radiate to the neck, left sternal border, and, in some cases, to the apex.

Signs and Symptoms

Syncope, angina, and dyspnea (remembered with the acronym *SAD*) on exertion are the classic symptoms of aortic stenosis. If syncope occurs with exertion, the aortic stenosis is typically severe. Angina may be present because of decreased perfusion of the left ventricle due to left ventricular hypertrophy (LVH) rather than CAD, but both exist in many cases.

Associated physical findings include the following: an early ejection click, a diminished S_2, a heave or sustained apical impulse with LVH, crackles at the lung bases with left ventricular failure, jugular venous distension, hepatomegaly, and peripheral edema that may be associated with right ventricular failure. Treatment includes medical and/or surgical intervention.

Diagnostic Studies

- **Chest x-ray**—X-ray is helpful for outlining the heart border in LVH. Calcification of the aortic valve may be visible on x-ray.
- **12-lead EKG**—An EKG may show evidence of LVH. On examination, look for other signs of LVH, such as a left ventricular heave and an S_4.
- **Echocardiography**—This diagnostic can determine the presence or absence and the severity of aortic stenosis.
- **Graded Exercise Test**—This is helpful in determining the severity of aortic stenosis.
- **Cardiac catheterization**—The definitive study for the severity of aortic stenosis, cardiac catheterization measures systolic blood flow across the aortic valve along with pressure differences between the left ventricle and the aorta.

PULMONIC STENOSIS

Pulmonic stenosis, less common than aortic stenosis, is heard best at the third left intercostal space. It is the second most common form of congenital heart disease. It is more common in women, and about two-thirds of adults are hemodynamically insignificant.

Signs and Symptoms

A crescendo–decrescendo systolic ejection murmur is associated with pulmonic stenosis. The quality of the murmur is harsh, of medium pitch, and, if loud, may be associated with a thrill. In patients with severe pulmonic stenosis, dyspnea, cyanosis, syncope on exertion, palpitations, and right HF can occur.

Diagnostic Studies

- **Chest x-ray**—Unless right ventricular failure occurs, the heart may not appear enlarged on x-ray. Pulmonary artery dilatation is commonly seen but does not reflect the severity of the disease.
- **12-lead EKG**—EKG changes in mild pulmonic stenosis are minimal, but in severe obstruction to right ventricular flow, peaked P waves can be seen and sometimes RBBB.

- *Echocardiography*—This study can be helpful in determining the degree of right ventricular hypertrophy and in distinguishing pulmonic stenosis from other lesions.
- *Cardiac catheterization*—As in aortic stenosis, cardiac catheterization is the definitive diagnostic test for the presence and severity of pulmonic stenosis.

HYPERTROPHIC CARDIOMYOPATHY (HCM)

HCM, a rare form of HF, has also been termed *idiopathic hypertrophic subaortic stenosis* or *asymmetrical septal hypertrophy*. The cause of HCM is unknown but is thought to be genetic. Manifestations may not be apparent until adulthood, and it is generally seen in conjunction with essential HTN.

Signs and Symptoms
The most common presenting symptoms are dyspnea on exertion and chest pain. Although the chest pain mimics that of angina, it is not relieved by sublingual nitroglycerin. Syncope is also a common complaint and may be more severe after exertion.

Clinical findings include an S_4 and a grade IV systolic murmur heard at the left sternal border that increases when upright and decreases with squatting. Both atrial and ventricular arrhythmias can occur and are problematic. Atrial fibrillation may occur as a result of a chronic elevation of left atrial pressure. Ventricular arrhythmias can cause sudden death, especially after extreme exertion. This illuminates the importance of a good history and physical examination for athletic screening. A family history of sudden death, dyspnea on exertion, syncopal episodes during or after exercise, and chest pain warrant diagnostic testing.

Diagnostic Studies
- *Echocardiography*—In the case of HCM, echocardiography is diagnostic, and more invasive studies generally are not necessary. Echocardiogram findings include asymmetric LVH, a hypercontractile left ventricle, and delayed diastolic filling of the left ventricle.
- *Cardiac catheterization*—This diagnostic procedure may be helpful but generally is not necessary for diagnosis.

MITRAL REGURGITATION

Mitral regurgitation is very common for most patients with HF, especially those with dilated cardiomyopathy. Complications include embolism, usually secondary to the atrial fibrillation. Bacterial endocarditis occurs most frequently (20%) in patients with mitral incompetence.

Signs and Symptoms
Dyspnea is the most common presenting symptom. Palpitations are common, and atrial fibrillation may develop. The murmur of mitral regurgitation is heard best in the apex, often with radiation to the left axilla. It is pansystolic,

high-pitched, and blowing and may be associated with a thrill. There may be a decreased S_1, an S_3, and a sustained apical impulse owing to LVH. Secondary left atrial enlargement results from systolic backflow into the left atrium.

Diagnostic Studies

- **Chest x-ray**—The left atrium and left ventricle are enlarged proportionate to the severity of the disease.
- **12-lead EKG**—Atrial arrhythmias are common, particularly atrial fibrillation. Right and left bundle branches are uncommon. The main change seen is higher voltage.
- **Echocardiography**—In addition to visualizing the diseased valve, echocardiography can assist in determining the size of the left atrium and left ventricle.
- **Cardiac catheterization**—In patients with hemodynamically significant mitral regurgitation, cardiac catheterization is the definitive choice for determining the need for surgical intervention.

MITRAL VALVE PROLAPSE (MVP)

MVP, also termed *click-murmur syndrome*, is a variant of mitral regurgitation and occurs in approximately 10% of young women. MVP generally is hemodynamically insignificant and characterized by normal heart size and dynamics, although the process can progress to hemodynamically significant mitral regurgitation.

Signs and Symptoms

Patients are usually asymptomatic but may complain of palpitations. Characteristically, a portion of the mitral valve balloons into the left atrium, giving rise to a midsystolic click followed by a soft grade I murmur that crescendos up to S_2. It is high-pitched and is heard best at the apex or left sternal border. Some patients with MVP have only a murmur and no click, and others have only a click and no murmur.

Diagnostic Studies

- **Echocardiography**—In addition to visualizing the diseased valve, echocardiography can assist in determining the size of the left atrium and left ventricle. No other diagnostics should be necessary for diagnosing MVP.
- **Holter monitor**—If the patient complains of frequent palpitations related to MVP, a Holter monitor might be indicated to determine if the palpitations are benign, and the patient can be reassured.

TRICUSPID REGURGITATION

The most common initiator of tricuspid regurgitation is pulmonary HTN; it may also be a secondary result of left ventricular HF. There also may be secondary right atrial enlargement owing to backflow into the right atrium. When right ventricular HF occurs, it results in jugular venous distension and possible liver enlargement.

Signs and Symptoms

Symptoms are consistent with the right ventricular low-output state (i.e., fatigue; fullness in the abdomen; ankle swelling; and, in late stages, ascites). Right upper quadrant discomfort may be present due to liver congestion. Atrial fibrillation or flutter occurs as the right atrium enlarges, giving rise to right ventricular failure.

The murmur of tricuspid regurgitation is heard best at the left sternal border and may radiate to the right of the sternum. The murmur is pansystolic, high-pitched, and blowing, and it increases with respiration. Tricuspid regurgitation may be associated with right ventricular hypertrophy resulting in a right parasternal lift.

Diagnostic Studies

- **Chest x-ray**—The right atrium and right ventricle are enlarged proportionate to the severity of the disease.
- **12-lead EKG**—Atrial arrhythmias, particularly atrial fibrillation, are common. Bundle branch blocks are uncommon. The main change seen is higher voltage.
- **Echocardiography**—In addition to visualizing the diseased valve, echocardiography can assist in determining the size of the right atrium and right ventricle.
- **Swan-Ganz pressure readings**—The v peak and the y trough are exaggerated during inspiration.

Physiological or Functional Murmurs

Physiological or functional murmurs are systolic murmurs caused by a temporary increase in blood flow rather than by a structural abnormality and include such conditions as anemia, hyperthyroidism, pregnancy, and fever.

Innocent Murmurs

This type of systolic murmur results from turbulent blood flow and is not associated with heart disease. Innocent murmurs occur commonly in children and young adults and reflect the contractile force of the heart that results in greater velocity of flow during early systole. They are heard best in the second and third left interspaces along the left sternal border or at the apex. They are short, heard in early systole, and are less than grade III. Innocent murmurs often disappear with the patient in a sitting position.

DIASTOLIC MURMURS

Unlike some physiological causes of functional or innocent systolic murmurs, diastolic murmurs almost always indicate pathology. They are low-pitched and often very faint and difficult to hear.

MITRAL STENOSIS

Mitral stenosis results from thickening and stiffening of the mitral valve, usually secondary to rheumatic fever, which is rare in the United States due to the use of effective antibiotics to prevent infections.

Signs and Symptoms

The most common presenting symptoms are dyspnea on exertion and hemoptysis due to pulmonary congestion. The pulmonary congestion is caused by increased left atrial pressure related to the decrease in left atrial emptying. Crackles may be heard at the lung bases but are not present in all patients with pulmonary congestion. Orthopnea may be present because the lungs become more congested in the recumbent position. When the heart rate is increased as a result of fever, exertion, anxiety, or infection, congestion worsens and pulmonary edema may result. In addition, atrial fibrillation often develops in patients with mitral stenosis, which in turn worsens the pulmonary congestion. Over time, increased pulmonary vascular resistance may lead to right ventricular hypertrophy.

The murmur is generally grade I to IV and low-pitched; therefore, it is heard better with the bell at the apex in the left lateral recumbent position. The first heart sound (S_1) is loud, followed by S_2 and a loud opening snap that precedes the murmur.

Diagnostic Studies

- *12-lead EKG*—Broad, notched P waves will provide evidence that mitral stenosis exists, but the EKG is not helpful in determining the severity. If right ventricular hypertrophy is present, it is manifested by right axis deviation.
- *Chest x-ray*—The heart size may be normal, or the left atrium may be enlarged, but enlargement of the pulmonary artery is usually not seen until the pressures in the pulmonary artery are high. Radiographic changes in the chest that signify chronic pulmonary congestion are Kerley B lines, which are seen as thickened, interlobular septa, particularly at the outer edges of the lungs.
- *Echocardiography*—In addition to visualizing the diseased valve, echocardiography can assist in determining the size of the left atrium and left ventricle.
- *Cardiac catheterization*—Heart catheterization is the definitive diagnostic study to determine the severity of the mitral stenosis.

TRICUSPID STENOSIS

Tricuspid stenosis is most often caused by rheumatic fever and almost always accompanies the dominant mitral stenosis. The right atrium becomes hypertrophied with a small right ventricle.

Signs and Symptoms

Patients complain of fatigue and possibly right upper quadrant discomfort related to an enlarged liver. There is an accentuated *a* wave in the jugular venous pulse.

Examination findings include a low-pitched, rumbling mid-diastolic murmur, heard at the left sternal border in the fourth interspace and increasing with inspiration. The duration of the murmur is related to the severity of the stenosis and the stroke volume.

Diagnostic Studies

- *12-lead EKG*—The EKG will show peaked P waves in the inferior leads because of an overload of the right atrium.
- *Chest x-ray*—An enlarged superior vena cava and enlarged right atrium are revealed.
- *Echocardiography*—In addition to visualizing the diseased valve, echocardiography can assist in determining the size of the left atrium and left ventricle.
- *Cardiac catheterization*—Catheterization is helpful in determining the pressure gradients across the tricuspid valve and the severity of the valvular stenosis.

AORTIC INSUFFICIENCY/REGURGITATION

Aortic regurgitation results from failure of the leaflets of the aortic valve to close completely during diastole. This causes a backflow of blood from the aorta into the left ventricle. Volume overload of the left ventricle occurs because of the backflow of blood, which can lead to LVH. In this case, the apical impulse is accentuated and a left ventricular heave is seen. The most common cause of aortic insufficiency is infective endocarditis associated with rheumatic fever. In acute infectious destruction of the aortic valve, dyspnea, orthopnea, and cough are the most common presenting cardiac symptoms, resulting from pulmonary edema. This is often life-threatening, and prompt treatment is necessary.

Signs and Symptoms

In chronic aortic regurgitation, patients often complain of palpitations. If these are caused by ventricular arrhythmias, a thorough investigation is necessary to avoid a lethal ventricular arrhythmia. If LVH and failure develop, the symptoms typically are dyspnea and chest pain. An unexplained symptom of patients with aortic incompetence is increased sweating, which is thought to involve the cholinergic sympathetic vasodilator fibers. The greater volume of blood being pumped out of the ventricle increases the systolic pressure, causing a widened pulse pressure.

The murmur of aortic regurgitation is caused by increased blood flow across the aortic valve. The murmur is heard best in the second, third, and fourth interspaces, just to the left of the sternum. The quality is blowing, high-pitched, and usually grade III or less. It may radiate to the apex; having the patient sit and lean forward aids in hearing the murmur.

Diagnostic Studies

- *12-lead EKG*—In patients with hemodynamically significant aortic regurgitation, LVH is reflected on the EKG by increased height of the R waves in the left-sided chest leads, increased depth of the S waves in the right-sided chest leads, and associated ST changes.
- *Chest x-ray*—In chronic, severe aortic regurgitation, the chest x-ray shows an enlarged left ventricle and aortic dilatation. Confirmation with EKG is prudent.

- *Echocardiography*—In addition to visualizing the diseased valve, echocardiography can assist in determining the size of the left atrium and left ventricle.
- *Cardiac catheterization*—Catheterization is preferred over echocardiography for definitive diagnosis of aortic valve disease causing rapid aortic runoff. It is also useful in determining heart pressures and pulmonary vascular resistance.

PULMONIC INSUFFICIENCY/REGURGITATION

Pulmonary insufficiency rarely occurs in patients without pulmonary HTN and is usually seen in conjunction with right ventricular hypertrophy.

Signs and Symptoms

Pulmonary regurgitation rarely occurs except in conjunction with pulmonary HTN, and the symptoms are consistent with cor pulmonale. Progressive exertional dyspnea is present in the majority of cases. This diastolic murmur of pulmonic regurgitation is high-pitched, heard best at the base, and difficult to distinguish from aortic incompetence.

Diagnostic Studies

See Diagnostic Studies under "Aortic Insufficiency/Regurgitation."

VENTRICULAR SEPTAL DEFECT

Ventricular septal defect (VSD) is a congenital heart defect in which oxygenated blood is shunted from a higher-pressured left ventricle to a lower-pressured right ventricle through an abnormal opening in the ventricular septum. This left-to-right shunt causes an increased blood flow across the pulmonic valve. The signs and symptoms depend on the size of the defect and the age of the patient.

Signs and Symptoms

Adult patients with large defects usually complain of dyspnea on exertion. In children, VSDs are often accompanied by other congenital anomalies and can be life-threatening if not surgically repaired. Small defects can be clinically insignificant and may become smaller or even close as the child grows.

Characteristic of a VSD is a loud, harsh, pansystolic murmur at the lower left sternal border usually accompanied by a thrill. If the shunt is large, there is a mid-diastolic murmur of mitral flow heard at the apex, elevated pulmonary artery pressure, and possible HF.

Diagnostic Studies

- *12-lead EKG*—The EKG initially shows signs of LVH (tall R waves and inverted T waves in leads II, III, aVF, and V_6), but as right ventricular and pulmonary artery pressures increase, changes consistent with right ventricular hypertrophy are seen (tall R wave in V_1, small R wave in V_6, prominent S wave in V_6, and right axis deviation).

- *Chest x-ray*—Left and right ventricular enlargement, cardiomegaly, and an enlarged pulmonary artery are seen on x-ray.
- *Echocardiography*—In addition to visualizing the diseased valve, echocardiography can assist in determining the size of the left atrium and left ventricle.
- *Cardiac catheterization*—A heart catheterization is necessary prior to corrective surgery to determine the size and location of the VSD, the severity of the pulmonary vascular resistance, and the presence of other congenital anomalies, such as patent ductus arteriosus or coarctation of the aorta.

ATRIAL SEPTAL DEFECT

ASD is a congenital abnormality in which oxygenated blood is shunted from a higher-pressured left atrium to a lower-pressured right atrium through an abnormal opening in the atrial septum. This causes an increased right ventricular stroke volume and increased blood flow across the tricuspid valve and to the lungs.

Signs and Symptoms

ASDs are often accompanied by other congenital heart defects, but in an uncomplicated lesion, patients are often asymptomatic until early adulthood, when they present with dyspnea on exertion or palpitations resulting from atrial arrhythmia. Because patients may be asymptomatic for many years, right HF can be the first sign, and patients may present with edema and ascites. Some patients may present with stroke at a young age without having been formally diagnosed with ASD.

A pulmonic systolic ejection murmur is present owing to the increased blood flow through the pulmonary valve. Tricuspid stenosis likewise develops as a result of the increased diastolic flow across the tricuspid valve, producing a diastolic murmur. There is fixed splitting of the second heart sound. A visible pulsation over the second and third left intercostal space may be seen due to increased right ventricular stroke volume. Atrial arrhythmias, especially atrial fibrillation, are common in the adult population with ASD.

Diagnostic Studies

- *12-lead EKG*—A majority of patients with ASD have a right ventricular conduction defect, and in older patients, a prolonged P-R interval is also common. Evidence of right ventricular hypertrophy may be present.
- *Chest x-ray*—The heart is usually enlarged, and the pulmonary artery and branches are dilated. The right atrium and ventricle are enlarged, although right atrial enlargement can be difficult to determine.
- *Echocardiography*—These studies are helpful to visualize right ventricular enlargement and movement of the mitral and tricuspid valves.
- *Cardiac catheterization*—Although the preceding studies are helpful in diagnosis, cardiac catheterization is essential for confirmation of ASD.

■ Elevated Blood Pressure

The 2017 ACC/AHA guidelines for the prevention, detection, evaluation, and management of high BP is as follows:

Hypertension Classifications

BP Category	Systolic Blood Pressure, mm Hg*		Diastolic Blood Pressure, mm Hg*
Normal	Less than 120	and	Less than 80
Elevated	120–129	and	Less than 80
Hypertension Stage 1	130–139	or	80–89
Hypertension Stage 2	≥140	or	≥90

Note that if the patient's systolic BP falls in a different category than the diastolic BP, by default the patient will be categorized in the higher category. Also, the BP measurement is based on an average of two or more carefully measured readings on two or more occasions.

Blood Pressure Goals as Recommended by the 2017 ACC/AHA Guidelines

Clinical Condition(s)	Blood Pressure Goal
*No clinical CVD and 10-year ASCVD risk <10%	<130/80
Clinical CVD or 10-year ASCVD risk ≥10%	<130/80
Older persons (≥65 years of age; noninstitutionalized, ambulatory, community living)	Systolic BP <130
Diabetes, chronic kidney disease, HF, stable CAD, secondary stroke prevention, peripheral arterial disease	<130/80

As recommended by the 2017 ACC/AHA guidelines, if the patient is outside the BP goal, pharmacological treatment with BP-lowering medications along with lifestyle modifications is recommended.

   *Although the BP goal for a patient without clinical CVD and a 10-year ASCVD risk of less than 10% is <130/80, the threshold for starting BP-lowering medication is at ≥140/90 mm Hg.

History

It is important to determine whether there is a medical history or family history of HTN. Identify the medications the patient is taking, especially over the counter, including pain medications. Ask about lifestyle behaviors, such as the patient's activity level, and the use of tobacco, alcohol, and/or drugs. Inquire about the presence of chronic disease in the patient or family that may cause or contribute to HTN. At diagnosis, most patients do not have subjective complaints.

Physical Examination

The BP should be measured in both arms while the patient is sitting in a chair with feet on the floor with the back supported. Ensure that the patient has emptied the bladder and has been without caffeine, exercise, or smoking for at least 30 minutes prior to having the BP measured. All clothing covering the location of the BP cuff placement should be removed. It is also important that the patient and the clinician refrain from talking during the BP measurement. At the first visit, the BP should be taken and recorded in both arms, using the arm with the higher reading for future measurements. Repeated measurements should be at least 1 to 2 minutes apart, using the average of two or more readings on two or more occasions to estimate the patient's BP level.

If orthostatic hypotension is suspected, then BP and pulse should also be taken with the patient in three different positions (in this order: lying, sitting, and standing) with measurements separated by 1 to 2 minutes. As the patient moves into the standing position, it is important to monitor the patient for lightheadedness to avoid injury should the patient fall during the procedure.

Measure temperature, pulse, and respirations, and note fever, tachycardia, or tachypnea. Upper and lower extremity pulses should be compared to look for coarctation. The abdomen should be auscultated for aortic and renal artery bruits. The heart should be examined for an S_3 or S_4, indicating decreased compliance of the left ventricle and ventricular hypertrophy, a systolic ejection murmur that might indicate aortic stenosis or the diastolic murmur of aortic insufficiency. The eyes should be examined for exophthalmos and the retinas inspected for such hypertensive changes as hemorrhages, exudates, A-V nicking, copper or silver wire appearance, or papilledema, which might point to a more serious neurological cause.

PRIMARY (ESSENTIAL) HYPERTENSION

Based on the revised cut-points of stage 1 HTN in the 2017 guideline, approximately 46% of adults in the United States have HTN, and of that group, 95% have primary HTN. The pathophysiology of primary HTN is varied. Genetic factors are significant contributors, especially if both parents have HTN. Other factors include sympathetic nervous system hypersensitivity, decreased ability to balance sodium and calcium, and a renin-angiotensin-aldosterone imbalance. Factors that may exacerbate the predisposition to develop HTN include a sedentary lifestyle, obesity, smoking, alcohol use, sodium intake in some individuals, low potassium intake, polycythemia, and long-term use of NSAIDs.

Signs and Symptoms

In primary HTN, most patients are asymptomatic. Some patients complain of a throbbing headache that is usually worse in the morning. Some patients state that they can hear their heart beating in their ears when it is quiet or when they go to bed at night.

Diagnostic Studies
- **TSH, T$_3$, and T$_4$**—These hormones are measured to identify thyroid disease.
- **Electrolytes**—If chronic kidney disease (CKD) is a comorbid condition, potassium may be increased.
- **Serum renin and aldosterone levels**—These are used to rule out hyperaldosteronism.
- **Fasting blood glucose**—Hyperglycemia is seen in diabetes, a common comorbidity, or in pheochromocytoma.
- **Renal chemistries**—These studies identify renal parenchymal disease.
- **Urinalysis**—This test is used to determine specific gravity, proteinuria, hematuria, or casts that might indicate renal parenchymal disease.
- **24-Hour urine for catecholamines**—The presence of urine catecholamines assists in the diagnosis of pheochromocytoma.
- **Echocardiography**—Structural or functional heart abnormalities are identified by echocardiography studies.
- **Renal Doppler ultrasound**—This procedure identifies renal vascular disease.
- **Renal arteriography**—Renal arteriography is used to identify renal vascular disease.
- **CT scan or MRI**—These procedures can identify renal vascular disease, adrenal adenoma, adrenal hyperplasia, or pheochromocytoma.
- **Chest x-ray**—Coarctation of the aorta is revealed on x-ray.
- **EKG or echocardiography**—These procedures can identify ventricular hypertrophy or valvular disease in patients with known cardiac disease.

SECONDARY HYPERTENSION

Only 5% or less of patients have specific, identifiable causes of HTN, particularly those who develop HTN at an early age with no family history, those whose previously controlled HTN suddenly becomes uncontrolled, and those who first develop HTN after age 50. There are several causes of secondary HTN, including renal parenchymal disease, such as glomerulonephritis, pyelonephritis, tuberculosis of the kidney, or scarring from trauma; renal arterial disease, such as renal artery stenosis, aneurysm, embolism, or infarction; renal tumors; coarctation of the aorta; endocrine disorders, such as pheochromocytoma, primary aldosteronism, Cushing's syndrome, thyroid disease, or acromegaly; hypercalcemia; pregnancy; neurological disorders, such as tumor or trauma causing increased intracranial pressure; chronic alcohol use or abuse; obstructive sleep apnea; and medications, such as hormone replacement therapy, oral contraceptives, prolonged use of corticosteroids, NSAIDs, theophylline, or cold preparations containing ephedrine. Illegal drug use such as amphetamines and cocaine can cause immediate and long-term HTN.

Signs and Symptoms
In secondary HTN, the symptoms are consistent with the underlying etiology. Assess for complaints such as nervousness, diaphoresis, palpitations, dyspnea, tremor, muscle weakness, polyuria, nocturia, nausea, or vomiting.

Diagnostic Studies

See Diagnostic Studies under "Primary (Essential) Hypertension."

■ Elevated Lipids

Dyslipidemia is a disproportionate amount of deleterious lipids in the blood leading to an increase in ASCVD. For primary and secondary prevention of ASCVD, three lipoproteins seem to be of most importance when evaluating a patient's risk for ASCVD: low-density lipoprotein cholesterol (LDL-C), high-density lipoprotein cholesterol (HDL-C), and apolipoprotein B (apoB). Generally, lower is better for LDL-C, non-HDL-C (total cholesterol minus HDL-C), and apoB. Non-HDL-C and apoB should be considered in addition to LDL-C in patients with triglycerides (TGs) greater than 150 mg/dL to improve the prediction of ASCVD events. Current recommendations from the 2020 American Association of Clinical Endocrinologists and the American College of Endocrinology (AACE) base treatment decisions on the risk category of the patient.

Thus, the aim for primary prevention is to keep LDL-C levels below 130 mg/dL. Based on the recommendations in patients with known ASCVD or patients with increased risk factors including diabetes, the target cholesterol levels are more stringent, with LDL-C goals ranging from <100 to <55 based on risk category (Handelsman et al., 2020). Based on the 2020 recommendations, first-line treatment for patients at moderate to extreme risk includes a moderate- or high-intensity statin (based on risk category) in addition to

ASCVD Risk Categories and Treatment Goals Based on the 2020 AACE Guidelines

Risk Category	Treatment Goals (mg/dL)			
	LDL-C	*Non-HDL-C*	*Apo B*	*TG*
Extreme risk[a]	<55	<80	<70	<150
Very high risk[b]	<70	<100	<80	<150
High risk[c]	<100	<130	<90	<150
Moderate risk[d]	<100	<130	<90	<150
Low risk[e]	<130	<160	Not recommended	<150

[a]Extreme risk defined as progressive ASCVD including unstable angina; established clinical ASCVD in patients with diabetes, CKD stage ≥3 (estimated GFR ≤59 mL/min/1.73 m²), or heterozygous familial hypercholesterolemia.
[b]Very high risk defined as established or recent hospitalization for ACS, carotid, or PVD; a 10-year risk >20%; diabetes or CKD stage ≥3 with one or more risk factors.
[c]High-risk defined as two or more risk factors and 10-year risk <10%.
[d]Moderate risk defined as less than two risk factors and 10-year risk <10%.
[e]Low-risk defined as no risk factors.

lifestyle modifications. In addition to lowering LDL, statin therapy reduces TG as much as 35%. Raising HDL (above 40 mg/dL for men and above 50 mg/dL for women) and lowering TG (below 150 mg/dL) are important components of treatment in addition to lowering LDL, especially for those with ASCVD risk factors. The complete guidelines for management of dyslipidemia can be found in the AACE lipid guidelines (Handelsman et al., 2020).

Women older than 44 and men older than 34 should be screened at least every 5 years, unless there are comorbid conditions such as diabetes, kidney disease, or heart disease, which would necessitate yearly screening. Elevated lipids should be treated aggressively with diet and exercise, weight loss, and lipid-lowering drugs when necessary. The relationship of dyslipidemia to heart disease lessens with age; therefore, patients older than 75 years without heart disease or other risk factors are treated less aggressively.

History

The history includes screening for the risk factors listed in Box 8.3 in addition to any history of elevated LDL-C, non-HDL-C, triglycerides, and/or apoB.

Physical Examination

The physical examination includes measuring height and weight to calculate body mass index (BMI). The formula for calculating BMI is $wt(kg)/ht(m^2)$. A waist/hip ratio is also an indicator for risk of heart disease. A ratio greater than 0.85 for women and greater than 0.95 for men is considered to place individuals at increased risk, especially if accompanied by hyperinsulinemia or diabetes. These are part of a constellation of symptoms termed *syndrome X* or *metabolic syndrome* that indicates the greatest risk for the development of heart disease.

Box 8.3

Risk Factors for Dyslipidemia

- Obesity
- Sedentary lifestyle
- Diabetes
- Positive family history
- High-fat diet
- Alcohol use
- Tobacco use
- Hypothyroidism
- Chronic kidney disease
- Obstructive liver disease
- Cushing's disease
- Medications, particularly progestins, androgenic steroids, beta blockers

SYNDROME X OR METABOLIC SYNDROME

When occurring together, a cluster of risk factors known as syndrome X, or metabolic syndrome, seems to dramatically increase the risk for CAD, diabetes, and stroke. Lack of physical activity and poor dietary habits lead to a positive energy balance, increased body fat, and insulin resistance. Therefore, obesity may be the underlying factor causing the regulation defect in the insulin receptor, thus promoting insulin resistance. The more calories consumed, the more insulin needed to store the glucose and break down protein and fat. As fat cells become full, they become less sensitive to insulin, increasing the amount of insulin needed to perform the same work. Eventually, the body loses its ability to increase insulin secretion. Decreased secretion and insulin resistance impair sugar storage, leading to increased circulating glucose and a tendency for the increased sugar to be converted to fat, thus increasing the risk for type 2 diabetes and dyslipidemia, which leads to ASCVD.

Treating only one of these risk factors does not lower morbidity and, in some cases, makes other risk factors worse. Weight loss, through diet and exercise, is the most important factor in preventing the progression of this syndrome. Insulin sensitivity increases with weight loss and is thought to be due to the loss of visceral fat. The target BMI is less than 22 kg/m^2 for women and less than 27 kg/m^2 for men. Weight loss will also reduce HTN and improve the lipid profile. Aerobic and resistance exercise assists in weight loss and improves carbohydrate and lipid metabolism. Medication for HTN and dyslipidemia may be necessary in patients who do not make the needed lifestyle changes or who are slow to make significant improvement.

Risk Factors for Metabolic Syndrome

Risk Factor	Defining Level
Abdominal Obesity	Waist Circumference
Men	>102 cm (>40 in)
Women	>88 cm (>35 in)
Triglycerides	>150 mg/dL
HDL Cholesterol	
Men	<40 mg/dL
Women	<50 mg/dL
Blood Pressure	≥130/85 mm Hg
Fasting Glucose	≥100 mg/dL

At least three of the five metabolic risk factors above are needed to meet the diagnosis of metabolic syndrome.

GENETIC HYPERLIPIDEMIA

Two genetic disorders that result in dyslipidemia are familial hypercholesterol-emia and familial hyperchylomicronemia, which cause extremely high levels of LDL-C and TG, respectively. Persons with familial hypercholesterolemia may develop ASCVD in childhood and CAD between ages 30 and 40. Persons with familial hyperchylomicronemia may develop recurrent pancreatitis and hepato-splenomegaly in childhood.

Signs and Symptoms

Generally, patients are made aware of their dyslipidemia based on results from laboratory blood tests. Occasionally, lipid plaque, called *xanthelasma*, develops around the eyes, but it is not apparent until dyslipidemia has been present for some time.

Diagnostic Studies

- *Lipid panel*—The lipid panel measures total cholesterol, TG, HDL-C, LDL-C, and a total cholesterol/HDL ratio as a risk for heart disease. More sophisticated lipid profiles measure particle size, such as apoB, which gives a more accurate picture of cardiac risk.
- *Glucose*—Fasting glucose should be measured because type 2 diabetes is often responsible for dyslipidemia (especially increased TG or decreased HDL).
- *Insulin*—Insulin levels are not part of a routine workup, although they are helpful in detecting hyperinsulinemia and early type 2 diabetes.
- *Thyroid panel*—Hypothyroidism affects lipid levels and should be ruled out before placing a patient on lipid-lowering drugs.
- *Genetic testing*—Children with significant dyslipidemia may warrant genetic testing.

■ Difficulty Breathing and Shortness of Breath

Dyspnea, or shortness of breath, has many causes, including cardiac or pulmo-nary disease, anxiety, obesity, and anemia. Patients with a cardiac cause may also complain of increased symptoms with exertion and dyspnea that wake them up at night and are relieved by sitting up. This paroxysmal nocturnal dyspnea (PND) is one of the early signs of HF and therefore is more specific for cardiac disease. Dyspnea caused by cardiac disease results most commonly from left ventricular dysfunction and/or valvular disease.

History

The history should inquire about respiratory disease, HF, MI, heart murmur, arrhythmias, rheumatic fever, angioplasty, or cardiac surgeries. Inquire about other serious illnesses or hospitalizations and about current medicines, both pre-scription and over the counter. The review of systems should include chest pain, HTN, palpitations, dyspnea on exertion, PND, cough, fatigue, weight gain or loss, and most recent EKG. A thorough respiratory review of systems should also be done, which includes history of productive cough, asthma, wheezing, pleurisy, bronchitis, pneumonia, hemoptysis, tuberculosis, last chest x-ray, and purified protein derivative tuberculin test. A smoking history is also essential.

Physical Examination

The general survey includes any acute respiratory distress at rest, cyanosis, anxiety, restlessness, or confusion. Monitor vital signs for tachycardia, tachypnea, hypotension, or narrow pulse pressure, which could indicate ventricular dysfunction. A thorough examination of the lungs, heart, neck, abdomen, and extremities should be done. Auscultate the lungs for adventitious sounds, particularly crackles at the bases, which might indicate HF, although it is important to note that up to 20% of patients with acute HF will have clear lung sounds. Other adventitious sounds could indicate a respiratory condition (pneumonia, for example) rather than pulmonary edema from a cardiac cause. Keep in mind that obstructive lung disease is often complicated by cardiac disease, so there may be more than one disease process occurring. Percuss the lungs for areas of dullness, indicating fluid or solid mass, such as pneumonia, pleural effusion, cancer, or pulmonary fibrosis. If possible, pulse oximetry provides valuable information about oxygenation. Inspect the precordium for a parasternal lift or accentuated apical impulse, indicating ventricular hypertrophy. Palpate the precordium for a thrill, indicating at least a grade IV murmur. Auscultate all cardiac areas for murmurs, indicating valvular heart disease, an S_3 related to volume overload and HF, an S_4 usually heard in diastolic failure, and any arrhythmias that could be either a cause or a result of HF. Examine the neck for jugular venous distension (JVD) with the patient's head elevated to 30 degrees. This is a sign of right-sided HF. Auscultate the carotids for bruits or murmurs that may radiate into the neck, usually aortic in origin. Palpate the thyroid for enlargement or nodules because both hyper- and hypothyroidism can cause HF. The abdomen should be examined particularly for right upper quadrant discomfort related to hepatic congestion and enlargement secondary to right HF. Check for hepatojugular reflux by placing sustained (10 seconds or more) firm pressure on the liver while observing for JVD. In right HF, ascites may also be present. Examine the extremities for edema (which may be pitting) seen in HF.

Diagnostic Studies

- *CBC*—A CBC should be done to check for anemia, which could cause or worsen dyspnea and HF.
- *Chemistry panel*—A chemistry panel should be ordered to check kidney function, liver function, and electrolyte balance—particularly hypokalemia, which can cause arrhythmias.
- *Thyroid profile*—It is wise to rule out hyper- or hypothyroidism.
- *Brain natriuretic peptide (BNP) or pro-BNP*—For patients with comorbid respiratory disease, BNP or pro-BNP can help differentiate a cardiac from a respiratory etiology of dyspnea.

- *Chest x-ray*—Most importantly, the x-ray reveals the presence of cardiomegaly, which can assist in the diagnosis of HF as a cause of the dyspnea. Look for fluid at the bases, flattening of diaphragms in chronic obstructive pulmonary disease (COPD), tumors in cancer, increased markings, interstitial edema, atelectasis, or pneumonia. Pulmonary vasculature may be normal, especially in chronic HF. Pleural effusions indicate HF or metastatic cancer, and thoracentesis is indicated to examine the fluid for malignant cells.
- *Echocardiography*—This diagnostic test shows the size and function of the ventricles if HF is thought to be the cause of the dyspnea. It can also be helpful in detecting shunts and pericardial effusion and for visualizing the heart valves for abnormalities.
- *Cardiac catheterization*—This procedure may be necessary only when valvular heart disease is thought to be causing the dyspnea or if left ventricular heart dysfunction is caused by myocardial ischemia and revascularization is a treatment consideration.

HEART FAILURE

HF can occur at any age, depending on underlying diseases, but as a primary diagnosis, it is more common in older patients. There are four main determinants of HF with reduced ejection fraction (previously referred to as systolic function):

1. *Myocardial contractility*—A decrease in contractility can result from a loss of functional muscle caused by MI or other diseases affecting the myocardium. A decrease in contractility results in decreased stroke volume.
2. *Heart rate*—When the stroke volume decreases, the heart attempts to compensate by increasing heart rate. When increased heart rate cannot compensate, cardiac output decreases, leading to HF. Bradycardia can occur in a number of cardiac conditions, which are outlined in this chapter under "Bradyarrhythmias." Also, bradycardia in a nonathlete can lead to decreased cardiac output and ensuing HF.
3. *Preload*—Preload is determined by the end-diastolic stretch of the ventricular muscle fibers. This is equal to the end-diastolic volume or pressure. If preload is excessively elevated, pump failure can result. This occurs with valvular regurgitation. Starling's law states that the force of the heartbeat is determined by the length of the fibers constituting the muscular wall—that is, an increase in diastolic filling increases the force of the heartbeat.
4. *Afterload*—Afterload is the ventricular wall tension during systole, which determines the impedance to ejection of blood from the left ventricle. If afterload is excessive, the heart cannot pump adequately against increased resistance. This can be seen in severe HTN or aortic stenosis.

HF can also occur in patients with preserved ejection fraction (previously referred to as diastolic dysfunction). In patients with this type of HF, the ejection fraction is 50% or higher. In addition, HF can occur when supply cannot meet

Classes of Heart Failure

Class I	No limitation of physical activity. Ordinary physical activity does not cause undue fatigue, dyspnea, palpitation, or anginal discomfort.
Class II	Slight limitation of physical activity. Comfortable at rest, but ordinary physical activity results in symptoms of fatigue, dyspnea, palpitation, or anginal discomfort.
Class III	Marked limitation of physical activity. Comfortable at rest, but less than ordinary activity causes symptoms of fatigue, dyspnea, palpitation, or anginal discomfort.
Class IV	Unable to engage in any physical activity without discomfort, and symptoms of cardiac insufficiency are present at rest. If any physical activity is undertaken, symptoms increase.

Data from https://www.heart.org/HEARTORG/Conditions/HeartFailure/AboutHeartFailure/Classes-of-Heart-Failure_UCM_306328_Article.jsp

demand as a result of high output states, such as severe anemia and thyrotoxicosis. Other, less common causes of high output states are arteriovenous shunting and Paget's disease of the bone.

The American Heart Association classifies HF into four functional categories, according to the limitation on activity.

Signs and Symptoms

The three most common symptoms of HF are dyspnea with exertion or rest, orthopnea, and edema. Patients also may complain of nonproductive cough and fatigue. Signs include ankle or pretibial edema, rapid weight gain caused by fluid retention, bibasilar crackles, tachycardia with a gallop rhythm, and hypoxia. Left ventricular failure is most commonly characterized by dyspnea on exertion, cough, fatigue, orthopnea, PND, cardiac enlargement, crackles, gallop rhythm, and pulmonary congestion. Right ventricular failure is more commonly characterized by dependent edema, elevated venous pressure, hepatomegaly, and possibly ascites. Although left and right failure can occur independently, they often occur together, and left ventricular failure is the most common cause of right ventricular failure.

RESPIRATORY DISEASE

Dyspnea is a symptom in many respiratory diseases, which are covered in Chapter 9. A holistic look at the patient—including age, history, smoking, and alcohol use, and comorbid conditions—can assist the practitioner in differentiating a cardiac from a respiratory origin for dyspnea.

LIVER DISEASE

Severe liver diseases, resulting in ascites, can cause venous congestion and dyspnea. These symptoms generally occur in end-stage liver disease and are secondary to the more serious symptoms of liver disease, such as jaundice, bleeding, right upper quadrant pain, and encephalopathy. Liver disease is easily diagnosed by laboratory tests, ultrasound, and biopsy. See Chapter 11.

KIDNEY DISEASE

As in liver disease, dyspnea is a secondary symptom in kidney failure as a result of fluid retention. Kidney failure can be a cause of HF, and dyspnea is one of the early symptoms. Laboratory testing for kidney function and urinalysis will assist in diagnosis. See Chapter 12.

■ Acute and Subacute Bacterial Endocarditis

Bacterial endocarditis is a microbial infection of the endocardium. The most common causative organisms are *Staphylococcus aureus*, group A streptococcus, pneumococcus, and gonococcus. Although the incidence of subacute bacterial endocarditis has been fairly stable over the last few decades, it has increased in the older population owing to stiff, sclerotic valves. Other risk factors include intravenous drug use, dental disease, and invasive diagnostic procedures. Nosocomial infections have increased in open-heart surgery patients. The disease may be acute or subacute, and recurrences are not uncommon. If untreated, bacterial endocarditis is fatal because of a variety of complications. Prompt referral and hospitalization are necessary for antibiotic therapy and other supportive measures. As prevention against bacterial endocarditis, patients who are considered at highest risk for endocarditis should have antibiotic prophylaxis prior to certain dental or surgical procedures. Those at highest risk include patients with a history of infectious endocarditis, a prosthetic heart valve or a valve repair with prosthetic material, and congenital heart disease or certain congenital heart defects.

Signs and Symptoms

Initially, the signs and symptoms are similar to those of other systemic illnesses, including fever, chills, arthralgias, malaise, and fatigue. Petechiae, anemia, weight loss, new or worsening heart murmur, and emboli alert the examiner to a more serious disease process. Emboli may cause life-threatening events such as stroke or MI. Hematuria or proteinuria may result from a renal embolism or acute glomerulonephritis. Endocardial vegetation may occur, causing valvular incompetence or obstruction.

Diagnostic Studies

- *Blood cultures*—Cultures will confirm the diagnosis. Three blood cultures should be taken, 1 hour apart, before starting antibiotics.
- *Chest x-ray*—Underlying cardiac disease and/or pulmonary infiltrates are revealed on x-ray.
- *Echocardiography*—Echocardiography is helpful to identify which valves are affected and the presence of valve vegetations and valve ring abscesses.

PERIPHERAL VASCULAR SYSTEM

The assessment of the peripheral vascular system includes the following:

- Inspection and palpation of the peripheral pulses for strength and quality
- Inspection and palpation of the skin for color, texture, and temperature changes
- Inspection of the extremities for edema, open sores, ulcers, and pressure areas
- Auscultation of the arteries for bruits
- Questioning of the patient for subjective complaints of discomfort or pain at rest and with exercise

Note that arterial and venous insufficiency present with different signs and symptoms (Table 8.4).

Differential Diagnosis of Chief Complaints

▪ Peripheral Edema

In ambulatory patients, fluid collects dependently in the lower extremities; in nonambulatory patients, it collects in the sacral area. Nonpathological causes of edema include poor venous return in prolonged standing or sitting. Pathological causes of edema result from right and left HF, kidney disease, liver disease, or tumors that obstruct venous return. One of the early signs of HF is pretibial and ankle edema. Kidney failure causes fluid retention, and hepatic disease may cause ascites, which contribute to peripheral edema.

HEART FAILURE

See pp. 288–289 in this chapter.

KIDNEY DISEASE

See p. 290 in this chapter.

Table 8.4		
Differentiation of Arterial and Venous Insufficiency		
Sign	Arterial Insufficiency	Venous Insufficiency
Pulse	Decreased/absent	Normal
Edema	Absent or mild	Significant
Pain	Severe	Absent/mild
Temperature	Cool	Normal
Color	Pallor with elevation; dusky red on dependency	Hyperpigmented; cyanotic on dependency
Skin	Thin, atrophic; risk of gangrene	Thick; risk of stasis ulcers

LIVER DISEASE

See p. 290 in this chapter.

History

The age and general health of the patient can lead to either a high or a low index of suspicion for cardiac causes of edema. Older patients and those with comorbid conditions have a greater risk of a cardiac cause for the edema. Ask the patient about history of respiratory, cardiac, kidney, liver, or vascular disease. A history of HF makes a recurrence likely. Ask about any history of cancer, particularly abdominal or genitourinary. Ascites can occur with these cancers, causing lower extremity edema. Determine how many pillows the patient sleeps on at night, and ask about the presence of PND, another early sign of HF. Inquire about daily activities, exercise, and occupation to determine a simple, mechanical cause of the edema. Psychosocial data is important, such as assessment of alcohol intake and high-risk sexual practices, which might lead to suspicion of a possible hepatic cause. A positive smoking history is a significant contributing factor in PVD. Note any symptoms of intermittent claudication, such as complaints of cramping, aching, or pain in the ankle, calf, or thigh that occur with exercise and are promptly relieved with rest.

Physical Examination

Assess the extent and magnitude of the edema. Assess whether the edema is confined to the ankles, or whether it extends up the leg to include pretibial edema or higher. Grade the edema on a scale of 1+ to 4+, or mild to pitting. Assess the peripheral pulses and major arteries—the abdominal aortic, renal, iliac, and femoral arteries—for bruits. Stenosis or occlusion of any of these arteries can affect distal pulses. Assess capillary refill time and pallor or rubor of the skin on elevation and dependence.

Assess the skin integrity as you look for thinning, ulcers, or necrosis, which often occur in PVD. Hyperpigmentation and atrophic skin changes are common in venous insufficiency. Note any change in temperature of the skin. Cellulitis can sometimes mimic PVD and causes increased temperature. Coolness of the skin suggests circulatory impairment. Ulceration or necrosis are serious signs of circulatory impairment and must be promptly treated to avoid amputation.

Many people have dependent edema in the absence of heart disease that is due to prolonged sitting and standing or poor venous return, but a thorough examination of the heart, lungs, and abdomen is warranted. If the edema is accompanied by HF, crackles may be heard at the lung bases. Listen for other adventitious sounds, such as wheezes or decreased breath sounds that might indicate obstructive lung disease, often complicated by right HF. Auscultate all cardiac areas for murmurs that would indicate valvular heart disease, an S_3 related to volume overload and HF, an S_4 usually heard in HF with preserved ejection fraction, and any arrhythmias that could be either a cause or a result of HF. Palpate the precordium for a thrill that would indicate at least a grade

IV murmur. Inspect the precordium for a parasternal lift or accentuated apical impulse, indicating ventricular hypertrophy. Examine the neck for JVD with the patient's head elevated to 30 degrees. This is a sign of right-sided HF. Auscultate the carotids for bruits or murmurs that may radiate into the neck, usually aortic in origin. Palpate the thyroid for enlargement or nodules because hyper- and hypothyroidism can both cause HF. The abdomen should be examined particularly for right upper quadrant discomfort related to hepatic congestion and enlargement secondary to right HF. Check for hepatojugular reflux by placing sustained firm pressure on the liver while observing for JVD. In right HF, ascites may also be present.

Diagnostic Studies

- *CBC*—A CBC should be done to check for anemia, which could cause or worsen HF, of which edema is a symptom.
- *Chemistry panel*—This study should be ordered to check kidney function, liver function, and electrolyte balance.
- *Thyroid profile*—It is wise to rule out hyper- or hypothyroidism.
- *Chest x-ray*—Most importantly, the x-ray reveals the presence of cardiomegaly, which can assist in the diagnosis of HF as a cause of the edema. Look for fluid at the bases, flattening of diaphragms in COPD, pleural effusion, tumors in cancer, increased vascular markings, interstitial edema, atelectasis, or pneumonia. Pulmonary vasculature may be normal, especially in chronic HF. Pleural effusions indicate HF or metastatic cancer, and thoracentesis is indicated to examine the fluid for cancer cells.
- *Echocardiography*—These studies show the size and function of the ventricles if HF is thought to be the cause of the edema. Echocardiography can also be helpful in detecting shunts and pericardial effusion and for visualizing the heart valves for abnormalities.

■ Leg Pain

Consider a vascular origin for leg pain that is not musculoskeletal in nature. Pain or weakness that occurs in the calves, and sometimes the thighs or buttocks, with exercise and dissipates at rest is most likely related to PVD. If it is related to arterial insufficiency, the pain comes on rapidly during exercise, is quickly relieved by rest, and usually increases as the intensity and duration of the exercise increases. This is termed *intermittent claudication*. If the leg pain is due to venous insufficiency, the picture is quite different. The onset of the pain is gradual and may not occur immediately after exercise. There is greater variability of the pain in response to duration and intensity of exercise. The pain tends to be a constant ache that may last hours to days. A potentially life-threatening complication of venous insufficiency is thrombophlebitis.

History

The most important question to ask is if there is a history of previous blood clots in the lower extremities. Also inquire about other blood clotting disorders.

Ask about recent trauma to the lower extremities, history of abdominal cancers, prolonged immobility or travel, cardiovascular or cerebrovascular disease, chronic spinal conditions, paresthesias, weakness in the lower extremities, or calf pain during walking or exercise.

Physical Examination

The physical examination should include temperature, color, condition of the skin, and presence of arterial pulses in the lower extremities. Note any calf redness or edema. Evaluate the patient's ability to differentiate sharp and dull sensation in the lower extremities as well as deep tendon reflexes. Note any weakness or evidence of discomfort with ambulation.

THROMBOPHLEBITIS/DEEP VEIN THROMBOSIS (DVT)

In addition to arteriovenous insufficiency, other risk factors for thrombophlebitis include immobility, orthopedic surgery, malignancy, HF, smoking, pregnancy, oral contraceptive or hormone use, advanced age, and clotting disorders. The majority of cases occur in the deep veins of the calf, and the remainder occur in the iliac or femoral veins. The prognosis of thrombophlebitis is good, unless the patient develops a PE. Recurrent PE may occur. DVT can be a result or a cause of chronic venous insufficiency. Anticoagulant therapy should be instituted to prevent PE and to avoid the complication of chronic venous insufficiency.

Signs and Symptoms

The signs and symptoms of DVT include swelling, tenderness, and inflammation of the calf and often pain with ambulation. In about 50% of cases, symptoms are absent and PE may be the first sign. PE should be suspected with a complaint of acute onset of shortness of breath, chest pain, or hemoptysis in a person with any of the above risk factors. Preventive measures include early mobilization of postsurgical patients, raising the foot of the bed, and antiembolism hosiery, especially for patients who have a history of venous insufficiency and for people traveling long distances by airplane.

Diagnostic Studies

* **Calf measurement**—A simple measurement with a measuring tape of both calves for comparison should always be performed in the clinical setting. DVT causes swelling and redness of the affected leg.
* **D-dimer laboratory**—D-dimer is one of the protein fragments produced when a blood clot gets dissolved in the body. It is normally undetectable or detectable at a very low level unless the body is forming and breaking down blood clots. Then, its level in the blood can significantly rise. A negative test can reliably rule out a DVT, but the test has low specificity and cannot be used exclusively to diagnose DVT. Other causes of an elevated D-dimer include recent surgery, trauma, infection, heart attack, and some cancers or conditions in which fibrin is not cleared normally, such as liver disease. Imaging studies are necessary to confirm a diagnosis of DVT.

- *Duplex Doppler ultrasound*—Because of its sensitivity, specificity, and noninvasive method, duplex ultrasound is the recommended diagnostic test for venous thrombosis. It gives segmental readings on blood flow both distal and proximal to the thrombus. It is most accurate for clots in the veins proximal to the popliteal; however, it is not a reliable indicator of small thrombi in the calf veins.
- *Venography*—Contrast venography remains the most accurate diagnostic procedure for DVT. It gives information regarding location, extent, and degree of attachment of the thrombus. Venography is particularly useful when there is a strong clinical suspicion of a calf thrombosis and when Doppler ultrasound has not given adequate information.

ARTERIAL INSUFFICIENCY

Patients with peripheral arterial disease often have underlying atherosclerosis. Other diseases, such as diabetes, HTN, CAD, carotid or renal artery disease, CKD, and obesity, should also raise the index of suspicion for arterial insufficiency. Smoking is a strong risk factor for all vascular disease. Patients older than 50 are at increased risk for peripheral arterial disease. A history of significant trauma or surgeries may be a risk factor.

Wells Model of the Clinical Pretest Probability for Deep Vein Thrombosis

Score

1	Active cancer treatment or palliation within previous 6 months
1	Paralysis, paresis, or recent plaster immobilization of the lower extremity
1	Recently bedridden for >3 days or major surgery within 12 weeks
1	Localized tenderness along the distribution of the deep venous system
1	Entire leg swollen
1	Calf swollen >3 cm as compared to asymptomatic leg (measured 10 cm below tibial tuberosity)
1	Pitting edema (greater in the symptomatic leg)
1	Collateral superficial veins present (nonvaricose)
1	Previous documentation of DVT
–2	Alternative diagnosis as likely or more likely than that of DVT

If both legs are symptomatic, score the more severe side:
High Risk = scored 3 or more (probability of DVT 53%)
Moderate Risk = 1 or 2 (probability of DVT 17%)
Low Risk = 0 or less (probability of DVT 5%)

Wells P. Wells' criteria for DVT. MDCalc. mdcalc.com. Available at: https://www.mdcalc.com/wells-criteria-dvt

Signs and Symptoms

Intermittent claudication is present in approximately 50% of patients with peripheral arterial disease. Other symptoms include numbness or pain at rest. Some patients are asymptomatic. In severe cases, ulceration may lead to gangrene and amputation. See Table 8.4 for the signs and symptoms of arterial insufficiency.

Diagnostic Studies

The ankle-brachial index (ABI) is currently the easiest and least expensive noninvasive method for diagnosing PVD and is particularly helpful in office and home settings. The ABI is obtained by the following steps:

1. Obtain brachial systolic pressure in both arms. Select the higher of these two values.
2. Use a Doppler stethoscope to obtain systolic pressure in the dorsalis pedis or posterior tibialis vessel.
3. Divide ankle pressure by the higher brachial pressure.

The index should be 1.00 or higher. If it is less than 0.5, blood flow impairment is significant. An abnormal ABI indicates the need for a vascular consult.

The ABI may be falsely elevated in diabetic patients because calcification of the vessels raises the pressure, especially in the ankle. Doppler ultrasound is also helpful but requires specialized equipment.

Duplex Doppler ultrasound is a relatively inexpensive, accurate method for diagnosing arterial insufficiency, often making arteriography unnecessary. Flow velocity can be measured, and arterial stenosis and occlusion can be detected.

CHRONIC VENOUS INSUFFICIENCY

Chronic venous insufficiency can be a long-term complication of venous thrombosis owing to the destruction of valves in the deep veins. The calf muscle pump that returns blood from the lower legs is damaged, increasing ambulatory pressure in the calf veins. A constellation of symptoms is set up: aching or pain in the lower legs, edema, thinning and hyperpigmentation of the skin, superficial varicosities, venous stasis, and ulceration. Ankle edema is often the earliest sign. Other causes of chronic venous insufficiency include trauma and pelvic neoplasm, and it is occasionally secondary to superficial venous disease. Prompt treatment of DVT with anticoagulants decreases the risk for chronic venous insufficiency and PE as a complication. General measures for symptom management include the following: elevation of the legs intermittently during the day and at night, avoidance of prolonged sitting or standing, and wearing of support or compression stockings. Wearing an Unna boot is valuable and successful in the treatment of stasis ulcers.

Signs and Symptoms

Stasis dermatitis and stasis ulcers are common in chronic venous insufficiency. See Table 8.4 for signs and symptoms of venous insufficiency.

Diagnostic Studies

- ***Duplex Doppler ultrasound***—Owing to its sensitivity, specificity, and non-invasive method, duplex ultrasound is recommended for the diagnosis of venous disease. It gives segmental readings on blood flow and is accurate for the diagnosis of occlusion. It is most accurate for clots in the veins proximal to the popliteal; however, it is not a reliable indicator of small thrombi in the calf veins.
- *Venography*—Contrast venography remains the most accurate diagnostic procedure for venous disease. Venography is particularly useful when there is a strong clinical suspicion of a calf thrombosis and when Doppler ultrasound has not given adequate information. It gives information regarding location, extent, and degree of attachment of the thrombus.

VARICOSE VEINS

Often a precursor to chronic venous insufficiency, varicose veins are usually caused by occupations that involve prolonged standing or sitting in one place, overweight, pregnancy, or a familial tendency. They may increase the patient's risk for DVT, or they may occur secondary to a DVT. Blockage to lymphatic flow can cause varicosities as seen with pelvic neoplasm. They appear as long, dilated, tortuous veins in the lower extremities.

Signs and Symptoms

Although cosmetically unsightly, varicose veins may be completely asymptomatic, or the patient may complain of aching or fatigue in the legs, particularly with standing. The same general measures should be applied that are used with chronic venous insufficiency.

Diagnostic Studies

Usually the physical examination is enough for the diagnosis, but ultrasound or venography may be warranted if thrombosis is suspected. Excision of the varicosity and ligation of the vein are possible for symptom relief or for cosmetic reasons and rarely to prevent complications. For small varicosities, compression sclerotherapy is helpful.

REFERENCES

American College of Cardiology. (2019). ASCVD 10-year Risk Estimator Plus. Retrieved July 8, 2021 from https://tools.acc.org/ASCVD-Risk-Estimator-Plus/#!/calculate/estimate/

Arnett, D. K., Blumenthal, R. S., Albert, M. A., Buroker, A. B, Goldberger, Z. D., Hahn, E. J., Himmelfarb, C. D., Khera, A., Lloyd-Jones, D., McEvoy, J. W., Michos, E. D., Miedema, M. D., Muñoz, D., Smith, Jr., S. C., Virani, S. S., Williams, Sr., K. A., Yeboah, J., Ziaeian, B. (2019). 2019 ACC/AHA guideline on the primary prevention of cardiovascular disease: A report of the American College of Cardiology/American Heart Association Task Force on Clinical Practice Guidelines. *Circulation, 140,* e596–e646. https://doi.org/10.1161/CIR.0000000000000678

Handelsman, Y., Jellinger, P. S., Guerin, C. K., Bloomgarden, Z. T., Brinton, E. A., Budoff, M. J., Davidson, M. H., Einhorn, D., Fazio, S., Fonseca, V. A., Garber, A. J., Grunberger, G., Krauss, R. M., Mechanick, J. I., Rosenblit, P. D., Smith, D. A, & Wyne, K. L. (2020). Consensus statement by the American Association of Clinical Endocrinologists and American College of Endocrinology on the management of dyslipidemia and prevention of cardiovascular disease algorithm–2020 executive summary. *Endocrine Practice, 26*(10), 1196–1224. https://doi.org/10.4158/CS-2020-0490

Jellinger, P. S., Handelsman, Y., Rosenblit, P. D., Bloomgarden, Z. T., Fonseca, V. A., Garber, A. J., Grunberger, G., Guerin, C. K., Bell, D. S. H., Mechanick, J. I., Pessah-Pollack, R., Wyne, K., Smith, D., Brinton, E. A., Fazio, S., & Davidson, M. (2017). American Association of Clinical Endocrinologists and American College of Endocrinology guidelines for the management of dyslipidemia and prevention of cardiovascular disease. *Endocrine Practice, 23*, 1–87.

Maddox, T. M., Januzzi, Jr., J. L., Allen, L. A., Breathett, K., Butler, J., Davis, L. L., Fonarow, G. C., Ibrahim, N. E., Lindenfeld, J., Masoudi, A. F., Motiwala, S. R., Oliveros, S., Patterson, H., Walsh, M. N., Wasserman, A., Yancy, C. W., & Youmans, R. Q. (2021). 2021 Update to the 2017 ACC Expert Consensus Decision Pathway for Optimization of Heart Failure Treatment: Answers to 10 pivotal issues about heart failure with reduced ejection fraction: A report of the American College of Cardiology Solution Set Oversight Committee. *Journal of the American College of Cardiology, 77*(6), 772–810. https://doi.org/10.1016/j.jacc.2020.11.022

Pulvarth, S., Gurram, M. K. (2014). Effectiveness of D-dimer as a screening test for venous thromboembolism: An update. *North American Journal of Medical Sciences, 6,* 491–499. https://doi.org/10.4103/1947-2714.143278

Wells, P. Wells' criteria for DVT. MDCalc. mdcalc.com. Accessed July 5, 2021, from https://www.mdcalc.com/wells-criteria-dvt

Whelton, P. K., Carey, R. M., Aronow, W. S., Casey, D. E., Collins, K. J., Himmelfarb, D. D., DePalma, S. M., Gidding, S., Jamerson, K. A., Jones, D. W., MacLaughlin, E. J., Muntner, P., Ovbiagele, B., Smith, S. C., Spencer, C. C., Stafford, R. S., Taler, S. J., Thomas, R. J., Williams, K. A., Williamson, J. D., & Wright, J. T. (2018). 2017 ACC/AHA/AAPA/ABC/ACPM/AGS/APhA/ASH/ASPC/NMA/PCNA guideline for the prevention, detection, evaluation, and management of high blood pressure in adults: a report of the American College of Cardiology/American Heart Association Task Force on Clinical Practice Guidelines. *Hypertension, 71,* e13–e115. https://www.ahajournals.org/doi/10.1161/HYP.0000000000000065

Yancy, C. W., Jessup, M., Bozkurt, B., Butler, J., Casey, D. E., Colvin, M. M., Drazner, M. H., Filippatos, G. S., Fonarow, G. C., Givertz, M. M., Hollenberg, S. M., Lindenfeld, J., Masoudi, F. A., McBride, P. E., Peterson, P. N., Stevenson, L. W., & Westlake, C. (2017). 2017. ACC/AHA/HFSA Focused Update of the 2013 ACCF/AHA Guideline for the Management of Heart Failure: A report of the American College of Cardiology/American Heart Association Task Force on Clinical Practice Guidelines and the Heart Failure Society of America. *Circulation, 136*(6), e137–e161. https://doi.org/10.1161/CIR.0000000000000509

Chapter 9

Respiratory System

Anna Jessup ·
Mary Jo Goolsby ·

R espiratory complaints are common in most health-care settings. Chronic obstructive pulmonary disease (COPD), composed of emphysema and chronic bronchitis, affects over 16 million adults in the United States and is now the fourth leading cause of death (American Lung Association, 2018). Pneumonia, with influenza, is currently the eighth leading cause of death in the United States and the greatest cause of infection-related deaths (CDC, 2021). The prevalence of asthma is also increasing. There are 19.2 million adults (7.7% of the population) and 5.5 million children younger than 18 years (7.5% of the population) with asthma, accounting for 9.8 million office visits in the United States (CDC, 2022).

Respiratory complaints, such as dyspnea and cough, can be vague and quite nonspecific. In addition, many extrapulmonary systems, such as cardiac, neurological, or the upper airway, may be the source of pulmonary signs and symptoms. A careful and detailed history and physical examination, with attention first to the respiratory system, enable accurate diagnosis. For instance, the history of uncontrolled hypertension and previous myocardial infarction in a nonsmoker, paired with the complaint of cough or sudden onset of dyspnea, direct the examiner to consider the potential for congestive heart failure, whereas a similar complaint in an otherwise healthy-appearing teen is more likely to suggest asthma or bronchitis.

History

■ Symptom Analysis

Regardless of the chief complaint, a thorough symptom analysis is warranted. It is important to understand when the complaint started and how the onset occurred. Determine how it has evolved, starting with the initial episode or awareness of the problem. Ask whether the problem is constant or intermittent. Determine whether a similar problem has been experienced in the past. It is important to learn whether factors such as emotions, exposure to outdoor allergens, or fatigue tend to precipitate or accelerate the complaint. Also determine if the symptoms tend to be tied to any particular time of day, such as night, early morning, or immediately following a meal. Another timing-related issue involves whether the complaint has continued essentially unchanged, worsened, or improved since first noticed.

The quality of the symptom is important. For chest discomfort, it is important to determine whether the pain or discomfort is sharp, dull, or aching. If the complaint is a cough, the potential qualities include whether the cough is mild and tickling or sharp and paroxysmal. For some complaints, such as wheezing and tightness or pain, it is also necessary to determine the exact location of the symptom and whether the patient has noticed any radiation to other sites and how it relates to respirations. Pleuritic chest pain may indicate pulmonary embolism. The severity is always important to establish.

As with other symptoms, it is always important to ask about self-treatment the patient may have tried and the response. For instance, determine what the patient has done to minimize the symptoms, including whether the patient has altered normal activity or taken any medications (prescribed or over-the-counter [OTC]). Include questions to identify herbal agents, illicit drugs, and complementary therapies tried.

When asking about the existence of associated symptoms, perform a review of pulmonary symptoms. There is a long list of symptoms that should be explored during this part of the history. Determine whether the patient has experienced any shortness of breath, nausea, or sweating, and if so, record the amount of work or effort that causes this symptom. Cardiac involvement must be ruled out. Ask about nocturnal orthopnea or related difficulty sleeping. Specifically, ask about the number of pillows the patient uses to sleep and about the sleeping position. A patient may use no pillows yet only rest comfortably in a recliner. Determine whether the patient has had a cough and whether any cough has been associated with the production of sputum or with hemoptysis. Also ask about wheezing, chest tightness, and sense of congestion. Ask whether the patient has had a fever, chills, or night sweats. In addition to asking about symptoms related to the lower respiratory tract, other systems should be explored based on the presenting symptom and symptom analysis.

■ Past Medical and Family History

The medical history should identify history of allergies, COPD, chronic bronchitis, asthma, pneumonia, recent or recurrent upper respiratory infections, and tuberculosis. Ask about the history of malignancy. Conditions stemming from other systems are often important to specifically address, including heart failure, gastroesophageal reflux disease (GERD), and allergies. During this part of the history, determine the approximate date of the patient's last chest x-ray and skin test for tuberculosis and the results of the test. The family history should be explored. Ask whether there is a family history of the conditions just mentioned.

■ Habits

The patient's habits are important in the assessment of respiratory complaints. Always establish the patient's smoking history, calculating pack years, and use of vaping products. Also determine any occupational or recreational exposures to toxins. Travel history is often significant, particularly for exposure to various infectious disorders affecting the lungs. Knowledge of the patient's exposure to pets is important because it can suggest exposure to infectious diseases or allergens. Identify all medications/drugs taken, including prescribed, OTC, and recreational, as well as any herbal or alternative therapies.

Physical Examination

The history should guide attention within the physical examination. However, regardless of the complaint, a thorough and orderly approach is recommended. In addition to the respiratory examination, a more comprehensive approach is usually necessary, regardless of whether the symptoms are mild or severe, acute or chronic. Other systems that should often be included are cardiac, musculoskeletal, neurological, and upper respiratory (ear, nose, and throat).

The examination actually starts during the history, as the examiner observes the patient's general condition. For instance, note whether the patient is able to provide a history without respiratory discomfort. Notice the patient's demeanor and apparent energy level. Assess the patient's breathing pattern and general coloring as the patient talks.

In assessing the lungs and chest, it is important that the patient be disrobed from the waist up and examined in an area with good lighting. The assessment of the chest involves all four components of physical assessment: inspection, palpation, percussion, and auscultation.

■ Inspection

Start by observing the patient's quiet respirations. Notice the rate, rhythm, depth, and amount of effort required. Check for obvious use of accessory muscles, as might be seen in several pulmonary conditions, including asthma, COPD, and pneumonia. Notice the movement of the chest and whether it is symmetrical. Identify any intercostal inspiratory retractions or expiratory bulges, which may indicate asthma or COPD. The chest configuration should be determined, including whether the chest is symmetrical and noting the ratio of the anterior-to-posterior (AP) diameter compared with the transverse chest diameter. A symmetric chest abnormality, such as pectus excavatum, or an asymmetric configuration, such as is often seen in scoliosis or kyphosis, may restrict respiratory effort. Increased AP diameter is indicative of COPD and pectus carinatum.

■ Palpation

Following inspection, gently palpate any area of discomfort or pain. Examples include intercostal tenderness, which could indicate inflamed pleurae, and costal-sternal border pain, which could indicate costochondritis. Next, palpate any area of visible deformity. Determine the respiratory excursion, or expansion, by placing hands around the patient's posterior rib cage with the thumbs approximately at the level of the 10th rib, thumbs touching, then asking the patient to take a deep breath while you observe the movement of the hands. The motion should be symmetrical. Less-than-anticipated movement occurs with advanced

COPD and many restrictive processes, such as interstitial lung disease. Asymmetry of movement occurs with atelectasis, lobar collapse, pneumothorax, and several other conditions.

The quality of tactile fremitus is determined by palpating symmetrical areas with the palmar surface of the hands and fingers, as the patient is directed to speak, usually repeatedly saying "99" or "1-2-3" in a loud and a low-pitched voice. This maneuver provides only a rough estimate of lung condition but is useful in guiding further assessment. Areas of increased fremitus should raise the suspicion of conditions resulting in increased solidity or consolidation in the underlying lung tissue, such as in pneumonia or pulmonary fibrosis. Conversely, areas of decreased fremitus raise the suspicion of abnormal fluid- or air-filled spaces, such as occurs with pleural effusion, pneumothorax, or emphysema. In the instance of an extensive bronchial obstruction, no palpable vibration is felt in the related field.

■ Percussion

Percussion provides an estimate of the relative amounts of air, fluid, and solid matter in a space and is helpful in identifying the margins of organs, including the lungs. The lung fields should be percussed posteriorly, starting from the superior-most areas and then proceeding inferiorly to the level of the diaphragm. Hyperresonance suggests air trapping, which occurs with COPD or tension pneumothorax. Dullness is detected over the actual site of consolidated lung or pleural fluid. Dullness is found with pneumonia, severe atelectasis, or pleural effusion.

■ Auscultation

The most helpful assessment maneuver involves auscultation of the lung fields. The general lung fields should be auscultated, with special attention paid to any areas where previous abnormalities were detected. With the patient breathing fully through an open mouth, a full inspiratory and expiratory cycle should be assessed at each site. During auscultation, the examiner should first notice the qualities associated with the breath sound, then assess for the presence of any adventitious lung sounds.

Breath sounds vary in intensity, volume, and duration, depending on the site along the tracheobronchoalveolar system. In the upper part of the respiratory tree, over the trachea, breath sounds should be "bronchial," meaning they are loud, and the inspiratory component is shorter than the expiratory component. Over the bronchi, the bronchovesicular sounds are of a medium intensity, and the inspiratory and expiratory components are of equal duration. Finally, the vesicular sounds over the peripheral lung tissue are, by comparison, softer in volume and have a shorter expiratory phase. Increased breath sounds over peripheral lung regions indicate consolidation, which may occur with pneumonia. Decreased, or softer, peripheral breath sounds indicate bronchial obstruction or pleural effusion.

Table 9.1	
Adventitious Sounds	
Description	Significance
Crackles	
Coarse, medium, or fine; early, mid-, or late-inspiratory	Atelectasis, bronchiectasis, congestive heart failure, pulmonary fibrosis
Rhonchi, Wheezes	
Low- or high-pitched; inspiratory or expiratory	COPD, acute and chronic bronchitis, asthma, bronchiectasis, pneumonia
Friction Rub	
Loud, grating; late inspiratory–early expiratory	Inflamed pleura; pneumonia, pleuritis, malignancy

Adventitious breath sounds are extra, abnormal sounds detected in addition to the expected breath sounds. Terms such as *rhonchi*, *wheezes*, and *crackles* are used to describe these adventitious sounds. The term *rales* is confusing and has largely been replaced with the more explanatory term *crackles*. Regardless of the terminology used, it is important to provide as many descriptors as possible relative to the adventitious sound. Descriptors can include details of the detected pitch, amplitude, and quality of the sound. For instance, crackles can be described as loud or soft, coarse or fine. Wheezes, or rhonchi, can be described as loud or soft, high- or low-pitched, coarse/sonorous, squeaking, or hissing/sibilant. Another important characteristic to note is whether adventitious lung sounds occur early or late in the respiratory cycle. All of these characteristics are helpful in determining the cause. Table 9.1 describes potential adventitious sounds tied with some respiratory disorders.

Because mobile bronchial secretions can cause adventitious sounds, ask the patient to take a deep breath and cough if these sounds are detected. This often clears the airway and eliminates or changes the adventitious sounds. The effect of cough (or lack of cough) on the adventitious sounds is important to record. Failure to have the patient clear the airway of mobile secretions could result in a misdiagnosis.

A final adventitious sound is the pleural friction rub, typically a loud, grating sound produced when the two inflamed and roughened surfaces of the visceral and parietal pleurae rub together. A friction rub is usually noted in the late inspiratory and early expiratory phases and in the lower anterolateral lung fields. Examples of conditions that result in a pleural rub include pneumonia and malignancy.

Depending on the findings associated with the examination up to this point, the examiner can decide whether to proceed with auscultated spoken sounds: bronchophony, egophony, and/or whispered pectoriloquy. If the examination is normal up to this point, there is no need to proceed with spoken sounds. However, if an abnormality is detected, this maneuver may provide valuable data that will help to narrow the assessment. As with tactile fremitus, the patient is again directed to repeatedly say "99" or "1-2-3" as the examiner auscultates the lung fields. The expected norm is that the volume and clarity of the transmitted speech sounds are uniform throughout the lung fields. An increased volume in one area is called *bronchophony*, suggesting an area of consolidation or effusion. Whispered sounds are also auscultated as the patient whispers "99" or "1-2-3." Any area of increased clarity is positive for whispered pectoriloquy, another indication of consolidation. Finally, the lung fields can be auscultated as the patient repeats "E-E-E." If the detected sound is heard as "A-A-A" with a nasal quality over a particular area, indicating egophony, this is a final indication of consolidation.

■ Diagnostic Studies

Diagnostic studies are often helpful in making a definitive diagnosis for pulmonary conditions. Spirometry provides a range of information about the lung function and is important in differentiating among causes of respiratory complaints. A number of portable and accurate devices are available. Pulse oximetry provides a portable, simple method to determine the percentage of hemoglobin saturated with oxygen. Arterial blood gases, rarely obtained in outpatient settings, provide data on a patient's acid–base balance and whether disturbances stem from respiratory or metabolic derangements.

■ Imaging Studies

A wide range of imaging studies are useful in assessing respiratory complaints. In addition to plain films, computed tomography (CT) scans, ultrasounds, and, on occasion, positron emission tomography (PET) scans provide noninvasive ways to assess pulmonary tissue and space.

DIFFERENTIAL DIAGNOSIS OF CHIEF COMPLAINTS

■ Cough

Cough is an extremely common and potentially nonspecific complaint. Whereas the cough serves as an important defense mechanism, it is often the major reason a patient seeks diagnosis and treatment of many self-limiting and minor complaints as well as many life-threatening ones. Cough is classified as acute (less than 3 weeks in duration), subacute (lasting 3 to 8 weeks), and chronic (8 or more weeks in duration), and these distinctions help to narrow the potential differential diagnoses. However, patients with chronic cough may present acutely as some component of their problem is exacerbated.

The history and physical examination are essential in eliminating potential causes and identifying the most likely causes of cough. For instance, when a person presents with a cough after being prescribed an angiotensin-converting enzyme (ACE) inhibitor, a thorough history and physical examination help the provider ensure that there is no other likely coexisting problem triggering and/ or causing the cough.

History

The history should include a thorough analysis of the cough, including a determination of how long it has persisted. It is essential to identify any associated symptoms, including shortness of breath, wheezing, orthopnea, fever, chills, chest pain or discomfort, sputum production, postnasal drainage, and hemoptysis. The medical history should be comprehensive, with a particular focus on the potential for asthma, COPD, chronic or acute bronchitis, heart failure, GERD, or recent upper or lower respiratory infections. The medication history will not only exclude the potential for ACE inhibitor–induced cough but will also identify other problems for which medications are taken. The patient's prior self-treatment or prescribed treatment of cough should be explored, including the response and tolerance of the treatment. Family history should be established.

Physical Examination

A thorough examination of the lungs should be performed as described earlier in this chapter. Note the patient's general appearance and any distress as the history is provided. Vital signs should be evaluated for respiratory rate, pulse, and temperature. Note the respiratory excursion as deep breaths are taken and whether a cough is triggered. If tactile fremitus is conducted, be attentive to areas of increased or decreased vibration. Carefully assess breath sounds and note the characteristics of any adventitious sounds. Observe any sputum that can be produced for color and consistency. Depending on the history and physical findings to this point, additional assessment may be warranted and may include, for example, the upper respiratory, cardiac system, or gastrointestinal (GI) systems.

Diagnostic Studies

Diagnostic studies are often not indicated. Depending on the presentation, spirometry or chest x-ray are the studies most likely to be indicated.

UPPER AIRWAY COUGH SYNDROME

Postnasal discharge or drainage is the most common cause of chronic cough, which is diagnosed as upper airway cough syndrome (UACS).

Signs and Symptoms

The patient complains of a chronic cough often associated with a sensation of drainage in the back of the throat and the need to clear the throat frequently. There may be accompanying hoarseness. Depending on the cause of the UACS, the patient will have symptoms consistent with allergic rhinitis, chronic sinusitis, or another condition, such as a cold or viral upper respiratory infection. Although no sputum is produced, there is a potential that secretions will be cleared from the posterior pharynx by the coughing effort. Common signs include throat clearing, drainage on the posterior pharynx, and hyperemia and cobblestoning of the posterior pharynx, with a negative chest examination.

Diagnostic Studies

No studies are usually warranted initially. Response to treatment for UACS provides presumptive diagnosis. Depending on the patient's risk factors, specific diagnostic studies can be considered to rule out other causes, which could coexist with UACS, and contributing factors. These include allergy testing and radiographs of the sinuses or chest.

ASTHMA

Asthma is a chronic condition that involves inflammation of the airways, with varying degrees of airway obstruction and hyperresponsiveness. The incidence of asthma is increasing in the United States, and it affects people of all ages. Although typically associated with wheezing, a cough may be the primary complaint associated with asthma.

Signs and Symptoms

The patient complains of intermittent sensation of chest tightness, cough, shortness of breath, and wheezing. The cough is typically nonproductive. The symptoms may become relatively persistent and affect quality of life. Symptoms often worsen with activity, viral infections, exposure to allergens, or other triggers. The Expert Panel Report 3 (EPR3) is the most recent report from National Heart, Blood, and Lung Institute (2007) to address assessment and diagnosis of asthma. The EPR3 provides several tables defining the characteristics to use to stage asthma according to levels of severity. The history is an important aspect because the frequency of various symptoms, nighttime awakenings, use of a short-acting beta agonist, and interference with activities are used, along with spirometry, in staging asthma. Examination may reveal wheezes. Deep respiratory effort may trigger paroxysmal coughing. Respiratory effort may require use of accessory respiratory muscles. However, absence of physical findings does not rule out the presence of asthma. In addition to respiratory findings, patients with asthma often have other signs of atopy, including allergic rhinitis or atopic dermatitis.

Diagnostic Studies

Pulmonary function tests or spirometry provide diagnosis; diminished forced expiratory volume in 1 second (FEV_1)/forced vital capacity (FVC) ratio and diminished FEV_1 indicate obstructed outflow. Some degree of reversibility occurs with the administration of bronchodilators. Chest films are generally within normal limits unless there is significant air trapping. Peak flow meters should not be used as diagnostic tools. They are appropriate for monitoring ongoing symptoms and determining the response to therapy, particularly once a patient's "personal best" is determined.

CHRONIC OBSTRUCTIVE PULMONARY DISEASE (COPD)

COPD is most commonly caused by smoking, with the onset of symptoms typically beginning in middle age. When younger patients or nonsmokers develop findings consistent with COPD, alpha-1 antitrypsin deficiency should be suspected. COPD is actually made up of two related and often coexisting problems: chronic bronchitis and emphysema. The condition is frequently progressive, with little reversibility.

Signs and Symptoms

Common symptoms of COPD include chronic cough and dyspnea. Cough, usually the earliest symptom, generally develops following years of smoking and with variable sputum production. Dyspnea, a key symptom of COPD, is progressive and often becomes debilitating. The symptoms are worse on exertion and are usually progressive over time. There is often a history of exacerbations, during episodes of acute bronchitis. On physical examination, lung sounds are diminished. The patient develops a "barrel chest" in which the AP chest diameter is greater than the lateral diameter as the COPD advances. However, physical examination is considered inadequate to definitively detect COPD. Advanced and progressive disease results in right heart failure or cor pulmonale with abdominal distension, liver tenderness, and peripheral edema.

Diagnostic Studies

Spirometry should be performed to confirm diagnosis and should include measure of FVC, FEV_1, and the FEV_1/FVC ratio.

The Global Initiative for Chronic Obstructive Lung Disease (GOLD, 2021) grading system addresses the frequency and severity of exacerbations and how COPD affects daily life. Recognizing the importance of symptom assessment in addition to spirometry, the Modified Medical Research Council (MMRC) Dyspnea Scale and the COPD Assessment Test (CAT) are included in the 2021 grading.

The degree of airflow obstruction is still considered for categorizing COPD into four stages of airflow limitation, ranging from mild to very severe. Each stage is characterized by a decreased ratio of FEV_1 to FVC to less than 70%. The percentage of predicted FEV provides further differentiation; this value varies from greater than 80% for stage I (mild) to less than 80%, less than 50%, and less than 30% for stages II (moderate), III (severe), and IV (very severe), respectively.

Chest radiographs reveal hyperinflation of the lungs with flattened diaphragm and should be used to confirm but not diagnose a patient with COPD. Currently, the American Thoracic Society (2003) recommends that all individuals with COPD or asthma with chronic obstructive changes be tested for alpha-1 antitrypsin deficiency. If alpha-1 antitrypsin deficit is suspected, a qualitative serum should be performed as a screen, followed by quantitative study, as indicated.

PNEUMONIA

Pneumonia involves inflammation and consolidation of lung tissue. Pneumonia is broadly categorized by whether it occurs outside of the hospital (community-acquired pneumonia) or within the hospital (nosocomial, or hospital-acquired, pneumonia). The cause is most often *Streptococcus pneumoniae, Haemophilus influenzae,* or *Staphylococcus aureus.* In 2020, COVID-19 arose as a cause of pneumonia and other respiratory distress (Box 9.1). Atypical pneumonia involves infection of mycoplasma, legionella, or chlamydia. However, pneumonia can be caused by a wide range of microorganisms, including other bacteria, viruses, and fungi.

Signs and Symptoms

The symptoms of pneumonia are quite varied. Commonly, the patient complains of cough associated with fever, malaise, shaking chills, rigors, and chest discomfort. The patient often appears ill. Abnormal vital signs include tachycardia and tachypnea and fever. There is uneven fremitus, and the area over the consolidation percusses dully. On auscultation, there are bronchial breath sounds, often with crackles. Bronchophony, egophony, and whispered pectoriloquy are often present.

Diagnostic Studies

Chest film typically reveals an area of infiltrate. It is a red flag if a pleural effusion is also visualized, in which case adequate follow-up to exclude development of an empyema is mandatory. This often involves prompt referral to a pulmonologist for possible thoracentesis. Cultures and Gram stains of sputum are usually not ordered for outpatients. The white blood cell count is often elevated. Use of the CURB-65 will help determine if the patient warrants hospitalization with this pneumonia (Box 9.2).

Box 9.1

COVID-19 Decision Rule

Trubiano et al. (2020) published the COVID-MATCH65 clinical decision rule, which provides a framework for stratifying the risk of COVID-19 among patients with associated acute respiratory syndrome. COVID-MATCH65 is a mnemonic-based tool that assigns or deducts points for each of the following: **C**OVID-19 exposure or international travel within past 14 days (+2.5), **M**yalgia/malaise (+1), **A**nosmia/ageusia (+2.5), **T**emperature/any reported fever (+0.5), **C**oryza/sore throat (–1), **H**ypoxia/oxygen saturation <97% on room air (+1), **65** years or older (+1).

Risk is estimated based on total points as follows: <1 point = low (0.5%) risk; 1–1.5 point = moderate (1.5%) risk; 2–3.5 points = high (6%) risk; 4–4.5 points = very high (20%) risk; ≥5 points = extreme (50%) risk.

Box 9.2

Community-Acquired Pneumonia Decision Rule

Decision Rule: CURB-65 provides framework for determining whether the patient diagnosed with community-acquired pneumonia can be safely monitored and treated at home. One point is awarded for each of the following factors present:

- **C**onfusion of new onset
- **B**UN >20 mg/dL*
- **R**espiratory rate of ≥30 breaths/minute
- **B**lood pressure <90 mm Hg systolic or diastolic ≤60 mm Hg
- Age **65** or older

Patients scoring 3 to 5 typically require hospitalization for observation and therapy. Scores of 0 to 1 indicate likelihood that outpatient management is appropriate. A score of 2 is inconclusive.

* If blood urea nitrogen (BUN) is unavailable, may omit and then adjust the scoring system.

ACUTE BRONCHITIS

Acute bronchitis is commonly encountered in ambulatory care and affects persons of all ages. It involves inflammatory processes of the bronchial smooth muscles and is associated with a wide range of microorganisms, usually viral.

Signs and Symptoms

Cough is the most common symptom of bronchitis and may persist for several weeks after the initial infection resolves. During the acute phase, the cough may be productive. There may be associated symptoms, including fever, malaise, chest discomfort, chills, and headache. The chills and chest discomfort are mild in comparison to the symptoms of pneumonia. There may be wheezes and/or rhonchi on auscultation, which disappear or alter with cough effort. Fremitus is equal, and there is no egophony.

Diagnostic Studies

No studies are necessary unless chest radiology is needed to rule out pneumonia. Spirometry can be performed to rule out asthma and monitor response to therapy.

CONGESTIVE HEART FAILURE

Congestive heart failure often results in cough associated with the other symptoms and findings common to congestive heart failure. See Chapter 8.

GASTROESOPHAGEAL REFLUX DISEASE

GERD is a common cause of chronic cough. The mechanism by which GERD causes cough usually involves vagal stimulation rather than aspiration. Although cough may be the only symptom of GERD, patients usually also complain of heartburn or other GI symptoms. See Chapter 11.

BRONCHIECTASIS

Bronchiectasis involves dilation of one or more bronchi. Congenital bronchiectasis affects infants and children. Acquired bronchiectasis involves older children and adults and stems from infections, bronchial obstruction, and cystic fibrosis.

Signs and Symptoms

There is usually a history of chronic, productive cough. Sputum is typically mucopurulent and produced in increased amounts. Other common findings include shortness of breath, wheezing, fatigue, and possibly hemoptysis. Physical examination reveals rhonchi and/or wheezing. In advanced disease, clubbing and cyanosis may be present.

Diagnostic Studies

Chest films reveal linear markings, atelectasis, and pulmonary cysts. To confirm diagnosis, a high-resolution CT scan is used. Sputum studies may include positive cultures. A complete blood count may identify either anemia or polycythemia and increased white blood cell count. Pulmonary functions vary. Diagnostic studies are further needed to identify the cause of the condition.

TUBERCULOSIS

Tuberculosis is caused by a mycobacterium and frequently affects the lungs, although other organs may be involved. Risk factors include low socioeconomic status, impaired immune system, and crowded conditions. Tuberculosis presents a significant public health threat, and early diagnosis and treatment are important.

Signs and Symptoms

Many times, patients with active tuberculosis are essentially symptom free. Some complain of malaise and/or fevers but have no significantly disruptive complaints. When respiratory symptoms occur with tuberculosis, cough is common; the cough is nonproductive at first and is later associated with sputum production. Additionally, patients with tuberculosis may experience progressive dyspnea, night sweats, weight loss, and hemoptysis.

Diagnostic Studies

Plain chest films reveal hilar adenopathy and multilobular granulomas, particularly of the upper lungs. For this reason, it is important to include a lordotic view with the usual AP and lateral views. Tuberculin skin testing is positive. Sputum reveals acid-fast bacilli. Sputum acid-fast bacilli culture requires up to 3 weeks for definitive diagnosis but should identify *Mycobacterium tuberculosis*. Active tuberculosis must be referred to the local public health department for treatment.

MALIGNANCY

Pulmonary malignancies may arise anywhere from the tracheobronchial tree to peripheral lung tissue.

Signs and Symptoms

There may be few symptoms until the condition is advanced. Common complaints include dyspnea, cough, hemoptysis, fatigue, wheezing, and chest discomfort. Suspicion of potential malignancy should be heightened in patients who present with cough and hemoptysis paired with history of recurrent respiratory infections. Physical signs depend on the area of involvement, and the examination may be entirely normal. However, patients with pulmonary malignancy may appear ill, have unexplained weight loss, and have a variety of abnormal pulmonary findings, including asymmetrical breath sounds, adventitious sounds, and stridor.

Diagnostic Studies

Pulmonary functions vary, depending on the location and size of the mass. Chest films are often nondiagnostic, although they may reveal a nodule, mass, or other abnormality. A CT scan of the chest is typically diagnostic. Diagnosis is made on biopsy and histopathology, with samples obtained by fine needle aspiration, bronchoscopy, mediastinoscopy, or thoracentesis.

PHARMACOLOGICAL AND ACE INHIBITOR–INDUCED COUGH

Although cough can be associated with a variety of other medications, including aspirin, ACE inhibitors are a common cause of chronic cough. ACE inhibitors allow kinins to accumulate in the respiratory tract, causing a cough in 10% to 20% of patients who are prescribed these agents.

Signs and Symptoms

The cough associated with ACE inhibitors is dry and intractable and often worst at night. Aspirin is a rare trigger of asthma, and a cough due to aspirin or NSAIDs is often tight and dry, accompanied by wheezing. The history reveals cough onset soon after a newly prescribed agent.

Diagnostic Studies

No studies are warranted except to rule out other causes. Diagnosis is typically made by discontinuing the offending agent. ACE-associated cough may persist for a considerable time following elimination of the agent.

■ Shortness of Breath and Dyspnea

Dyspnea is the subjective sense of discomfort or difficulty breathing. Commonly, patients with dyspnea may present with complaint of shortness of breath, chest tightness, or simply difficulty breathing or catching the breath. In addition to the history and physical specific to the respiratory system, a comprehensive assessment must be included, because the causes of dyspnea may stem from many extrapulmonary conditions.

■ History

It is essential that the symptom be thoroughly explored in order to help the patient definitively define the complaint. The setting in which the dyspnea occurs is important, including whether it occurs in specific situations or activities, is persistent or intermittent, and has any associated symptoms. The duration and progression are important to identify. Ask about how, if at all, the patient's routines have been affected by the dyspnea.

A variety of measures can be used to assess dyspnea. For instance, the patient can be asked to identify the point along a 10-cm visual analog scale that best depicts the dyspnea experienced, with one pole representing absence of shortness of breath or dyspnea and the other pole representing the worst dyspnea imaginable. Other scales depend on numerical rating or are specific to dyspnea related to a particular condition, such as asthma or cancer. A thorough medication history must be obtained along with a medical and family history. Habits such as tobacco use are important.

Physical Examination

A thorough respiratory and cardiac examination should be performed. Be attentive to signs of respiratory distress during the history or in response to the various maneuvers associated with the examination. Note any signs of edema.

Diagnostic Studies

The need for diagnostic studies is indicated by the patient's presentation. Examples of studies that might be warranted include spirometry, chest films, complete blood count, and thyroid function tests.

PNEUMONIA

Pneumonia often causes acute dyspnea. See previous discussion on pneumonia, pp. 308–309.

CONGESTIVE HEART FAILURE

Dyspnea is associated with congestive heart failure. See Chapter 8.

PLEURAL EFFUSION

Pleural effusions involve an abnormal collection of fluid in the pleural space. Effusions are usually secondary to another condition, such as malignancy, heart failure, cirrhosis, trauma, and infections.

Signs and Symptoms

Dyspnea is the most common symptom associated with pleural effusion, but effusion may be accompanied by cough, pain, and systemic symptoms, such as malaise and fever. Abnormal physical findings become evident as the effusion increases in volume. These include decreased lung sounds, dullness over the effusion, decreased fremitus, egophony, and whispered pectoriloquy. With extremely large effusions, the mediastinum and trachea may shift to the opposite side. The exception involves effusion related to malignancy, in which case the mediastinum and trachea may be pulled toward the malignancy.

Diagnostic Studies

Chest films reveal the fluid collection as an increased area of density, blunting of the costophrenic angle, and elevation of the hemidiaphragm. Plain films may also reveal a potential cause, including a mass or malignancy, infiltrates of pneumonia, or cardiomegaly of heart failure. A consultant may perform a thoracentesis to remove the effusion for observation and therapy. Observations include determining whether the fluid is purulent, bloody, milky, or malodorous. Testing could involve Gram stain, cell count with differential, culture and sensitivity, cytology, and chemical studies (protein, glucose, and lactate dehydrogenase).

PULMONARY EMBOLISM

Pulmonary emboli (PE) are life-threatening events stemming from venous thrombi. The symptoms associated with PE range from very dramatic to nonspecific, making them sometimes difficult to diagnose.

Signs and Symptoms

A history of immobility, surgery, pregnancy, hypercoagulability, deep venous thrombosis, or other conditions may be associated with the development of emboli. Dyspnea is common to PE, as is pleuritic chest pain. Patients may have no symptoms at all or only nonspecific dyspnea. However, in severe cases, the patient presents with a sudden onset of severe dyspnea associated with cough, chest pain, and, potentially, hemoptysis. While physical findings vary, assess for signs and symptoms of deep venous thrombosis. The patient may be tachypneic and tachycardic. There may be findings consistent with pleural effusion on the affected side (see preceding subsection).

Diagnostic Studies

Plain chest films are usually normal but may reveal atelectasis, pleural effusion, or infiltrates. Ventilation/perfusion scanning reveals a perfusion defect and should be used if intravenous contrast media is contraindicated. A CT pulmonary angiogram has high sensitivity and specificity for PE and should be ordered to visualize narrowing of blocked blood vessels, if there is concern for pulmonary embolism. A D-dimer blood test can be helpful, although it is nonspecific.

RESTRICTIVE LUNG DISEASE

Both pulmonary and extrapulmonary disorders can result in diminished lung capacity and restrictive lung disease. Pulmonary disorders that affect the compliance of the lung tissue result in decreased ventilation, as do extrinsic conditions, such as kyphosis and scoliosis. Onset may be gradual for lung problems, such as pneumonitis, pulmonary fibrosis, and sarcoidosis, as well as extrinsic causes, such as kyphosis or obesity.

Signs and Symptoms

There may be a family history of intrinsic restrictive lung disease or personal history of occupational exposure to toxins. Patients with neuromuscular disorders often have symptoms of generalized fatigue and weakness. With extrinsic conditions, such as kyphosis, scoliosis, or obesity, physical findings are usually evident. Examination reveals restricted respiratory excursion and, often, basilar crackles.

Diagnostic Studies

Appropriate studies vary, depending on the suspected cause of restricted airway disease. Spirometry reveals decreased FEV_1, total lung capacity, and/or FVC. The FEV_1/FVC ratio will be normal. If an unknown cause is suspected, a complete lung function test with lung volumes and a diffusing lung capacity is indicated.

PNEUMOTHORAX

Pneumothorax involves air in the pleural cavity. A pneumothorax can occur spontaneously in otherwise healthy individuals or can be secondary to trauma or intrinsic lung disease.

Signs and Symptoms

There is a history of sudden onset of shortness of breath associated with chest pain. The patient usually presents in great distress, with tachycardia and tachypnea, and is often splinting the chest. There is decreased fremitus and increased hyperresonance on the affected side. Lung sounds are diminished or absent. The trachea may shift away from the affected side if a large pneumothorax is present.

Diagnostic Studies

Plain chest films usually reveal the pneumothorax with an absence of lung markings in the affected area and a shift of the mediastinum. Prompt referral to the emergency department is warranted to ascertain if needle/catheter aspiration or chest tube placement is indicated.

ADULT RESPIRATORY DISTRESS SYNDROME

Adult respiratory distress syndrome (ARDS) involves pulmonary inflammation, increased membrane permeability, and edema. ARDS affects 190,000 in the United States annually, with 74,000 deaths (Griffiths et al., 2019). As the name implies, it is a syndrome, not a specific disease. It is associated with a diverse number of conditions such as pneumonia, sepsis, aspiration, inhalation of noxious agents, burns, trauma, and as a complication of significant surgical procedures (e.g., cardiac, neurological). Prognosis is mixed, and ARDS may lead to complications, including other organ failure. Progression may be rapid, requiring ventilator assistance. If ARDS is suspected in an ambulatory setting, emergent transport to critical care facility is important to prevent systemic complications.

Signs and Symptoms

Symptoms include acute onset of shortness of breath, cough, and white or frothy sputum. The symptoms progress rapidly with dyspnea, tachypnea, and tachycardia at rest. Other findings are specific to the underlying cause. Crackles may be present, with visible respiratory difficulty, hypotension, and cyanosis. Patients develop persistent hypoxia that fails to respond to oxygen therapy, and complete respiratory failure can rapidly develop.

Diagnostic Studies

Hypoxemia is common with abnormal blood gases. Radiological findings reveal bilateral pulmonary infiltrates. B-type natriuretic peptide less than 100 pg/mL supports ARDS diagnosis as opposed to cardiogenic pulmonary edema. Other laboratory abnormalities are dependent on the cause of onset (Griffiths et al., 2019). Blood cultures are warranted if sepsis is suspected.

FOREIGN BODY ASPIRATION

Aspiration of a solid or semisolid object can be life-threatening. Foreign body aspiration can occur at any age. However, young children, who have a tendency to put objects in their mouths, have the highest incidence of foreign body aspiration and associated mortality. The onset of symptoms may be sudden if the object obstructs the airway. However, if the airway is not significantly obstructed, symptoms may develop more slowly, as the aspiration results in pneumonia.

Signs and Symptoms

There may be a witnessed episode of sudden difficulty breathing or choking accompanied by inability to speak, cyanosis, coughing, and/or loss of consciousness. If the airway obstruction is complete, respiratory arrest occurs. If obstruction is partial, there will be varying degrees of coughing, wheezing, and stridor. If the obstruction is not significant, the patient may present with complaints of cough, increasing dyspnea, fever, and symptoms consistent with pneumonia. Physical findings depend on the degree of obstruction and can include stridor, wheezing, diminished lung sounds, cyanosis, and findings consistent with pneumonia.

Diagnostic Studies

Plain chest films may reveal air trapping or atelectasis as well as the radiolucent object. A CT scan may be necessary to identify radiopaque objects. A bronchoscopy may be necessary to identify and remove a foreign object.

MALIGNANCY

Pulmonary and nonpulmonary malignancies may result in difficulty breathing. See previous discussion, pp. 310–311.

ASTHMA

Shortness of breath or dyspnea is extremely common in asthma. See previous discussion, p. 306.

CHRONIC OBSTRUCTIVE PULMONARY DISEASE

Progressive dyspnea is a common finding of COPD. See previous discussion, p. 307.

ANEMIA

Anemia can result in dyspnea or a sense of "air hunger." See the discussion of anemia in Chapter 17.

■ Wheezing and Chest Tightness

Wheezing is an audible respiratory sound often associated with a sense of chest tightness and dyspnea. Many of the conditions included in the preceding discussions of cough and dyspnea also cause wheezing and chest tightness. For this reason, the history and physical assessment for this complaint are the same as for the other respiratory complaints and should be thorough.

LARYNGEAL OR TRACHEAL OBSTRUCTION

Obstruction of the large airways can occur with many conditions, including inflammation, malignancy, laryngospasm, and foreign body aspiration.

Signs and Symptoms

The symptoms and signs vary, depending on the condition responsible for the obstruction. The wheezing is evident over the major airways as a harsh stridor than typical wheezing.

Diagnostic Studies

Appropriate diagnostic studies depend on the suspected cause.

ASTHMA

Wheezing is commonly associated with asthma. See previous discussion, p. 306.

ACUTE BRONCHITIS

See previous discussion, p. 309.

CHRONIC OBSTRUCTIVE PULMONARY DISEASE

Wheezing often occurs with COPD, particularly chronic bronchitis. See p. 307.

MALIGNANCY

Bronchial and pulmonary tumors can present with wheezing. See pp. 310–311.

■ Hemoptysis

Hemoptysis can be associated with a wide range of pulmonary disorders, which have been described in this chapter. With presentation of a hemoptysis complaint, it is essential that the history identify associated symptoms in addition to the analysis of hemoptysis. Investigate recent exposures to other persons with infectious diseases. Patients living in proximity to others are at increased risk for contracting infectious respiratory disorders. A history of smoking is important; a history of tuberculosis or positive skin tests must be identified. A thorough examination of the respiratory system provides data important to narrowing the differential diagnosis. Diagnostic studies often include plain radiographs of the chest.

TUBERCULOSIS

Hemoptysis is a late symptom of tuberculosis, which is described on p. 310.

PNEUMONIA

Pneumonia may result in hemoptysis and is described on pp. 308–309.

MALIGNANCY

Malignancy should always be considered for patients with hemoptysis. See pp. 310–311.

BRONCHITIS

Bronchitis can result in hemoptysis. See p. 310.

PULMONARY EMBOLISM

See p. 313.

■ Pleuritic Pain

Pleuritic pain is associated with respiratory movements and breathing. Although the cause is often respiratory in nature, pleuritic pain is also associated with chest trauma and inflammation as well as with GI and cardiac disorders. Pleuritic pain can cause significant distress and anxiety. A thorough symptom analysis is necessary. Through the history, determine whether there have been recent symptoms of respiratory infection, trauma to the chest, or extrapulmonary symptoms consistent with musculoskeletal, GI, or cardiac problems. A comprehensive physical assessment is necessary.

COSTOCHONDRITIS

Costochondritis is pain at a costosternal cartilage site. It can follow trauma to the chest wall, but the cause is often not identifiable. The symptoms may follow a period of strenuous exercise or coughing.

Signs and Symptoms

The patient reports pleuritic pain that is affected by breathing or chest motion. The site of tenderness is limited, and the pain is reproducible with firm pressure to the site. On occasion, there are signs of inflammation at the tender area, but generally, the physical examination is otherwise negative.

Diagnostic Studies

Generally, no diagnostic studies are warranted.

PLEURISY

Pleurisy involves inflammation of the pleura and is often related to underlying infectious processes.

Signs and Symptoms

The patient complains of severe and sharp pleuritic pain with acute onset. The pain may be noted only with cough, respiration, or maneuvers that cause chest motion. However, there may be a sense of vague, consistent pain that becomes pronounced with respiratory motions. The patient often splints the chest and attempts shallow respirations to limit the discomfort. A pleural friction rub may be auscultated. Pleural effusion may develop, with physical findings of percussive dullness, decreased fremitus, egophony, and decreased breath sounds at the site.

Diagnostic Studies

The diagnosis is usually based on the history of definitive pleuritic pain and physical findings. However, chest films can be obtained and will vary from being within normal limits to revealing an infiltrate or pleural effusion.

CHEST TRAUMA

Direct trauma to the chest can result in pain that is worsened with respirations owing either to rib fracture or to injury to the intercostal muscles.

Signs and Symptoms

The history should reveal the offending trauma, with physical findings consistent with the injury.

Diagnostic Studies

Diagnostic studies should be determined by the history of trauma.

PERICARDITIS

Pericarditis involves inflammation of the pericardium. Pericarditis can be associated with an infectious disorder and a variety of other conditions. See the discussion in Chapter 8.

PULMONARY EMBOLISM

See previous discussion, p. 313.

MALIGNANCY

See previous discussion, pp. 310–311.

REFERENCES

American Lung Association. (2018). COPD Prevalence. Retrieved March 9, 2021, from https://www.lung
.org/research/trends-in-lung-disease/copd-trends-brief/copd-prevalence

American Thoracic Society/European Respiratory Society. (2003). American Thoracic Society/European
Respiratory Society statement: Standards for the diagnosis and management of individuals with alpha-1
antitrypsin deficiency. *American Journal of Respiratory Critical Care Medicine, 168*(7), 818–900.

Centers for Disease Control and Prevention. (2022). Asthma. Retrieved March 23, 2003 from http://www
.cdc.gov/nchs/fastats/asthma.htm

Centers for Disease Control and Prevention (2021). Leading Cause of Death. Retrieved March 6, 2021,
from https://www.cdc.gov/nchs/fastats/leading-causes-of-death.htm

GOLD. (2021). Global strategy for diagnosis, management, and prevention of COPD. Retrieved March 6,
2021, from https://goldcopd.org/wp-content/uploads/2020/11/GOLD-REPORT-2021-v1.1-25Nov20
_WMV.pdf

Griffiths, M., McAuley, D., Perkins, G., Barrett, N., Blackwood, B., Boyle, A., Chee, N., Connolly, B.,
Dark, P., Finney, S., Salam, A., Silversides, N., Tarmey, N., Wise, M., & Baudouin, S. (2019). Guidelines
on the management of acute respiratory syndrome. *BMJ Open Respiratory Research, 6*(1). https//doi
.org//10.1136/bmjresp-2019-000420

National Heart, Lung and Blood Institute. (2007). Expert panel report 3 (EPR3): Guidelines for the diagnosis
and management of asthma. Retrieved March 6, 2021, from https://www.nhlbi.nih.gov/guidelines/asthma

Trubiano, J., Vogrin, S., Smibert, O., Marhoon, N., Alexander, A., Chua, K., James, F., Jones, N., Grigg,
S., Xu, C., Moni, N., Stanley, S., Birrel, M., Rose, M., Gordon, C., Kwong, J., & Holmes, N. (2020).
COVID-MATCH65: A prospectively derived clinical decision rule for severe acute respiratory syndrome
coronavirus 2. *PLoS One 15*(12), e0243414. https:// doi.org/10.1371/journal.pone.0243414

Chapter 10

Breasts

- Anna Jessup
- Mary Jo Goolsby

Women in the United States have a one-in-eight (13%) chance of being diagnosed with breast cancer during their lifetime. The American Cancer Society (2019a) estimated the diagnosis of approximately 268,600 cases of female breast cancer, in addition to 48,100 cases of breast cancer in situ; approximately 2,670 new diagnoses of male breast cancer were estimated for 2019. It was estimated that 41,760 women and 500 men would die from breast cancer in 2019.

Although fewer than 1% of women have mutations in genes associated with breast cancer, such mutations significantly increase the risk of breast cancer. A family history of ovarian, pancreatic, or prostate cancer has been associated with an increase in breast cancer risk (American Cancer Society, 2019a). Compared to the 10% lifetime risk of breast cancer diagnosis for the general female population, the risk of developing breast cancer by age 80 years increases to 70% for those with genetic mutations of *BRCA1* and *BRCA2* (American Cancer Society, 2019a). Genetic mutations must be considered with family and personal history in establishing risk for future development of breast cancer. Further discussion regarding the genetics of breast cancer is provided in Chapter 4.

It is important to remember that the majority of breast complaints and findings are related to benign conditions. It is crucial to recognize and respond appropriately to potential signs of malignancy and to recognize the range of other common breast conditions and their indications.

History

In addition to intrinsic breast disease, the function and structure of the breasts are influenced by changes in many other body systems. For example, disorders of the musculoskeletal, respiratory, cardiovascular, or neurological systems can result in chest discomfort that is perceived as mastalgia, having breast origin. Endocrine problems, both reproductive and nonreproductive, may result in changes to breast tissue, comfort, and secretions. When assessing problems related to

Gail Model for Breast Cancer Risk Assessment

The Gail Model is a clinical prediction rule used to estimate a patient's risk for breast cancer. The model identifies the relative risk associated with three factors obtained through history: age at menarche, number of previous breast biopsies, and the age at first live birth. The model combines the three risks to determine the woman's overall relative risk for her current age. Although applying the model is somewhat cumbersome, electronic calculators based on the model, some with slight adaptations, are readily available. One source is the calculator available at the National Cancer Institute's Web site, where individuals and providers can enter the information pertaining to each identified risk factor and receive the patient's risk for developing breast cancer within the next 5 years and by age 90 years.

the breasts, it is important to consider the range of disorders that may influence breast health. Risk prediction rules are available to estimate a woman's risk of developing breast cancer at some point in time. One such tool that incorporates known genetic mutation is based on the Gail Model (Box 10.1) and is available through the National Cancer Institute at www.cancer.gov/bcrisktool (NCI, n.d.).

■ General History: Symptoms Analysis and Review of Systems

When obtaining a history related to a breast complaint, always complete a symptom analysis, using the PQRST mnemonic (palliative/provoking, quality, radiation, severity, timing) sequence. The analysis of individual symptoms is addressed in detail later in this chapter. When a patient complains of one breast symptom, it is important to obtain a complete review of other possible symptoms, including pain, mass, nipple discharge, skin changes, and recent nipple inversion. It is also important to ask about the presence of general and nonspecific symptoms, such as fatigue, fever, appetite change, and weight loss. These will often be helpful in identifying potential endocrine problems or malignancy, which may present with nonspecific complaints.

■ Past Medical History

Ask about reproductive and menstrual history, including, as appropriate, age at menarche and at menopause. Breast cancer risk increases with early menstruation or late menopause. There is a 20% risk of developing breast cancer with menarche before age 11 years or menopause after age 55 years (American Cancer Society, 2019a). Ask about pregnancies, including the age at each pregnancy and whether the pregnancy resulted in a live birth. Assess the history of breastfeeding. Identify all previous breast surgeries or procedures, including breast augmentation or reduction, biopsies, and diagnostic studies. Determine the history of trauma to the chest/breasts. Obtain a history of chronic or current acute illnesses, particularly those of the reproductive or endocrine system. If the patient complains of breast pain, ask about musculoskeletal, cardiac, and neurological disorders. Obtain a history of all medications prescribed for or taken by the patient, including hormonal birth control. Many pharmacological agents have the potential to affect breast function, including hormone replacements, contraceptives, antidepressants and psychoactives, and antihypertensives. Diethylstilbestrol (DES) exposure during pregnancy (as a pregnant patient or fetus) is associated with increased risk of breast cancer. The medication history may also help to identify a previously undisclosed health problem.

■ Family History

The family history should identify any breast problems and disorders that might influence the breasts. Ask about the history of breast or ovarian cancer, fibrocystic breasts, and any reproductive and endocrine disorders. Chapter 4 describes how to obtain a three-generation genetic history relevant to breast cancer.

■ Habits

Obtain a history of caffeine and alcohol intake as well as all over-the-counter and recreational drug use, smoking, physical activity, diet, environmental chemicals, and pollutants. Identify the level of physical activity and any occupational or recreational activities that might cause trauma to the chest area.

Physical Examination

Although the examination of the female breasts is described, the same assessment should be performed for all patients, particularly when the male patient presents with any of the symptoms described under "Differential Diagnosis of Chief Complaints."

■ Order of the Examination

Examination of the breasts typically includes only inspection and palpation. Inspect the breasts with the patient in both sitting and supine positions, and palpate once the supine position is assumed.

Inspection

Observe the breasts while the patient is at rest, comparing for symmetry of size and contour. While the breasts often differ in size, the difference is typically not excessive and is long-standing as opposed to a recent development. Continue to inspect the breasts as the patient moves her arms through various motions: raising the arms overhead, lowering the arms so that she presses palms together in front of her, and then pressing the hands downward against the hips. Finally, observe as the patient leans forward at the waist. Through each motion, inspect the breast contours individually, observing for retractions, dimples, and irregularities of contour while also comparing the breasts with each other for symmetry. If normal, the breasts should move freely, and the contours should remain smooth throughout the movement. The motions cause contraction of the breasts' underlying musculature, which may result in a "pulling" from any abnormal mass so that a retraction or dimple becomes evident.

Following this surface inspection, assist the patient in assuming a supine position. Inspect the breasts again for general symmetry, comparing one with the other. Then inspect each breast individually, noting the skin's color and apparent texture, the general contour and smoothness, vascular pattern, areola, and nipple. Carefully note any irregularities or suspicious areas for detailed palpation. Identify any areas of retraction, dimpling, swelling, skin lesions, or discharge. Recent nipple inversion, retraction, or excoriation should be identified. Observe for other skin changes, including the peau d'orange condition in which the skin of the breast is swollen so that the hair follicles look like "dimples" and the skin develops the texture of an orange peel.

Palpation

Before palpating either breast, ask the patient to raise her arm on the side to be examined, placing her hand behind her head so that her shoulder is extended to approximately 90 degrees. This position provides better access to the breast region because it flattens the breast tissue across the chest wall. Examination of the breast should include the region from the midsternal line to the midaxillary line, from the subclavicular to approximately the sixth to seventh rib, or the "bra line." Palpation of the breast should also include attention to the axillary and subclavicular lymph nodes. While several systems (e.g., vertical strip, circular) provide good coverage of the breast region, the vertical strip method is currently more widely accepted. Each practitioner should become comfortable and consistent in a sequence that ensures palpation of the full breast region.

Regardless of the approach used, light, medium, and deep pressure should be applied at each palpation point. Varying the palpation pressure is more likely to allow detection of masses—whether they are superficial or deep. Compress the area immediately beneath each areola, and gently squeeze each nipple. Ask the patient to inform you of any areas of tenderness or pain elicited with the examination.

Breast tissue may be normally somewhat nodular or irregular, but the texture should be generally consistent between the breasts. Note any masses, nodules, or areas of firmness. Any mass should be assessed for size, consistency, mobility, margins/borders, shape, and delineation. It is sometimes helpful to palpate symmetrical areas of breast tissue simultaneously to assess areas of thickening or fullness.

As you palpate each breast, identify any discharge, which is most likely to be produced with pressure over the areola and/or when the nipple is gently squeezed. If discharge is produced, notice whether it comes from one or multiple ducts. When there is discharge from multiple ducts, there is a higher likelihood of a cause such as fibrocystic change or galactorrhea. While malignancy should always be considered in the differential diagnosis for nipple discharge, the likelihood of malignancy increases when the discharge is from only one duct. Any discharge should be assessed for color, consistency, and odor. Collect the discharge by pressing a clean glass slide lightly against the nipple. In addition to facilitating the ability to judge the color and consistency of the discharge, the slide can also be used for cytology testing if warranted. The discharge should also be tested for blood, using a guaiac card.

■ Diagnostic Studies

Breast imaging, including mammography, ultrasound, magnetic resonance imaging (MRI), and tomosynthesis, is frequently conducted to assess breast complaints and findings. Clinicians should be familiar with the BI-RADS numbered categorization of mammography findings and recommended response.

The most common image used for women older than 40 years is the mammogram. While screening mammography includes standard views for all women, diagnostic mammography includes images specific to a patient's complaints or findings (e.g., mass, lymphadenopathy, discharge, pain) or as further evaluation of an abnormality detected during screening imaging. The newer digital breast tomosynthesis provides a more three-dimensional image of the breast compared to mammography. Described by the American College of Radiology (2014) as an advance to digital mammography, the now FDA-approved digital breast tomosynthesis is not currently considered the standard image. It is generally used to provide better images for women with dense breasts.

Breast ultrasounds, like mammograms, are used in screening and the diagnostic process. They are used most often in younger women or those with high breast density. While mammography reports have included statements regarding breast density, allowing clinicians to determine whether alternative imaging such as ultrasound was warranted, states increasingly are adopting laws requiring that imaging centers inform patients of breast density and promote dialogue with clinicians.

A number of laboratory tests are used in the diagnostic process, depending on the breast complaint and findings. These include evaluation of nipple discharge (as above), tumor markers, and biopsies.

The breast examination provides opportunity to educate the patient on relevant breast cancer screenings. Controversy exists regarding whether to encourage breast self-examination and to conduct regular clinical breast examinations, as well as regarding the frequency of screening mammography. Table 10.1 summarizes the recommendations provided by the U.S. Preventative Services (2016), American Cancer Society (2020), and the American College of Obstetricians and Gynecologists (2017) for women at average risk for breast cancer.

■ Special Considerations

Women for whom special consideration is warranted include those who have had a mastectomy or breast-sparing surgery, cosmetic or postmastectomy augmentation, or breast reduction surgery. In these cases, careful history and examination

Table 10.1

Breast Cancer Screening Recommendations

	U.S. Preventative Services	American Cancer Society	American College of OB/GYN
Mammography	50–74: Biennial screening* >75: Insufficient evidence *Women may opt to begin screenings 40-49	40–44: Optional annual screening 45–54: Annual >55: Option to continue annual *or* biennial screening* *Continue screening if life expectancy >10 years and good health	≥40: Annually (if not initiated in 40s), screening begins no later than age 50. 50–70: Every 1-2 years* *Continue screening until at least age 75
Breast Self-Examination	No recommendation for or against teaching breast self-examination	Recommend women become familiar with breasts' appearance and feel so as to be able to report changes immediately	Encourages breast self-examination awareness, i.e., the breasts' normal appearance and feel
Clinical Breast Examination	No recommendation for or against clinical breast examination	Not recommended due to lack of evidence	Offered as option 25–39: Every 1–3 years ≥40: Annually

relevant to the breasts are indicated. When mammograms or other imaging studies are ordered on a woman who has undergone any of these procedures, these details of the history should be clearly noted.

Women who have previously been diagnosed and treated for breast cancer may require more frequent clinical breast examination than is usually recommended. The unaffected breast should be examined using standard technique. Any remaining tissue on the affected side, including the axilla, should also be carefully examined.

Following breast augmentation, the ability to examine the breast tissue is somewhat dependent on the type and placement of the implant or augmentation.

RED FLAG **Warnings for Breast Complaints**

- *Hard, stone-like mass*
- *Immobile, fixed mass*
- *Inflammatory skin changes*
- *Thickening and/or dimpling of skin*
- *Palpable axillary nodes*
- *Bloody nipple discharge*
- *Systemic symptoms*

Ask about any difficulty the woman may have experienced at the time of the procedure or implant as well as current symptoms. Access to certain tissues may be occluded by the implant. Distortions of the breast may indicate capsular contraction, peri-implant fluid collection, or implant rupture.

Following breast reduction, deep scarring and adhesions may form, confounding the ability to palpate a mass. There may also be voids in the breast tissue, particularly in the tissue underlying the area of scarring, such that the normal and regular distribution of tissue is altered.

Differential Diagnosis of Chief Complaints

■ Breast Mass

Breast tissue is normally glandular and may have a rather nodular consistency. The degree of nodularity tends to fluctuate through the menstrual cycle in premenopausal women. A *dominant breast mass* is a mass that persists throughout a woman's hormonal cycles, is larger and firmer than any other irregularities, and differs from the rest of the breast tissue. Dominant masses typically fall into the following categories: fibroadenomas, cysts, fibrocystic changes, fat necrosis, and malignancy. Whenever a breast mass is identified, it should be followed to diagnostic resolution. Breast cancer is always included in the differential diagnosis, and diagnostic efforts should either rule out the existence of a malignancy or identify it in a timely manner. Missed or delayed diagnoses can have catastrophic results and are, in fact, consistently among the most frequent causes of malpractice suits.

History

It is essential to obtain a complete reproductive and menstrual history and to ascertain the symptoms associated with the discovery of the mass. Determine how long the mass has been present and whether it has changed since first noticed. If present for a while, ask whether any of its characteristics fluctuate in relation to the menstrual cycle. Identify any accompanying symptoms, such as pain, nipple discharge, or skin changes. Ask about recent trauma to the breast. The presence of systemic symptoms, including loss of energy, altered appetite, weight loss, and fever, is important because they may be signs of advanced breast cancer. Determine family history of breast disease, malignancies, and related conditions.

Physical Examination

It is important to perform a complete breast examination for any complaint of breast mass. Throughout the examination, be attentive for changes in the skin; the contours of the breasts, including dimpling or retractions; nipple discharge; eczematous or similar rash or erosions around the nipple; and palpable axillary or subclavicular lymph nodes. It is crucial to confirm the presence of a palpable mass, carefully noting its location and other characteristics.

The dimensions, mobility, consistency, and texture of each palpable breast mass are important in determining further diagnostic workup. For any mass, determine whether the consistency is soft, rubbery, firm, or hard; whether it is fixed and immobile or moves freely; whether it has smooth or irregular margins; and whether it is tender, painful, or painless. Determine whether the skin overlying an identified mass moves independently of the mass or, instead, is connected to the mass so that they move together. As the mass is palpated, try to determine whether it is cystic or solid. Any patient with a dominant breast mass should be referred for definitive diagnosis.

Diagnostic Studies

All patients with a palpable dominant breast mass should be referred for definitive diagnostic workup. Imaging and other studies, such as biopsies, are necessary to discriminate among potential causes when a breast mass is detected by either the patient or the provider.

When referring a patient with a breast mass for imaging or other diagnostic evaluation, it is critical to provide any descriptives of the finding possible (location, size, etc.). Unfortunately, palpation and mammography or ultrasound, alone or together, are inadequate to definitively identify the cause of a breast mass and to rule out malignancy. The "triple test" recommended for evaluation of a breast mass involves clinical examination, either ultrasound or mammogram, and aspiration and/or biopsy.

The American College of Radiology (2017a) guidelines determine the selection of an ultrasound or mammography based on age and other situations. The American College of Radiology recommends that women who are older than 40 years and have a palpable mass be assessed with mammography. Women younger than 30 years with a mass have denser breasts, and ultrasound is therefore often more useful than a mammogram. Women age 30 to 40 years can be assessed by either mammography or ultrasound initially. Ultrasounds are helpful in determining whether a mass that feels potentially "cystic" is fluid filled or solid. Regardless of the recommended image pursued, it is crucial that the woman understand that even a diagnostic imaging procedure is a screening tool and is never diagnostic regarding the existence or absence of a malignancy.

The patient should be referred to a surgeon for definitive diagnosis through fine needle aspiration (FNA) or core biopsy. If a FNA reveals only nonbloody aspirate and the mass appears to be resolved following aspiration, the surgeon may decide to recheck the patient in approximately 1 month. If the mass is still resolved at the follow-up visit, a decision may be made not to do any follow-up at that time but instead to perform serial examinations over time. If a FNA reveals bloody aspirate or reveals a solid mass (suggested by inability to aspirate the mass), or if the cyst returns following aspiration, a biopsy is indicated.

MALIGNANCY

In the United States in 2022, about 43,250 women are expected to die from breast cancer (BreastCancer.org). It is the most common form of cancer among women and the second leading cause of cancer deaths. The differential diagnosis should include malignancy when a woman complains of or the practitioner identifies a breast mass. A thorough history and careful physical examination are essential if breast cancer is suspected.

Signs and Symptoms

A breast lump is the most common presenting complaint in breast cancer and is usually the only presenting complaint. More rarely, the presentation may include complaint of discomfort, skin change, or discharge. If the cancer is advanced, the patient may have extra-breast symptoms, such as fatigue, weight loss, and bone pain. The typical malignant mass is solitary, nontender, hard, immobile or fixed, and poorly defined. It may be accompanied by nipple erosion or other inflammatory skin changes, as seen in Paget's disease; nipple discharge; skin thickening or dimpling; retraction; and palpable axillary nodes. Although most malignant masses are painless, associated discomfort does not exclude the potential for breast cancer.

Diagnostic Studies

Any breast mass, particularly those that are solitary, noncyclic, and nontender, should trigger a mammogram or ultrasound as well as a consultation with a surgeon who will determine the need for FNA, biopsy, or other diagnostic studies.

FIBROADENOMA

Fibroadenomas are common, benign neoplasms that usually occur in premenopausal women, appearing in the second or third decade. Women with fibroadenomas have a slightly higher-than-average lifetime risk of developing breast cancer.

Signs and Symptoms

There are usually no complaints other than the mass. Although fibroadenomas are usually solitary, they can be multiple. The lump is generally mobile, rubbery, and nontender; has discrete and smooth borders; and is less than 5 cm in diameter. However, fibroadenomas may also have irregular borders.

Diagnostic Studies

A mammogram or ultrasound is usually ordered to confirm the diagnosis and rule out malignancy. Even when a newly identified mass is consistent with a fibroadenoma and imaging supports the diagnosis, a surgical consult should be considered for definitive diagnosis. Newer diagnostics include 3D mammography, contrast-enhanced MRI mammography, positron emission mammography, and molecular breast imaging, also called scintimammography (American Cancer Society, 2019b).

FIBROCYSTIC CHANGE

Fibrocystic breast changes include a variety of histopathological variations, with fibrotic thickening often paired with the development of cysts. However, this condition is considered benign and/or physiological rather than pathological.

Signs and Symptoms

The nodularity is usually associated with tenderness. The nodularity and tenderness are both cyclic in nature, fluctuating with the menstrual cycle. The symptoms are usually most severe just before menses. The size and/or number of lumps or nodules may fluctuate during the cycle. The changes are usually bilateral. Breast discharge may also occur cyclically before menses and is usually serous.

Diagnostic Studies

Diagnostic studies are usually not warranted in young women who have lumpy breasts with multiple areas of thickening and a cyclic component, with or without tenderness. The patient should be instructed to complete a breast symptom calendar for at least 2 months, at which time the calendar can be studied to assess the cyclic nature of the symptoms. If there is a dominant mass identified or some other diagnostic uncertainty exists, a surgical consult should be obtained.

TRAUMA

Trauma to the anterior chest area may result in a palpable breast mass. An automobile accident with injury from the seat belt, air bag, steering wheel, or dashboard is a common source of breast trauma. The trauma may result in a variety of injuries, and deeper damage should be considered, with assessment for musculoskeletal and lung injury. When a palpable mass results from chest trauma, it typically represents either a hematoma or area of secondary fat necrosis. Even when a mass is identified subsequent to direct trauma, the provider must remain suspicious for the possibility of malignancy that preexisted but was undetected before the accident.

Signs and Symptoms

A palpable mass due to trauma typically is associated with chest wall and breast discomfort. There may be an area of ecchymosis or discoloration in the distribution of trauma. Patients with large breasts are more likely to develop fat necrosis than are those with small breasts. A palpable mass associated with trauma is often poorly defined and immobile. An area of fat necrosis is typically superficial and may develop calcified margins. It can be difficult to differentiate between isolated trauma and a potential for malignancy. Serial examinations should demonstrate resolution of any hematoma and/or no increase in mass size.

Diagnostic Studies

Because the potential for malignancy is not easily excluded, an ultrasound or mammogram should be considered. Additional imaging may include plain films to assess the condition of ribs and other bones and to exclude pneumothorax or hemothorax resulting from trauma.

▪ Breast Pain

Breast pain—mastalgia or mastodynia—is the most common breast complaint. The most common type of breast pain is cyclic mastalgia, which occurs in premenopausal women and is associated with hormonal fluctuations. In contrast, noncyclic breast pain is often unilateral and may be described in many ways, including sharp, burning, and aching. Many benign breast changes, including cysts, mastitis, trauma, abscess, duct ectasia, and fibroadenoma, are associated with noncyclic mastalgia. While breast pain usually tends to be mild, it can be quite severe. Both noncyclic and cyclic breast pain may be associated with certain variables, such as the intake of methylxanthine-/caffeine-containing products. Although pain is not commonly associated with the diagnosis of breast cancer, it may accompany malignancy and is sometimes the presenting complaint. A complaint of breast pain may also represent pain referred from another origin, usually related to some musculoskeletal or neuropathic disorder.

History

It is important to have the patient describe the pain in detail, through a symptom analysis, to identify palliative/provocative factors, the actual quality and type of pain, the primary region of pain and any radiation, the severity of the pain, any associated breast or systemic symptoms, and the timing. Any prior breast complaints, disorders, surgeries, and procedures should be determined. Ask whether the pain is associated with any particular physical activities. Determine whether there have been any other symptoms, such as fever or general malaise. The menstrual history is important. If the patient has an infant, determine the history of lactation. It may be appropriate to explore symptoms associated with other systems, including cardiac, neurological, and musculoskeletal. Identify any current medications, particularly hormonal contraceptives. The family history should include questions about breast cancer and fibrocystic breasts.

Physical Examination

A general survey should be completed to determine the patient's overall appearance. The examination should focus on the breasts and should be expanded as indicated. Observe for masses, skin texture changes, redness/inflammation, and discharge. Notice whether any of the motions involved in the inspection phase of the examination seem to elicit discomfort. Ask the patient to point to the area of discomfort. If the patient has complained of discomfort limited to a specific region, palpate the opposite breast first before proceeding to the nontender portion of the affected breast. Gently palpate the area of tenderness or pain, noting the boundaries of the discomfort, and assess the underlying tissue for any change in texture or for masses.

Diagnostic Studies

A variety of diagnostic studies may be appropriate for the assessment of breast pain. If the pain is cyclic in nature and related to menses, there is generally no indication to order diagnostic studies. A diary of the breast discomfort may prove helpful, however. If the patient is older than 30 years and has not had a recent mammogram, it is appropriate to order a routine mammogram as a part of normal care. If a solid mass or cyst is suspected, the pain is noncyclic, or the patient is postmenopausal, a surgical consult should be obtained. If the patient is younger than 30 years, an ultrasound is appropriate in lieu of the mammogram. If mastitis is suspected, a white blood count is indicated.

HORMONAL, CYCLIC MASTALGIA

Although it is broadly assumed that cyclic mastalgia is related to fluctuating hormones, the mechanisms resulting in the discomfort are unknown. There does not seem to be a direct correlation between fluid retention, for instance, and breast tenderness or pain. Women who experience cyclic mastalgia usually have onset as a teen or young adult. It is important to determine menstrual and reproductive history and to identify all pharmacological agents taken. A complete breast examination should be performed.

Signs and Symptoms

The pain associated with hormonal fluctuation most commonly occurs during the second half of the woman's cycle. The variability of the signs and symptoms is identified with a symptom calendar. The pain is typically poorly localized, bilateral, and nonspecific. It may be accompanied by a sense of breast fullness. The examination may identify the multiple, bilateral nodularities associated with fibroadenomas or fibrocystic changes.

Diagnostic Studies

The breast pain diary identifies the cyclic nature of the pain and its association with the menstrual cycle. A mammogram or ultrasound reveals no indication of malignancy or mass other than fibroadenomas or cysts.

FIBROADENOMAS AND FIBROCYSTS

Two benign causes of breast pain include fibroadenomas and fibrocystic breasts. Although fibroadenomas are not typically painful, they can be accompanied by discomfort. Both conditions are described in the previous section on breast masses.

MASTITIS

Mastitis is an inflammatory breast disorder, typically occurring in lactating women (puerperal mastitis) and caused by either a streptococcal or a staphylococcal infection. The cause likely stems from altered nipple/areola skin integrity with retrograde infection. Mastitis occurs rarely in nonlactating females, and in this situation, it often stems from duct ectasia (see later discussion on breast discharge) with an anaerobic microbe. It is important to recognize mastitis so that it can be promptly treated. Because mastitis is rare among nonlactating women, providers should remain suspicious of the potential for inflammatory breast cancer in women who are not nursing, particularly if there are no systemic symptoms of infection.

Signs and Symptoms

The patient typically complains of unilateral pain, redness, and swelling of one breast. Systemic symptoms include fever, chills, and myalgia. The examination reveals a wedge-shaped area of redness that is swollen and very tender. The patient is typically nursing, and there is often visible discharge of milk, which may be spontaneous as the breast becomes engorged once the breast becomes too painful to nurse.

Diagnostic Studies

A white blood count should be obtained and is usually elevated. Even though the breast milk can be cultured, this is not generally recommended. If the presentation is atypical—that is, the patient is not lactating—and there are no associated systemic signs or symptoms, a consultation should be obtained and mammography ordered to determine the definitive diagnosis and to rule out malignancy.

MALIGNANCY

Although pain is not a common complaint with breast cancer, the potential for a malignancy must always be considered in the differential diagnosis.

CHEST WALL PAIN AND COSTOCHONDRITIS

Costochondritis involves localized discomfort, often quite sharp in nature, along the costochondral and/or costosternal cartilages. Costochondritis is described in Chapter 9.

PENDULOUS BREASTS

Pain can be associated with pendulous breasts, which causes strain on the underlying muscles and Cooper's ligaments.

RADICULAR NERVE PAIN

Nerve root inflammation or impingement can result in pain that radiates or is experienced in the breast region. Thoracic lesions may radiate to the chest. Nerve pain typically is sharp or burning in nature. Nerve pain is described in Chapter 16, and herpes zoster pain is described in Chapter 4.

CARDIAC PAIN

Ischemic heart pain can be misinterpreted as breast pain. When the presentation involves atypical breast pain and/or occurs in a patient at high risk for cardiac disease, cardiac pain should be strongly considered in the differential diagnosis. Cardiac pain is described in Chapter 8.

■ Nipple Discharge

Although nipple discharge may occur without pathology, it may be indicative of serious disorders. Categories of nipple discharge include galactorrhea, physiological discharge, and pathological discharge. Galactorrhea can be caused by a variety of endocrine disorders. Causes of nonmalignant pathological discharge include ductal papilloma, duct ectasia, and fibrocystic changes. Discharge may be present

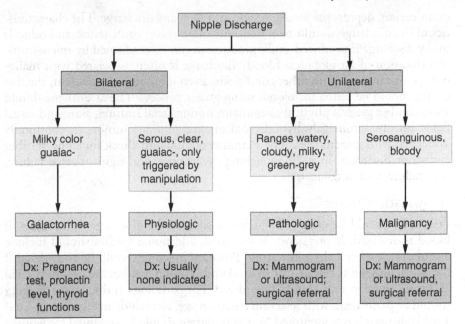

Figure 10.1 Nipple discharge algorithm.

at the diagnosis of breast cancer. However, the vast majority (95%) of nipple discharge cases are from benign causes. In more than 50% of female patients, a very small amount of discharge (one or a very few drops) can be produced by manipulating the breast and nipple, but this is not considered spontaneous. Figure 10.1 depicts an approach to differentiating cause of nipple discharge.

History

Determine whether the discharge is bilateral or unilateral and whether it comes from single or multiple ducts. Ask whether it comes from the same site on the nipple each time. Determine whether the discharge is spontaneous or comes only after breast manipulation. The color and consistency of the discharge should be determined, as should the presence of any other breast symptoms, including pain, retraction, skin changes, or mass. The menstrual, reproductive, and lactation histories are important. A thorough medication and substance history is crucial, as breast discharge can be caused by several agents. Because discharge can be a sign of other conditions, including renal, endocrine, and idiopathic disorders, ask about a history of headaches, visual changes, recent trauma, and thyroid symptoms or disorders. Determine whether the patient participates in high-intensity exercise and, if so, what type of bra is worn.

Physical Examination

The breast examination should be thorough and include manipulation intended to produce discharge. If no discharge is produced by the general breast examination, depress the areolar region and note any discharge. The characteristics of the discharge should be noted, including color, consistency, and odor. If milky discharge is produced, milk production can be confirmed by microscopic identification of fat globules. Bloody discharge is often associated with malignancy but can stem from other conditions. Even if blood is not evident, the discharge should be tested for blood, using guaiac process. The assessment should also include a general physical assessment, noting facial features, skin, and visual fields, because acromegaly, hypothyroidism, and pituitary tumors are commonly associated with galactorrhea. The examiner should also check for signs of other endocrine disorders, including Cushing's syndrome, and signs of renal failure, liver failure, and sarcoidosis.

Diagnostic Studies

Pregnancy should be excluded. Prepare a slide of the discharge for cytology if blood is detected. If pregnancy is excluded, additional studies should include a prolactin level and thyroid testing. Pituitary imaging should be considered if the prolactin level is elevated. If thyroid and pituitary studies are negative, renal and liver function tests should be ordered. For pathological discharge, imaging should be performed, with selection based on age, to exclude malignancy, even if a palpable mass is not identified. A mammogram should be obtained for women older than 40 years, an ultrasound for women younger than 30 years, and either mammogram or ultrasound for women age 30 to 40 years (American College of Radiology, 2017b).

GALACTORRHEA

Galactorrhea is characterized by bilateral and milky discharge from multiple ducts in a woman who is neither pregnant nor lactating. A variety of drugs could cause galactorrhea, as could an elevated prolactin level associated with pituitary tumor or hyperthyroidism. The drugs associated with galactorrhea include antidepressants (amitriptyline, imipramine), psychoactives (haloperidol, thioridazine), hormones (estrogens, progestogens), antiepileptics (valproic acid), and antihypertensives (verapamil). This list is not exhaustive.

Signs and Symptoms

If associated with prolactin elevation, there may be symptoms of a pituitary tumor, including headaches, vision change, relative infertility, and amenorrhea. The signs of thyroid disease or acromegaly may be present. If acromegaly is involved, the woman may admit to recent changes in shoe or ring size as well as other structural changes. The history may identify one or more of the medications commonly associated with galactorrhea. The breast examination is negative with the exception of possibly stimulating the production of milky, nonbloody discharge from multiple ducts.

Diagnostic Studies

Laboratory studies should include a pregnancy test, prolactin level, and thyroid functions.

PHYSIOLOGICAL DISCHARGE

As noted earlier, physiological discharge is not rare. It may be associated with fibrocystic breasts or gynecomastia, or it may exist with no other breast complaints. In addition to squeezing of the breast, physiological discharge may be caused by trauma or exercise. It may occur in response to hormonal changes at puberty or menopause.

Signs and Symptoms

Physiological discharge is not spontaneous but is triggered by manipulation and/ or excessive movement. It is bilateral, comes from multiple ducts, and is serous in appearance. The patient may complain of cyclic symptoms of mastalgia or lumpy breasts.

PATHOLOGICAL DISCHARGE

Pathological discharge is most often unilateral, spontaneous, and limited to one duct, although multiple ducts in a limited area may be involved. It can be intermittent and persistent. The color of pathological discharge ranges widely and can be watery, cloudy, bloody, serosanguineous, green-gray, or multicolored. In spite of the term *pathological*, the cause is usually benign and frequently includes duct ectasia or an intraductal papilloma. Duct ectasia results in dilation of one major breast duct and causes approximately one-third of the cases of pathological discharge. Papillomas are responsible for 44% of pathological discharge. Papillomas can occur singly or in multiples; the intraductal papilloma is generally located proximal to the nipple.

Signs and Symptoms

Because the discharge associated with ductal ectasia is often stagnant, the discharge is cheesy in appearance. It is often associated with noncyclic breast discomfort and a subareolar lump at the site of the dilated duct. Because one major duct is involved, the discharge comes also from one duct or nipple area. However, in contrast to the discharge associated with duct ectasia, papillomas cause discharge that ranges from serous to serosanguineous to bloody. A clean glass slide is used to collect discharge for inspection and any subsequent analysis.

Diagnostic Studies

A mammogram or ultrasound should be ordered, and it will reveal the dilated duct or the papilloma. Surgical consultation is indicated to determine the need for excision.

MALIGNANCY

Nipple discharge is also a potential sign of malignancy (11%). Up to 5% of women diagnosed with breast cancer have nipple discharge as part of their presentation, although it is rarely a solitary symptom or sign. Cytology of the discharge is diagnostic in only approximately 50% of cases in which cancer is present and is therefore not reliable in diagnosis. Mammography should be performed to begin discrimination among benign causes, such as mammary duct ectasia, cancer, and other possibilities. However, a negative mammogram does not exclude malignancy. In fact, of those women who presented with nipple discharge and were diagnosed with cancer, only approximately 50% had an abnormal mammogram. Thus, if a benign explanation is not identified for the discharge, the woman should be referred to a surgeon for further evaluation.

PAGET'S DISEASE

It is possible that spotting from nipple erosion of Paget's disease may be construed by a patient as discharge, which is described in the following section.

■ Skin Lesions of the Nipple and Areola

It is not common for skin conditions to involve the breast area, although it is possible for the skin overlying the breast to be involved with atopic rashes, herpes zoster, or other conditions. Paget's disease is a malignancy that involves skin changes of the nipple and, later, the areola, and should be considered when patients complain of a rash or other skin lesion on the breast.

History

The history for breast-related skin changes should include an analysis of the skin lesion. Ask when the patient first noticed the lesion and how, if at all, it has progressed since that time. Ask about associated symptoms such as pain, discharge, bleeding, or itching. Ask whether the patient has noticed any masses or other breast changes. Determine whether skin changes have been noticed elsewhere. Ask about any activities that might have caused the lesion. Explore whether the patient has experienced any general symptoms such as fatigue or fever. Ask about prior history of atopic diseases and malignancies. Similarly, review the family history for atopic diseases and malignancies.

Physical Examination

A thorough breast examination should be performed with assessment of any masses, nodules, or discharge, as described earlier in this chapter. Any skin lesions should be evaluated as described in Chapter 4, noting particularly the location and whether the nipple and areola are involved.

Diagnostic Studies

If the lesion involves the nipple or areola, a surgical consult and mammogram should be arranged. Otherwise, if the physical examination does not cause suspicion for malignancy, the diagnostic studies are likely not warranted but would be consistent with the differential diagnosis.

PAGET'S DISEASE

Paget's disease is responsible for a small percentage of breast cancers. The typical presentation involves skin changes of the nipple and/or areola, with the nipple being involved first. The condition does not always involve a palpable mass or nodule. Any patient with unexplained skin changes to the nipple and areola area should be evaluated by a surgeon. Even with another potential explanation for the condition, a surgical consult should be considered, or the patient should be scheduled for a timely reevaluation.

Signs and Symptoms

The patient may describe the persistence of skin changes for several months. The skin changes involving the nipple and, potentially, the areola, range from scaling redness to various degrees of ulceration. On occasion, the patient may provide a history of intermittent clearing with or without some prior self-treatment. There is often no palpable mass, and there may be no mammographic abnormality.

Diagnostic Studies

A mammogram or ultrasound should be ordered and a surgeon consulted for definitive diagnosis.

SKIN MALIGNANCY

It is possible that a skin malignancy, such as malignant melanoma or Bowen's disease, could involve the skin overlying the breast. Skin malignancies are described in Chapter 4.

HERPES ZOSTER

Herpes zoster can affect the skin overlying the breast, depending on the nerve root involved. Herpes zoster is described in Chapter 4.

OTHER SKIN CONDITIONS

Atopic diseases such as eczema, contact dermatitis, and infectious skin conditions could involve the breast area. See Chapter 4.

■ Male Breast Enlargement or Mass

As noted previously, although the risk for developing breast cancer is much lower in men than in women, 1% of all breast cancer is diagnosed in men. In addition to the potential for a malignancy, complaints of breast changes in men may indicate hormonal disturbances, adverse effects of medications, and systemic symptoms of liver or renal disease. Complaints of breast enlargement or mass should trigger careful investigation.

The general term for male breast enlargement is *gynecomastia*, which can be present in one or both breasts. Even though hormone-related gynecomastia is relatively common, particularly in pubertal and older adult males, it must be differentiated from adipose tissue, lipoma, hematoma, malignancy, and systemic conditions.

History

Obtain a full history of the breast enlargement, including when it was first noted, any subsequent changes in the area, and any associated symptoms. When asking about associated symptoms, include skin changes, discharge, pain or tenderness, and systemic symptoms that would indicate extramammary conditions. Identify any history of previous breast changes or procedures and the family history of breast disease. The medical history should be directed toward identifying all current and previous medical problems and a list of all medications/drugs currently taken.

Physical Examination

A complete examination of the breasts should be performed. The male breasts are best examined with the patient resting supine with his arm raised over his head. The same examination techniques used for women should be incorporated, including careful inspection for any skin changes, retractions, areas of thickening, bulges, or visible masses. The palpation should include comparison of breast tissue consistency between the breasts and identification of any palpable masses and their characteristics. The axillary nodes should be assessed. Obese men are more likely to have "fatty breasts" than true gynecomastia. It is often helpful to compare the consistency of the affected breast(s) with the consistency of the tissue in the anterior axillary fold region to determine whether adipose tissue is involved.

Diagnostic Studies

If a palpable mass is discovered that is not consistent with gynecomastia (see the following section), an ultrasound or mammogram should be obtained to determine the cause. Ultrasound is recommended for men younger than 25 years and mammogram for men 25 years or older (American College of Radiology, 2017c). A surgical consult should be obtained if a benign diagnosis is not certain.

GYNECOMASTIA

Gynecomastia most often occurs during infancy, puberty, and senescence. It is caused by an altered balance between estradiol and testosterone levels. Although it can be an indication of primary hypogonadism (see Chapter 13 on the male reproductive system), hyperthyroidism, cirrhosis, or renal disease, the majority of the cases are specific to hormonal changes of puberty, are drug induced, or are idiopathic. With the presentation of breast enlargement in a male, malignancy must always be considered.

Signs and Symptoms

The enlargement associated with gynecomastia presents as a disk-shaped rubbery area of tissue that is centered beneath the areola, extending out centrifugally. The thickened area of tissue may be tender, and there may be associated nipple discharge. Other times, there are no other findings or symptoms except for the area of enlargement. If the enlargement is drug induced, the patient may identify one of the many drugs known to cause gynecomastia, such as phenytoin, cimetidine, estrogens, calcium channel blockers, ACE inhibitors, spironolactone, finasteride, methyldopa, or marijuana. If the drug is eliminated, the enlargement may resolve. If related to cirrhosis or renal failure, other physical signs of the etiologic condition should be evident. A mass that is located remote to the areola or is hard, irregularly shaped, or immobile is not consistent with gynecomastia.

Diagnostic Studies

If the mass or enlargement is consistent with gynecomastia, there is no need to perform diagnostic studies. However, ultrasound or mammography should be considered, if necessary, for either definitive diagnosis or reassurance of the patient. The provider should be alert to the remote potential that the gynecomastia stems from cirrhosis or renal disease and determine whether renal or liver function studies should be ordered.

PSEUDOGYNECOMASTIA

Pseudogynecomastia refers to fatty deposits and enlargements of the breast related to obesity.

Signs and Symptoms

The patient will have no tenderness, discharge, discrete palpable masses, or other symptoms related to the breast enlargement. The area of enlargement will have a consistency similar to the patient's other fatty areas, such as the tissue in the immediate region of the anterior axillary fold.

There are no diagnostic studies indicated for pseudogynecomastia.

MALIGNANCY

Approximately 2,670 (1%) new diagnoses of male breast cancer were estimated for 2019, with 500 related deaths (American Cancer Society, 2019a). Men develop the same types of breast cancer as women. Therefore, it is important to include malignancy in the differential diagnosis when a man complains of breast enlargement, as men are more likely to be diagnosed with advanced (regional or distant stage) breast cancer. Factors that increase the risk of breast cancer in men include a previous history of breast or testicular disease, radiation, *BRCA1* and *BRCA2* gene mutations, diabetes, obesity, and Klinefelter's syndrome, as well as a family history of breast cancer. A history of gynecomastia is not associated with an increased risk for breast cancer.

Signs and Symptoms

The man may complain of breast tenderness, skin changes, and/or nipple discharge. There may be associated systemic symptoms of fatigue, weight loss, and so on. The mass may be more evident in a male patient who has less breast tissue than a woman. The mass will usually lie in a location inconsistent with gynecomastia. However, regardless of the site, any firm or hard mass should trigger investigation for malignancy. Nipple discharge associated with malignancy is often bloody.

Diagnostic Studies

As described above, an ultrasound or mammogram should be obtained for any male patient with breast enlargement that is not consistent with gynecomastia. Any nipple discharge can be evaluated using the same methods described earlier for females with nipple discharge.

REFERENCES

American Cancer Society. (2019a). Breast cancer facts & figures 2019-2020. https://www.cancer.org/content /dam/cancer-org/research/cancer-facts-and-statistics/breast-cancer-facts-and-figures/breast-cancer-facts -and-figures-2019-2020.pdf

American Cancer Society. (2019b). Newer and experimental breast imaging tests. https://www.cancer.org /cancer/breast-cancer/screening-tests-and-early-detection/experimental-breast-imaging.html. Retrieved 4/4/2021

American Cancer Society. (2020). American Cancer Society Recommendations for the Early Detection of Breast Cancer. https://www.cancer.org/cancer/breast-cancer/screening-tests-and-early-detection/american -cancer-society-recommendations-for-the-early-detection-of-breast-cancer.html

American College of Obstetricians and Gynecologists. (2017). Breast Cancer Assessment and Screening in Average-Risk Women. https://www.acog.org/clinical/clinical-guidance/practice-bulletin/articles/2017/07 /breast-cancer-risk-assessment-and-screening-in-average-risk-women

American College of Radiology. (2014). ACR statement on breast tomosynthesis. Retrieved https:// www.acr.org/About-Us/Media-Center/Position-Statements/Position-Statements-Folder/20141124-ACR -Statement-on-Breast-Tomosynthesis

American College of Radiology (2017a). ACR appropriateness criteria: Evaluation of the symptomatic male breast. Retrieved from https://acsearch.acr.org/docs/3091547/Narrative/

American College of Radiology (2017b). ACR appropriateness criteria: Nipple discharge. Retrieved from https://acsearch.acr.org/docs/3099312/Narrative/

American College of Radiology. (2017c). ACR appropriateness criteria: Palpable breast masses. Retrieved from https://acsearch.acr.org/docs/69495/Narrative/

BreastCancer.Org. Breast cancer facts and statistics. Retrieved from https://www.breastcancer.org/facts -statistics#section-us-breast-cancer-statistics

NCI (n.d.). Breast Cancer Risk Assessment Tool. Retrieved from https://www.cancer.gov/bcrisktool/

U.S. Preventative Services Task Force. (2016). Breast Cancer: Screening. https://uspreventiveservicestaskforce .org/uspstf/recommendation/breast-cancer-screening

Chapter 11

Abdomen

Mary Jo Goolsby ·
Laurie Grubbs ·

D igestive diseases encompass a vast range of acute and chronic conditions. Annually, a gastrointestinal (GI) diagnosis is responsible for over 54.5 million ambulatory visits and 3 million admissions in the United States. Abdominal pain was the common diagnosis in 16.5 million visits, with gastroesophageal reflux disease (GERD) and reflux esophagitis accounting for over 5.6 million visits. GI hemorrhage is the most common reason for hospitalization. Colorectal cancer remains the most frequent GI cancer, followed by pancreatic and liver cancers. There are an estimated 61 million upper endoscopies and 11 million colonoscopies performed annually. The 2018 cost for GI disease was almost $136 billion (Peery et al., 2019).

The causes of abdominal complaints can range from very mild, self-limited problems to those that can be disabling or result in mortality. In addition to digestive diseases, abdominal complaints may be indicative of musculoskeletal, neurological, genitourinary, reproductive, cardiovascular, or respiratory disorders.

History

■ General History

A general history for an abdominal complaint should include any reports of nausea and/or vomiting; current bowel habits, including diarrhea, changes in bowel or bladder habits, or constipation, and pain, weight loss or gain, change in appetite, bloating, excessive gas or belching, dysphagia, heartburn or indigestion, rectal bleeding, or black stools. Ask about history of jaundice, liver disease, hepatitis, gallbladder disease, fever, or malaise. As specific complaints are discussed subsequently in the chapter, further symptom analysis is described.

■ Past Medical History

A general past medical history should include any history of jaundice, liver disease, hepatitis, gallbladder disease, infectious diseases, peptic ulcer disease (PUD), GERD, bleeding or platelet disorders, trauma, or previous surgeries with the emphasis on abdominal surgeries.

■ Family History

Identify any family history of liver or gallbladder disease, hepatitis, or cancer. There is a familial predisposition to certain diseases of the digestive tract, such as inflammatory bowel disease, polyposis, and cancer of the colon. The risk of hepatitis is increased among family members in the same household, especially hepatitis C.

■ Habits

Habits may be particularly important for certain abdominal complaints, especially the use of tobacco, caffeine, and alcohol. Also important are a list of all medications/drugs, activity, exercise, and sleep patterns. Identify usual dietary intake. Explore sexual habits. Ask about travel patterns and recent exposures.

Physical Examination

The abdominal examination begins with inspection, followed by auscultation, percussion, and palpation while envisioning the expected underlying structures.

Abdominal Regions

RIGHT UPPER QUADRANT	EPIGASTRIC	LEFT UPPER QUADRANT
Liver	Stomach	Spleen
Gallbladder	Pancreas	Pancreas
Tip of right kidney		Tip of left kidney
Diaphragm		

RIGHT LUMBAR	UMBILICAL	LEFT LUMBAR
	Uterus	
	Bowel	
	Aorta	

RIGHT LOWER QUADRANT	SUPRAPUBIC	LEFT LOWER QUADRANT
Appendix	Bladder	Left Ovary
Right ovary	Uterus	Bowel
Bowel		

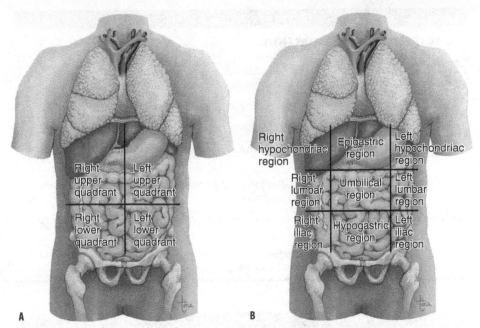

Figure 11.1 Areas of the abdomen: A. four quadrants. B. nine regions. (From Scanlon, V. C., & Sanders, T. [2014]. *Essentials of anatomy and physiology* [7th ed.]. Philadelphia: F. A. Davis. Reprinted with permission.)

Right upper quadrant
Left upper quadrant
Right lower quadrant
Left lower quadrant

Right hypochondriac region
Epigastric region
Left hypochondriac region
Right lumbar region
Umbilical region
Left lumbar region
Right iliac region
Hypogastric region
Left iliac region

A   B

Auscultating before percussion or palpation allows the examiner to listen to the abdominal sounds undisturbed. Moreover, if pain is present, it is best to leave palpation until last and to gather other data before possibly causing the patient discomfort. When examining the abdomen, it often helps to break the abdomen down into quadrants, or regions, in order to consider which organs are involved (Fig. 11.1).

■ Order of the Examination

Inspection

Inspect for scars, striae, venous pattern, rashes, contour, symmetry, masses, peristalsis, pulsations, or discolorations. Tangential lighting is helpful when observing for peristalsis and pulsations. See Table 11.1 for abnormalities found on inspection.

Auscultation

Perform auscultation before palpation to hear unaltered bowel sounds. It is important to listen to each area for 10 to 15 seconds. Listen for bruits over the aorta and the iliac, renal, and femoral arteries. Note the presence or absence of sounds, as well as the quality and magnitude of sounds. See Table 11.2 for abnormalities found on auscultation.

Table 11.1

Abnormalities on Inspection

Physical Finding	Cause
Scars	Indicates past surgery or trauma.
Striae	Includes obesity, ascites, pregnancy, tumor, Cushing's disease, and steroid use.
Venous pattern	May be prominent in fair-skinned people or due to congested portal circulation.
Discoloration	Consider jaundice, Addison's disease, von Recklinghausen's disease, trauma, or other rashes or lesions.
Visible peristalsis	In an older adult, consider bowel obstruction. In newborns, upper abdominal peristalsis is diagnostic for pyloric stenosis.
Pulsations	Visible aortic pulsations may be normal in thin individuals but in others may indicate aortic aneurysm.
Distention	For changes in contour or symmetry, consider the Fs of abdominal distention: fat, fluid, feces, fetus, flatus, fibroid, full bladder, fatal tumor, false pregnancy.

Table 11.2

Abnormalities on Auscultation

Physical Finding	Cause
Bruits	A swishing sound heard over the aortic, renal, iliac, and femoral arteries, indicating narrowing or aneurysm.
Pops/tinkles	High-pitched sounds suggesting intestinal fluid and air under pressure, as in early obstruction.
Rushes	Rushes of high-pitched sounds that coincide with cramping suggest intestinal obstruction.
Borborygmi	Increased, prolonged gurgles occur with gastroenteritis, early intestinal obstruction, and hunger.
Rubs	Grating sounds that vary with respiration. Indicate inflammation of the peritoneal surface of an organ from tumor, infection, or splenic infarct.
Venous hum	A soft humming noise often heard in hepatic cirrhosis that is caused by increased collateral circulation between portal and systemic venous systems.
Succussion splash	A splashing noise produced by shaking the body when there is both gas and fluid in a cavity or free air in the peritoneum or thorax.
Decreased/absent sounds	Occurs with peritonitis or paralytic ileus.

Percussion

In an orderly approach, percuss the abdomen for areas of dullness, indicating fluid or solid rather than air. Also note areas of resonance, hyperresonance, and tympany. Observe the patient for indications of discomfort with percussion. See Table 11.3 for normal percussion tones.

Table 11.3

Normal Tones Produced by Percussion

	Most Dense			Least Dense	
Tone	Flat	Dull	Resonant	Hyperresonant	Tympanic
Intensity	Soft	Medium	Loud	Very loud	Loud
Pitch	High	Medium	Low	Very low	High
Duration	Short	Medium	Long	Very long	Medium
Area	Muscle, bone	Liver, spleen	Lung	Emphysematous lung	Gastric air bubble

Palpation

Both light and deep palpation are necessary to detect tenderness, tumors, or changes in underlying abdominal structures. First, lightly palpate each quadrant, noting any detectable structures and indications of tenderness or pain. Repeat the sequence, using deeper palpation and avoiding painful areas until last. Note areas of tenderness, changes in contour, consistency of organs, and the presence of masses—and if masses are present, their consistency, size, shape, location, and delineation. See Table 11.4 for abnormalities found on palpation.

- Light palpation is helpful in detecting tenderness and guarding.
- Deep palpation is usually required to delineate masses.

Rectal Examination

A digital rectal examination is included in the abdominal examination. Note skin changes or lesions in the perianal region or the presence of external hemorrhoids. Insert the gloved index finger into the anus with the patient either leaning over or side-lying on the examination table, and note any internal hemorrhoids or fissures. Check the stool for occult blood. For male patients, the rectal examination is necessary for direct examination of the prostate.

■ Special Maneuvers

Rebound Tenderness

Rebound tenderness is tested by slowly pressing over the abdomen with your fingertips, holding the position until pain subsides or the patient adjusts to the discomfort, and then quickly removing the pressure. Rebound pain, a sign of peritoneal inflammation, is present if the patient experiences a sharp discomfort over the inflamed site when pressure is released.

Rovsing's Sign

Appendicitis is suggested when there is referred rebound pain in the *right* lower quadrant when the examiner presses deeply in the *left* lower quadrant and then quickly releases the pressure.

Table 11.4

Abnormalities on Palpation

Condition	Description	Characteristics
Hepatomegaly	Liver enlargement can be detected by percussion and/or palpation and can be caused by cirrhosis, hepatitis, right heart failure, cysts, and malignancy.	Cirrhosis produces an enlarged, firm, nontender liver. Hepatitis and right heart failure are characterized by a smooth, tender liver. Cysts may not be palpable but will produce right upper quadrant pain and tenderness. A malignancy typically produces a firm, irregular liver surface.
Splenomegaly	The causes of an enlarged spleen include infectious or inflammatory diseases, such as mononucleosis, infectious hepatitis, subacute bacterial endocarditis, psittacosis, tuberculosis, malaria, sarcoidosis, amyloidosis, and systemic lupus erythematosus; lymphoproliferative and myeloproliferative diseases, such as lymphoma, leukemia, polycythemia, and myelofibrosis; hemolytic anemias and hemoglobinopathies; splenic cysts; and storage diseases, such as Gaucher's, Niemann-Pick, and Hand-Schuller-Christian.	In addition to an enlarged and usually tender spleen, other symptoms are early feeding satiety, splenic friction rub, epigastric and splenic bruits, and cytopenias.
Aortic aneurysm	Arteriosclerosis is the most common cause of aortic aneurysm. Aging, cigarette smoking, and hypertension are contributing factors. Trauma; syphilis; congenital connective tissue disorders, such as Marfan's disease; and positive history of aneurysm also increase the incidence.	A prominent lateral pulsation suggests an aneurysm.
Tumor	Caused by any benign or malignant growth in any of the abdominal organs.	Vary according to the affected organ but include pain, bloating, obstruction, anorexia, and changes in bowel or genitourinary functioning.

Heel Strike

Ask the patient to stand with straight legs and to raise up on toes. Then ask the patient to relax, allowing the heel to strike the floor, thus jarring the body. A positive heel strike is indicative of appendicitis and peritoneal irritation. Alternatively, strike the plantar surface of the heel with your fist while the patient rests supine on the examination table.

Obturator Sign

Pain is elicited in appendicitis by inward rotation of the hip with the knee bent so that the obturator internus muscle is stretched.

Psoas Sign

Place your hand on the patient's thigh just above the knee and ask the patient to raise the thigh against your hand. This contracts the psoas muscle and produces pain in patients with an inflamed appendix.

Murphy's Sign

Pain is present on deep inspiration when an inflamed gallbladder is palpated by pressing the fingers under the rib cage. Murphy's sign is positive in cholecystitis.

Hepatojugular Reflux

Hepatojugular reflux is elicited by applying firm, sustained hand pressure to the abdomen in the mid-epigastric region while the patient breathes regularly. Observe the neck for elevation of the jugular venous pressure with pressure of the hand and sudden drop of the jugular venous pressure when hand pressure is released. Hepatojugular reflux is exaggerated in right heart failure.

Scratch Test

An alternative to palpation/percussion to determine hepatic size is the "scratch" test. It is performed by placing the stethoscope over the liver and then lightly scratching up the abdomen on the right side, using a fingertip or tongue depressor. The sound you hear through the stethoscope will be intensified over the liver.

Shifting Dullness

To differentiate ascites, test for shifting of the peritoneal fluid to the dependent side by rolling the patient side to side and percussing for dullness on the dependent side of the abdomen. Note: This maneuver is nonspecific and has, for the most part, been replaced by ultrasonography of the abdomen.

RED FLAG ◄ **Red Flags for Abdominal Pain**

- *Pain that awakens patient*
- *Pain that persists more than 6 hours and progresses in intensity*
- *Progressive abdominal distension*
- *Fever, leukocytosis, granulocytosis*
- *Pain that changes location*
- *Radiation of the pain to shoulder (cholecystitis) or back (pancreatitis/aneurysm)*
- *Pain worsened by movement, respirations*
- *Pain followed by vomiting or intractable vomiting*
- *Hematemesis*
- *Black, tarry stools*
- *Pain associated with signs of hypovolemic shock*
- *Associated syncope*
- *Decreased urine output*

DIFFERENTIAL DIAGNOSIS OF CHIEF COMPLAINTS

■ Abdominal Pain

Abdominal pain is one of the most common complaints in primary care and can be functional or organic in cause and acute or chronic in nature. Even though the causes of abdominal pain are often self-limiting, the pain can also indicate a life-threatening situation and must be carefully assessed.

When a patient complains of abdominal pain, it is essential to rule out indications for an emergency referral by carefully reviewing the history of the complaint, including the general description, quantity, quality, location, timing, and onset of the pain and associated symptoms. Although the physical examination may suggest the cause, the examination may be normal even with underlying pathology. Laboratory studies and diagnostic testing may be necessary to pinpoint the actual cause and rule out the more serious causes.

There are three major classifications of abdominal pain: visceral, somatoparietal, and referred. Referred pain is simply pain radiating or referring from a site external to the abdomen. See Table 11.5 for differentiating common characteristics of visceral and somatoparietal pain.

Table 11.5	
Differentiating Types of Abdominal Pain	
Visceral	**Somatoparietal**
Poorly localized	Localized
Vague	Intense
Often midline	Guarding
Crampy	Patient often still
Burning	
Patient often restless	
Associated with:	Worsened by:
Diaphoresis	Movement
Pallor	Respirations
Nausea	Cough
Caused by:	Caused by:
Inflammation or injury to solid or hollow organs	Inflammation of the parietal peritoneum

■ Right Upper Quadrant Pain

A complaint of right upper quadrant (RUQ) pain encompasses a variety of possible causes, most commonly diseases of the liver, gallbladder, pancreas, or lung. In the abdomen, it is important also to consider referred pain from a different area in the abdomen or from a different body system. Also consider diseases of the colon or kidney, or the gynecological system for women, which are covered in this chapter under Table 11.8 "Differential Diagnosis of Lower Abdominal Pain." Because the abdomen contains many structures and organs, a thorough history and physical examination is necessary, with special maneuvers, if warranted.

History

Begin with the exact location of the pain, onset, timing, quality, quantity, and alleviating or aggravating factors. It is particularly important to determine whether the pain is related to meals or movement. Ask if there has been any fever, nausea, vomiting, diarrhea, constipation, anorexia, or change in urine or stool color/consistency, which may indicate liver or gallbladder disease. A pleuritic cause for the pain should be considered; inquire about cough, shortness of breath, or fever. Include a smoking history. Ask about diet history, particularly regarding a high-fat diet or fad diets that might exclude food groups or be very low in calories, which may increase the likelihood of gallbladder disease. Inquire about sexual practices, alcohol, and drugs (prescription and illicit) that might alert you to an increased risk for liver disease, particularly hepatitis. Ask about foreign travel because hepatitis is endemic in some areas, and often the standards for food preparation are not the same elsewhere as in North America. Ask about patient and family history of breast or colon cancer, gallbladder or liver disease, and general disorders of the digestive tract.

Physical Examination

A thorough abdominal examination should be performed with particular attention to the RUQ, assessing for tenderness, rebound, masses, and organ enlargement or nodularity. A respiratory examination should include auscultation for adventitious breath sounds and the presence of friction rubs or voice sounds. Table 11.6 summarizes differential diagnosis for RUQ and left upper quadrant (LUQ) pain.

The conditions of the underlying organs are key to identifying the etiology of RUQ pain. Consider diseases of the gallbladder, liver, pancreas, or lung as the most likely cause of pain. In the case of the RUQ, laboratory testing can be most helpful in diagnosis (Table 11.7).

GALLBLADDER DISEASE

A mnemonic used to describe a common presentation for cholecystitis is "female, fat, and forty," although it can occur in much younger and older individuals after surgery, trauma, burns, sepsis, or critical illness. Young people have shown

Table 11.6

Differential Diagnosis for Right and Left Upper Quadrant Pain

Disease	History	Diagnostic Studies	Physical Findings
Cholecystitis	RUQ pain, anorexia, nausea, vomiting, fever	CBC, LFTs, amylase, gallbladder US, HIDA scan	↑ Neutrophilic leukocytes, ↑ AST/ALT, ↑ amylase with common duct obstruction; US will show nonvisualization of the gallbladder and wall thickening
Liver disease	RUQ pain, sexual practices, travel, alcohol use, history of malignancy, nausea, vomiting, anorexia, drugs, raw shellfish ingestion, change in color of urine or stools, weight loss, abdominal distention	LFTs, hepatitis profile, abdominal US or CT	↑ LFTs, ↑ IgM, and specific antigens will be present for hepatitis A, B, and C; US or CT may show cysts or tumors, obstruction
Pancreatitis	Epigastric pain, alcohol abuse, liver or gallbladder disease, jaundice, hyperlipidemia	Amylase, lipase, LFTs, plain abdominal films, abdominal US or CT, chest x-ray	↑ Amylase and lipase, ↑ LFTs, ↑ WBC, epigastric tenderness, pancreatic or biliary obstruction on US or CT
Pleurisy	Respiratory disease, such as upper respiratory infection or pneumonia, shortness of breath, chest trauma, other systemic disease	Chest x-ray	If there is air or fluid in the pleural space, investigate other more serious diagnoses
Hypersplenism	LUQ pain, anorexia, fever, fatigue, weight loss, recent infection, bruising or bleeding, lymphadenopathy, jaundice	CBC, platelet, SPE, amylase, B_{12}, uric acid, bone marrow aspiration, abdominal CT	Vary depending on underlying cause: cytopenias or myeloproliferation or lymphoproliferation, ↑ B_{12} in leukemias and polycythemia, ↑ uric acid in proliferative disorders, monoclonal gammopathy or ↑ immunoglobulins on SPE, abnormalities on CT and bone marrow aspirate

ALT = alanine aminotransferase; AST = aspartate aminotransferase; CBC = complete blood count; CT = computed tomography; HIDA = hepatobiliary iminodiacetic acid; IgM = immunoglobulin M; LFT = liver function tests; LUQ = left upper quadrant; RUQ = right upper quadrant; SPE = serum protein electrophoresis; US = ultrasound.

an increased incidence of cholecystitis if they are adhering to drastic weight-loss diets that are extremely low in fat and calories.

Signs and Symptoms

Initially, acute colicky pain is localized in the RUQ and is often accompanied by nausea and vomiting. Murphy's sign is frequently present. Fever is low grade, and the increase in neutrophilic leukocytes in the blood is slight. Acute cholecystitis improves in 2 to 3 days and resolves within a week; however, recurrences are

Table 11.7

Laboratory Studies for Upper Abdominal Pain

Study	Description
Complete blood count (CBC)	CBC determines elevated white blood cells in infection; decreased hematocrit and hemoglobin, indicating the possibility of a gastrointestinal bleed; and cytopenic or myeloproliferative disorders, indicating hepatic or splenic involvement.
Platelet count	Thrombocytopenia or thrombocytosis may indicate diseases involving the liver or spleen.
Alanine aminotransferase (ALT)	ALT primarily helps diagnose liver disease but also detects biliary obstruction.
Aspartate aminotransferase (AST)	AST primarily helps diagnose liver disease; however, elevations are also associated with acute common bile duct obstruction. AST levels may be affected by statin drugs, acetaminophen, and alcohol.
Alkaline phosphatase	Alkaline phosphatase is used as a tumor marker and an index of liver and bone disease or metastasis in correlation with other findings.
Gamma glutamic transpeptidase (GGT)	GGT determines liver cell dysfunction and detects alcohol-induced liver disease. The GGT can be helpful as a confirmatory test.
Lactate dehydrogenase (LDH)	LDH is a widely distributed enzyme that is elevated with cellular damage of the liver, kidney, skeletal muscle, and heart.
Bilirubin	Bilirubin evaluates liver function, biliary obstruction, and hemolytic anemia.
Albumin	Albumin is influenced by nutritional state and hepatic and renal function.
Amylase	Amylase helps distinguish pancreatitis from other causes of abdominal pain.
Lipase	Lipase helps diagnose pancreatitis and stays elevated longer than amylase. However, lipase is not specific and may also be elevated in biliary and hepatic disease, diabetes mellitus, and gastric malignancy.
Hepatitis profile	A hepatitis profile detects acute or chronic, active and previous disease, carrier state, and immunity to hepatitis A, B, and C.
Prothrombin time (PT)	An increased PT indicates clotting dysfunction, which may be attributed to liver disease.
Serum protein electrophoresis (SPE)	An SPE is an evaluation of proteins (e.g., albumin, alpha globulins, beta globulins, and gamma globulins) present in the serum. SPE may help diagnose autoimmune liver disease, cirrhosis, and a_1-antitrypsin deficiency.
Helicobacter pylori	H. pylori is a serum blood test that detects common bacteria causing peptic ulcer disease.

common. If acute cholecystitis is accompanied by jaundice and cholestasis (arrest of bile excretion), suspect common duct obstruction, which generally requires surgical or endoscopic procedure.

Diagnostic Studies

Suggested laboratory tests include alanine aminotransferase (ALT), aspartate aminotransferase (AST), amylase, and lipase. A diagnosis can usually be made with ultrasound or hepatobiliary iminodiacetic acid (HIDA) scanning.

Decision Rule

Ebell (2001) reports a decision rule for common bile duct lithiasis developed by Houdart and colleagues (1995). The prediction rule was developed on a sample of 503 patients and validated on a group of 279 patients. They found that patients were at low risk (0.6%) for common bile duct lithiasis if they presented with no jaundice and normal transaminases, had a common bile duct diameter of less than 8 mm, and had no ultrasound-demonstrated intrahepatic duct enlargement. In contrast, patients who had jaundice, abnormal transaminases, a common bile duct diameter of greater than 8 mm, and intrahepatic duct enlargement were categorized as "at risk" (39%).

If the signs and symptoms do not typically point to cholecystitis (e.g., there is no fever or elevated white blood cell [WBC] count) and an abdominal ultrasound is negative, magnetic resonance imaging (MRI) or a computed tomography (CT) scan is recommended. A chest x-ray is recommended if respiratory involvement is suspected.

LIVER DISEASE

Liver diseases include viral hepatitis (hepatitis A, B, C, D, E, F [not confirmed], and G), alcohol-related hepatitis, nonalcoholic steatohepatitis, fatty liver, cirrhosis, hepatic cysts, and malignancy (primary or metastatic).

Signs and Symptoms

The major clinical manifestations of liver disease include jaundice, hepatomegaly, cholestasis, portal hypertension, ascites, and encephalopathy. Symptoms vary with the cause, but many are insidious, especially with hepatitis. Liver disease is often discovered on routine examination or laboratory testing.

Diagnostic Studies

If liver disease is suspected, begin with liver function tests (ALT, AST, alkaline phosphatase, albumin, bilirubin, and total protein) and a hepatitis profile. These tests provide valuable information on most liver diseases, except hepatic cysts, which generally do not alter liver functions. If cirrhosis, malignancy, fatty liver, or a hepatic cyst is suspected or should be eliminated, include an abdominal ultrasound or CT scan. A liver biopsy is sometimes warranted to confirm the diagnosis.

Those found to have hepatitis B or C should be referred to a gastroenterology or infectious disease specialist. Hepatitis A is usually self-limiting and can be managed by the primary care provider.

PANCREATITIS

Biliary tract disease and alcoholism account for most pancreatitis admissions. The most common cause of pancreatitis is alcohol abuse. Other causes include hyperlipidemia, drugs, toxins, infection, structural abnormalities, surgery, vascular disease, trauma, hyperparathyroidism and hypercalcemia, renal transplantation, and hereditary pancreatitis.

Signs and Symptoms

Pancreatitis is characterized by severe abdominal pain, often with radiation to the back, and is usually accompanied by nausea and vomiting. The pain is steady and boring (piercing, penetrating), often refractory to opioid pain medicines, and persistent for many days. Fever is present within a few hours, and other signs include tachycardia, rapid and shallow respirations, postural hypotension, diaphoresis, blunted sensorium, abdominal distention, tenderness, hypoactive bowel sounds, and possibly ascites.

Diagnostic Studies

There is no single test to diagnose pancreatitis, but several tests support the clinical impression, including serum amylase and lipase, WBC, chest x-ray, and ultrasound. Lipase and amylase are usually quite elevated, as is the WBC. Ultrasound imaging will detect an enlarged pancreas as well as gallstones and biliary obstruction. A CT scan can be used in lieu of ultrasound to image the pancreas, but it is less helpful in identifying gallstones as the potential cause.

PLEURISY

Pleurisy may result from (1) an underlying lung process, (2) an infection or irritation in the pleural space, (3) the transport of an infectious or other disease agent or neoplastic metastases to the pleura, and (4) trauma, especially rib trauma. Basilar pleurisy may produce referred pain to the abdomen.

Signs and Symptoms

Pleurisy is differentiated from abdominal disease by chest x-ray or evidence of a respiratory origin, such as increased pain with deep breathing and coughing, shallow or rapid breathing, the absence of nausea or vomiting, or a tendency toward relief of pain with pressure on the chest wall or abdomen. A pleural friction rub is pathognomonic.

Diagnostic Studies

Pleurisy may not be evident on any thoracic imaging, and diagnosis may be made by history and physical examination. A chest x-ray or CT of the chest showing inflammation or pleural thickening is helpful in some cases. See also Chapter 9.

■ Left Upper Quadrant Pain

Diseases and disorders of the spleen, stomach, and pancreas are the most likely causes of LUQ pain (see Table 11.6). Also consider colon and kidney disease, which are covered in this chapter under Table 11.8 "Differential Diagnosis of Lower Abdominal Pain." For disorders of the spleen and pancreas, laboratory evaluation is helpful, along with the history and physical. For the stomach, more definitive diagnostic tests may be needed.

History

LUQ pain is often associated with causes that are outside the abdomen. Hematopoietic malignancies, such as lymphomas and leukemias, and other hematologic disorders, such as thrombocytopenia, polycythemia, myelofibrosis, and hemolytic anemia, often cause enlargement of the spleen, leading to LUQ pain. In addition to questions about the specific characteristics of the pain, it is important to ask the patient about fever, unusual bleeding or bruising, recent diagnosis of mononucleosis, fatigue, malaise, lymphadenopathy, cough, arthralgias, anorexia, weight loss, jaundice, high blood pressure, and headache.

Physical Examination

A thorough abdominal examination is necessary with special attention to the LUQ. A respiratory examination should be included to rule out referred pain. A hematopoietic cause can be explored only through laboratory tests (see Table 11.7).

HYPERSPLENISM

Hypersplenism, an overactive spleen, is associated with the spleen's increased filtering and destruction of red blood cells, as well as WBCs and platelets. Splenomegaly is a main feature of the condition. Hypersplenism is almost always secondary to other primary disorders, most commonly cytopenic hematologic disorders such as lymphoma, leukemia, thrombocytopenia, polycythemia, myelofibrosis, and hemolytic anemias. Other causes include portal or splenic vein thrombosis; infection, such as mononucleosis, infectious hepatitis, subacute bacterial endocarditis, psittacosis, miliary tuberculosis, malaria, brucellosis, and syphilis; sarcoidosis; amyloidosis; connective tissue diseases, such as systemic lupus erythematosus and rheumatoid arthritis; lipoid and nonlipoid storage diseases; and splenic cysts. The degree of associated splenomegaly is usually consistent with the degree of cytopenia and results from an increase in splenic workload by the trapping and destruction of abnormal blood cells or diverse abnormal circulating organisms.

Signs and Symptoms

The signs and symptoms are highly variable and relate to the underlying cause. The patient may complain of early satiety or abdominal fullness and LUQ pain. If the cause is infectious, fatigue and/or fever are common. On physical examination, splenomegaly is present. An epigastric or splenic bruit may be present. The complete blood count (CBC) may identify anemia, leukopenia, thrombocytopenia, or any combination of the three.

Diagnostic Studies

Several laboratory studies may be needed to diagnose the numerous underlying causes of hypersplenism. Begin with a CBC and platelet count, which will likely provide the most information on how to proceed. If abnormal, a bone marrow biopsy is indicated. Other tests to consider are serum protein electrophoresis, liver function tests, B_{12}, amylase, and CT or MRI of the abdomen.

PLEURISY

See p. 353.

PANCREATITIS

See pp. 352–353.

■ Epigastric Pain

The epigastric region is a very common site of discomfort stemming from many digestive structures. Epigastric pain can represent the heartburn or dyspepsia often associated with GERD as well as several other diseases, including malignancies. Heartburn, often from GERD, is a very common complaint; patients may use alternative terms to describe this sensation, including "indigestion" or "sour stomach." *Dyspepsia* covers a variety of complaints that include heartburn, fullness, bloating, and upper abdominal pain. Because pain in this region provides little specificity on its own, the history is crucial in narrowing the differential diagnosis.

The physical examination is most helpful in eliminating some of the rarer causes of epigastric pain; the common causes are typically associated with benign physical findings. A change in vital signs can point to cardiac or respiratory disturbances and to potential fevers and infections. A positive hemoccult on rectal examination may indicate an upper GI bleed or malignancy. Malignancy should also be suspected if there is weight loss and/or a palpable abdominal mass. Listen for adventitious abdominal sounds, such as succussion splash, indicating air or fluid in the thorax or peritoneum, or aortic bruit heard with abdominal aneurysm. Be alert for a positive Murphy's sign, which is seen in cholecystitis. Note any abnormalities in skin tone and/or color that could indicate liver disease, cholecystitis, or hypoxia owing to respiratory or cardiac disease.

Common Causes of Epigastric Pain

- GERD
- Gastric or duodenal ulcer
- Gastric or duodenal malignancy
- Esophageal spasm
- Cholecystitis
- Pancreatitis
- Hepatitis/liver disease
- Medication intolerance
- Ischemic heart disease
- Pregnancy

History

To differentiate among the causes of epigastric pain, have the patient clearly describe the complaint, particularly the characteristics (e.g., sharp, dull, nagging, burning, steady, cramping, boring), and point to the exact location of the pain. Discomfort stemming from a serious disorder is often constant and intense and may radiate to the back. Determine what factors worsen and/or improve the discomfort, particularly any relationship to meals or activity. In addition to rating the severity of the pain, determine what, if any, behaviors the pain has limited, including intake or physical activities. Establish the type of onset and progression, including whether the discomfort is intermittent, gradually increasing in severity, and so on. Finally, determine what, if any, associated symptoms the patient has noticed. Important considerations include vomiting, regurgitation, diaphoresis, dysphagia, blood in the stool or emesis, shortness of breath, fatigue, weight loss, and radiation to other sites (intra- and extra-abdominal). Obtain a respiratory and cardiac history. Ask about any new or current medications.

Physical Examination

A thorough examination of the entire abdomen is necessary, with special attention to the epigastric area. Tenderness can be present with PUD and pancreatitis. Auscultating for bruits in this area is vital; an abdominal aortic aneurysm may present with epigastric pain. It is a life-threatening and possibly emergent problem. Vital signs and weight need to be recorded. Look for any signs of infection, blood loss, or weight loss in the case of malignancy. A rectal examination for occult blood can add important information. In addition, a thorough respiratory and cardiac examination should be performed because the pain may be referred. Depending on history and cardiovascular risks, consider an electrocardiogram to rule out a cardiac source for the pain (see Table 11.7 for related laboratory tests).

GASTROESOPHAGEAL REFLUX DISEASE

GERD is the most common organic cause of heartburn. Lower esophageal sphincter control can be decreased by several medications (e.g., theophylline, dopamine, diazepam, calcium channel blockers), foods and beverages (e.g., caffeine, alcohol, chocolate, fatty foods), and tobacco use. When lower esophageal sphincter tone is lower than normal, secretions are allowed to reflux into the esophagus, causing discomfort. Reflux is also promoted by weight gain and other variables causing greater pressure against the lower esophageal sphincter.

Signs and Symptoms

The most common symptom of GERD is heartburn, which typically occurs after meals and is often relieved by antacids. Other symptoms include belching, regurgitation, and/or water brash. Respiratory and ear, nose, and throat symptoms may develop, including cough, wheeze, aspiration, hoarseness, and globus sensation (fullness in the throat). Symptoms may occur primarily at night, when patients recline following a meal. See Box 11.1 for common triggers of GERD.

BOX 11.1

Common Triggers for GERD

- Tomato products
- Citrus
- Spicy foods
- Coffee
- Fatty foods
- Peppermint
- Chocolate
- Alcohol
- Smoking

Diagnostic Studies

Diagnosis can often be made by the history, although the degree of symptoms may not be consistent with the degree of esophageal injury. When GERD is the most likely cause of acute epigastric discomfort, empiric treatment may include avoiding any triggers and prescribing antacids and/or antisecretory agents, particularly for a young, otherwise healthy patient without known risk factors for more serious disorders. However, the risk of delaying the definitive diagnosis and treatment must be weighed when considering this route. Endoscopy provides direct visualization of the esophagus and evidence to rule out other disorders. Ambulatory esophageal pH monitoring may help to identify association between symptoms and reflux. Barium swallows and upper GI x-ray can assist in ruling out hiatal hernia but may have a high potential of missing esophageal damage.

PEPTIC ULCER DISEASE

PUD includes both gastric and duodenal ulcers. *Helicobacter pylori* and NSAIDs are common causes of both disorders, along with some probable genetic predisposition. Zollinger-Ellison syndrome commonly results in gastric ulcer development. The incidence of gastric ulcer is higher in persons who smoke and those with certain chronic diseases, including cirrhosis, hyperparathyroidism, chronic renal failure, and lung disease.

Signs and Symptoms

Epigastric pain is common with both gastric and duodenal ulcers and is described as a gnawing or burning sensation. Whereas the pain of gastric ulcer is usually worsened by intake, a duodenal ulcer usually causes pain on an empty stomach. It is not uncommon for the pain of duodenal ulcer to awaken the patient from sleep at 1 a.m. to 2 a.m. Antacids typically offer relief for both types of ulcer. Pain may be episodic with symptom-free intervals. Pain may radiate to the back. Associated symptoms include bloating, belching, nausea, and loss of appetite. The physical examination is not usually positive other than potentially identifying some degree of abdominal tenderness. As the mucosa erodes, bleeding may occur. If rupture occurs, pain acutely changes character and is intractable.

Diagnostic Studies

Stool guaiac should be performed on any patient with epigastric pain. PUD should be suspected in any patient with dyspepsia/epigastric pain who does not fit the profile associated with GERD, is older than 50 years, and has associated weight loss or loss of appetite. For these patients, direct endoscopy should be ordered, during which biopsies will be taken of any erosive site to rule out gastric malignancy. If PUD is diagnosed, testing for *H. pylori* should be performed. When patients with gastric ulcers have neither *H. pylori* nor a history of NSAID use, serum gastrin level should be determined, assessing for Zollinger-Ellison syndrome.

HIATAL HERNIA

Hiatal hernias are common and often asymptomatic, although they may be associated with more severe symptoms of acid reflux and esophagitis in patients with GERD. Hiatal hernias are found in one-fourth of patients with GERD, and the majority of patients with erosive esophagitis and Barrett esophagus (McQuaid, 2018). Risk factors for hiatal hernia include age older than 50 years and obesity.

Signs and Symptoms

Most small hiatal hernias cause no signs or symptoms. However, larger hiatal hernias may cause symptoms similar to those of GERD, including heartburn, belching, dysphagia, chest or abdominal pain, and feeling of fullness.

Diagnostic Studies

A hiatal hernia can be diagnosed with a barium swallow (esophagram), endoscopy, and/or esophageal manometry. Conservative treatment is recommended with medication for esophageal reflux. Surgery is rarely recommended but may be helpful in patients for whom medication and lifestyle changes are unsuccessful.

GASTRIC MALIGNANCY

Although the incidence of gastric cancer is lower than in the past, it has remained relatively steady for several years. It was estimated that approximately 26,560 adults would be diagnosed in the United States in 2021, with 11,180 deaths (American Cancer Society, 2021a). Suspected contributing factors, including excess salt intake and chronic gastritis, as is seen with *H. pylori*, can lead to gastric cancer. The early stage of the disease is asymptomatic, and diagnosis is made usually only after significant advancement. The 5-year survival rates for localized, regional, and distant stomach cancers are 70%, 32%, and 6% respectively (American Cancer Society 2021b).

Signs and Symptoms

Cancers of the stomach are rarely symptomatic until the disease has progressed. Symptoms may be mild and consistent with heartburn or include more definitive abdominal pain. Other symptoms include nausea and vomiting, diarrhea, constipation, fullness, anorexia, fatigue, and weight loss. Although the abdominal examination may be negative, tenderness, and/or a palpable mass may be present.

Diagnostic Studies

The patient should be referred for endoscopy. A CBC should be ordered, anemia assessed, and stool guaiac performed.

PANCREATITIS

See pp. 352–353.

CHOLECYSTITIS

See pp. 349–350.

HEPATITIS

See pp. 352, 385.

■ Right and Left Lower Quadrant Abdominal Pain

Lower abdominal pain can have a multitude of causes, including diseases or disorders of the appendix, colon, kidney, bladder, ureter, ovary, uterus, and prostate. Pinpointing the specific location of the pain is crucial to beginning the differential diagnosis. However, caution is recommended because abdominal pain can be referred from areas of the abdomen other than the point of origin. Because of the complexity of the differential diagnosis for lower abdominal pain, diagnostic tests are often necessary to confirm the findings of the history and physical examination.

History

There are a multitude of etiologies for lower abdominal complaints. It is important to begin with a thorough history. Although abdominal pain can often radiate to other areas or can present a vague and confusing picture, pinpointing the location of the pain is a prudent place to start—have the patient point to the site. Question the patient about the onset of the pain and the progression since onset. Determine whether it is accompanied by fever, anorexia, nausea, or vomiting, which might suggest appendicitis, gastroenteritis, or obstruction. It is imperative to ask about the last menstrual period and about birth control methods to rule out ectopic pregnancy. A history of miscarriages and/or sexually transmitted infections (STIs) can give more clues for the risk of ectopic pregnancy. Sex practices and the number of sexual partners can alert the practitioner to the risk for pelvic inflammatory disease (PID). Ovarian tumors can go undetected for months, so the examiner must be alert to vague symptoms such as bloating, gas, dyspepsia, and pressure-type pain that might indicate a need for further investigation. In a postmenopausal patient, these complaints should not be trivialized. A positive family history of ovarian cancer in a patient presenting with these complaints is a red flag. Urinary symptoms such as dysuria, hematuria, and a history of kidney stones indicate a risk for kidney stones. Persistent, asymptomatic hematuria is concerning for bladder inflammation or malignancy. If the patient complains of pain with movement or exercise and gives a history of heavy lifting, hernia may be suspected. Sudden onset of severe lower abdominal pain, nausea, and vomiting in a young male patient should alert the examiner to the possibility of testicular torsion. A complaint of fatigue, weakness, weight loss, or change in bowel or bladder habits is worrisome, and a malignancy should be on the top of the list of differential diagnoses. Occasionally, hip disorders can present as lower abdominal pain.

Physical Examination

A thorough abdominal and genitourinary examination is necessary in all patients but is of particular importance in female patients. *No complaint of lower abdominal pain in a female patient should be evaluated without performing a pelvic examination.* A rectal examination should be performed for occult blood, as well as palpation of the uterus or prostate and a check for the presence of masses or tenderness. Although musculoskeletal causes of lower abdominal pain are unusual, a musculoskeletal history and examination should be included, particularly when the pain is in the groin or hip area.

For clarity, the lower abdominal complaints are broken down into the following regions: right lower quadrant (RLQ), left lower quadrant (LLQ), periumbilical, and suprapubic. For an overview and summary of the differential diagnosis of lower abdominal pain as well as laboratory studies, see Tables 11.8 and 11.9.

APPENDICITIS

Other than hernia, appendicitis is the most common cause of acute abdominal pain. It occurs most commonly between the ages of 10 and 30 years. Gangrene, perforation, and peritonitis can develop within 36 hours of onset, if untreated; historically, approximately 15% of patients sent to surgery with a clinical diagnosis of appendicitis are falsely positive. Ultrasound and CT have decreased the incidence of overdiagnosis, although sometimes laparotomy or laparoscopy still are required for a definitive diagnosis and treatment. Gynecological disorders and gastroenteritis are the most common causes of misdiagnosis.

Signs and Symptoms

The pain of appendicitis usually evolves over a few hours and initially is poorly localized, midline, vague, and associated with some degree of nausea and/or loss of appetite. In a matter of hours, the pain migrates to the RLQ, becoming more intense and localized, and may increase with coughing or walking. Low-grade fever typically develops. The various tests for peritoneal irritation (i.e., rebound tenderness, Rovsing's sign, heel strike, psoas, and obturator) are positive.

Table 11.8

Differential Diagnosis of Lower Abdominal Pain

Disease	History	Diagnosis	Findings
Appendicitis	Anorexia, nausea, vomiting, fever, midline or RLQ pain worsening with cough or walking	CBC, abdominal CT or US	+ Rebound tenderness, fever, leukocytosis of 10,000–20,000/mL, US or CT may be positive for perforation/abscess
Ectopic pregnancy	Amenorrhea, severe RLQ or LLQ pain	Pelvic US, urine and serum hCG	A pregnancy outside the uterus, usually the tube, + hCG, + US, + rebound tenderness
Colorectal cancer	Weight loss, fatigue, change in bowel habits, anemia, + hemoccult	Hemoccult, CBC, CEA, flexible sigmoidoscopy, colonoscopy	+ Hemoccult, ↑ CEA, ↓ hematocrit and hemoglobin, + flexible sigmoidoscopy or colonoscopy
Urinary calculi	+ History of stones, severe colicky flank pain	U/A, plain abdominal x-ray, renal US, IVP	Hematuria, + stone visualization with x-ray or US
Ovarian tumor	+ Family history, abdominal bloating, pain, or heaviness	Pelvic examination, pelvic US, CT, CA-125	↑ CA-125, mass on examination, CT, or US
Hernia	History of straining or heavy lifting, previous abdominal surgery, lower abdominal or groin pain	Physical examination or US	Palpable mass in the inguinal ring or femoral area
Intestinal obstruction	History of abdominal surgery or inflammatory bowel disease, radiation, or impaction; abdominal pain or distention, vomiting; obstipation	Flat and upright abdominal x-ray, BE, CBC, electrolytes, BUN, creatinine, U/A	+ Mass on examination, BE, or x-ray; tinkles, rushes, borborygmi, or absent bowel sounds, ↑ SG, ↑ BUN and creatinine; electrolyte imbalance; leukocytosis
Diverticulitis	+ History of diverticulosis	CBC, flexible sigmoidoscopy, BE, abdominal CT	Leukocytosis, abdominal mass, stricture, hypertrophy of colonic musculature, possible free air in the abdomen
Gastroenteritis	Sudden-onset diarrhea, abdominal cramping, nausea, vomiting, fever	CBC, stool for ova and parasites, culture and sensitivity	Abdominal tenderness, borborygmi, possibly positive stool culture

BE = barium enema; BUN = blood urea nitrogen; CA-125 = cancer antigen 125; CEA = carcinoembryonic antigen; CBC = complete blood count; CT = computed tomography; hCG = human chorionic gonadotropin; IVP = intravenous pyelogram; LLQ = left lower quadrant; RLQ = right lower quadrant; SG = specific gravity; U/A = urinalysis; US = ultrasound.

Table 11.9

Laboratory Studies for Lower Abdominal and Suprapubic Pain

Study	Description
Complete blood count	White blood cell (WBC) count is elevated in appendicitis and diverticulitis, and the hematocrit and hemoglobin may be decreased in colon cancer.
Serum/urine pregnancy	In ectopic pregnancy, human chorionic gonadotropin may not be at the levels appropriate for the number of weeks as estimated by last menstrual period.
Urinalysis (U/A)	A dipstick or complete U/A identifies WBCs and blood, indicating infection, renal calculi, or malignancy; increased specific gravity with dehydration.
Prostate-specific antigen (PSA)	A PSA is a useful screening and diagnostic tool for prostate disease; if elevated, a prostate ultrasound and biopsy is recommended.
Wet prep, gonococcal/chlamydia culture	A wet prep can identify WBCs, but a culture is necessary to identify the offending organism. A gonococcal/chlamydial culture may be positive in salpingitis/pelvic inflammatory disease (PID). If positive for STI, other test considerations include rapid plasma reagin, HIV, and hepatitis profile.
Carcinoembryonic antigen (CEA)	The CEA will be elevated in colon cancer.
Cancer antigen 125 (CA-125)	A CA-125 is a tumor marker for progression or regression of ovarian tumors but can be helpful for initial diagnosis. False negatives occur in approximately 20% of patients with ovarian cancer. False positives can occur in patients with endometriosis, benign ovarian cysts, first-trimester pregnancy, PID, cirrhosis, and pancreatic cancer. It is more specific in postmenopausal than premenopausal women.
Celiac panel	Tissue transglutaminase (tTG) IgA is a common screening for celiac disease. Endomysial antibody IgA is an effective confirmation for a positive tTG test as it looks for a type of antibody that is highly specific to celiac disease.

Diagnostic Studies

An elevated WBC and the physical examination are the two most important diagnostic tools. If the diagnosis is still uncertain, an abdominal CT with contrast is helpful, with ultrasound as an alternative.

ECTOPIC PREGNANCY

A pregnancy is considered ectopic if implantation takes place outside the uterus, with 98% of those occurring in the fallopian tube (i.e., tubal pregnancy). Conditions that predispose a patient to an ectopic pregnancy are those that prevent the migration of the fertilized ovum to the uterus; approximately 50% are due to a previous tubal infection. Other risk factors include a history of infertility, PID, previous abdominal or tubal surgery, previous tubal pregnancy, and the use of an intrauterine device.

Signs and Symptoms

The most obvious sign of ectopic pregnancy is amenorrhea followed by spotting and sudden onset of severe lower quadrant pain. A stat pregnancy test should be performed. Backache may be present. There is tenderness on pelvic examination, and a pelvic mass may be palpated. Blood is present in the cul-de-sac. Shock and hemorrhage occur if the pregnancy ruptures and abdominal distention with peritoneal signs will ensue. Immediate laparoscopy or laparotomy is indicated because this condition is life-threatening.

Diagnostic Studies

The diagnosis of ectopic pregnancy can be made with urine human chorionic gonadotropin (hCG) or stat serum hCG, pelvic ultrasound, and if necessary, culdocentesis to detect blood in the cul-de-sac.

COLORECTAL CANCER

Colorectal cancer is the second leading cause of death from malignancies in the United States. Over half of the lesions are located in the rectosigmoid region and are typically adenocarcinomas. Risk factors include a history of polyps, positive family history of colon cancer or familial polyposis, ulcerative colitis, granulomatous colitis, and a diet low in fiber and high in animal protein, fat, and refined carbohydrates.

Signs and Symptoms

The cancer may be present for several years before symptoms appear. Complaints include fatigue, weakness, weight loss, alternating constipation and diarrhea, a change in the caliber of stool, tenesmus, urgency, and hematochezia. Physical examination is usually normal except in advanced disease when the tumor can be palpated or if hepatomegaly is present owing to metastatic disease.

Diagnostic Studies

Stool for occult blood is recommended, and a colonoscopy is diagnostic. Recommended laboratory studies include a CBC and carcinoembryonic antigen (CEA) test. A positron emission tomography (PET) scan may be valuable for tumor origin and metastasis.

URINARY CALCULI

Urinary calculi can occur anywhere in the urinary tract. Men are more frequently affected by urinary calculi, with a ratio of 4:1, until the sixth or seventh decade, when the risk equalizes. Many factors contribute to the formation of stones, including geographic, diet, genetic, and occupational factors. Stones occur more frequently in people living in hot, humid climates. Diets high in salt and protein and, in some cases, oxalate and purines can increase the risk of calculi. Despite previous beliefs, a diet high in calcium is a contributing factor only in some individuals. Some stones, particularly cystine stones, may be genetically linked, and persons in sedentary occupations are more likely to develop stones than are manual laborers. The most common types of stones are made of calcium (calcium oxalate and calcium phosphate); the other three types are struvite, uric acid, and cystine.

Signs and Symptoms

The location of pain varies based on a stone's location. It can originate in the flank or kidney area, radiating into the RLQ or LLQ, and then to the suprapubic area as the stone attempts to move down the tract. The pain is severe, acute, and colicky, and it may be accompanied by nausea and vomiting. If the stone becomes lodged at the ureterovesical junction, the patient will complain of urgency and frequency. Blood will be present in the urine.

Diagnostic Studies

The urinalysis typically shows hematuria. Infection must be ruled out because a combination of infection and obstruction requires prompt intervention to prevent pyelonephritis and kidney damage. A renal ultrasound or plain flat plate of the abdomen is often helpful in diagnosing stones. However, not all stones are visible on x-ray. If diagnosis remains uncertain, a noncontrast CT is indicated. Alternatively, an intravenous pyelogram should be ordered if a CT is not available. Pain medicine is imperative if patients are to undergo lengthy diagnostic testing.

OVARIAN CYST AND TUMOR

Although there are no hard-and-fast rules, ovarian cysts are more likely to occur in the younger patient, whereas ovarian cancer has a greater incidence in the postmenopausal patient. Women with a positive family history of ovarian cancer have a 5% lifetime risk versus a 1.6% risk in those with no family history. The long-term use of oral contraceptives may decrease the risk of ovarian cancer.

Signs and Symptoms

Ovarian masses are often asymptomatic, but symptoms may include pressure-type pain, heaviness, aching, and bloating. Cysts tend to be more painful than malignant tumors and often spontaneously resolve with the onset of the menstrual cycle. Masses are typically detected on pelvic examination. In advanced malignancies, ascites is often present.

Diagnostic Studies

An elevated cancer antigen 125 (CA-125) result indicates the likelihood that the mass is malignant. A transvaginal pelvic ultrasound has a higher diagnostic sensitivity than a transabdominal ultrasound for ovarian masses. If diagnosis is unclear, a CT, MRI, or PET scan can be performed. A laparoscopy or exploratory laparotomy is necessary for staging, tumor debulking, and resection. Certain types of ovarian cancers, such as germ cell or stromal tumors, may require additional laboratory tests, including alpha-fetoprotein, hCG, lactic dehydrogenase, serum estrogen and testosterone, and/or inhibin. Endometriosis is a common noncancerous cause of elevated CA-125.

INGUINAL AND FEMORAL HERNIA

In the majority of hernia cases, a history of heavy physical labor or heavy lifting can be elicited. Young children and individuals with a history of abdominal surgery are also at increased risk.

Signs and Symptoms

RLQ or LLQ pain that may radiate into the groin or testicle is typical. The pain is usually dull or aching unless strangulated, in which case the pain is more severe. The pain increases with straining, lifting, or movement of the lower extremities. Physical examination reveals a bulge at the femoral area or inguinal ring, often with tenderness. The bulge appears as the patient coughs or bears down and disappears when relaxing or lying down.

Diagnostic Studies

The physical examination is often all that is necessary for diagnosis, but ultrasound or pelvic CT may be helpful.

INTESTINAL OBSTRUCTION

The most common causes of mechanical obstruction are adhesions, almost exclusively in patients with previous abdominal surgery, hernias, tumors, volvulus, inflammatory bowel disease (e.g., Crohn's disease, colitis), Hirschsprung's disease, fecal impaction, and radiation enteritis. Additional information can be found under the sections on nausea and vomiting and diarrhea.

Signs and Symptoms

Initially, the patient complains of a cramping periumbilical pain that eventually becomes constant. Abdominal distention, vomiting that may lead to dehydration, diarrhea in partial obstruction, and obstipation occur when obstruction is complete. Physical examination reveals mild, diffuse tenderness without peritoneal signs, and possibly visible peristaltic waves. In early obstruction, tinkles, rushes, and borborygmi can be heard. In late obstruction, bowel sounds may be absent. There is minimal or no fever. Carefully inspect and palpate for hernias and masses.

Diagnostic Studies

A flat and upright abdominal film may reveal bowel distention and the presence of multiple air–fluid levels. A CT or MRI may be necessary for confirmation. CBC and electrolytes are recommended to look for leukocytosis and electrolyte imbalance; blood urea nitrogen (BUN), creatinine, and urinalysis are performed to detect extracellular volume loss.

DIVERTICULITIS

Diverticular disease is prevalent in patients older than 60 years. It is seen more commonly in Western countries and is thought to be due to raised intraluminal colonic pressures. Since the sigmoid colon has the smallest diameter of any portion of the colon, it is the most common site for the development of diverticula. Patients with connective tissue disease, such as scleroderma, Marfan's syndrome, and Ehlers-Danlos syndrome, are at increased risk. Chronic constipation can be an aggravating factor due to straining, which increases intraluminal pressures.

Signs and Symptoms

Although the pain can be generalized, it typically localizes with time to the left lower abdomen and is accompanied by tenderness, fever, and leukocytosis. These symptoms in a person with a known history of diverticulosis make the diagnosis almost certain for diverticulitis. Other symptoms can include constipation or loose stools, nausea, vomiting, and positive stool occult blood. With diverticulitis, there is an increased risk of perforation, which presents with a more dramatic clinical picture of peritonitis. Early signs of peritonitis, such as a positive heel strike test and/or rebound tenderness, may be present. Sepsis may ensue if peritonitis is due to perforation; therefore, prompt referral to a surgeon is necessary.

Diagnostic Studies

A CBC will show mildly elevated WBC. Plain abdominal films are limited in establishing diverticulitis in the absence of abscess or perforation. In comparison, a CT without contrast is more sensitive.

Acute medical management is indicated, and after 7 to 10 days, a flexible sigmoidoscopy and/or barium enema with water-soluble contrast is recommended. These should not be done in the acute stage because the risk of perforation increases during the procedure.

GASTROENTERITIS

See sections on nausea and vomiting and diarrhea, pp. 367, 373.

■ Pelvic or Suprapubic Pain

The following possible etiologies for pelvic pain/suprapubic pain are varied and are covered in detail in Chapters 12 to 14:

- Inguinal and femoral hernia
- Testicular torsion
- Prostatitis
- Prostate cancer
- Epididymitis
- Urinary tract infection
- PID/salpingitis
- Renal calculi
- Pyelonephritis

History

Ask about urinary symptoms, such as dysuria and frequency; heavy lifting; contact sports; sexual practices; the presence of vaginal or penile discharge; and a history of STIs, kidney stones, or prostate disease.

Physical Examination

The physical examination should include a thorough abdominal examination, a pelvic and genital examination, and a rectal examination, including prostate for male patients.

◼ Nausea and Vomiting

Nausea and vomiting usually stem from GI infections but may reflect many categories of problems, including other infections, actual or functional GI obstruction, metabolic disorders, central nervous system disorders, drugs, pain, pregnancy, and psychiatric disorders. A detailed list of potential causes is provided in Table 11.10. This section describes the basic approach to nausea and vomiting to differentiate among major potential causes. Table 11.10 summarizes common findings for each condition listed and will help narrow your diagnosis and limit your work-up appropriately. The approach to nausea and vomiting should be determined by the patient's age, overall health, and medical history.

Table 11.10		

Causes of Nausea and Vomiting

Cause	Examples	Typical Signs and Symptoms
Infection	Gastroenteritis (viral or bacterial), hepatitis, PID, viral syndrome, upper respiratory infection	Abrupt onset, spontaneous vomiting, often accompanied by fever, malaise, and diarrhea
Food poisoning	Bacterial sources: *Clostridium botulinum*, *Staphylococcus* Nonbacterial sources: mushrooms, poisonous plants, fish, chemicals	Symptoms occur hours to days after exposure, severe nausea and vomiting often with diarrhea, neurological symptoms, liver involvement
Gastrointestinal obstruction	Gastric outlet obstruction related to PID, GERD, malignancy, esophageal stricture, pyloric stenosis, or intestinal obstruction related to malignancy, intussusception, adhesions, and motility disorders	Emesis containing undigested food, upper or lower abdominal pain and tenderness, absent bowel sounds, x-ray or CT showing bowel loops, ileus, mass, or stricture
Metabolic disorders	Renal disease with uremia, hyperglycemia, ketoacidosis, Addison's disease, hyperthyroidism	Mild nausea rarely accompanied by vomiting; fatigue, weakness, muscle cramping, skin changes, hypotension or hypertension, neuropathic changes, abnormal renal or endocrine laboratory studies
Medication	Cardiac medicines, especially digitalis and quinidine; antihypertensives; antibiotics; bronchodilators, especially aminophylline; antineoplastic drugs; NSAIDs; monoamine oxidase inhibitors; antidepressants; antiretrovirals; oral hyperglycemics	Symptoms may be from central trigger zone stimulation or irritation to the gastric mucosa. Reactions to medicine generally cause a persistent nausea. If from gastric irritation, the nausea will worsen soon after medication administration. With trigger zone stimulation, nausea is often delayed. If related to cardiac medicines or bronchodilators, there may be changes in heart rate and electrocardiogram readings.

(cont. on page 368)

Table 11.10

Causes of Nausea and Vomiting—cont'd

Cause	Examples	Typical Signs and Symptoms
Central nervous system disorders	Meningitis, increased intracranial pressure, migraines, space-occupying lesion or fluid, Ménière's disease, cerebellar disorders	Central nervous system–related vomiting is often projectile and not preceded by nausea. Vomiting caused by a space-occupying lesion is often worse upon arising due to a recumbent increase in intracranial pressure. Depending on the cause, accompanying symptoms include headache, visual disturbances, nystagmus, ataxia, and, in meningitis, nuchal rigidity.
Cardiac disease	Myocardial infarction, congestive heart failure	Often nausea only, but vomiting may occur in myocardial infarction with severe pain. In congestive heart failure, the nausea is vague and persistent, accompanied by pain, diaphoresis, shortness of breath, and edema.
Pregnancy	Due to either hormonal or emotional changes	Typically nausea without emesis, often in the morning but may present with persistent or intermittent vomiting, missed or irregular menses, and positive human chorionic gonadotropin.
Psychogenic	Anorexia, bulimia, anxiety	Usually promptly follows eating, may remit on hospitalization, and is more common in young women.
Cholecystitis/pancreatitis	Due to infection, inflammation, or obstruction of the pancreas or gallbladder	Nausea and vomiting is intermittent and usually accompanied by RUQ or epigastric pain.

History

A thorough symptom analysis should identify any triggering events, such as meals, offensive odors, motion, position changes, and pain. Determine what, if anything, relieves the symptoms, including any attempted self-treatments. Determine what is meant by a complaint of "nausea": loss of appetite, queasiness, sense of imminent vomiting, or retching. When vomiting has occurred, determine the color, amount, presence of bile or undigested food, and frequency/ number of episodes. The severity of the nausea can be rated. The presence of associated symptoms (e.g., fever, diarrhea, diaphoresis, syncope, pain) is an important consideration. When determining the temporal sequence, establish the relationship to meals, activity, or travel; the time of day when symptoms are the worst; when the symptoms were first noticed; sudden or gradual onset; and whether the patient has been exposed to others who are ill. Whereas nausea is commonly intermittent in nature, medications can cause unrelenting symptoms.

Because many substances can cause nausea, the complete drug history is essential and should include prescribed, over-the-counter (OTC), and recreational drugs and alcohol. For women, date and duration of last menstrual period is essential. Table 11.10 lists specific causes of nausea and vomiting and the common descriptions. The current and past health history may identify comorbid disorders that might cause nausea (e.g., renal failure with metabolic disturbances, diabetes with gastroparesis) as well as treatment modalities that might contribute to the nausea or vomiting.

Physical Examination

The physical examination should start with a general survey and vital signs. Pulse and blood pressure, including postural changes, provide important information about hydration status, and a fever may suggest infection; weight helps to determine any changes associated with decreased intake and/or significant vomiting. Assess skin turgor and coloring (e.g., jaundice). A thorough abdominal examination should be performed, noting distention, signs of obstruction, surgical scars, bowel sounds, organomegaly, masses, and tenderness.

VIRAL INFECTION

Viral gastroenteritis is the most common cause of nausea, vomiting, and diarrhea. At least 50% of cases of gastroenteritis as food-borne illness are due to norovirus. Another 20% of cases, and the majority of severe cases in children, are due to rotavirus. Other significant viral agents include adenovirus and astrovirus.

Signs and Symptoms

Nausea and vomiting associated with acute infections (viral and bacterial) may be accompanied by fever and diarrhea and by other commonly associated symptoms, including malaise and fatigue. Nausea and vomiting from infections generally have a very abrupt onset; spontaneous vomiting may occur when the patient is unable to reach the toilet. The patient may be able to identify exposure to other persons with similar symptoms or other persons who ate the same meal and then developed nausea and vomiting. If hepatitis is involved, the predominant symptoms are usually nausea and/or anorexia, although vomiting may occur. Fever might be present. With dehydration, the patient may complain of light-headedness or dizziness; the pulse may be elevated and the blood pressure positive for postural changes. Mucous membranes may be dry, and skin turgor is diminished. Bowel sounds are often exaggerated even without diarrhea; borborygmi may be present. The abdomen may be tender and/or distended.

Diagnostic Studies

Typically, common viral causes of nausea and vomiting require no diagnostic studies because they resolve within 72 hours. If the vomiting is severe, baseline laboratory tests such as CBC, urinalysis, and electrolytes are indicated to assess for infection, electrolyte balance, and hydration status. If the nausea is accompanied by severe or prolonged diarrhea, suspect a bacterial cause and obtain a

CBC, stool cultures for ova and parasites (O&P), culture and sensitivity (C&S), and *Clostridium difficile*.

BACTERIAL INFECTION

Food poisoning can have either an infectious or a noninfectious cause. Noninfectious causes occur when one eats food contaminated with chemicals or food that contains naturally occurring toxins, such as mushrooms or fish. The range of infectious causes is broad and includes *Staphylococcus, Clostridium botulinum, Clostridium perfringens, Escherichia coli, Salmonella, Shigella,* and *Yersinia enterocolitica*. These infections can be contracted through food but generally are due to poor handwashing since it is a fecal–oral transmission. Some sources of the infection are improperly prepared food, reheated meat dishes, seafood, dairy, and bakery products. Other risk factors include travel or residence in areas of poor sanitation. Onset of symptoms is hours to days, depending on the organism, and symptoms include fever, headache, malaise, and diarrhea.

Signs and Symptoms

The presentation of food poisoning varies, depending on the offending agent. Symptoms include headache and fever, abdominal pain, and diarrhea. Although the disturbance is usually self-limited, severe fluid and electrolyte disturbances may occur. In contrast, a botulism-related attack usually begins with severe nausea, vomiting, and/or diarrhea, but these symptoms are often followed by neurological symptoms. Staphylococcal food poisoning may result in fever, whereas vital signs usually remain normal with botulism. *E. coli* infections can be severe and occasionally fatal. When noninfectious poisons are involved, the symptoms may progress to profound neurological findings, liver damage, and even death, depending on the offensive toxin.

Diagnostic Studies

When food poisoning is suspected, serum or stool culture for the offending organism should be performed. The food may be tested, as might the vomitus.

GASTROINTESTINAL OBSTRUCTION (REAL AND FUNCTIONAL)

GI obstructions cause vomiting when contents cannot pass distally. Gastric outlet obstruction may be related to PUD. Intestinal obstruction often occurs from adhesions from prior surgical procedures; other causes include malignancy and intussusception. Functional obstruction can develop from motility disorders, such as gastroparesis, when smooth muscle contraction is diminished.

Signs and Symptoms

The contents of the vomitus commonly vary according to the level of obstruction. Gastric outlet obstruction is associated with emesis containing undigested food. Proximal small intestinal blockage is likely to be bile-stained. Distal intestinal blockage is more likely to contain fecal matter. Proximal blockage may result in a large volume of emesis, as the stomach produces up to 1.5 L of secretions per 24 hours. When real obstruction is involved, pain often builds in a crescendo fashion and is then intermittently relieved or lessened following emesis. The degree of cramping and pain is often related to the proximity of the obstruction, so that obstructions of the lower intestines may have less severe cramping, vomiting, and/or pain. Bowel sounds often are high pitched and metallic sounding but may later become absent. Tenderness may be localized or diffuse. Distention as well as a succussion splash may be present.

Diagnostic Studies

Flat and upright plain films of the abdomen typically depict dilated loops of bowels, free air, gas, or ileus. A CT scan or MRI would determine the presence of an ileus or mass. Endoscopy can identify strictures associated with PUD and esophageal disorders. A barium swallow can monitor motility.

PREGNANCY

Hormonal changes associated with pregnancy are believed to contribute to nausea and vomiting, particularly in the first trimester.

Signs and Symptoms

Although pregnant patients may well present with persistent or intermittent vomiting episodes, pregnancy more commonly causes nausea without emesis. The nausea can occur at any time of the day but occurs most often in the morning and without regard to meals. Although this may be the presenting symptom of pregnancy, the patient will have recently missed or had an irregular period. Pregnancy-related nausea and vomiting are also discussed in Chapter 20.

Diagnostic Studies

Perform urine or serum hCG.

METABOLIC DISORDERS

A variety of metabolic disorders can present with nausea and/or vomiting. Common examples include renal disease associated with uremia and many endocrine problems, such as hyperglycemia, ketoacidosis, Addison's disease, and hyperthyroidism.

Signs and Symptoms

Nausea is more common than vomiting with metabolic disorders. With uremia of renal failure, other common symptoms are muscle cramping, neuropathic changes, hypertension, and skin changes. With diabetes, the patient may present with the classic symptoms of hyperglycemia. With adrenal insufficiency, or Addison's disease, common early symptoms include fatigue, weakness, hypotension, and skin changes. With hyperthyroidism, symptoms include hypertension, tachycardia, weight loss, tremor.

Diagnostic Studies

The diagnosis depends on the suspected metabolic disorder. Consider BUN/creatinine, which will be elevated in renal disease. Order blood glucose, serum bicarbonate, and urine ketones if diabetes is suspected with or without ketoacidosis. Sodium, potassium, cortisol, and adrenocorticotropic hormone (ACTH) can assist in a diagnosis of Addison's disease. Order TSH/T4 hyperthyroidism is suspected.

CENTRAL NERVOUS SYSTEM DISORDERS

The range of neurological disorders that result in nausea and/or vomiting is broad. Included are meningitis, increased intracranial pressure, migraines, space-occupying lesions, and Ménière's disease.

Signs and Symptoms

Central nervous system–related vomiting is often projectile and may not be preceded by nausea. Associated complaints and findings depend on the causative lesion. Papilledema may accompany increased intracranial pressure. Neurological deficits may be evident with increased intracranial pressure, space-occupying lesions, and meningitis. Nuchal rigidity is a classic finding for meningitis. With Ménière's or other forms of labyrinthitis, nystagmus and/or ataxia may be present. Migraines may be preceded with the classic visual disturbance or other auras and are typically unilateral (see Chapter 17).

Diagnostic Studies

A CT scan of the head is warranted in most cases, and if meningitis is suspected, a lumbar puncture may be necessary.

MEDICATIONS

Drugs are very common causes of nausea and vomiting. The nausea associated with medications may stem from either central trigger zone stimulation or irritation to the gastric mucosa. Drugs commonly associated with nausea and vomiting are listed in Table 11.10.

Signs and Symptoms

Drugs, like other toxins, generally cause a persistent nausea. There may be associated findings related to the toxic level. For instance, with excessive levels of digitalis, vision may be altered and bradycardia evident. With excessive aminophylline, tachycardia and tremors may be manifested.

Diagnostic Studies

The primary diagnostic study would be a level of the suspected agent.

PSYCHOGENIC CAUSES

Emotional disturbances may result in either chronic or recurrent episodes of vomiting. Examples include bulimia and extreme anxiety responses.

Signs and Symptoms

Usually, psychogenic vomiting promptly follows eating and may occur during the meal; it is more common in young women. This vomiting is not urgent and can usually be suppressed; it may remit on hospitalization. The patient may show little concern regarding the vomiting. The patient may be very thin, but often in the case of bulimia, the patient is of normal weight. In other patients, vomiting occurs when there is acute anxiety associated with stressful situations or events, such as public speaking, interviews, and tests.

Diagnostic Studies

When no organic cause is found to explain recurrent or chronic vomiting, a psychiatric history should be performed.

CARDIAC CAUSES

Depending on the patient's health history and/or risk factors, you may include cardiac-related disorders in your differential diagnosis for nausea and vomiting. These can be associated with both myocardial infarction and congestive heart failure (see Chapter 8). Another potential cardiac-related source, mentioned previously, includes cardiac medications.

GASTROESOPHAGEAL REFLUX DISEASE

See pp. 356–357.

PEPTIC ULCER DISEASE, GASTRITIS

See pp. 357–358.

CHOLECYSTITIS

See pp. 349–350.

■ Diarrhea

The causes of diarrhea are numerous and include bacterial, viral, organic, and functional. The mechanisms are due to (1) abnormal transport mechanisms; (2) a change in the osmotic mechanism, resulting in variations in absorption; (3) increased motility; and (4) exudative blood or pus, which decreases absorption.

Most cases are self-limiting and resolve within days without medical intervention. When high fever, intractable vomiting, or severe dehydration is present, prompt attention is necessary, and hospitalization frequently is required—especially in children or geriatric patients.

History

Symptoms vary according to the cause of the diarrhea. A thorough symptom analysis should identify the time of onset, whether onset was sudden or gradual, and the duration of the symptoms. Determine severity according to whether the diarrhea is intermittent or persistent and according to the number of stools per day. Inquire as to associated symptoms, such as abdominal pain, fever, nausea, or vomiting, as well as whether there is any relation to meals. Ask the patient to describe the color of the stool, looking for reports of dark or bloody stools; the consistency (i.e., formed, watery, fatty, or greasy); and the presence of mucus or odor. It is important to ask about recent meals or travel and if accompanying others may have similar symptoms; recent antibiotics or other new medications, either prescription or OTC; and history of alcohol abuse or PUD that could indicate a GI bleed. Dehydration and electrolyte depletion are concerns, and the volume of fluid intake should be determined. If diarrhea has been chronic, changes in weight or appetite should be recorded. Stress or anxiety may be a causative factor; therefore, psychosocial issues should be investigated.

Physical Examination

The physical examination should begin with vital signs, particularly determining the presence of fever, which might indicate infection, and tachycardia or orthostatic hypotension, which might indicate dehydration. Other signs of dehydration include dry mucous membranes, light-headedness, syncope, lethargy, and oliguria. If there is accompanying electrolyte imbalance, cardiac arrhythmias, muscle weakness, tetany, or vascular collapse may occur, particularly in young children, older patients, or patients who are already debilitated. Listen for hypoactive or hyperactive bowel sounds, which could indicate early obstruction; palpate for abdominal tenderness, indicating infection or inflammation; and perform a digital rectal examination, checking for heme-positive stool. A CBC showing anemia might indicate malignancy; leukocytosis might indicate inflammatory bowel disease. Significant unexplained weight loss should be investigated. Sigmoidoscopy or colonoscopy is warranted if symptoms persist.

INFECTIONS (VIRAL AND BACTERIAL)

For a general discussion on causes and risk factors, see the earlier section on nausea and vomiting, pp. 367–370.

Signs and Symptoms

Diarrhea associated with acute infections (viral and bacterial) may be accompanied by fever, nausea, and vomiting; other commonly associated symptoms include malaise, fatigue, weakness, and light-headedness. Diarrhea from infections generally has a very abrupt onset; spontaneous diarrhea may occur, and the patient is unable to reach the toilet. The patient may be able to identify exposure to other persons who had similar symptoms or who ate the same meal or traveled to the same area and then developed the diarrhea. If the diarrhea is severe, dehydration may ensue, causing tachycardia and postural hypotension. Mucous membranes may be dry and skin turgor diminished. Bowel sounds are often exaggerated even without diarrhea; borborygmi may be present. The abdomen may be tender and/or distended.

Several viruses have been identified as causing diarrhea: norovirus, rotavirus, adenovirus, and enterovirus, with the latter two sometimes associated with respiratory symptoms. Common bacterial causes of diarrhea either from toxins or from mucosal invasion and ulceration include *Vibrio cholerae*, *Salmonella*, *Shigella*, *E. coli*, *Clostridium*, *Yersinia*, and *Campylobacter*. A botulism-related attack usually begins with severe nausea, vomiting, and/or diarrhea, but these symptoms are often followed by neurological symptoms, such as diplopia, loss of accommodation, diminished pupillary reflex, and dysphagia. *E. coli* infection is characterized by acute onset, severe abdominal cramps and watery/bloody diarrhea. Fever may be present. *E. coli* infection can be complicated by hemolytic-uremic syndrome, which is characterized by hemolytic anemia, thrombocytopenia, and acute renal failure. The prognosis in these cases is grave. *E. coli* infection can result in death with or without these complications, especially in children and older patients. When noninfectious poisons are involved, the symptoms may progress to profound neurological findings, liver damage, and even death, depending on the toxin.

Diagnostic Studies

Typically, common viral causes of nausea, vomiting, and diarrhea require no diagnostic studies and will resolve within 72 hours. If the diarrhea is severe or prolonged, baseline laboratory tests such as CBC, urinalysis, and electrolytes are indicated to assess for infection, electrolyte balance, and hydration status. If a bacterial cause is suspected, obtain stool cultures for O&P, C&S, and, specifically, the offending organisms.

PARASITIC INFECTION

Parasitic infections are common in rural or developing areas of Africa, Asia, and Latin America and less common in industrialized areas. In industrialized areas, parasitic infections also may affect immigrants and people who are immunocompromised. The infections may occur in institutions with poor sanitation and unhygienic practices (e.g., day-care centers, nursing homes). Parasites causing diarrhea usually enter the body through the mouth. They are swallowed and can remain in the intestine or burrow through the intestinal wall and invade other organs.

Signs and Symptoms

Certain parasites, most commonly *Giardia lamblia*, transmitted by fecally contaminated water or food, can cause diarrhea, bloating, flatulence, cramps, nausea, anorexia, weight loss, greasy stools because of its interference with fat absorption, and occasionally fever. Symptoms usually occur about 2 weeks after exposure and can last 2 to 3 months. Often the symptoms are vague and intermittent, which makes diagnosis more difficult. There is no chemoprophylaxis, but boiling water deactivates the *Giardia* cysts. Anti-infectives are available for treatment. Other parasites that cause diarrhea include tapeworm and roundworm, but they are uncommon in humans.

Diagnostic Studies

Serial stool samples for O&P should be ordered because a single sample may not reveal the offending parasite. Stool microscopy remains the standard for testing and successfully identifies *Giardia* in 90% of infected patients. Stool antigen enzyme-linked immunosorbent assays (ELISA) also are available and can be used in addition to stool microscopy. ELISA has a sensitivity of 88% to 98% and a specificity of 87% to 100%. Duodenal contents can be sampled by the Entero-Test, which collects the sample by having the patient swallow a nylon string with a weight on the end and then removing the string after a certain amount of time. This is more reliable than stool cultures, but the procedure is not desirable to the patient.

AMEBIC DYSENTERY

This particular type of dysentery is common in tropical climates but rare in temperate climates.

Signs and Symptoms

It is characterized by semifluid stools containing mucus, blood, and active trophozoites. This form of dysentery may become chronic, and the symptoms are recurrent abdominal cramping and soft stools. In the chronic state, weight loss is significant, and anemia is present.

Diagnostic Studies

The diagnosis is made by stool cultures, and three to six specimens may be needed before an accurate diagnosis can be made.

MEDICATION REACTION/SENSITIVITY

Drugs are a very common cause of diarrhea. The diarrhea associated with medications may stem from either a generalized allergic reaction or irritation of the intestinal mucosa. Many drugs can cause diarrhea, but among the drugs commonly associated are quinidine, digitalis, antibiotics, metformin, and many selective serotonin reuptake inhibitors. A late sequela of antibiotic treatment—particularly with clindamycin, ampicillin, cephalosporins, erythromycin, tetracycline, and sulfamethoxazole/trimethoprim—is pseudomembranous colitis resulting from C. difficile. An antibiotic-induced change in the intestinal flora is the predisposing factor. C. difficile has been implicated in much of the nosocomial cases of diarrhea in hospitals and nursing homes. In some instances, necrotizing colitis may ensue.

Signs and Symptoms

Drugs, like other toxins, generally cause persistent diarrhea. Drugs that affect the lower GI tract often affect the upper GI tract as well, and it is common to find associated nausea or vomiting.

Diagnostic Studies

A history of a new medication gives a high likelihood of that being the causative agent. A stool culture specifically for C. difficile is necessary. Stopping the drug or replacing it with another category of drug should resolve the diarrhea.

MUCOSAL DISEASES

Several diseases can cause mucosal inflammation and ulceration, resulting in intermittent and often severe diarrhea. These diseases include ulcerative colitis, Crohn's disease, regional enteritis, GI tuberculosis, and carcinomas.

Signs and Symptoms

The symptoms and severity of the diarrhea vary according to the underlying cause. The symptoms of carcinomas are generally insidious. The diarrhea is mild and intermittent. Often malignancies are found on routine hemoccult test, sigmoidoscopy, or colonoscopy. There should be a high index of suspicion with unexplained weight loss or new-onset iron-deficiency anemia in a patient older than 40 years. With colitis, enteritis, Crohn's disease, and tuberculosis, the onset of the diarrhea may be sudden and severe with fever and significant abdominal tenderness, or it may be slow in onset with mild cramps and the urge to defecate. The stool is frequently bloody with pus and/or mucus. Malaise, fever, and weight loss are common. Initially, a history and stool examination are helpful in making a diagnosis. The stool is heavy with red blood cells and WBCs, and usually overt blood and pus are present. Because bouts are recurrent, a positive history of these diseases supports an exacerbation. There is a risk of bowel perforation and resultant peritonitis, and in these cases, mortality may be as high as 40%.

Diagnostic Studies

A CBC and erythrocyte sedimentation rate (ESR) should be performed. Colitis is often accompanied by leukocytosis, anemia, and an elevated sedimentation rate. In malignancies, anemia is often the first sign found on routine laboratory studies. A variety of diagnostic tests may be helpful in making a definitive diagnosis, including abdominal CT, barium enema, sigmoidoscopy, or colonoscopy.

IRRITABLE BOWEL SYNDROME

Irritable bowel syndrome (IBS) is a functional motility disorder involving the upper and lower GI tracts. The exact cause is unknown. It is three times more prevalent in women and accounts for more than half of all GI referrals. Diarrhea or constipation may predominate, or they may be mixed (classified as IBS-D, IBS-C, or IBS-M, respectively). IBS may begin after an infection (postinfectious, IBS-PI) or a stressful life event. It is highly correlated with emotional factors, particularly anxiety and stress, which can result in a heightened sensitivity to food, and parasympathomimetic drugs, causing abnormalities in transit—increased in the diarrhea-predominant group and decreased in the constipation-predominant group.

There is no cure for IBS, and treatments focus on symptom management through dietary adjustments, medication, and psychological interventions. Other GI disorders may present with symptoms similar to IBS, including celiac disease, parasitic infections, several inflammatory bowel diseases, functional chronic constipation, and chronic functional abdominal pain. The exact cause of IBS is unknown, but it is hypothesized that it is a disorder of the interaction between the brain and the gut.

Signs and Symptoms

IBS is characterized by mild to severe abdominal pain, discomfort, bloating, and alteration of bowel habits. It causes intermittent nausea, distention, flatulence, diarrhea, and/or constipation. Symptoms usually occur in the waking hours and may be worsened or triggered by meals. In some cases, the symptoms are relieved by bowel movements.

Diagnostic Studies

Diagnostic studies include digital rectal examination and 3-day hemoccult tests for occult blood; stool for O&P and C&S; CBC to check for anemia, which might indicate a malignant cause of the symptoms; and ESR, chemistry panel, amylase, and urinalysis to rule out inflammatory, hepatic, pancreatic, or renal causes. IBS is primarily a diagnosis of exclusion, and blood tests have been developed—immunoglobulin A antibody (IgA) and tissue transglutaminase IgA antibody (tTG-IgA)—to assist in differentiating celiac disease from IBS. Sigmoidoscopy or colonoscopy is recommended to rule out malignancy or more serious inflammatory causes.

CARBOHYDRATE INTOLERANCE

More commonly known as lactose intolerance, this condition actually represents a symptom complex resulting from a lack of intestinal enzymes (usually lactase) necessary to break down disaccharides. Unsplit disaccharides in the intestine retain water and result in diarrhea.

Signs and Symptoms

Symptoms include nausea, diarrhea, abdominal cramps, borborygmi, bloating, and flatulence, which generally occur within 1 to 2 hours after eating the offending food, usually dairy products. Diarrhea may be severe, but the duration is relatively short.

Diagnostic Studies

Acid stools with a pH less than 6 are suspicious. The hydrogen breath test, if available, is easy and reliable. A lactose or glucose challenge is diagnostic when diarrhea occurs in about 30 minutes. Jejunal biopsies are generally not performed because they are invasive and expensive.

INTOLERANCE TO SUGAR ALCOHOLS

Natural sugars have been replaced with sugar alcohols in numerous foods, drinks, energy bars, candies, and gum. The most common sugar alcohols are xylitol, erythritol, sorbitol, mannitol, lactitol, and maltitol. Sugar alcohols are identified as FODMAP carbohydrates—fermentable oligosaccharides, disaccharides, monosaccharides and polyols. They are touted as adjuncts to weight loss and reduced blood sugar, but artificial sweeteners do not eliminate sugar cravings, have little or no effect on blood sugar levels, and can cause unwanted gastrointestinal symptoms, especially when consumed in large quantities. Other sugar substitutes such as saccharin, sucralose, and stevia may not have the same sensitivity side effects as the sugar alcohols but may have other negative side effects such as glucose intolerance and increase in risk for obesity and diabetes.

Signs and Symptoms

Sugar alcohols can cause gas, bloating, diarrhea, constipation, and other digestive symptoms in people who are sensitive to them.

Diagnostic Studies

There are no diagnostic tests for sensitivity to sugar alcohols. Patients should be aware of the many zero-calorie products on the market and read labels carefully. Trial and error will usually make the diagnosis of sugar alcohol sensitivity.

LAXATIVE USE AND ABUSE

Laxative abuse is often seen in older patients, as caused by chronic or overtreatment of constipation. It is also seen in eating disorders, particularly bulimia, as a water and weight loss aid.

Signs and Symptoms

Misuse of laxatives may cause muscle weakness, lethargy, weight loss, electrolyte depletion, cardiac arrhythmias, changes in the intestinal mucosa, and bleeding.

Diagnostic Studies

The diagnosis of laxative abuse is made by history. Those treating constipation should be educated regarding dietary changes, adequate fluid intake, and the proper use of bulking agents so as to avoid the need for laxative use. Overdependence on laxatives for regular bowel movements only compounds the constipation problem. Rarely does this type of laxative use cause serious electrolyte imbalance. In patients with an eating disorder, however, the abuse is significant and can lead to serious complications. CBC and electrolytes will identify anemia or electrolyte depletion. Psychological counseling is necessary for patients with an eating disorder.

GASTROINTESTINAL SURGERY

Any surgery that affects intestinal transit, such as large bowel resection, gastric resection, gastric or intestinal bypass, pyloroplasty, or vagotomy, may cause diarrhea. A history of any of these procedures suggests the surgery as the causative factor. Because malabsorption, malnutrition, vitamin deficiency, and anemia may result, patients need education on vitamin and mineral supplementation.

■ Constipation

Constipation is a common complaint generally used to describe excessively dry, small, or infrequent stools. According to a more specific definition, constipation is the presence of more than one of the following conditions for at least 3 months:

• Straining with bowel movements more than 25% of the time
• Hard stools more than 25% of the time
• Incomplete evacuations more than 25% of the time
• Fewer than three bowel movements per week

The term *constipation* covers more than infrequent stools and must be addressed from the patient's viewpoint. Constipation is often a chronic condition. Patients often self-treat both real and perceived constipation; its presence may be identified when the history reveals frequent or chronic use of laxatives or cathartics. Lifestyle factors (e.g., nutritional and fluid intake, activity) often contribute to chronic constipation. The altered colonic transit time may also be associated with medications, endocrine disorders, neurological deficits, and various GI disorders; constipation may be one sign of an eating or psychiatric disorder. Acute-onset constipation may stem from bowel obstruction or ileus.

History

Establish what the term *constipation* means to the patient. Ask how long it has existed and whether it is constant or intermittent. Determine how, if at all, the patient's previous bowel patterns differed. Explore the current bowel history: frequency of bowel movements; changes in caliber, color, quantity, or consistency (are the movements hard?); the need to strain; and whether there is complete evacuation. Ask about associated symptoms: abdominal bloating/fullness, rectal pain or bleeding, blood or mucus in the stool, altered appetite, and abdominal pain. Establish whether the constipation alternates with normal bowel pattern or diarrhea or is progressive. Find out whether the patient has experienced any weight loss because the potential for a malignancy must be considered. Establish the presence of any associated complications: hemorrhoids, fissures, or fecal incontinence. Obtain a history of endocrine, neurological, or GI problems; abdominal surgeries; and currently prescribed or OTC medications. Obtain a history of dietary and fluid intake, activity, and recreational drug use.

Physical Examination

The physical examination should start with a general survey: Note the patient's overall appearance and whether the patient appears healthy or ill, has any obvious deficits, or exhibits physical signs of systemic disorders. Obtain a weight. Observe the skin and mucous membranes for signs of dehydration. Depending on the history and your general survey, you should examine other systems. Otherwise, the examination can focus on the abdomen and rectum.

Inspect and auscultate the abdomen first, noting any scars, distention, visible masses, and discoloration. If bowel sounds are not immediately evident, continue listening for at least 15 seconds in each quadrant before you conclude that they are absent; if sounds are present, determine the pitch and frequency. Identify areas of dullness over organs and estimate organ size. Note any areas of dullness over the bowel. Palpate superficially at first, noting any guarding, rigidity, or tenderness. Palpate more deeply to assess organs and any other areas of firmness or mass. For any palpable mass, determine the consistency, size, shape, mobility, and margins. Perform an anorectal examination, inspecting the anus for tone, fissures, external hemorrhoids, or other defects. Palpate the rectum for masses and stool, noting the consistency of anything palpated; perform guaiac on any palpated stool.

COLONIC MOTILITY DISORDERS

Disorders of the smooth muscle of the colon can cause hypotonia and decreased motility; examples include congenital and acquired myopathies and enteric nerve disorders, such as Hirschsprung's disease. The result can be slowed transit time with greater intervals between evacuations, the development of bowel dilation, or pseudo-obstruction.

Signs and Symptoms

The history may identify a familial tendency to constipation. The patient may have previously attempted increasing dietary fiber and fluids and maintaining a reasonable activity level, without improvement.

Diagnostic Studies

A barium enema can identify areas of colon dilation. Measurements of whole-gut transit time are available; serial radiographs identify the position of ingested radiopaque marker(s) over time. A variety of specialized tests, performed by a gastroenterologist, provide information regarding bowel motility and tone.

INTESTINAL OBSTRUCTION

Obstructions of the colon cause a progressive constipation, which may be associated with pain, nausea, or other symptoms. In older patients, constipation may be the presenting symptom of obstruction. Malignancy must be considered.

Signs and Symptoms

There may be a history of the stool having become smaller in diameter, known as "pencil" stool, as well as a history of decreasing frequency of bowel movements and/or blood in the stool. Obstipation—extreme obstruction—leads to the failure to pass even gas. If a volvulus is the cause, the symptoms may or may not include pain and discomfort. Abdominal distention is marked in colonic obstruction. As the problem progresses, the patient may develop signs of shock. A palpable mass may be evident in volvulus or malignancy. The degree of tenderness is variable. There may be high-pitched bowel sounds or borborygmi until a late stage, at which time bowel sounds are absent.

Diagnostic Studies

Plain films of the abdomen should be ordered, looking for dilated loops of bowel, air–fluid levels, and the absence of colonic gas. The nature of an obstruction can be identified with a barium enema, CT scan, or colonoscopy/flexible sigmoidoscopy. If the obstruction is due to strangulation, the CBC may show a leukocyte shift to the left. Never order a barium upper GI series until colonic obstruction has been ruled out.

RECTOCELE AND PROLAPSE

Structural disorders of the anorectum and/or pelvic floor can cause constipation. A rectocele occurs when the rectovaginal septum bulges anteriorly. Weakness of the pelvic floor results in a widened anorectal angle and thereby a weakened perineal body. The pelvic floor may be weakened during childbirth, trauma, or repeated straining during bowel movements (thus, the cause and effect are blurred). Once weakened, the pelvic floor resistance is lessened and the stool is not directed/extruded through the anal canal. Both problems are more common among female patients.

Signs and Symptoms

Patients may complain of general constipation but may also note that the problem is more related to the act of defecation, which is difficult. Women who have developed a rectocele may perceive that there is weakness in the perineal area and that a mass is evident at the introitus when they strain; some learn to support the introitus to facilitate defecation. The physical signs of rectocele are determined during the vaginal examination; refer to Chapter 14.

Diagnostic Studies

A barium enema provides evidence of rectocele with lateral view but is usually not warranted, as the physical examination identifies the change. When bleeding from a fistula or hemorrhoid occurs, a proctoscopic examination should be performed to ensure there is not also a malignancy or other mass.

MEDICATIONS

Many medications can cause or contribute to constipation. The medications most commonly associated with constipation are listed in the Medications Causing Constipation box.

Signs and Symptoms

Constipation related to medications can be acute or chronic, either following the initial introduction of a new drug or after some time period has elapsed. The appearance of the abdomen and the presence of bowel sounds are usually not altered. Depending on the severity of the constipation, the abdominal examination may be within normal limits; however, feces may be palpable, and there may be some tenderness with deep palpation. The anorectal examination will typically be normal, although you may palpate hard, dry feces.

◆ MEDICATIONS CAUSING CONSTIPATION

- Analgesics/ narcotics
- Antacids containing aluminum
- Anticonvulsants
- Antidepressants
- Antihypertensives (calcium channel blockers, beta blockers)
- Antiparkinsonian agents
- Antispasmodics/ anticholinergics
- Calcium supplements
- Diuretics
- Iron supplements
- Sedatives/ tranquilizers

Diagnostic Studies

There are usually no studies necessary. A common diagnostic effort is to discontinue the suspected offending drug; however, it is not always possible to discontinue a medication in order to confirm the relationship (thus, other treatments/recommendations must be made to minimize the constipating effects of necessary drugs). If obstruction is suspected, refer to the earlier section on intestinal obstruction.

PSYCHIATRIC DISORDERS AND EATING DISORDERS

Constipation has been associated with depression. Patients with eating disorders commonly develop constipation unless they are also using laxatives. Patients with various psychiatric disorders may deny having bowel movements and fictitiously report constipation.

Signs and Symptoms

The history is very important in order to determine the actual pattern of bowel movements. Patients may give a history of frequency and characteristics of bowel habits that are well within normal range, but they may indicate dissatisfaction or concern over some specific characteristic, such as the color or caliber, in spite of no report of a recent change. When a psychogenic cause is suspected, a psychiatric history is warranted. Look for indications of depression or obsessive-compulsive disorder. Perform a thorough overall history and physical examination to ensure that an organic cause is not missed. Ask specifically about antidepressant medications that might be contributing to the constipation. Recognize also that patients who initially develop real or perceived constipation associated with psychogenic causes often begin to use laxatives and cathartics progressively and develop a dependence on these agents.

Diagnostic Studies

A patient might underestimate the frequency of bowel movements. Consider having the patient monitor bowel movements over several days, using a diary card. The patient should document each bowel movement and the volume and form of the stool. Although no specific diagnostic studies are necessary, you should, on the basis of presentation and history, order those necessary to exclude major organic causes. Possible studies include thyroid studies, electrolytes, CBC, abdominal imaging, sigmoidoscopy, and colonoscopy.

ENDOCRINE DISORDERS

Both hypothyroidism and diabetes can contribute to or cause constipation by decreasing motility. In hypothyroidism, myxedematous tissue may infiltrate the gut, resulting in megacolon. Diabetes should be considered as contributory to constipation when patients have other signs of autonomic neuropathy. The hypercalcemia associated with hyperparathyroidism may cause constipation. A thyroid profile and/or Hgb A1c are diagnostic for thyroid disease and diabetes mellitus, respectively.

NEUROLOGICAL DISORDERS

Many neurological disorders, including Parkinson's disease, multiple sclerosis, and spinal cord injuries, can alter bowel patterns. It is unknown whether the neurological changes caused in the brain of a patient with Parkinson's disease also affect the enteric nerves or if constipation is the result of decreased pelvic floor muscle tone. Multiple sclerosis is believed to contribute to slow transit time and altered pelvic floor muscle tone. The degree to which a spinal cord lesion affects bowel function depends on the level of injury; injuries may alter distal transit time as well as sphincter responsiveness. See Chapter 15.

IRRITABLE BOWEL SYNDROME

See previous discussion, pp. 377–378.

■ Jaundice

Jaundice, a yellow discoloration of skin and mucous membranes, stems from an elevation of either unconjugated or conjugated bilirubin. Causes of unconjugated hyperbilirubinemia include both bilirubin overproduction, as occurs in several hemolytic disorders, and impaired bilirubin uptake, associated with inherited disorders. Conjugated hyperbilirubinemia is more common and stems from either impaired hepatic excretion or extrahepatic obstruction. Hepatitis is the most common cause of jaundice (75%) among persons younger than 30 years. Obstruction is the most common etiology of jaundice (60%) after age 60 years, and the causes include gallstones, tumors, or strictures from past surgeries. Other relatively common causes in older adults include congestive heart failure (10%) and metastatic malignancy (13%). Jaundice may be the presenting sign of serious disease in all age groups. With appropriate history, physical examination, and early diagnostic studies, the cause of jaundice usually can be correctly identified as either obstructive or nonobstructive.

History

The patient's age is an important consideration in differentiating among potential causes of jaundice. Find out when the discoloration was first noticed and whether other symptoms have developed or been associated with this finding. Important associated symptoms include pruritus, malaise, fever/chills, nausea, anorexia, change in the color of urine or feces, and abdominal pain. The medical history must address previous hepatic or biliary diseases, malignancy, hemolytic disorders, and surgeries as well as other potential contributing disorders, including congestive heart failure. Obtain a family history of hemolytic, biliary, and hepatic disorders. Obtain a thorough medication history, including OTC and herbal agents; determine the use of alcohol and recreational drugs, particularly intravenous drug use, and social risk factors for hepatitis, including sexual practices.

Physical Examination

The physical examination should include a general survey of the skin and mucous membranes, observing for discoloration, dryness, spider angiomas, petechiae, and xanthomas, as well as excoriations indicative of pruritus (see Chapter 4). The general survey should also consider the patient's mental status as an indicator of liver disease. The lungs and heart should be assessed briefly to identify overall health and indications of heart failure (see Chapter 8). Unless otherwise indicated by the history, the remainder of the physical examination should focus on the abdomen. Carefully observe for scars from previous surgical procedures. Percuss to determine organ size and any unexpected areas of dullness indicative of a possible mass. As you percuss, note any areas of tenderness, particularly over the liver. Palpate to further assess abdominal organs. As you palpate for the liver, be attentive for a positive Murphy's sign. If the liver is palpable, note the consistency and margins in addition to the size.

HEPATITIS

Jaundice causing injury to the liver can have many potential sources; viruses and hepatotoxins are the most common causes. Viral diseases that can cause hepatitis include the identified hepatitis viruses (A, B, C, D, E, F [not confirmed], and G), Epstein-Barr, and cytomegalovirus. Hepatotoxins include numerous prescribed and OTC medications, such as acetaminophen, methyldopa, isoniazid, and phenytoin; immune modulators; herbal remedies; alcohol; and, more rarely, chemical exposures. Explore potential sources of viral illness, including exposures to blood and body secretions and toxins through occupational, sexual, and/ or recreational activities. Obtain a complete list of all drugs and herbal agents ingested as well as the use of alcohol.

Signs and Symptoms

Viral causes of hepatitis with jaundice often have accompanying symptoms of the virus, including malaise and myalgia, as well as RUQ discomfort and anorexia. There may be a history of previous episodes of viral hepatitis or other hepatic injury. Nonhepatic signs of viral illness, including fever, splenomegaly, and lymphadenopathy, may be present. Hepatomegaly with tenderness may be present.

Diagnostic Studies

Obtain a CBC; liver functions, including ALT and AST; amylase; lipase; hepatitis screen; total and direct bilirubin levels; and prothrombin times. Consider abdominal/liver ultrasound or CT to evaluate organomegaly or mass. Referral for liver biopsy may be warranted.

HEPATIC AND PANCREATIC CANCERS

Primary or metastatic cancers of the liver and/or pancreas can cause obstructive hyperbilirubinemia and jaundice. Jaundice may be the initial sign of a malignancy or may follow the development of other symptoms. Review the medical history of malignancies and family history of cancer. A previous malignancy should raise suspicion for a recurrent malignancy in the differential diagnosis for unexplained jaundice. If hepatic or pancreatic cancer is suspected, a prompt, thorough physical examination is warranted owing to the potential for metastatic disease and the need to identify the primary site. During the abdominal examination, carefully palpate the area of the liver and the remainder of the abdomen, checking for masses or unexpected findings.

Signs and Symptoms

Associated symptoms may include RUQ discomfort, nausea, fever, back pain, weight loss, ascites, fatigue/weakness, white chalky stools, and pruritus. None of these symptoms are specific to malignancy; however, other causes of jaundice are less likely to be associated with weight loss. Hepatomegaly and tenderness, including gallbladder discomfort, may be present.

Diagnostic Studies

In addition to a CBC, liver functions, amylase, lipase, and bilirubin levels, abdominal CT and/or ultrasound should be ordered promptly.

CIRRHOSIS

Cirrhosis develops with the replacement of normal liver tissue by regenerative, fibrotic nodules and may occur in the late phase of a variety of disorders that damage the liver, such as chronic viral hepatitis, Wilson's disease, and drug and alcohol toxicity.

Signs and Symptoms

Symptoms may be subtle at first or dramatic. A patient may present with jaundice and describe an associated, progressive pattern of pruritus, weakness, anorexia, nausea, and weight loss. Alternatively, a patient with undiagnosed cirrhosis may present with jaundice and also with acute onset of ascites, bleeding varices, and/or severe RUQ discomfort. Hepatomegaly may be evident with tenderness and pronounced vascular patterns visible over the abdomen. Edema of lower extremities is common. Mental status changes may be evident on examination due to elevated ammonia levels in the blood.

Diagnostic Studies

In addition to AST and ALT, diagnostic studies should include a CBC, alkaline phosphatase, bilirubin, albumin, ammonia, and prothrombin time tests. An ultrasound or CT of the abdomen should be done to further evaluate the liver size and structure.

CHOLECYSTITIS, CHOLELITHIASIS, AND CHOLANGITIS

Occlusion of the common bile duct may occur with disorders of the gallbladder and/or bile duct. See also the section on cholecystitis earlier in the chapter.

Signs and Symptoms

All three conditions are generally accompanied by RUQ discomfort, anorexia, and nausea. Charcot's triad, which includes jaundice, RUQ pain, and fever/chills, is common to problems resulting in obstructions of the bile duct. Identify any history of biliary surgery. Assess the abdomen, noting the condition of the liver, and test for Murphy's sign. Observe the skin for xanthomas.

Diagnostic Studies

Obtain an ultrasound of the gallbladder and biliary structures. When there is a high index of suspicion for obstructive causes of jaundice, either endoscopic retrograde cholangiopancreatography or percutaneous transhepatic cholangiography are appropriate initial imaging studies.

HEMOLYTIC DISORDERS

A variety of conditions causing hemolysis of the red blood cells can result in jaundice: acquired hemolytic anemia, sickle cell anemia, hemolytic drug reactions, autoimmune disorders, HELLP (hemolysis, elevated liver enzymes, and low platelets) syndrome, leukemia and lymphoma, and others.

Signs and Symptoms

If hemolytic anemia is involved, the history may also include weakness, fatigue, dyspnea, palpitations, or other symptoms common to anemia. Other symptoms may include abdominal pain, fever, and chills if hemolysis has been rapid. Patients with sickle cell disorder usually can provide a history of recurrent episodes of symptoms, including severe pain, weakness, dyspnea, swollen joints, and/or skin lesions—often requiring serial hospitalizations. The medication survey may identify medications with hemolysis as a potential adverse effect, such as cephalosporins, the penicillin derivatives levofloxacin and nitrofurantoin, NSAIDs, and methyldopa. Assess for splenomegaly and hepatomegaly. Observe skin and mucous membranes for lesions, purpura, and/or pallor. Assess joints for swelling, inflammation, or tenderness. Assess heart and lungs; determine the presence of any associated cardiomegaly.

Diagnostic Studies

Order a CBC, noting the hematocrit, red blood count and indices, hemoglobin, and reticulocyte count. Tests for hemoglobinopathies may be indicated, as might an indirect Coombs' test for levels of antibodies to the red blood cells. A bone marrow test may be warranted depending on laboratory results.

Serum studies that are less common but are appropriate for certain causes of jaundice include iron, transferrin, ferritin, antimitochondrial antibodies, antinuclear antibodies, and ceruloplasmin.

PANCREATITIS

See earlier discussion, pp. 352–353.

■ Gastrointestinal Bleeding

Patients with GI bleeding may complain of hematemesis, melena, or hematochezia. Alternatively, they may have occult bleeding and be unaware of the problem. When a patient presents with GI bleeding, the first step must be to determine hemodynamic stability. Stability is assessed, to a large extent, by consideration of the patient's vital signs and general appearance. This discussion does not apply to patients who present with significant acute blood loss or who otherwise require urgent stabilization and treatment. Rather, this section describes the approach for patients who appear stable and who present with a history of blood in emesis or stool as well as those in whom occult bleeding is suspected or confirmed. It is important to narrow the differential diagnosis to allow for a focused approach.

History

It is important to obtain a thorough symptom analysis of any complaint of GI bleeding, including the timing, progression, and description of the blood. Whether the blood is noticed in emesis and/or in stool determines the amount, color, odor, and any other characteristics of the emesis and stool. The ability to differentiate between melena and hematochezia is helpful. When melena is present, the blood is likely to have been present for over 14 hours; therefore, the site of bleeding is most likely distant from the rectum (upper GI). When hematochezia is present, the blood is less likely to have remained in the bowel long enough for the hemoglobin to degrade it, and thus the source is more likely to be nearer the rectum, usually in the colon. However, rapid upper GI bleeding can result in hematochezia. Establish the history of bowel movements and previous episodes of emesis and/or retching. Identify other indications of bleeding, including bleeding gums, bruising, or epistaxis. Associated symptoms such as pain, weakness, constipation, or diarrhea must be identified. Prior GI conditions, malignancies, bleeding disorders, comorbidities, and current medications must be determined. A review of habits should include diet, alcohol intake, and tobacco use. A history of any prior GI diagnostic studies and their results should be determined.

Physical Examination

The physical examination must start with a general survey and accurate vital signs. Observe the patient's general overall appearance and any signs of pallor, weakness, or dyspnea. Obtain pulse and blood pressure while the patient is lying, sitting, and standing, and note any postural changes. The heart and lungs, as well as any compensatory changes related to bleeding, should be assessed to determine general well-being. Finally, unless otherwise indicated, the examination should focus on the abdomen. Note any areas of discomfort, organomegaly, palpable masses, and unexpected dullness to percussion. A rectal examination must be performed, noting the presence of hemorrhoids or masses and testing for occult blood.

MALLORY-WEISS TEAR

Upper GI hemorrhage may result from a tear at the gastroesophageal junction, known as a Mallory-Weiss tear. A patient may develop more than one tear.

Signs and Symptoms

These tears are most common in alcoholic patients following an episode of vomiting or retching. If a laceration/tear of the mucosa causes GI bleeding, the patient may demonstrate alterations in hemodynamic status and possibly shock.

Diagnostic Studies

A stat CBC is necessary as a baseline. Consider ordering an ethanol level if alcohol is suspected as a contributing factor. The bleeding associated with a laceration is considerable, and the patient must be referred immediately for evaluation and endoscopic visualization of the lesion.

GASTRITIS

Although gastritis is not commonly associated with major GI bleeding, it may lead to chronic blood loss and anemia. More often, bleeding occurs after an area of gastric mucosal injury has ulcerated.

Signs and Symptoms

Explore symptoms of epigastric and/or periumbilical discomfort. Identify potential causes of gastric mucosal injury—the most common being NSAID use and stress. Stress-related mucosal damage may follow a major surgery, burn, or severe medical illness—that is, a disorder that has caused the patient to become extremely ill rather than a mild, transient condition. Currently, stress-related gastritis is less common because at-risk patients are often prophylactically treated with agents to alter the gastric pH.

Diagnostic Studies

A CBC is warranted to identify the amount of blood loss, if any. An upper endoscopy will illuminate the cause of the gastric symptoms and/or bleeding.

MALIGNANCY

Even though cancer can cause a major bleeding episode, it more commonly causes chronic, slower bleeding. When occult blood or other signs of GI bleeding are present, a malignancy must be considered in the differential diagnosis, with a likely site dependent on the presentation.

Signs and Symptoms

Determine the history of malignancies and risk factors for malignancy. Bleeding caused by cancer is usually painless but may have associated symptoms, such as altered bowel patterns, fatigue, and so on. A palpable mass may be present. There is usually no tenderness on examination. Rectal examination may detect a palpable mass. Consider the patient's overall appearance and determine whether there has been significant weight loss.

Diagnostic Studies

A CBC should be drawn to check for anemia, which may be the first sign of a malignancy, and a chemistry profile should be done for distant metastases. Colonoscopy is necessary for diagnosis and biopsy. Upper endoscopy is necessary for diagnosis and biopsy of gastric malignancies. An ultrasound or abdominal CT with contrast will identify organ tumors. A PET scan may assist in pinpointing the site of malignancy and the presence of metastasis. A CEA is an important marker for the diagnosis and treatment monitoring of colon cancer.

HEMORRHOIDS

The most common cause of lower GI bleeding is hemorrhoids. The bleeding associated with hemorrhoids is usually evident as red blood on the formed stool, in the toilet bowl, or on the toilet tissue following a bowel movement.

Signs and Symptoms

Patients with hemorrhoids often complain of rectal discomfort as well as the contributing factors for hemorrhoid development, including constipation. Inspect the perianal rectal tissue. Anoscopy may be indicated. Perform a digital rectal examination to assess internal hemorrhoids.

Diagnostic Studies

No diagnostic studies are generally indicated. Hemorrhoids can usually be visualized with anoscopy. Consider flexible sigmoidoscopy for internal hemorrhoids. The patient should be reassessed following treatment of the hemorrhoids to ensure there is no continued bleeding to investigate.

DIVERTICULA

Most diverticula do not commonly cause GI bleeding; however, diverticula are quite common. Because the incidence of diverticula is so high and they have the potential to bleed, diverticula actually account for a great percentage of lower GI bleeding that is not related to malignancy or hemorrhoids.

Signs and Symptoms

Diverticular bleeding is usually painless. Diverticula should be considered if the patient gives the history of sudden onset of bright red blood in a large amount. Chronic, small bleeding is not associated with diverticula. The physical examination is usually unremarkable.

Diagnostic Studies

Because the amount of bleeding is significant, the patient should be referred, and a colonoscopy will likely be performed to identify the site of bleeding.

PORTAL HYPERTENSION

Patients with portal hypertension may develop GI bleeding from varices of the esophagus, stomach, intestines, or other sites. Portal hypertension is most commonly associated with cirrhosis, usually caused by alcohol abuse or hepatitis.

Signs and Symptoms

Because the incidence of esophageal and gastric variceal bleeding is greater than that associated with the intestines, it is important to assess the history of liver disease in any patient presenting with upper GI bleeding. Determine whether there have been previous episodes of variceal bleeding. Rule out risk factors for the development of liver disease and portal hypertension. Check for signs of liver disease, including jaundice, cirrhosis, telangiectasia, hepatomegaly, and RUQ tenderness.

Diagnostic Studies

Laboratory studies should include a CBC to assess for anemia and a prothrombin time and partial thromboplastin time to determine coagulation status. A CT scan or MRI and upper endoscopy will assist in the varices diagnosis.

OSLER-WEBER-RENDU DISEASE

Osler-Weber-Rendu disease, also known as hereditary hemorrhagic telangiectasia, is an autosomal dominant, hereditary disease caused by vascular malformation. It affects men and women equally. A thorough family history will aid in the diagnosis.

Signs and Symptoms

Arteriovenous malformations can occur at any age and affect the brain, liver, lungs, and bowel. Epistaxis usually begins in childhood, and telangiectasias of the lips, tongue, and skin appear in late childhood and adolescence. Patients may have a family or personal history of hypertension. GI bleeding, caused by mucosal vascular malformations, generally does not occur until the middle-adult years.

Diagnostic Studies

Diagnosis is usually made by history and physical examination. MRI and CT arteriography will detect arteriovenous malformations. Molecular analysis to identify the gene mutations responsible for hereditary hemorrhagic telangiectasia is currently available.

PEPTIC ULCER DISEASE

PUD causes more than 50% of GI bleeding, with the most common site being the duodenum. The use of NSAIDs is the most important risk factor for the development of bleeding from PUD, although the risk can be increased further by the use of anticoagulants, by *H. pylori*, and by increased acid as in conditions such as Zollinger-Ellison syndrome. See pp. 357–358 for more information.

ESOPHAGITIS AND HIATAL HERNIA

It is rare for patients to develop a significant bleeding episode related to esophagitis or a hiatal hernia. Either may cause a chronic blood loss with occult blood in the stool and anemia. For further information, see p. 358.

COLITIS

See Mucosal Diseases, pp. 376–377.

REFERENCES

American Cancer Society. (2021a). Key statistics about stomach cancer. Retrieved August 17, 2021, from https://www.cancer.org/cancer/stomach-cancer/about/key-statistics.html

American Cancer Society. (2021b). Stomach cancer survival rates. Retrieved August 17, 2021, from https://www.cancer.org/cancer/stomach-cancer/detection-diagnosis-staging/survival-rates.html

Ebell, M. H. (2001). *Evidence-based diagnosis: A handbook of clinical prediction rules.* Springer.

Houdart, R., Perniceni, T., Dame, B., Salmeron, M., & Simon, J. F. (1995). Predicting common bile duct lithiasis: Determination and prospective validation of a model predicting low risk. *American Journal of Surgery, 170*(1), 38–43.

McQuaid, K. R. (2018). Gastrointestinal disorders. In S. J. McPhee & S. J. M. A. Papadakis (Eds.), *Current medical diagnosis and treatment* (57th ed.). McGraw-Hill.

Parker, S. (2008). Digestive disease: The facts. Retrieved November 23, 2013, from www.healthguidance.org/entry/6328/1/Digestive-Diseases-The-Facts.htm

Peery, A. F., Crockett, S.D., Murphy, C. C., Lund, J. L., Dellon, E. S., Williams, J.L., Jensen, E. T., Shaheen, N. J., Barritt, A. S., Lieber, S.R., Kochar, B., Barnes, E.L., Fan, Y. C., Pate, V., Glanko, J., Baron, T. J., & Sandler, R. S. (2019). Burden and cost of gastrointestinal, liver, and pancreatic diseases in the United States: Update 2018. *Gastroenterology, 156*(1), 254–272.e11. doi: 10.1053/j.gastro.2018.08.063

Chapter 12

Genitourinary System

Susanne A. Quallich •
Michelle Lajiness •

T he assessment of a genitourinary (GU) complaint should lead the practitioner to a differential diagnosis narrowed through further evaluation. Symptom analysis of lower urinary tract complaints can be aided by objective psychometric instruments, which can reliably reflect a change (improvement or worsening of the condition) in symptoms over time. Many of the disease entities can significantly affect a patient's quality of life and overall social functioning. GU conditions can impact a variety of patient behaviors, including travel, social functions, entertainment pursuits, sexual activity, sleep, and activities around the home. This chapter focuses on groups of complaints that are unique to the GU system, and it presents the most common differential diagnoses in each category.

Throughout life, hormonal influences and age-related structural changes in anatomy and tissue consistency cause variances in voiding function that affect the quality of life. In infancy, the emptying of the bladder is reflexive. As we age into puberty and adulthood, unless there is a congenital anomaly, trauma, or an intervening illness or surgery that directly affects our ability to maintain urinary control, voiding function is taken for granted. Middle adulthood and later adulthood are times when hormonal influences and anatomical changes are noted. At this time, the degree to which one is able to remain continent of urine and to comfortably empty the bladder begins to affect quality of life.

In men, the prostate is under the influence of testosterone over the entire life span. The prostate gradually undergoes hypertrophy, causing obstructive symptoms, as though liquid flowing through a tube were being slowly held back. An assessment of urinary function for men should include the International Prostate Symptom Score, a validated, reliable instrument designed to objectively measure how much urinary symptoms affect the overall quality of life for men (Barry et al., 1992).

In women, estrogen influences tissue elasticity and bacterial populations. Birth trauma and surgery with the resulting scar tissue may change the anatomical relationships and musculature of the pelvis and therefore have a role in future urinary function.

> **RED FLAG** ◀ **Red Flags in the Assessment of the Genitourinary System**
>
> - *Gross hematuria must be referred urgently to a urologist, with accompanying studies arranged and, if possible, completed before the appointment.*
> - *Abrupt onset or worsening testicular pain, regardless of patient age (see Chapter 13).*
> - *Anuria and oliguria require aggressive evaluation and/or admission for management.*
> - *Acute urinary retention must be referred to the nearest emergency department immediately.*
> - *Large kidney masses—particularly when accompanied by the classic triad of gross hematuria, flank pain, and a palpable mass—must be referred emergently to a urologist.*
> - *Pain associated with any GU structure that awakes the patient or prevents sleep.*
> - *A toxic-appearing patient with poor urine output.*

Although lower urinary tract symptoms (LUTS) arise from different causes in men and women, the signs and symptoms can be very similar. Over the life span, storage function and bladder outlet obstruction vary more than bladder contractility. The discussion of presentation, symptoms, and diagnostic workup are directed at the evaluation of these clinical entities in the adult or geriatric patient. See the Red Flag box relative to the assessment of the adult GU system. Evaluation of the pediatric patient with GU complaints, although similar, does vary and is not addressed in this chapter.

History

■ General History

The general history for a patient who presents with GU complaints should begin with questions regarding a previous history of any similar complaints. A sexual history is appropriate, including recent changes in partners and an assessment of general sexual habits. The history should include a discussion of any recent (within the last 6 months) systemic illness; recent weight gain or loss; smoking, alcohol consumption, and illicit drug use; recent nausea, vomiting, fever, chills, or other constitutional symptoms; and exposure to chemicals or dyes. A general history of the GU tract must also include a list of current prescription and over-the-counter, homeopathic, or naturopathic medications. Ask what remedies have been tried prior to presentation. As each presenting complaint is listed, additional specific history-taking points are discussed.

▪ Patterns of Pain

Knowledge of the potential sources of GU pain and a range of pain syndromes is important to accurately assess complaints of pains. These are reviewed in Table 12.1.

▪ Past Medical and Surgical History

The GU-related medical and surgical history should include any surgeries to the GU tract or reproductive structures, prostate surgery, bladder reconstructions, and previous treatment for reproductive or GU malignancies, as an infant, child, or adolescent. It is vital to elicit an accurate history of any surgery that may affect the vascular or nerve supply to the urinary tract or bladder, including pelvic surgery, retroperitoneal surgery, or back surgery. Obtain a previous history of nephrolithiasis or urolithiasis or treatment for other GU conditions, including urinary tract infections (UTIs). Previous pregnancies, live births, birth trauma, and manner of delivery should also be assessed.

▪ Family History

Family history is important because it can help establish a patient's risk for various GU conditions. Include a history of GU malignancies, prostate or bladder problems, family history (particularly first-degree relatives) of nephrolithiasis or urolithiasis, incontinence (particularly female relatives), or complaints similar to the patient's. It is recommended that the family history be as specific as possible, noting the relationship to the patient, to provide further insight into congenital or hereditary risk factors.

▪ Sexual History

The degree of detail regarding sexual history is guided by the patient's presenting complaints. Sexual history should include activity from adolescence through adulthood and should include the patient's sexual orientation. The number of current and lifetime sexual partners should be discussed along with any history of sexually transmitted infections (STIs) and the treatment received. A history of intravenous drug use and the date and results of the patient's last HIV test should also be noted.

Questions regarding safe sex and condom use (serial monogamy risk) and specifics about sexual practices are also relevant. The patient's preferred method of birth control should be noted. Questions regarding erectile dysfunction, premature ejaculation, change in libido, pelvic pain, or incontinence during sexual activity can also provide insight into disease pathology (see Chapters 13 and 14 on the male and female reproductive systems for details on these topics).

Table 12.1

Sources of Pain

Source of Pain	Spinal Level	Presentation
Kidney/renal pain	T10–12, L1	Dull, constant ache to the CVA, lateral to sacrospinalis muscle and just below 12th rib Can spread to subcostal area toward umbilicus or LLQ Results from distension of renal capsule
Pseudorenal pain	T10–12	Caused by mechanical derangement of costovertebral or costotransverse joints, resulting in pressure on costal nerves Mimics renal pain or ureteral colic Can cause costovertebral pain May radiate to ipsilateral LQ Pain is positional, acute, absent on arising, and increases during the day Pain exacerbated with heavy work
Ureteral pain	*Upper ureter:* T11–12	Due to acute obstruction
	Mid-left ureter: T12, L1	Pain due to hyperperistalsis and smooth muscle spasm as ureter tries to overcome obstruction Back pain from renal capsular distension and colicky pain (from ureteral muscle and renal pelvic spasm): • Radiates to CVA, toward LQ, along the course of the ureter • In men, also pain to bladder, scrotum, testicle • In women, also pain to vulva *Upper ureter stone:* pain radiates to testicle (nerve supply similar to kidney and upper ureter) *Mid-right ureter stone:* pain referred from McBurney's point and can present like appendicitis *Mid-left ureter stone:* mimics pain to descending and/or sigmoid colon *Stone close to bladder:* edema and inflammation to ureteral outlet with resulting vesical (bladder) irritability
Vesical (bladder) pain	No corresponding level	*Overdistention:* suprapubic pain; other suprapubic pain is likely not bladder in origin *Pain with UTI:* usually referred to distal urethra (terminal dysuria)
Prostatic pain	S2–4	Pain directly from prostate is uncommon Acute inflammation: may have discomfort or fullness to perineal and/or rectal area Possible lumbosacral backache Can cause dysuria, frequency, urgency
Epididymal pain	No corresponding level	Due to acute infection Pain in scrotum Begins as pain in groin or LQ abdomen Can reach costal angle and mimic stone pain Inflammation of testicle possible
Testicular pain	No corresponding level	Very severe, felt locally Can radiate along spermatic cord to lower abdomen and/or CVA Varicocele can cause dull ache that worsens after heavy exercise (see Chapter 13)

CVA = costovertebral angle; LLQ = left lower quadrant; LQ = lower quadrant; UTI = urinary tract infection.

Physical Examination

■ General History

Inspection

Look for suprapubic fullness and fullness at the costovertebral angle (CVA). Examine for any visible striae or truncal obesity. Refer to Chapters 13 and 14 for the specifics of genital inspection. The male patient should be standing and facing the examiner.

Auscultation

The examiner can auscultate the scrotum to distinguish loops of bowel from scrotal mass if a hernia is suspected. Listen over the renal artery to rule out renal artery aneurysm; otherwise, perform the usual auscultation of the abdomen as described in Chapter 11.

Percussion

Perform percussion at the CVA and flank to elicit and identify pain that may be associated with hydronephrosis or pyelonephritis. This can also help to localize or outline a suspected renal mass and to determine whether it is tender. The percussion of the abdomen is as indicated in Chapter 11.

Palpation

The specifics of palpation relative to the GU system pertain to the palpation of the kidneys and the inguinal regions for hernia or adenopathy as well as digital rectal examination (DRE). Palpation of the GU system is described in Table 12.2.

Table 12.2	

Palpation of Genitourinary System

Procedure	Technique
Digital rectal examination	Gloved, lubricated finger is inserted into anus. Sweep back and forth across the surface of the prostate. Sweep the anal ring and the rectal walls 360 degrees. The examination can result in a sensation of pressure and possibly an urge to urinate. The prostate should be symmetric (but asymmetry is a normal variant); nontender; free of nodules; approximately the size of a walnut; and have a smooth, rubbery consistency. The examination also involves an assessment of anal sphincter tone and an estimate of prostate size in grams. This examination can be done with the patient standing and bent over, side-lying, or in dorsal lithotomy position.
Examination for inguinal hernia	The index finger is inserted into the scrotum and invaginates the scrotum into the external inguinal ring (scrotum should be invaginated in front of testicle); fingertips of other hand should then be placed over internal inguinal canal and patient should be asked to cough. If present, a hernia will be felt as a bulge that descends against the index finger with Valsalva maneuver.
Palpation of kidneys	With the patient lying supine, for the right kidney, the examiner should place the left hand, palm up, under the tenth to twelfth ribs and place the right hand on top of the abdomen, just below the right costal margin. For the left side, the examiner should reverse the hands so the right hand is under the patient's left costovertebral angle. Ask the patient to take a deep breath. When the breath is fully drawn, ask the patient to exhale. As the diaphragm moves into the thoracic cavity, the lower pole of the kidney may be felt slipping across the fingertips of the hand beneath the tenth and twelfth ribs.

Diagnostic Studies

■ Laboratory Evaluation

Urinalysis

Significant urinalysis findings are described in Table 12.3. Urinalysis is not sufficient alone to diagnose a suspected UTI. A culture is necessary for accurate treatment.

Urine Cultures

Laboratory cultures of the urine are indicated with suspected UTI and are particularly important for recurrent UTIs or a UTI that seems refractory to treatment.

Cytology

Urine cytology is part of a gross hematuria workup, and a positive cytology may indicate bladder, ureteral, or renal pelvic malignancy. This test should be sent from a patient's first voided morning urine on three separate days, if possible, for the greatest degree of accuracy. Urine cytology is an inexpensive means of screening for cancer in a patient with irritative lower urinary tract complaints.

Serum Creatinine and Blood Urea Nitrogen

Serum creatinine and blood urea nitrogen (BUN) provide information regarding kidney function. They are useful with suspected disease and possible obstruction due to benign prostatic hypertrophy (BPH), kidney stones, or ureteral stones. Other laboratory tests are ordered at the clinician's discretion to evaluate the suspected cause of disease; they are discussed in the diagnosis sections of specific conditions.

Table 12.3	
Urinalysis Findings	
Urinalysis Component	**Interpretation**
Color	Bright red if urological or anatomic cause
	Tea-colored or brown urine may be due to old clots, glomerulonephritis, or other medical cause
Specific gravity	May see low specific gravity with hydronephrosis, intrinsic renal disease
Protein	Values 3–4 or higher may indicate glomerulonephritis or other decline in kidney function
Leukocyte esterase	If positive, suggests presence of white blood cells (does not localize source of infection); 80% to 90% sensitive; approximately 95% specific
Erythrocyte casts	Indicates glomerular source for hematuria (medical hematuria)
Crystalluria	May indicate stone disease
Nitrite	If positive, suggests presence of bacteria (does not localize source of infection); 50% sensitive; approximately 95% specific.

Table 12.4

Age-Specific Prostate-Specific Antigen Reference Ranges

Age Range	Blacks	Asians	Whites
40–49 y	0–2 ng/mL	0–2 ng/mL	0–2.5 ng/mL
50–59 y	0–4 ng/mL	0–3 ng/mL	0–3.5 ng/mL
60–69 y	0–4.5 ng/mL	0–4 ng/mL	0–4.5 ng/mL
70–79 y	0–5.5 ng/mL	0–5.0 ng/mL	0–6.5 ng/mL

Adapted with permission from Richardson, T. D., & Oesterling, J. E., 1997.

Prostate-Specific Antigen Testing

Prostate-specific antigen (PSA) is a measurable protein produced by the prostate gland. It is commonly used as a marker for the presence of prostate cancer, but it is not specific to this. The PSA can be elevated by infection, ejaculation within the 48 hours prior to testing, GU instrumentation, or increased gland volume, such as that seen with BPH. Guidelines for normal range are presented in Table 12.4 and are based on age and ethnicity. Recent attempts have been made to make this test more specific to prostate cancer by establishing additional variables such as PSA velocity: If the PSA rises more than 0.75 ng/mL per year, the risk for prostate cancer is increased, and urology referral should be initiated. Pharmacotherapy with finasteride and dutasteride is associated with a >50% decrease in PSA, which must be considered when evaluating results on patients so treated. Consult current guidelines from organizations such as the American Urological Association or American Cancer Society.

▪ Radiological Evaluation

Uroradiological Study

The simplest uroradiological study is the KUB (kidney, ureters, bladder). It can be helpful as a screening or preliminary test, especially if clinical suspicion points to possible renal or ureteral lithiasis or if there is suspicion for constipation contributing to symptoms. A KUB study often shows calcified abnormalities in both the urinary tract and the skeletal system, and it may also demonstrate large soft tissue masses. A KUB is routinely used to track the progress of ureteral stones as they are passed and to provide a rapid method for evaluating the asymptomatic stone patient for recurrence.

Ultrasonography

Ultrasound is a noninvasive, relatively inexpensive, and widely available procedure that avoids radiation exposure and the risk of intravenous contrast. It is widely used to image all parts of the GU system. Ultrasound is superior to intravenous pyelography (IVP) for the evaluation of small lesions, and it is more sensitive than IVP in the evaluation of renal masses. It has limited utility for upper tract filling defects but can be useful for differentiating between medical renal (e.g., stemming from renal parenchyma) and urological renal (e.g., stemming from urological sources such as obstructive uropathy) disease. Ultrasound is also limited by the patient's body habitus and the skill of the operator. Since the development of renal ultrasound and computed tomography (CT), IVP is used infrequently.

Ultrasound is excellent for examination of the scrotum and its contents, and it can definitively distinguish between extra- and intratesticular pathologies.

Computed Tomography

An unenhanced helical CT (no contrast) scan is superior for the evaluation of suspected or actual stone disease because slices 3-mm thin are used (Rodger, Roditi, & Aboumarzouk, 2018). The advantages of CT include quick scanning time, wide field of view, good cross-sectional views, and ability to detect subtle differences in tissues. The disadvantages of CT include radiation dose, low soft tissue resolution, need for contrast media, and images limited to the transaxial plane.

Magnetic Resonance Imaging

Magnetic resonance imaging (MRI) has wide application in the evaluation of GU patients. It provides excellent images of the retroperitoneum, bladder, prostate, testes, and even the penis. The use of gadolinium as a contrast media has broadened the use of MRI further because it is well tolerated even by patients with compromised renal function. An MRI with contrast can provide increased characterization of renal masses and is clearly superior to CT in imaging the pelvis. When MRI is combined with angiography, renal vessels, renal vein thrombosis, and congenital abnormalities can be demonstrated.

The advantages of MRI include imaging in any plane, excellent soft tissue characterization, and lack of exposure to radiation. Its disadvantages include slow scanning time, decreased imaging clarity compared with CT, heat generation, and claustrophobia for the patient.

Computed Tomography Urography

A CT urogram is a CT test done with the addition of radiopaque dye, and it can image both the renal parenchyma and the urothelium (the lining of the ureters, bladder, and urethra) with a single examination. It combines the sensitivity and specificity of a CT scan for urinary calculi and small renal masses with the sensitivity and specificity of intravenous urography for urothelial abnormalities (Bishoff & Art, 2016). Some authors (Perlman et al., 1996) report that CT urography further characterizes masses seen on IVP and better detects small renal cell carcinomas (RCCs). Its sensitivity and specificity are superior to the IVP, and it can provide a safe and more precise evaluation. It is the preferred initial study in the evaluation of hematuria.

Magnetic Resonance Urography

Magnetic resonance (MR) urography is another emerging technology in the evaluation of GU pathologies. Similar to MR cholangiopancreatography, images are taken after the administration of intravenous gadolinium contrast. It is especially helpful in imaging patients with dilated tracts (Bishoff & Art, 2016). This study is currently limited by the poor spatial resolution of the resulting images and its poor record with calculi detection. However, it provides another method for detecting urinary tract dilatation, ureteric obstruction, duplicated renal collecting systems, and urothelial tumors. The sensitivity of MR urography is currently considered to be similar to that of the CT urogram.

DIFFERENTIAL DIAGNOSIS OF CHIEF COMPLAINTS

GENERAL COMPLAINTS

■ Flank Pain and Renal Colic

The kidney and ureters are described as the upper tracts. Symptoms in this anatomical area are a subjective indicator of change in the urinary outflow system. Upper tract symptoms arise from irritation in the kidney and/or blockage of urinary outflow. Causes of upper tract symptoms include kidney stones, urothelial cell carcinoma, and, rarely, RCC.

History

Presentation can vary widely, and the onset of complaints may be acute or insidious. A description of the pain is critical. Complaints can include a dull renal pain or a constant ache in the CVA area that can radiate laterally to the sacrospinalis muscle and just below the 12th rib. Pain can spread to the subcostal area toward the umbilicus or left lower quadrant. The patient may describe only back pain, which is the result of renal capsular distension, or colicky pain from the ureteral muscle and renal pelvic spasm. There may also be concurrent constitutional symptoms (e.g., nausea, vomiting, fever) and associated weight loss or gross hematuria. Determine the history of self-treatment, prior episodes of similar or other GU conditions, and most recent health status. Family history should be established.

Physical Examination

General appearance should be noted, as patients with complaints of flank pain may have widely varying presentations ranging from toxic or cachectic to only mild discomfort. A thorough GU examination and a general abdominal examination should be completed. Presence of CVA tenderness should be elicited. Palpation may reveal a palpable renal mass if the patient is thin or the mass is large enough. A pelvic examination should be completed as complaints warrant (e.g., in female patients who also complain of lower abdominal pain).

RENAL CELL CARCINOMA

RCCs have been referred to as the "internist's tumor" and as one of the great masqueraders in medicine. A patient with RCC presents with extraordinary variation, from a small asymptomatic lesion found on a CT or MRI scan during an evaluation for another complaint to a full-blown paraneoplastic syndrome with liver function derangements and hypercalcemia. RCCs can secrete biologically active substances, such as gonadotropins and adrenocorticotrophic hormone (ACTH). Laboratory findings can include normochromic anemia, an elevated erythrocyte sedimentation rate, and hematuria on urinalysis. Risk factors for RCC include smoking, environmental exposure to heavy metals, and hereditary conditions such as von Hippel-Lindau disease.

Signs and Symptoms

The signs and symptoms are described as in the preceding history subsection. The patient may present with obvious symptoms or vague constitutional complaints.

Diagnostic Studies

The workup is dictated by the patient's presentation and complaints. Initial laboratory work can include a urinalysis, urine cytology, complete blood count (CBC), liver function tests, and serum electrolytes. Imaging studies can include an IVP or renal ultrasound, CT scan, or MRI; the CT scan remains the gold standard for detection of RCC. Referral to a urology specialist is indicated; the more symptomatic the patient, the more urgent the referral. A biopsy is required for staging and treatment.

NEPHROLITHIASIS

Kidney stones are more common in men and rank as the third most common condition of the urinary tract. Kidney stones affect up to 5% of the worldwide population, with a lifetime risk of passing a kidney stone of about 8% to 10% and the incidence and prevalence increasing worldwide among adults. Several varieties of stones can be formed, the majority of which are radiopaque, and after an initial episode, the recurrence rate can be up to 50%. Most stones present with acute-onset pain due to the obstruction of the upper urinary tract. The symptoms associated with a kidney stone are due to the inflammation, edema, and hyperperistalsis of the GU tract, particularly the ureter. The number or size of the stone(s) correlates poorly with the degree of pain. Risk factors include a history of crystalluria, low fluid intake or dehydration (such as living in a hot, dry climate), socioeconomic factors (in industrialized countries), and a family history of stones. Over time, it has been noted that the chance of passing a stone spontaneously is based on the stone size and stone location. The smaller the stone and the more distally in the ureter the stone is located, the greater the likelihood of spontaneous passage. Smaller stones also will pass more quickly than

Decision Rule

Yallappa and colleagues (2018) completed a cumulative analysis using 70 studies and a total of 6642 patients with a median age of 46 years and a range of 18–74 years. The authors noted that 64% of patients successfully passed their stones spontaneously. About 49% of upper ureteral stones, 58% of midureteral stones, and 68% of distal ureteral stones passed spontaneously. Almost 75% of stones <5 mm and 62% of stones ≥5 mm passed spontaneously. The average time to stone expulsion was about 17 days (range of 6 to 29 days). The authors concluded that patients with a stone of ≤6 mm will pass the stone spontaneously without intervention (Yallappa et al., 2018).

---

larger stones. About 50% of patients with a stone <10 mm will spontaneously pass the stone (Assimos et al., 2016).

Signs and Symptoms

Patients will appear notably uncomfortable as they try to find a resting position that is not painful. They may also experience nausea and vomiting; other systemic indicators of renal colic may be noted, such as tachycardia. If a patient appears septic, referral to the nearest emergency department is mandatory.

Diagnostic Studies

Historically, the initial study recommended was a KUB or IVP; however, many facilities can perform a stone protocol spiral CT, a much more definitive test for the evaluation of kidney stones. Urinalysis usually shows some degree of hematuria or inflammation, may indicate infection, and may show crystals that can be a clue to the diagnosis of stone type. Referral to a urology specialist for management is indicated. Recurrent stone formers should also undergo a 24-hour urine collection for electrolytes (calcium, uric acid, phosphate, oxalate, phosphate uric acid) to evaluate for a metabolic condition that may be amenable to medical management.

UPPER URINARY TRACT OBSTRUCTION OR HYDRONEPHROSIS

This condition could be caused by an obstructing stone, ureteral stricture, prostatic hyperplasia, or renal or abdominal tumor that prevents the kidney from draining. The obstruction can be unilateral or bilateral, symptoms can be sudden or gradual in onset, and progressive renal damage will occur with time.

Signs and Symptoms

Flank pain may radiate along the course of the ureter and may be accompanied by a variety of constitutional symptoms. More severe or bilateral obstruction may cause weight loss and eventual uremia. A distended kidney may be noted on palpation, and CVA pain may be present if there is infection. GU, abdominal, pelvic, and rectal examinations are indicated.

Diagnostic Studies

The workup is the same as for the evaluation of kidney stone or renal tumor. Imaging studies are the key to determining the etiology.

PYELONEPHRITIS

Pyelonephritis is a bacterial infection of the renal pelvis and parenchyma, typically caused by *Escherichia coli* ascending from the lower urinary tract. Risk factors include vesicoureteral reflux, neurogenic bladder, stones of any part of the GU tract, immunosuppression, diabetes mellitus, or a new sexual partner (for women).

Signs and Symptoms

The patient will have bilateral or unilateral flank pain, fever, chills, nausea, and vomiting. LUTS, such as dysuria, may also be present. The patient will appear ill on presentation, with fever and tachycardia commonly noted. Palpation and/or percussion over the infected side is painful. There may be accompanying abdominal discomfort or abdominal distension.

Diagnostic Studies

A CBC will show leukocytosis, often with a shift to the left. Urinalysis will also demonstrate leukocytosis, red blood cells, protein, and bacteria. Urine culture will be positive with heavy growth; blood cultures may be necessary. BUN and creatinine suggest decreased renal function. Imaging studies should be considered if the patient appears ill or does not respond to initial outpatient management (CT scan or renal ultrasound to assess for urinary obstruction). Assessment must include the determination of whether or not the patient requires inpatient management.

AUTOSOMAL DOMINANT POLYCYSTIC KIDNEY DISEASE

A family history of autosomal dominant polycystic kidney disease (ADPCKD) should raise the level of suspicion if a renal mass is palpated. Adult-onset ADPCKD is uncommon under the age of 40 years.

Signs and Symptoms

Back or flank pain (60%), gross hematuria (30%), and renal stones (20%) are the most common symptoms. There may be infections in the cysts, hypertension, and decreasing renal function associated with the initial presentation. A CT scan may also reveal liver cysts concurrent with renal cysts that may begin to appear at age 30 years. During palpation of the abdomen, cysts on either or both kidneys may be evident.

Diagnostic Studies

A family history of liver or renal cysts will aid in diagnosis even in the absence of palpable masses. A renal ultrasound may reveal cystic lesions; a CT examination is more sensitive in the evaluation of cysts but also more costly. Once the diagnosis is established, imaging studies need not be routinely performed unless new symptoms require evaluation. Patients with an established diagnosis of ADPCKD should be followed by a urology and/or nephrology specialist for monitoring pyelonephritis, nephrolithiasis, and renal function. Severe renal dysfunction can lead to hypertension, heart disease, and stroke, so careful monitoring is necessary.

BLUNT RENAL TRAUMA

Blunt trauma typically causes damage in the transverse plane of the kidney. Damage to the kidney represents the most common injury to the GU tract. Trauma can be the result of a motor vehicle accident or contact sports and is usually seen in men and boys.

Signs and Symptoms

The patient usually has evidence of abdominal trauma, such as fractured ribs, with complaints of pain that localize to the affected side. If the injury is severe, there may be signs of shock.

Diagnostic Studies

History may be sufficient to establish that renal injury is likely. Urinalysis will show some degree of hematuria. The initial imaging study is an IVP; a CT urogram is indicated for evaluation if the kidney is poorly visualized on the IVP. The patient should be referred to a urologist for further evaluation and management or to the nearest emergency department if the injury appears severe.

■ Gross Hematuria

A sudden, noticeable change in the color of urine is usually quite alarming to a patient. Gross hematuria results from a sufficient number of erythrocytes in the urine for the patient or clinician to perceive a color change in the urine. Painless, gross hematuria may be ignored by some patients, resulting in a significant delay before presentation for evaluation. Gross hematuria is often the only indication of a urological malignancy; a malignancy is found in up to 40% of gross hematuria cases.

Therapeutic anticoagulation should not lead to either gross or microscopic hematuria. Hematuria may result if a patient becomes excessively anticoagulated. However, patients who are anticoagulated may also have coexisting urological malignancies, and an episode of gross hematuria in an anticoagulated patient warrants an evaluation.

History

Obtain a history of the hematuria, including the urine color and any accompanying symptoms. The urine color may range from pink to red or simply look like blood is being urinated. The episode is usually painless, but it can be associated with flank pain, nausea, vomiting, or generalized dysuria with or without other

Table 12.5

Possible Significance of Timing of Blood in the Urinary Stream

Description of Hematuria	Possible Site	Possible Cause
Microscopic hematuria	Any site within upper or lower urinary tract	UTI, prostatitis, urethritis, medical renal disease, bladder/ureteral/renal malignancy, stone disease
Initial gross hematuria	Anterior urethra	Stricture, meatal stenosis, urethritis, urethral cancer
Total gross hematuria	Source above bladder neck: bladder, kidney, ureter	Renal/ureteral/bladder stone or tumor; trauma; vigorous exercise; renal tuberculosis; hemorrhagic cystitis; interstitial cystitis; sickle cell disease; nephritis; ADPCKD; poststreptococcal glomerulonephritis
Terminal gross hematuria	Bladder neck, prostate, posterior urethra	BPH, regrowth BPH posttransurethral resection, bladder neck polyps, posterior urethritis, tuberculosis

ADPCKD = autosomal dominant polycystic kidney disease; BPH = benign prostatic hyperplasia; UTI = urinary tract infection.

LUTS. Ask about prior GU conditions, related family history, and habits. There may be an extensive smoking history or history of exposure to chemicals through the patient's job. It is vital to try to establish the timing of blood in the urinary stream, which can help predict the source of bleeding (Table 12.5).

Physical Examination

A routine GU examination and a pelvic examination for female patients (see Chapter 14 for pelvic examination methodology) are mandatory. The physical examination is often unremarkable except in the case of a kidney stone or ADP-CKD, in which case a large, boggy kidney may be palpated.

Selected Causes

Box 12.1 lists many of the most common causes of gross hematuria; it is commonly due to anatomic causes (nonglomerular bleeding).

Diagnostic Studies

Laboratory studies can include CBC, urinalysis, serum electrolytes, urine electrolytes, and urine cytology; studies are guided by the patient's presentation, risk factors for such GU diseases as bladder cancer, and comorbidities. Urine cultures are indicated with suspected UTI. Coagulation studies are performed as appropriate in anticoagulated patients. An imaging study (CT or ultrasound) will aid in evaluating an anatomical cause for the microscopic hematuria. The patient should be referred urgently to a urology specialist with the following studies completed before the visit: IVP, CT, or ultrasound; BUN and creatinine; urinalysis; and at least one urine cytology.

Box 12.1

Selected Causes of Gross Hematuria

- Arteriovenous malformation
- Autosomal dominant polycystic kidney disease (ADPCKD)
- Benign prostatic hypertrophy (BPH)
- Bladder neck polyps
- BPH regrowth posttransurethral resection
- Contamination from menstruation
- Hemorrhagic cystitis
- Interstitial cystitis
- Meatal stenosis
- Nephritis
- Posterior urethritis
- Poststreptococcal glomerulonephritis
- Renal tuberculosis
- Renal/ureteral/bladder stone
- Renal/ureteral/bladder tumor
- Sickle cell disease
- Trauma
- Tuberculosis
- Urethritis
- Urethral cancer
- Urethral stricture
- Vigorous exercise

■ Suprapubic Pain

The differential for complaints of midline lower quadrant pain includes many conditions that are not specific to the GU system. The key in evaluation of this complaint is a careful history and physical examination to localize the complaints to the actual structures involved.

History

A thorough history is indicated. Complaints on presentation may include pain to the midline lower abdomen that is constant or intermittent. The onset of the discomfort may have been acute or gradual. There may be associated complaints of perineal fullness, irritative voiding symptoms, or urinary retention. There may also be a variety of constitutional symptoms, including fever, chills, nausea, or vomiting.

Physical Examination

A routine GU examination is mandatory, including a DRE. An abdominal examination and a pelvic examination (in female patients) are also suggested. Physical examination may demonstrate pain on palpation of the suprapubic

Table 12.6

Selected Causes of Suprapubic Pain

Urethral	Prostate	Vesical
• Urethral syndrome • Urethral stenosis	• Acute or chronic bacterial prostatitis • Nonbacterial prostatitis • Prostatodynia	• Bladder cancer • Bladder stone • Interstitial cystitis • Urinary retention • Urinary tract infection
Distal Ureteral	**Large or Small Bowel (See Chapter 11)**	**Gynecologic (See Chapter 14)**
• Ascending infection • Foreign body • Stone	• Appendicitis • Diverticulitis • Inflammatory bowel disease • Malignancy	• Ectopic pregnancy • Endometriosis • Pelvic inflammatory disease • Uterine fibroids

region, and the bladder may be palpable. There may be global abdominal discomfort if gastrointestinal structures are involved. The patient may have CVA tenderness.

Selected Causes

Localization of the source of pain after physical examination, coupled with the history, aids in diagnosis of the potential cause. See Table 12.6 for examples.

Diagnostic Studies

The suspected cause guides the diagnostic workup. Laboratory studies can include CBC, urinalysis and culture, and urine cytology. The initial imaging study, if indicated, could be either a KUB or a CT scan, with any further workup dictated by initial findings of the laboratory studies and imaging. The patient may require urgent referral to a urologist, general surgeon, or gynecologist.

■ Anuria, Oliguria, and Renal Failure

Although anuria and oliguria are unusual as acute complaints, the course toward renal failure can be predicted in many patients, and patients should be questioned to elicit a report of decreasing urine. It remains important to establish the causes contributing to the renal dysfunction because many patients with severe kidney dysfunction will need a variety of support services, including dietitian consultations and dialysis, and select patients may be candidates for a renal transplant.

History

The history is the key to evaluating the suspected cause. The patient may report decreasing urine output over time or a recent change in medications. This can be complicated if the patient has a solitary kidney or previous renal transplant. Associated symptoms (e.g., flank pain, nausea, vomiting) must be noted; also note a history of recent intravenous dye administration. A thorough GU history as well as a general history and review of systems should be obtained.

Physical Examination

A complete physical examination, including routine GU examination, is required. The signs and symptoms depend on the cause and are not restricted to the GU system: flank pain if stone obstruction, murmur if endocarditis, palpable bladder if BPH, and generalized edema if myocardial failure.

Selected Causes

Table 12.7 lists many common causes, categorized as prerenal and postrenal.

Table 12.7

Selected Causes of Renal Failure, Anuria, and Oliguria

Prerenal	Postrenal
Decreased Vascular Volume	Upper Urinary Tract Obstruction
• Third spacing	• Kidney stone (unilateral vs. bilateral)
• Gastrointestinal losses	• Obstructing retroperitoneal mass
• Hemorrhage	• Pregnancy
• Reduced cardiac output	
• Septic shock	
• Severe dehydration	
• Spinal shock	
Myocardial Failure	Lower Urinary Tract Obstruction
• Cardiomyopathy	• Benign Prostatic Hypertrophy
• Ischemic heart disease	• Carcinoma (bladder, prostate)
• Tamponade	• Neuropathic bladder
• Valvular heart disease	• Prostatitis
	• Urethral stricture
Renal/Glomerular Causes	
• Acute glomerulonephritis	
• Vasculitis	
Vascular	
• Renal vein thrombosis	
• Renal artery occlusion	
Medication Related	
• Anticonvulsants	
• Antihypertensives	
• Chemotherapeutic agents	
• Diuretics	
• Radiographic contrast media	

Diagnostic Studies

The suspected cause and physical presentation guide the diagnostic workup. Laboratory studies can include CBC, urinalysis, serum electrolytes, and urine electrolytes. Initial imaging studies can include a renal or bladder ultrasound, and further workup is dictated by initial findings of the laboratory studies and imaging. A patient presenting acutely with anuria, oliguria, or renal failure requires an emergent referral for further evaluation and appropriate management based on the suspected cause.

■ Asymptomatic Microscopic Hematuria

Asymptomatic microscopic hematuria (AMH) is rarely a patient complaint; it is usually found on evaluation, such as during a routine medical examination or monitoring of a patient's kidney function. Opinions differ as to the appropriate long-term follow-up of the patient with persistent AMH, and ultimately the follow-up is guided by the patient's overall medical conditions and medication profile. AMH is defined as three or more red blood cells per high-power field on a properly collected urinary specimen in the absence of an obvious benign cause (e.g., UTI, injury). An AMH diagnosis cannot be based on a urine dipstick alone and must be confirmed by a microscopic evaluation (American Urological Association, 2016). Confirmed microscopic hematuria should be referred to a urologist.

History

A GU history should be obtained, as described earlier in this chapter. Usually there is no history of an associated complaint; the patient may give a history of recurrent stones, recent UTI, long-standing diabetes, or other medical renal disease. The patient may be taking prescription medication that can cause renal damage when used long term, and all over-the-counter and prescribed agents should be identified.

Physical Examination

A routine GU examination is required, including pelvic examination for female patients. AMH is often found incidentally on routine screening urinalysis, and there are no related signs.

Selected Causes

A detailed discussion of each potential differential diagnosis is beyond the scope of this chapter, and in many cases, a referral for further urological and/or nephrology evaluation is warranted. Box 12.2 lists many common causes of medical or renal hematuria. AMH is due to a physiological process (glomerular bleeding). Small, asymptomatic stones within the GU tract can cause intermittent AMH. Excessive anticoagulation has been known to lead to AMH.

Diagnostic Studies

Laboratory studies can include CBC, renal function, urinalysis, serum electrolytes, and urine electrolytes. Hemoglobin and hematocrit are not routinely indicated except as part of the CBC: AMH rarely causes significant blood loss. Urine cultures are indicated with suspected UTI. Order coagulation studies as

BOX 12.2

Selected Causes of Medical/Renal Hematuria

- Arteriovenous fistula
- Benign familial hematuria
- Berger's disease (IgA nephropathy)
- Bleeding disorder
- Bleeding dyscrasias/sickle cell disease
- Diabetes mellitus
- Drug-induced interstitial disease
- End-stage renal disease
- Exercise (marathon running)
- Familial glomerulonephritis
- History of analgesic abuse
- HIV
- Infections (e.g., hepatitis)
- Mesangioproliferative glomerulonephritis
- Postinfectious glomerulonephritis
- Systemic lupus erythematosus
- Vascular disease (e.g., renal artery embolism)

appropriate in anticoagulated patients. An imaging study will aid in ruling out an anatomical cause for AMH. The preferred method of imaging is a CT urogram to evaluate the renal parenchyma; MRI is an alternative method for those who cannot tolerate a CT. See Figure 12.1.

■ Prostate Nodule, Elevated Prostate-Specific Antigen, and Asymmetric Prostate

An asymmetric prostate is typically asymptomatic and not necessarily diagnostic of prostate cancer; asymmetry can be a normal finding on DRE but should be followed periodically to monitor for changes. A questionable finding on DRE should be referred to a urology specialist.

An elevated PSA is relative to an individual's baseline PSA value or is a value that lies outside the established norms for race and age (see Table 12.4). PSA velocity is also a valuable way to gauge the significance of the PSA value; it describes the rapidity of increase in PSA over time. Generally, an increase in the PSA value of 0.75 ng/mL or more over 12 months should trigger referral for a transrectal ultrasound-guided prostate biopsy for a histological evaluation for prostatic carcinoma.

Age-specific reference ranges for PSA (see Table 12.4) should be used as a guide when there is no previous PSA for comparison. A prostatic nodule found on DRE necessitates a referral to a urologist or radiologist for transrectal ultrasound-guided prostate biopsy and may well be the first indication of the presence of a cancer.

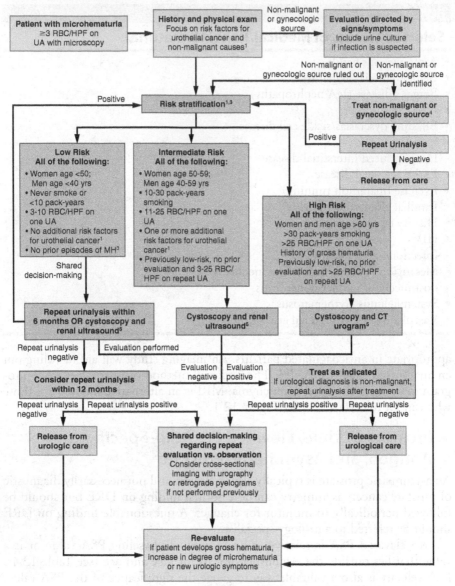

Figure 12.1 AUA algorithm for microscopic hematuria. (From Barocas, D., Boorjian, S., Alvarez, R., Downs, T., Gross, C., Hamilton, B., Kobashi, K., Lipman, R., Lotan, Y., Ng, C., Nielsen, M., Peterson, A., Raman, J., Smith-Bindman, R., & Souter, L. [2020]. Microhematuria: AUA/SUFU Guideline. *The Journal of Urology*, 204, pp. 778–786. Figure 1, p. 780.)

1. Main risk factors for urothelial cancer are those in the AUA risk stratification system (age, male sex, smoking, degree of microhematuria and history of gross hematuria). Additional risk factors for urothelial carcinoma include but are not limited to irritative lower urinary tract voiding symptoms, history of cyclophospharnide or ifosfamide chemotherapy, family history of urothelial carcinoma or Lynch Syndrome, occupational exposures to benzene chemicals or aromatic amines, history of chronic indwelling foreign body in the urinary tract.
2. If medical renal disease is suspected, consider nephrologic evaluation, and pursue concurrent risk-based urological evaluation.
3. Patients may be low-risk at first presentation with microhematuria, but may only be considered intermediate or high-risk if found to have persistent microhematuria.
4. There are non-malignant and gynecologic sources of hematuria that do not require treatment and/or may confound the diagnosis of MH. Clinicians can consider catheterized urine specimen in women with vaginal atrophy or pelvic organ prolapse. Clinicians must use careful judgment and patient engagement to decide whether to peruse MH evaluation in the setting of chronic conditions that do not require treatment, such as the aforementioned gynecologic conditions, non-obstructing stones or BPH.
5. Clinician may perform cross-section imaging with urography or retrograde pyelograms if hematuria persists after negative renal ultrasound.
6. MR Urogram or non-contrast imaging plus retrograde pyelograms if contraindications to CT urogram.

History

History should include analysis of any recent voiding symptoms, discomfort, or other GU symptoms. Family history of prostate or other malignancies should be determined. Usually there is no history of related symptoms unless BPH is present, as prostatic asymmetry or enlargement may be a finding on a routine physical examination. There may be a history of mild or moderate LUTS with obstructive features.

Physical Examination

A routine GU examination, including DRE, is required. On examination, a normal prostate is smooth with a rubbery surface (the posterior surface of the gland is palpated through the rectal wall), and the lateral lobes and median sulcus as well as the base and apex of the prostate can usually be appreciated. The seminal vesicles should not be palpable. Documentation should reflect the gland's size (estimated in grams), consistency, and symmetry and the presence or absence of nodules. Other abnormalities found during the DRE can include hemorrhoids, condyloma, and anal fissures.

Diagnostic Studies

As noted earlier, the PSA is assessed relative to the patient's age, race, and prior levels. PSA can be decreased during α-5 reductase use. Recent ejaculation has no clinically significant effect on the PSA value. Men should not be asked to abstain from sexual activities before a PSA screening test (Stenner et al., 1998), unless there is a history of elevated PSA (Herschman, Smith, & Catalona, 1997). Prostate biopsy is necessary and performed in a urology setting.

BENIGN PROSTATIC HYPERTROPHY

BPH is a nonmalignant enlargement of the transition zone of the prostate gland; the precise etiology is unclear. Risk factors are simply advancing age and normal androgen status, although there may be an additional genetic predisposition. The terms *BPH* and *obstructive symptoms* have traditionally been used to describe a collection of complaints associated with prostate overgrowth. In 2002, the International Continence Society assigned these symptoms under the term *lower urinary tract symptoms* (detailed later in this chapter). Prostate size correlates poorly with the degree of symptoms—that is, a larger size does not automatically mean worse symptoms, in part due to the subjective impressions of the patient.

Signs and Symptoms

LUTS associated with bladder outlet obstruction secondary to an enlarged prostate include urinary urgency, frequency, hesitation in getting the stream started, decreased caliber and force of stream, and nocturnal frequency of urination that is bothersome. This collection of symptoms has also been termed *prostatism*. A patient with BPH shows symmetric or asymmetric enlargement and a firm, smooth, nontender gland.

Diagnostic Studies

If the PSA level is elevated relative to the age-specific reference, or if there has been a rise greater than 0.75 ng/mL in less than 12 months, the patient should be referred to a urology specialist for discussion and management, including possible prostate biopsy or surgery to improve the urinary outlet (transurethral resection of the prostate).

PROSTATE CANCER

Early-stage prostate cancer is largely asymptomatic and is found as a result of screening for prostate cancer by DRE and PSA. Histological evaluation of biopsy specimens obtained during transrectal ultrasound-guided biopsy of the prostate provides a tissue diagnosis of prostate cancer and a Gleason score, which aids in deciding treatment options. Increased risk for prostate cancer is associated with more than two first-order relatives diagnosed with prostate cancer (Albertsen, 2018). Family members, such as grandfathers, with prostate cancer should raise the index of suspicion.

Signs and Symptoms

An asymmetric prostate, a prostatic nodule, or an elevated PSA level may be found during a routine physical examination. There may be a history of mild or moderate LUTS with obstructive features. A prostate suspicious for malignancy will demonstrate nodular areas and/or overall hardness.

Diagnostic Studies

Definitive diagnosis is made via prostate biopsy. Routine or urgent referral to a urologist is indicated, depending on the degree of PSA elevation or the degree to which it has risen since the previous value in conjunction with any suspicious findings on the rectal examination.

PROSTATITIS

Prostatitis is an acute or chronic infection of the prostate gland. Acute bacterial prostatitis is usually the result of infection by aerobic gram-negative rods (coliform bacteria or *Pseudomonas*). *Enterococcus faecalis*, an aerobic gram-positive bacteria, can also cause prostatitis. Routes of infection are ascent from the urethra, reflux of infected urine into the prostatic ducts, direct extension of bacteria, and migration via the lymphatic and vascular system. It may be associated with acute cystitis and may result in urinary retention.

Signs and Symptoms

Acute symptoms commonly include fever, low back and perineal pain, possible penis pain, urinary urgency and frequency, nocturia, dysuria, and muscle and joint aches. Transrectal palpation of the prostate reveals a very tender, boggy, swollen prostate. Urine may smell strong and be cloudy. Gross or microscopic hematuria may be present. CBC will be positive for leukocytosis and a shift to the left. Chronic prostatitis manifests as recurrent episodes of irritative symptoms of dysuria, nocturia, frequency, and urgency. Febrile episodes, gross hematuria, and hematospermia are rare. A tender, indurated epididymis can be associated with chronic prostatic infection.

Diagnostic Studies

Low back pain in the sacral area differentiates prostatitis from pyelonephritis, which manifests as flank pain. A urine culture will reveal the offending pathogen. Presentation of sudden, severe onset rather than milder, recurrent episodes differentiates acute from chronic prostatitis.

CHRONIC INFLAMMATION AND PROSTATODYNIA

The etiology of male urological chronic pelvic pain syndrome is still not certain, although an autoimmune process has not been ruled out. Further research is required to determine the putative autoantigen, the immune responses of patients, the role of bacteria in the inflammatory process, and the patient's pain response to GU insults. As yet, no diagnostic tests (other than to eliminate other pathology) and few treatments for urological chronic pelvic pain syndrome can be recommended on the basis of scientific evidence (Clemens et al., 2015).

Signs and Symptoms

The signs and symptoms are often similar to those of BPH or prostatitis, and patients may have focal pain to the genitals or rectum. Sexual function complaints may be present, and overall symptoms can wax and wane.

Diagnostic Studies

Chronic inflammation can be diagnosed only via prostate biopsy. Prostate cancer must be ruled out. Routine referral to a urologist for biopsy is indicated.

▪ Proteinuria

Proteinuria is another clinical entity that is discovered during an evaluation rather than presenting as a GU complaint. Proteinuria is an indicator of parenchymal disease of the kidney and is commonly seen in patients with conditions such as diabetic nephropathy, nephritic syndrome, autoimmune disease, multiple myeloma, and acute inflammation of the urinary tract. It can also be the result of prolonged use or abuse of NSAIDs.

History

A thorough GU-specific and general health history should be obtained if proteinuria is present. Determine whether there is a family history of potentially contributory conditions or kidney disease. Proteinuria is likely to be present with no structural abnormalities found and is almost always painless. It is important to establish the timing of proteinuria (relative to the patient's medical history): transient, intermittent, or persistent, or whether it is the initial episode.

Physical Examination

A routine GU examination is required. Other aspects of the examination are guided by the suspected cause (flank bruit, pericardial rub, skin lesions, edema). There are typically no signs or symptoms other than those resulting from the causative medical condition. A general physical examination should be completed.

Selected Causes

The medical/renal disease is glomerular, tubular, overflow, or tissue proteinuria.

Diagnostic Studies

Proteinuria is usually found on routine urinalysis; it may be falsely positive in the context of dilute urine. No further studies are indicated unless there are new progressive symptoms or the patient appears toxic or is manifesting other symptoms of renal or contributory conditions. Renal ultrasound or IVP studies can be considered in these cases (if the renal function can withstand contrast media). Referrals to a nephrologist for all persistent proteinuria and to an oncologist, as appropriate, are recommended.

LOWER URINARY TRACT SYMPTOMS

LUTS include a variety of complaints that help in the clinical identification of a potential diagnosis. Not all patients experience all symptoms, and the symptoms may be present in varying degrees at varying times. The symptoms are much more descriptive of lower urinary tract pathology in men and can be graded using a tool such as the AUA symptom score. Box 12.3 lists the components of LUTS.

Box 12.3

LUTS

- Acute retention (suprapubic pain, severe urgency)
- Chronic retention (much hesitancy starting stream, reduced force/caliber of stream)
- Cystitis
- Hesitancy (strains to force urine)
- Interruption of stream (can be accompanied by pain radiating down urethra)
- Loss of force/decreased caliber of stream (urethral resistance increases despite increased intravesical pressure)
- Sense of residual urine
- Terminal dribbling
- Urgency (strong, sudden desire to urinate owing to hyperactivity and irritability of the bladder)

The following presenting complaints represent common manifestations of disorders of the lower urinary tract. As part of the diagnosis, a measurement of a postvoid residual volume can be included with each differential that follows in this section if the clinical environment has the appropriate equipment. This measure will confirm that the patient is actually emptying the bladder or can provide a baseline against which to gauge interventions if the bladder is not being emptied.

■ Dysuria

Complaints of dysuria (burning, pain, or discomfort on urination) are more common in women than in men, largely as a result of the shorter urethral length in women. Infection is the most common cause of dysuria, and its presentation depends on which structure of the GU tract is affected. The infection can be secondary to an anatomical abnormality or abnormality of function, including postmenopausal status or prostatic hypertrophy. The patient may have undergone recent GU instrumentation or catheter placement, leading to a mechanical cause for the dysuria.

Dysuria can also be an indicator of other systemic conditions, such as diabetes mellitus, renal calculi, GU neoplasms, or depression. Debate exists over treating complaints of dysuria empirically with antibiotics, particularly when it is a recurrent complaint for a patient. The most common causes for dysuria are presented here as differentials.

History

The history should explore current voiding symptoms and history of GU problems. The patient may report pain, hesitancy, urgency, frequency, and discomfort on urination and may describe bladder fullness. There is usually a negative history of fever, chills, or other constitutional symptoms. The patient may also report a color change in urine or the presence of a strong odor to the urine. The timing of pain with urination (external, initial, during, terminal) may provide clues to the cause. Patients may have associated vaginal symptoms; everyone should be asked about their risk for STIs. The patient should also be asked about herbal, homeopathic, or vaginal hygiene remedies that may have been tried since symptom onset. Male patients should be specifically queried about the presence of LUTS, and women should be queried about incontinence and postintercourse symptoms.

Physical Examination

A routine GU examination is required, including DRE and pelvic as indicated, based on the patient's sex. A CVA examination and general abdominal examination should also be performed. The patient's general appearance should be noted, including whether the patient appears toxic.

UNCOMPLICATED URINARY TRACT INFECTION

Uncomplicated UTI is one of the most common infections seen in a primary care setting and occurs among patients of all ages, but it is more commonly seen in women. The etiology of UTIs is affected by a patient's comorbidities, including age, use of catheters, or neurological disease. The most common pathogen causing acute, uncomplicated UTIs is *E. coli*, followed by *Staphylococcus saprophyticus*, *Klebsiella*, *Enterobacter*, and *Proteus* species. Risk factors for the development of a UTI are well established and include increasing age, recent sexual intercourse, a history of UTI, use of a diaphragm or cervical cap, and anatomical abnormalities.

Signs and Symptoms

The signs and symptoms are as described in the preceding History subsection; onset is typically sudden and without other constitutional symptoms. Burning with urination, urinary frequency, suprapubic pain, and hematuria are considered classic symptoms of a UTI (Nicolle et al., 2019). Older female patients may be asymptomatic or have atypical symptoms such as confusion, dizziness, fatigue, or loss of appetite. Undiagnosed UTI can lead to urosepsis, particularly in this population.

Diagnostic Studies

According to the Infectious Disease Guidelines, the only accurate method to determine a UTI is with a urine culture when the patient is symptomatic (Nicolle et al., 2019). In women whose symptoms suggest uncomplicated UTI, a culture of greater than 10^2 CFU/mL is indicative of cystitis in a clean-catch specimen. If anatomical causes are suspected, diagnostic imaging, such as KUB or CT, should be arranged based on the suspected cause and patient's presentation. Blood for CBC and electrolytes should be considered based on the overall clinical presentation.

ASYMPTOMATIC BACTERIURIA

Using antibiotic stewardship principles, it is important to treat patients for a UTI only if they are symptomatic. Asymptomatic bacteriuria (ASB) is defined as one or more species of bacteria (greater than 100,000) with or without pyuria (white blood cells in the urine) in the absence of clinical symptoms of a UTI. Typical symptoms of an infection include dysuria, hematuria, increased frequency, and increased urgency (Nicolle et al., 2019). The treatment of ASB in nonpregnant adults is common, potentially detrimental, and has no clinical benefit (Nicolle et al., 2019). The prevalence of ASB is summarized in Table 12.8.

PAINFUL BLADDER SYNDROME/INTERSTITIAL CYSTITIS

Painful bladder syndrome (PBS)/interstitial cystitis (IC) is a poorly understood entity with a suspected cause related to a variety of factors that include autoimmune, allergic, and infectious components. PBS/IC is defined by the Society for Urodynamics and Female Urology (Hanno & Dmochowski, 2009) as an unpleasant sensation (pain, pressure, discomfort) perceived to be related to the urinary bladder, associated with LUTS of more than 6 weeks duration, in the absence of infection or other identifiable causes. Patients with IC suffer from chronic symptoms that include a combination of suprapubic pain, chronic pelvic pain, dyspareunia, dysuria, and negative urine cultures. Patients may become

Table 12.8	

ASB Prevalence

Population	Prevalence %
Healthy women	
Premenopausal	1–5
Postmenopausal (age 50–70 y)	2.8–8.6
Adults with diabetes	
Women	10.8–16
Men	3.6–19
Older adults in the community	
Women	10.8–16
Men	3.6–19
Older adults in long-term care	
Women	25–50
Men	15–50
People with spinal cord injury (using intermittent self-catheterization)	23–69
People with indwelling catheters	
Short term	3%–5%/catheter day (day one 3%–5% chance, day two 6%–10% chance)
Long term	100

Adapted from Nicolle et al., 2019.

debilitated by this disease; they may make up to 40 trips to the bathroom in 24 hours. IC is also marked by periods of remission and flare-up throughout a patient's lifetime. The prevalence of this disorder is not known. The actual diagnosis by a clinician is low (200/100,000 population), with the estimated prevalence of symptoms at 5,000/100,000 population. Typical age at onset varies from 30 to 70 years, and most patients visit an average of five physicians and wait 4 years before the correct diagnosis is made.

Signs and Symptoms

Patients describe a history of irritative voiding symptoms: urinary urgency, frequency, and pain. They may also complain of suprapubic pain, dyspareunia, and chronic pelvic pain. Symptoms may worsen in the week preceding menstruation and have often been present for a period of several months or years.

Diagnostic Studies

Urine culture will eliminate a UTI as the cause of these complaints. In order to diagnose IC, all other potential etiologies should be ruled out, including carcinoma or medication-induced cystitis. A cystoscopy may be necessary to rule out other causes, and referral to a urologist is indicated.

SEXUALLY TRANSMITTED INFECTION–RELATED URETHRITIS

Presentation of STI-related dysuria varies by sex, with female patients usually more affected than male patients. Consult the most updated Centers for

Disease Control and Prevention guidelines for details regarding identification and management.

Signs and Symptoms

See specific signs and symptoms in male and female patients in Chapters 13 and 14, respectively. Some STIs may be accompanied by complaints of constitutional symptoms or malaise.

Diagnostic Studies

STIs can be diagnosed with the appropriate cultures, Gram stains, swabs, and serological studies. Unless a patient appears ill and a white blood cell count seems indicated, no additional laboratory work or imaging studies are indicated. Treatment is often begun before the results of diagnostic tests are received; it is imperative to simultaneously treat the partner(s). Many STIs must be reported to the local health department.

COMPLICATED URINARY TRACT INFECTION

Defined as a UTI in a context that increases the likelihood of treatment failure or recurrent infection, this condition is seen in patients with GU anatomy abnormalities (e.g., BPH) or functional abnormalities (e.g., neurogenic bladder) and diabetes or other metabolic derangements. Other risk factors for a complicated UTI include male sex, pregnancy, extremely old or young age, or immunocompromised status. A complicated UTI can also be indicated when multiple organisms are present on culture. Complicated UTIs can evolve into more serious conditions, such as pyelonephritis.

Signs and Symptoms

Patient complaints are typically the same as for an uncomplicated UTI but often include constitutional symptoms. Symptom onset may be sudden or insidious. Prostatic symptoms may be present in patients with prostate enlargement, or there may be symptoms of concurrent prostatitis (see the sections on BPH and prostatitis). Complaints may also indicate upper tract involvement (see the section on pyelonephritis).

Diagnostic Studies

Initially, infected urine will be noted on urinalysis. Urine culture and sensitivity are required for diagnosis, particularly if the presentation is recurrent or refractory UTI, and appropriate laboratory work (CBC, serum electrolytes, blood cultures) should be ordered according to the patient's overall presentation and other comorbidities. Imaging studies are indicated on the basis of suspicion for anatomy abnormalities or obstruction. Hospital admission may be necessary depending on the overall clinical picture, comorbidities, hydration status, and need for further evaluation.

VAGINITIS

Vaginitis can be accompanied by irritation to adjacent structures as well as vaginal discharge and vulvar irritation. See Chapter 14 for additional discussion.

POSTMENOPAUSAL STATUS

Dysuria seen in patients after menopause can be accompanied by stress urinary incontinence (UI) and urinary frequency. All result from the mucosal thinning of the urethra and bladder in the absence of estrogen.

Signs and Symptoms

The signs and symptoms are similar to the complaints seen with a UTI but without constitutional symptoms. Patients may also experience vaginal dryness and related symptoms. Vaginal and urethral areas will appear pale owing to the diminished vascularity.

Diagnostic Studies

A history and physical examination are usually sufficient; a urinalysis will rule out a UTI.

GENITOURINARY NEOPLASM

Bladder cancer in particular can be accompanied by complaints of bladder irritability or LUTS, along with either gross or microscopic hematuria. Symptoms of bladder irritation are also common with both BPH and prostate cancer.

Signs and Symptoms

Patients with bladder cancer may have unremarkable physical findings unless there is a large-volume invasive tumor, in which case there may be a palpable thickness to the bladder. Patients who have prostate cancer may also describe LUTS and general bladder irritability; other physical findings are typically unremarkable.

Diagnostic Studies

A urinalysis is required to confirm or investigate the presence of blood. Urine cytology is needed to evaluate for malignant cells, although this will not determine the source of the abnormal cells (bladder, ureter, renal pelvis). If malignancy is suspected or confirmed, a staging CT scan should be ordered before urgent/emergent referral to a urology specialist for further management.

ANATOMIC ABNORMALITY

Anatomic abnormality includes such conditions as a ureteral or urethral stricture, duplication of the collecting system, meatal stenosis, phimosis, or vesicovaginal fistula. These conditions may become apparent after surgical procedures that promote scar tissue in the urethra, prolonged catheterization, and surgeries to the pelvic region.

Signs and Symptoms

Patients may describe a gradual onset of changes to their pattern of urination, such as spraying, painful urination, frequency, and the need to push in order to urinate. Physical examination includes a pelvic examination for women and special attention to the foreskin and meatal opening in men.

Diagnostic Studies

Physical examination alone may provide the diagnosis. Urinalysis may show some degree of contamination or a UTI. Suspicion of a structural abnormality requires referral to a urologist for further evaluation; depending on the suspected location of the abnormality, a retrograde urethrogram or IVP may be considered.

■ Difficulty Urinating or the Inability to Urinate

Urinary difficulties often occur insidiously, with few complaints from the patient until the situation is advanced or has created a social difficulty. However, when a patient has difficulty urinating or emptying the bladder, there is a motivation to seek evaluation sooner rather than later.

History

A detailed GU history is indicated, including family history, lifestyle habits, and review of symptoms. A patient may describe recurrent or persistent UTIs, dysuria, and varying LUTS, including difficulty starting the stream or nocturia. There may be a history of recent GU instrumentation, indwelling Foley catheter, or surgery. The patient may also describe a history of declining bladder control.

Physical Examination

A routine GU examination is required, including DRE in men and a pelvic examination in women.

BENIGN PROSTATIC HYPERPLASIA

See p. 413.

PROSTATITIS

See p. 414.

NEUROGENIC AND NEUROPATHIC BLADDER

Neurogenic (or neuropathic) bladder is the failure of the bladder to store or to empty. There may be spontaneous and uncoordinated contractions of the bladder when it is filling, or the bladder and sphincter may not work in concert, preventing the bladder from effectively emptying. Risk factors include spinal cord injury, trauma to the central nervous system, diabetes mellitus, spina bifida, multiple sclerosis, spinal disk disease, and pelvic surgery, among many others.

Signs and Symptoms

A variety of urinary complaints may occur, including incontinence, dribbling, and retention as well as disorders of bladder sensation. Associated complaints may reflect changes in bowel habits, sexual function, or lower extremity sensation. Physical examination involves not only a routine GU and pelvic examination but also a full neurological examination.

Diagnostic Studies

Order a urinalysis with a culture and sensitivity to rule out UTI as a treatable cause that would contribute to the complaints. Conduct other laboratory studies as suspicions dictate (such as an evaluation for diabetes). Consider an evaluation of the upper tracts with IVP or renal ultrasound. Referral to a urologist is warranted for further specialized testing.

POSTOPERATIVE URINARY RETENTION

The bladder may recover sluggishly after anesthesia, requiring a patient to embark on a short-term regimen of intermittent catheterization. A history of recent surgery that required bladder catheterization should be sufficient to confirm the diagnosis. This is more commonly seen in men.

URETHRAL LESIONS

Urethral cancer is a rare condition, but it can change the quality of the urinary stream. Some STIs can cause lesions within the urethra, resulting in pain and changes in the urinary stream.

Signs and Symptoms

The patient may complain of a splayed or intermittent urinary stream. The symptoms may be gradual in onset. There may be a history of STI, recent urethral trauma or instrumentation, or previous urethral stricture. Inspection may show visible lesions at the meatus.

Diagnostic Studies

Visual inspection may be sufficient to confirm the presence of lesions. Referral to urology for cystoscopic examination of the urethral tissue is recommended because lesions may indicate a urethral carcinoma.

BLADDER CALCULI

In the United States, bladder calculi are most frequently due to bladder outlet obstruction (e.g., BPH). They can also be caused by an elevated bladder neck in combination with an increased postvoid residual, which results in stagnant urine.

Signs and Symptoms

The presentation may be completely asymptomatic; there may be various complaints, including urinary retention, recurrent UTI, bladder pain, microscopic or gross hematuria, dysuria, urgency, or nocturia. The bladder may be palpable due to distension. Physical examination involves palpation of the bladder and, in women, pelvic examination.

Diagnostic Studies

A urine cytology and urine cultures may be considered if the patient is symptomatic. The initial imaging study can be a KUB or pelvic ultrasound, which will demonstrate the presence of one or more stones. Referral to a urology specialist for management is indicated.

■ Decreased Force of Stream or Spraying With Urination

Any change in the pattern of urination to which a patient is accustomed can be upsetting. Some of these complaints have causes that are easily remedied and may simply be related to age or pelvic floor weakness.

History

The history should include prior GU and gynecological conditions and procedures, and a general health history should be determined. The patient will give a history of decreased force and caliber of stream. Establish acute versus gradual onset and rule out genital trauma as a contributing factor. There may be a complaint of spraying with urination. Pain is not typically associated with this complaint.

Physical Examination

A routine GU examination is required, with attention to the location of the urethral opening, and DRE.

BENIGN PROSTATIC HYPERPLASIA

See p. 413.

EPISPADIAS AND HYPOSPADIAS

These conditions are more commonly diagnosed in infancy and have varying degrees of severity. Severe hypospadias in the infant can be confused with an intersex condition. In a female patient, leaving an epispadias untreated can result in incontinence as an adult. It is not uncommon for an adult male patient (hypospadias occurs in 1 of every 300 births assigned as male) to have a slight displacement of the urethral opening that was not surgically corrected during infancy or childhood. There is also an increased incidence of undescended testes with hypospadias; other consequences include infertility and upper urinary tract damage.

Signs and Symptoms

A patient may complain of a displaced urethral opening or the inability to direct the urinary stream. Patients may also complain of chordee (curvature of the penis caused by tethering of the skin and dartos fascia). A careful scrotal examination should be performed to confirm the presence of both testicles and to rule out an inguinal hernia. Rarely, the patient may present with complaints of infertility.

Diagnostic Studies

Physical examination should be sufficient to make the diagnosis. The patient should be referred to a urology specialist for further evaluation and management.

LESIONS RELATED TO SEXUALLY TRANSMITTED INFECTIONS

See discussions in Chapters 13 and 14.

DISTORTED FEMALE PELVIC ANATOMY

Cystocele, prolapse of the uterus, and failed continence surgery can all affect pelvic floor anatomy and cause urinary changes, including incontinence and changes to the quality of the urinary stream. See Chapter 14 for descriptions of these conditions.

■ Frequency, Urgency, and Hesitancy

Urinary complaints that involve frequency, urgency, or hesitancy can be seen by patient and provider alike as part of the aging process. However, in many cases, these complaints may have treatable or even reversible causes. A thorough history will sometimes uncover the cause, such as with radiation cystitis.

History

In addition to GU, gynecological, and general health history, it is important to explore the association with daily activities and the impact of the complaint on the patient's activities. All medications should be identified. These complaints may have an acute or insidious onset, particularly if irritative and obstructive symptoms are involved. The patient may provide a history of some degree of incontinence or dysuria.

Physical Examination

A routine GU examination is needed; other system examinations are dictated by history and accompanying complaints. Patients may have a palpable bladder on examination.

INTERSTITIAL CYSTITIS

See p. 418.

URINARY TRACT INFECTION

See p. 417.

BENIGN PROSTATIC HYPERPLASIA

See p. 413.

NEUROGENIC OR NEUROPATHIC BLADDER

See p. 422.

VOLUME- OR METABOLIC-RELATED CAUSE

The kidneys receive roughly 20% of cardiac output and have a major role in the volume and electrolyte homeostasis of the body. Changes to the fluid and electrolyte balance of the body can directly affect urinary output, such as in the osmotic diuresis seen with poorly controlled or undiagnosed diabetes mellitus.

Other examples include diabetes insipidus, metabolic acidosis and alkalosis, renal insufficiency, and congestive heart failure.

Signs and Symptoms

Volume- or metabolic-related conditions often involve varying GU complaints along with frequency, urgency, and hesitancy. Other systemic complaints representative of the particular endocrinopathy or underlying disease process will occur. The physical examination involves a routine GU examination and additional system examinations as indicated by presentation and history.

Diagnostic Studies

Urinalysis should be performed to rule out a UTI as a treatable cause contributing to the complaints. Other laboratory studies can be ordered as suspicions dictate (such as evaluation for diabetes), particularly electrolytes. Referral to the appropriate subspecialty may be needed for further diagnosis and management.

DRUG-INDUCED EFFECTS

Patients may complain of frequency that they associate with a particular medication. Alternatively, this association may not be clear until a complete list of the patient's medications is available.

Signs and Symptoms

Signs and symptoms are primarily frequency and urgency, both of which may be complicated by coexisting GU conditions, such as BPH, some type of incontinence, or mobility issues.

Diagnostic Studies

A review of a patient's medications and administration schedule should be sufficient to determine that a diuretic is a contributing cause. Consider urinalysis to rule out a UTI.

NEOPLASTIC (BLADDER OR RENAL CANCER)

See pp. 402, 421.

■ Nocturia

As nocturia persists, patients become more likely to seek evaluation and treatment. They begin to suffer fatigue from sleep interruption and deprivation, as there may be 45 minutes or less between urges to urinate.

History

The duration of the problem may be difficult to gauge because the onset may have occurred over several months. The patient's overall disposition and energy level should be noted. The patient should be asked to estimate the average number of episodes per night, and the presence of associated LUTS should be queried.

Physical Examination

A routine GU examination is needed; a pelvic examination or full physical examination may be indicated by history.

BENIGN PROSTATIC HYPERPLASIA

See p. 413.

INTERSTITIAL CYSTITIS

See p. 418.

VOLUME- OR METABOLIC-RELATED DISORDER

See p. 425.

EXCESSIVE FLUID INTAKE IN EVENING

When questioned, the patient will describe a pattern of increased fluid intake later in the day. History is usually sufficient to confirm the cause.

PHARMACOLOGICALLY INDUCED

This problem can present when a patient times the administration of a diuretic late in the afternoon or evening, with consequent complaints of urinary frequency late into the night. A review of medications and their timing should be sufficient to confirm this cause.

■ Urinary Incontinence

UI is a prevalent and costly public health problem. In population-based studies, overactive bladder prevalence rates range from 7% to 27% in men and 9% to 43% in women. Men can experience UI after pelvic surgery or owing to prostate enlargement. Women may experience UI after pelvic surgery, from numerous pregnancies and deliveries, or from a prolapsed uterus and/or bladder. The prevalence of UI increases as age increases; approximately 50% of older people in extended care are incontinent of urine, and 33% are incontinent all or most of the time. Given the increase in numbers of the aging population, UI will continue to affect large numbers of the population. Added costs arise from complications of UI, such as loss of wages, poor quality of life, depression, and loss of self-esteem, which increases the financial burden of UI even further (Lightner et al., 2019).

As a result of the constant production of urine and the bladder's finite storage capacity, incontinence will occur in anyone who does not have timely access to facilities, regardless of age, mobility, or sex. Box 12.4 lists several recognized patterns of urine loss.

The bladder has several functional features that contribute to normal continence: its normal capacity of 400 to 500 mL; the fullness sensation; the ability to accommodate various volumes without changes in intraluminal pressure;

Box 12.4

Patterns of Incontinence

- *Stress incontinence*, or the loss of urine with activities that cause changes in intra-abdominal pressure, such as sneezing, lifting, or exercise.
- *Urge incontinence*, or the loss of urine that results from detrusor overactivity at unusually low volumes of urine; symptoms can include involuntary loss of urine preceded by an urgent and compelling desire to void.
- *Mixed incontinence*, or a combination of both stress and urge incontinence.
- *Functional incontinence*, or the inability to make it to the toilet before losing control and/or an inability to undress properly; commonly influenced by both cognitive and functional status.
- *Overflow incontinence*, or a bladder that does not empty completely owing to outlet obstruction or neurogenic causes and subsequently spills urine when full.

---

the ability to initiate and sustain contraction until the bladder is empty; and a response to the voluntary inhibition of voiding despite the inherent involuntary nature of the organ.

The bladder receives afferent and efferent innervation from both the autonomic and the somatic nervous systems. Parasympathetic innervation arises from sacral segments 2–4 and projects to the pelvic plexus, supplying both the bladder and sphincter. Sympathetic control originates at the T10–L2 level. Somatic innervation originates from S2–S3 and travels via the pudendal nerve to the external urethral sphincter and permits the sensation of fullness, inflammation, or pain, depending on the specific pathway. Damage or other pathologies that affect these areas of the spine (herniated disk, spinal stenosis, degenerative changes in the vertebrae, or metastatic disease) can result in changes to bladder function and sensation. Diseases that result in neuropathies (e.g., diabetes mellitus, multiple sclerosis) can contribute to the dysfunction of bladder sensation and function.

Sex-specific anatomy may explain some of the difference in the incidence of UI. Female sex assigned at birth greatly increases the risk for UI, as does childbearing. Age is a risk factor but is not causative; some age-related changes associated with the urinary tract are normal. The most significant age-related changes in women are related to decreased estrogen influence. As estrogen levels decline, the epithelium and supporting tissues of the pelvis atrophy, resulting in friable mucosa and possible prolapse of the pelvic structures. The change in relationship of the pelvic structures results in hypermobility of the bladder base, pelvic muscle weakness, and urethral weakness, resulting in stress UI in women. The decreased glycogen content of the vaginal epithelium causes decreased lactic acid metabolism by Döderlein's bacillus, an increased pH of vaginal secretions, and therefore an increased risk for a UTI.

A variety of history and assessment points aid in narrowing the etiology of a patient's specific complaints.

History

Obtain a thorough GU history, including a detailed description of the type of incontinence experienced. Ask about activities that seem to trigger urine loss and any efforts the patient has taken to avoid or adapt to the incontinence. The patient will report some pattern of involuntary loss of urine; this may occur under specific circumstances or be nearly continuous. Detailing the context in which the urine loss occurs will aid with diagnosis. A general history is important, as existing comorbidities and surgical history provide additional clues to the etiology of the incontinence.

Physical Examination

A routine GU examination, including DRE, and, in women, a pelvic examination are needed.

Selected Causes

See Table 12.9.

Diagnostic Studies

The initial evaluation should include a urinalysis to rule out reversible causes of incontinence, such as a UTI. Consider a urine culture based on urinalysis results, BUN, and creatinine, as history and comorbidities indicate, and measurement of a postvoid residual volume to help distinguish the type of incontinence. If an imaging study is needed, the initial choice is renal ultrasound. Refer to a urology or urogynecology specialist as needed for specialized testing and concerns regarding an anatomic basis for the incontinence.

Table 12.9

Selected Causes of Urinary Incontinence

Female	Male	All
• Childbirth • Cystocele • Estrogen deficiency (atrophic vaginitis or urethritis) • Failed previous surgery to correct incontinence • Hysterectomy • Rectocele • Vesicovaginal fistula	• Prostatic hypertrophy • Prostatitis • Post-radical prostatectomy	• *Anatomical* (constipation; urinary retention; pelvic, back, or retroperitoneal surgery) • *Irritative* (interstitial cystitis, urinary tract infection) • *Metabolic* (diabetes mellitus, diabetes insipidus, aging) • *Neurological* (dementia, peripheral or autonomic neuropathy, spinal cord trauma or lesions, multiple sclerosis, diabetes) • *Pharmacological* (diuretics, sedatives, anticholinergics, alpha-adrenergic blockade) • *Vascular* (stroke)

REFERENCES

Albertsen, P. C. (2018).Prostate cancer screening with prostate-specific antigen: Where are we going? *Cancer,* *124*(3), 453–455. https://doi.org/10.1002/cncr.31140

American Urological Association. (2016). Diagnosis, Evaluation and Follow-up of Asymptomatic Microhematuria (AMH) in Adults. https://www.auanet.org//guidelines/asymptomatic-microhematuria-(amh)-guideline

Assimos, D., Krambeck, A., Miller, N. L., Monga, M., Murad, M. H., Nelson, C. P., Pace, K. T., Pais, V. M., Pearle, M. S., Preminger, G. M., Razvi, H., Shah, O., & Matlaga, B. R. (2016). Surgical management of stones: American Urological Association/Endourological Society guideline, part I. *The Journal of Urology.* https://pubmed.ncbi.nlm.nih.gov/27238616/

Barry, M. J., Fowler, F. J. Jr., O'Leary, M. P., Bruskewitz, R. C., Holtgrewe, H. L., Mebust, W. K., & Cockett, A. T. (1992). The American Urological Association symptom index for benign prostatic hyperplasia. *Journal of Urology, 148*(5), 1549–1557.

Bishoff, J. T. R., & Art, R. (2016). Urinary tract imaging: basic principles of computed tomography, magnetic resonance imaging, and a plain film. In: A. J. Wein, L. Kavoussi, A.W. Partin, & C. A. Peters (Eds.), *Campbell-Walsh urology* (11th ed. pp. 26–62e3). Elsevier.

Clemens, J. Q., Clauw, D. J., Kreder, K., Krieger, J. N., Kusek, J. W., Lai, H. H., & Landis, J. R. (2015). Comparison of baseline urological symptoms in men and women in the MAPP research cohort. *The Journal of Urology, 193*(5), 1554–1558.

Herschman, J., Smith, D., & Catalona, W. (1997). Effect of ejaculation on serum total and free prostate-specific antigen concentrations. *Urology, 50*(2), 239–243.

Hanno, P., & Dmochowski, R. (2009). Status of international consensus on interstitial cystitis/bladder pain syndrome/painful bladder syndrome: 2008 snapshot. *Neurology and Urodynamics, 28*(4), 274–286.

Lightner, D. J., Gomelsky, A., Souter, L., & Vasavada, S. P. (2019). Diagnosis and treatment of overactive bladder (non-neurogenic) in adults: AUA/SUFU Guideline amendment 2019. *Journal of Urology, 202;* 558.

Nicolle, L., Gupta, K., Bradley, S., Colgan, R., DeMuri, G. P., Drekonja, D., & Siemieniuk, R. (2019). Clinical practice guidelines for the management of asymptomatic bacteriuria: 2019 update by the Infectious Diseases Society of America. *Clinical Infectious Diseases, 68,* e83–e110.

Perlman, E. S., Rosenfield, A. T., Wexler, J. S., & Glickman, M. G. (1996). CT urography in the evaluation of urinary tract disease. *Journal of Computer Assisted Tomography, 20*(4), 620–626.

Richardson, T. D., & Oesterling, J. E. (1997). Age-specific reference ranges for serum prostate specific antigen. *Urological Clinics of North America, 24*(2), 339–351.

Rodger, F., Roditi, G., & Aboumarzouk, O. M. (2018). Diagnostic accuracy of low and ultra-low dose CT for identification of urinary tract stones: A systematic review. Urologia Internationalis, *100*(4), 375–385. https//doi.org/10.1159/000488062

Stenner, J., Holthaus, K., Mackenzie, S. H., & Crawford, E. D. (1998). The effect of ejaculation on prostate-specific antigen in a prostate cancer-screening population. *Urology, 51*(3), 455–459.

Yallappa, S., Amer, T., Patrick Jones, P., Francesco Greco, F., Thomas Tailly, T., Bhaskar, K., Somani, B. K., Nkem Umez-Eronini, N., Aboumarzouk, O. M. (2018). Natural history of conservatively managed ureteral stones: Analysis of 6600 patients." *Journal of Endourology, 32*(5), 371–379. doi:10.1089/end.2017.0848

Chapter 13

Male Reproductive System

Susanne A. Quallich ·

K nowledge of the anatomy and the ability to focus the history on the pre-senting complaint are the keys to accurately assessing complaints related to the male reproductive system (Fig. 13.1). Most of the information needed to arrive at an accurate diagnosis is gained through inspection, palpation, and a precise history. Because not all assessment points are relevant to every complaint, taking a problem-focused history is vital.

History

■ General History

In order to confirm normal physiological male development, the patient's general history relative to reproductive or genital complaints should first establish that puberty started in the early or middle teens. The history should include any past reproductive complaints; a discussion of any recent (within the last 6 months) systemic illness; recent weight gain or loss; new-onset pain to any of the reproductive organs; and smoking, alcohol consumption, and illicit drug use. It must also include a listing of current prescription and over-the-counter medications. As each complaint is discussed in this chapter, additional general and specific history-taking points are presented.

■ Past Medical History

The evaluation should proceed to a history of any condition that would affect the penis, testes, or hormones (including cryptorchidism, hypothyroidism, pituitary malfunction); any history of genitourinary (GU) surgeries (e.g., orchidopexy; YV plasty to bladder neck; inguinal hernia repair as infant, small child, or adult; epispadias or hypospadias repair; prostate surgery; bladder reconstructions; bladder surgeries; testicular surgeries); previous treatment for testicular or GU malignancies; and a history of vasectomy and when it was performed.

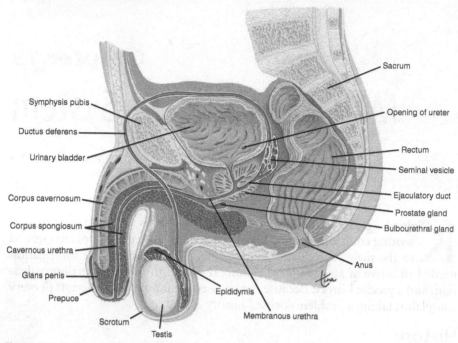

Figure 13.1 Anatomical structure of the male reproductive system. (From Scanlon, V. C., & Sanders, T. [2015]. *Essentials of anatomy and physiology* [7th ed.]. Philadelphia, PA: F. A. Davis. Reprinted with permission.)

▪ Family History

The family history should include a discussion of testicular or other GU malignancies, prostate or bladder problems in other family members (including female relatives with bladder conditions), other members of the family with complaints similar to the patient's presenting complaint, and a history of maternal medication or drug use while pregnant if known.

▪ Sexual History

A sexual history is particularly relevant when the main complaint involves the GU system. The history should include recent changes in sexual partners and sexual orientation, overall pattern of sexual activity, recent treatment for sexually transmitted infection (STI), history of having previously fathered any children, libido, erectile function, and evaluation and treatment of a partner that may have preceded the patient's current visit. Providers may also inquire about BDSM (bondage, discipline, domination, submission) practices as appropriate to presenting complaints.

▪ Habits

This discussion will include any activity that puts the groin area at risk for trauma (e.g., football, hockey, cycling, motocross, riding three- or four-wheeled vehicles). It also includes any potential exposure to environmental toxins.

Physical Examination

Examination of the male patient is best done in a warm room in order to avoid exaggeration of the cremaster reflex. For the purposes of this chapter, a routine genital examination involves inspection and palpation of the male genitalia, and a routine GU examination involves the routine genital examination and digital rectal examination (DRE). Specialized examination maneuvers are indicated as needed.

■ Order of the Examination

Inspection

Look for age-appropriate development of male secondary sex characteristics; lesions or scarring of the penis, scrotum, or groin; discoloration of the penis, scrotum, or groin; asymmetry of testicles; gynecomastia; location and size of the opening of the meatus; and presence of scars in the abdomen, groin, or inguinal areas. The tone of the dartos muscle governs the size of the scrotum; in a cool environment, as it causes the scrotum to contract.

Auscultation

Auscultate the abdomen as indicated (refer to Chapter 11). Auscultation is rarely indicated in the evaluation of male reproductive complaints except with a suspected herniation of bowel into the scrotum or as part of a complete physical.

Percussion

Percuss the abdomen as indicated (refer to Chapter 11). Percussion is rarely indicated in the evaluation of male reproductive complaints except as part of a complete physical. See the box for red flag presentations.

Palpation

Palpation is the most important part of the physical examination. The examination requires palpation of all suspected intrascrotal masses—that is, masses that may arise from the surface of the testicle or adjacent to or separate from the testes, scrotal skin, or scrotal wall. Table 13.1 reviews the palpation of the male reproductive structures.

RED FLAG ◄ **Red Flags in the Assessment of the Male Reproductive System**

- *Sudden onset of acute testicular pain*
- *Cellulitic or necrotic changes to the skin of the scrotum, penis, perineal region*
- *Erection lasting more than 60 minutes after cessation of sexual activity, without a decrease in turbidity*
- *Inability to urinate*
- *New mass, painful mass, or previously identified mass that is newly painful in the scrotum*

Table 13.1

Palpation of Male Reproductive Structures

Male Reproductive Structure	Normal Findings on Palpation	Abnormalities and Possible Significance
Penis	• Soft and pliable along length of shaft • Meatus midline and central to glans • Foreskin should retract and draw forward easily	• Areas of fibrous plaque along shaft—Peyronie's disease • Tenderness—possibly secondary to a urethral stricture • Difficulty with foreskin retraction—phimosis, edema, balanitis, balanoposthitis • Difficulty moving foreskin forward—paraphimosis, edema • Entire shaft of penis fibrous and with reduced pliability—previous priapism • Meatus not midline or central to glans—hypospadias, epispadias
Scrotum	• Loose sac of skin partially covered with hair	• Areas of erythema or nodularity—infected sebaceous glands or hair follicles • Unilateral, uncomfortable swelling of the scrotum—hydrocele, hematoma, varicocele
Testes	• Two testes, freely movable within the scrotum • Palpate between thumb and first two fingers of the hand • Firm, smooth, rubbery consistency • Average 6 cm × 4 cm in size • Symmetrical • Right testicle may be slightly anterior to left • Separate from epididymis	• Mass associated with testicle—tumor, hydrocele, spermatocele • Solitary testes—nondescent of testicle or previous surgical removal • Small, soft testicle(s)—Klinefelter disease, history of infection, late orchidopexy
Epididymis	• Soft ridge of tissue longitudinally posterior to the testicle • Separate from testicle	• Cystic or nodular—spermatocele, previous or current infection, history of vasectomy • Large and fluctuant—spermatocele • Localized pain—epididymitis, postvasectomy pain syndrome
Vas deferens and spermatic cord	• Soft, rubbery consistency • Smooth along its length • Able to trace vas deferens from epididymis to inguinal canal	• Absence of vas bilaterally or unilaterally—cystic fibrosis or a variant • Sperm granuloma—postvasectomy • Congested veins unilaterally or bilaterally—varicocele • Beading/nodularity of the cord—obstruction of epididymis, tubercular infection of the epididymis

■ Special Maneuvers

Table 13.2 outlines several physical examination maneuvers specific to the assessment of male reproductive complaints.

DIFFERENTIAL DIAGNOSIS OF CHIEF COMPLAINTS

GENERAL COMPLAINTS

■ Testicular or Scrotal Pain

Pain in the testicles or scrotum can present as an acute, nauseating pain after trauma to the area; a dull ache with a progressive onset; and the sharp, focused pain associated with an infection. A focused history and targeted examination often provide the necessary clues to diagnosis.

Table 13.2

Physical Examination Maneuvers for Assessment of Male Reproductive Complaints

Maneuver	Description
Cremasteric reflex	Brushing or touching the skin of the scrotum in a downward direction will result in the prompt elevation of the testicle on the same side. This reaction can be aggravated by a cool room—the reflex may have engaged before any contact with the examiner.
Digital rectal examination	Gloved, lubricated finger is inserted into the anus and swept across the surface of the prostate; prostate should be symmetrical, nontender, free of nodules, approximately the size of a walnut, and have a smooth, rubbery consistency. Examination also involves estimation of anal sphincter tone.
Examination for hernia	Index finger is inserted into the scrotum and invaginated into the external inguinal ring (scrotum should be invaginated in front of the testicle); fingertips of other hand should then be placed over the internal inguinal canal and patient should be asked to Valsalva. A hernia will be felt as a bulge that descends against index finger with Valsalva maneuver.
Neurological examination	Testing of superficial anal reflex (perianal sensation)—stroking the anus with a cotton swab will result in reflexive contraction of the external anal sphincter ("anal wink"). Testing of bulbocavernosus reflex—inserting a gloved finger into the anus and squeezing the glans penis will result in contraction of the anal sphincter and bulbocavernosus muscles. (These tests are most helpful when evaluating complaints of erectile and ejaculatory dysfunction.)
Transillumination of hydrocele	Light source shined through mass; hydrocele will glow reddish, may feel as though it surrounds testicle, and may feel turbid or tense.
Transillumination of spermatocele	Light source shined through mass; should palpate testicle as separate from the spermatocele; note that the epididymis may not be palpated separately from the spermatocele; the mass feels connected to testicle at testicle's superior aspect.
Valsalva maneuver to evaluate for varicocele	Performed with patient standing and in a warm room; having patient perform Valsalva will reverse the flow into the pampiniform plexus and result in palpable distension of the vessels ("bag of worms" if varicocele is of sufficient size).

History

Trauma may precede the complaint of pain in the testes or scrotum; it is important to establish the mechanism of injury if possible. The patient may report acute pain or progressive pain and tenderness after the insult. There may be a history of a sudden onset of acute pain and elevation of the affected testicle. The onset of the discomfort also may have occurred over time and could be associated with lesions or drainage from the scrotum; in such a case, the patient may also provide a history of recurrent scrotal infections and current constitutional symptoms, such as fever, chills, malaise, and nausea. Sudden onset of testicular pain may also be related to a musculoskeletal cause or radicular source and present in conjunction with back, sacroiliac, or hip pain.

Physical Examination

A thorough examination of the genitals is vital despite the fact that it may cause additional discomfort to the patient. Examination may reveal generalized tenderness of the scrotum and its contents, unilateral scrotal swelling, localized tenderness to one or more of the scrotal structures, or painful and edematous genitalia. If mild or moderate trauma is involved, ecchymotic areas or abrasions may be observed. In the case of radicular contributors, the pain may not localize to a specific scrotal or genital structure.

TESTICULAR TORSION

Testicular torsion is most commonly diagnosed in early puberty and results in the loss of blood flow to the affected testicle. Compromised blood flow results in swelling and tissue necrosis after 6 to 8 hours. There are no established risk factors, but it is more common during adolescence possibly due to the rapid growth of the testes.

Signs and Symptoms

Patients experience an acute and sudden onset of pain that localizes in the affected testicle, but it may also radiate to the inguinal areas or abdomen. This pain is often accompanied by abdominal discomfort, nausea, and vomiting. Asymmetric scrotal swelling is apparent on physical examination, with the affected testicle being somewhat elevated. The affected testicle may also have a somewhat horizontal lie. Traditional landmarks within the scrotum may be difficult to assess because of edema, and the cremaster reflex may be absent on the affected side. A history of a sports injury may be reported by the patient.

Diagnostic Studies

Testicular torsion is a true urological emergency that must be identified quickly. If it is suspected, the patient must be immediately referred to the closest emergency department for evaluation, imaging, and probable surgery to try to preserve the testicle (Box 13.1).

Box 13.1

Decision Rule: Testicular Torsion

Waldert and colleagues (2010) looked at color-flow with Doppler ultrasonography and its utility in evaluating testicular torsion. Their retrospective review was of 298 boys who presented with possible testicular torsion. The scrotal ultrasound sensitivity and specificity for identifying testicular torsion were 96.8% and 97.9%, respectively. Positive and negative predictive values were 92.1% and 99.1%, respectively. There is the potential for false negative with ultrasound in this group, especially if it is early in the natural history of torsion or in the setting of incomplete torsion.

FOURNIER'S GANGRENE

Fournier's gangrene is a progressive necrotizing fasciitis of the genitals and perineum, most commonly seen in males in their sixth decade, and usually caused by a combination of aerobic and anaerobic organisms. It can progress to involve the entire perineal area, abdominal wall, and buttocks. Risk factors for its development include poor personal hygiene with or without obesity, phimosis, undiagnosed or poorly controlled diabetes, alcoholism, malnutrition, chemotherapy or radiation treatment, perirectal or perianal infections, and local trauma to the genitals or perineal area (such as surgery).

Signs and Symptoms

There may be a prodromal period of generalized discomfort followed by erythema and edema in the affected areas. Cellulitic changes are apparent on physical examination and may be accompanied by crepitus, dark purple coloration, necrosis, eschar, and a foul odor. Often there are constitutional complaints of fever, chills, nausea, and vomiting, and the patient may progress to frank sepsis. Specific urological complaints may be noted as well, including dysuria, urethral discharge, or urethral obstruction.

Diagnostic Studies

A scrotal ultrasound can be helpful in defining areas of crepitus, but this should not delay referral. If Fournier's gangrene is suspected, the patient must be immediately referred to the closest emergency department for evaluation and probable admission. This is a true urological emergency that must be identified quickly.

INCARCERATED INGUINAL HERNIA

See Chapters 11 and 12.

TESTICULAR MASS OR TUMOR

Malignant tumors of the testes are uncommon, usually present for those between the ages of 15 and 35, are slightly more common on the right side, and arise from germ cells. The greatest risk factor for the development of a testicular tumor is cryptorchidism, with an overall incidence of 7% to 10% in the patient with a history of unilateral or bilateral undescended testes. Increased screening and early detection have significantly decreased the mortality from this malignancy, but up to 10% of patients present with pain and/or constitutional or pulmonary complaints that indicate metastasis.

Signs and Symptoms

A patient or his partner may have noticed a painless swelling of the testicle or a distinct nodule on self-examination. Minor trauma may have occurred to the affected side and initiated the onset of pain and/or swelling. The testicle gradually enlarges over time with some associated heaviness. Patients can complain of acute pain as their presenting symptom but usually present with history of a dull ache or heaviness that localizes to the affected side. Physical examination reveals a distinct mass or diffuse enlargement of the affected testicle; the mass may be firm, smooth, nodular, or fixed; the scrotum itself may feel warm and be erythematous. Palpation of the inguinal, supraclavicular, and axillary areas may show evidence of enlarged lymph nodes; examination of the abdomen may also demonstrate bulky retroperitoneal disease. In advanced disease, gynecomastia resulting from hormonal changes and wheezing due to lung metastasis may be observed.

Diagnostic Studies

The ultrasound is considered an extension of the physical examination in the case of a suspected testicular mass; a scrotal ultrasound can quickly and accurately distinguish a tumor from other intrascrotal pathologies. Lactate dehydrogenase (LDH), α-fetoprotein (AFP), and beta human chorionic gonadotropin (β-hCG) are the biochemical markers required to diagnose and classify testicular masses. In addition to routine chemistries and a white blood cell count, a chest x-ray and computed tomography (CT) scan of the chest, abdomen, and pelvis complete the metastatic workup. Removal of the testicle is necessary for an accurate pathological diagnosis. The patient should be referred urgently to a urologist; in many cases, the removal of the testicle and prompt treatment of the associated adenopathy can be curative, depending on the stage of the disease.

EPIDIDYMITIS

This inflammation of the epididymis is caused by the spread of an infection from the bladder or urethra owing to an alteration in the urethral closure mechanism. Uncircumcised men and men with indwelling catheters, benign prostatic hypertrophy, recent GU instrumentation, or prostatic surgery are at risk for epididymitis. In heterosexual men younger than 35, the causative organisms are likely to be *Neisseria gonorrhoeae* and *Chlamydia trachomatis*. In gay men, the causative organism is usually *Escherichia coli*. In cases where an organism associated with an STI is suspected, the exposure to the organism can significantly predate the development of epididymitis. If epididymitis is left unrecognized and untreated, it can progress to an abscess or chronic infection with resulting fibrosis, chronic scrotal pain, and infertility.

Signs and Symptoms

Complaints usually involve a sudden onset (over 24 to 48 hours) of painful swelling in the scrotum, which can be unilateral or bilateral. Pain may decrease with elevation of the scrotum (Prehn's sign), although this is an unreliable indicator. There may be an associated urethral discharge and/or fever, and complaints of urethritis, cystitis, or prostatitis are possible. On physical examination, the pain will localize to the affected epididymis with palpation, which will be swollen and indurated. The spermatic cord is usually tender and swollen, and pain may radiate to the inguinal canal and/or flank. Examination can be difficult, as inflammation can distort the anatomy, and manipulation is likely to increase the patient's complaints of pain.

Diagnostic Studies

An ultrasound will differentiate between testicular torsion and epididymitis, and it can be helpful in establishing the correct diagnosis in cases of the acute onset of pain (e.g., epididymitis versus torsion). Laboratory tests are not usually necessary, although the patient may exhibit an elevated white blood cell count with a fever. If an STI is suspected on the basis of history, a Gram stain of a urethral smear or urine culture can be ordered, and the partner must also be treated to prevent recurrent episodes. Treatment should follow the most recent Centers for Disease Control and Prevention (CDC) recommendations.

ORCHITIS

Orchitis is usually caused by the extension of an infection from the epididymis to the testicle and rarely exists independent of epididymitis. The risks and causative organisms are the same as for epididymitis. Orchitis may also occur as a sequela of mumps and occurs in up to 30% of prepubertal male patients with mumps.

Signs and Symptoms

The signs and symptoms are the same as those for epididymitis. On physical examination, the pain localizes to the affected testicle, and it may not be possible to distinguish the separation between the epididymis and the testicle owing to inflammation. A reactive hydrocele may form.

Diagnostic Studies

The diagnostics are the same as those for epididymitis, although an ultrasound is not typically needed.

HYDROCELE

A hydrocele is a collection of fluid between the layers of the tunica vaginalis, which surrounds the testicle, or fluid along the spermatic cord. The fluid is primarily water with some albumin. It often occurs unilaterally, and its origin is idiopathic in adult men, although there appears to be some decreased absorption of this fluid by the tunica itself. The fluid collection may be large enough to completely encompass the testicle.

Signs and Symptoms

Hydroceles are not usually painful, and they frequently present as a unilateral swelling of the scrotum that may extend into the inguinal canal. Men may report that there is less pronounced swelling early in the day that worsens as they go about their daily activities. There may be associated heaviness or discomfort during specific activities, such as prolonged standing, prolonged sitting, or bicycling. It may not be possible to feel the testicle during a physical examination if the hydrocele is large enough, and it is possible for the scrotal skin to suffer excoriation and erythema. A hydrocele can be confirmed with transillumination. A large hydrocele can distort the position of the other scrotal structures, particularly the epididymis, and make their identification challenging.

Diagnostic Studies

A scrotal ultrasound is not necessary but will definitively confirm a hydrocele and rule out any testicular pathology if the testicle cannot be palpated.

VARICOCELE

A varicocele is a palpable or visible dilation of the vessels of the pampiniform plexus in the scrotum; retrograde reflux of venous blood in the internal spermatic vein dilates the pampiniform plexus. Varicoceles are more common on the left, owing to the greater distance the internal spermatic vein must traverse to the left renal vein when compared with the right. The etiology of varicoceles remains unclear, and there are no specific risk factors. It is unusual for males to exhibit a varicocele before adolescence, and most varicoceles are asymptomatic. Varicoceles are commonly diagnosed during a routine health maintenance examination or during a urology or male infertility evaluation (semen parameters are often decreased; varicoceles represent a common cause of secondary male infertility) or less commonly during an evaluation for scrotal pain or a scrotal mass. If a varicocele is painful, the pain may increase with prolonged standing, exertion, or sitting; pain is rare after prolonged recumbency or sleeping. A varicocele typically presents unilaterally on the left side. The acute onset of a painful varicocele, on the left or right, may indicate obstruction of the spermatic or renal vein and warrants more urgent evaluation.

Signs and Symptoms

Most varicoceles are asymptomatic, but the patient may complain of a dull ache, fullness, pain that does not radiate, or pulling to the affected side of the scrotum. If the varicocele is large enough, it typically results in scrotal swelling that is noticeable to the patient, along with a bluish discoloration beneath the scrotal skin. Primary or secondary male infertility may be the presenting symptom. The varicocele can be exaggerated during physical examination by asking the patient to perform the Valsalva maneuver while standing; any distension of the pampiniform plexus should disappear when the patient lies down. A long-standing varicocele may cause testicular atrophy. If the varicocele is large, it may be visible during inspection ("bag of worms").

Diagnostic Studies

A scrotal ultrasound is not necessary but will definitively confirm a varicocele and rule out any testicular or scrotal pathology. The ultrasound must be specifically ordered to "r/o varicocele" to ensure that the test is done correctly for this finding. A solitary right-sided varicocele can be a sign of right renal vein obstruction, and an abdominal CT scan should be ordered to rule out any pathology. The patient can be routinely referred to a urology provider for further assessment and management, particularly if there are fertility concerns.

SPERMATOCELE

A spermatocele is usually a painless mass in the head of the epididymis that contains fluid and sperm. Since sperm are not produced until puberty, this lesion is never seen in preadolescents. Patients may complain of a scrotal mass that feels like "a third testicle" if it is sizable. If the mass is small, it can also be termed an epididymal cyst.

Signs and Symptoms

The spermatocele usually presents as a nontender mass that is clearly distinct from and above the testicle on palpation. Larger spermatoceles may present as a turbid mass; smaller lesions may feel more nodular. A spermatocele can sometimes be transilluminated.

Diagnostic Studies

Diagnostic studies are usually not necessary. A scrotal ultrasound is not necessary but will definitively confirm a spermatocele and rule out any testicular pathology. Lesions as small as 2 mm can be detected by ultrasound.

■ Testicular Mass

Any complaint of a testicular mass is considered malignant until proven otherwise.

History

The patient may report sudden or acute onset of a painful or tender testicle. Most patients are unable to report the length of time the lesion has actually been present. If the patient has felt a palpable mass, he may give history of increasing size and/or tenderness over a period of weeks or months. In addition to the history of how the mass has developed and any associated changes such as pain or discomfort, explore the patient's general health and review of systems, assessing urinary symptoms and presence of any systemic symptoms.

Physical Examination

A thorough examination of the genitals is vital, despite the fact that it may cause discomfort to the patient. Pain or tenderness may be noted on the examination and may localize to the testicle, where a palpable mass can be felt either continuous with the testicle or adjacent to it. There may or may not be inguinal adenopathy associated with the testicular pain.

TESTICULAR TUMOR

See pp. 437–438.

TESTICULAR TORSION

See p. 436.

HYDROCELE

See pp. 439–440.

SPERMATOCELE

See p. 441.

VARICOCELE

See pp. 440–441.

HEMATOMA

The patient describes a steadily enlarging, firm, and possibly painful mass located unilaterally in the scrotum. The mass can be of varying sizes. The key point is a recent history of some invasive procedure, such as a vasectomy, hydrocelectomy, spermatocelectomy, or trauma sustained during sports activities or a motor vehicle accident.

Signs and Symptoms

The patient will complain of an enlarging mass that became noticeable within a few days after his surgical procedure. Physical examination will usually show a unilateral firm mass that is nontender on palpation. Pain is caused by distortion and displacement of the surrounding structures.

Diagnostic Studies

A scrotal ultrasound is not necessary but will definitively confirm a hematoma and rule out any other pathology. Small hematomas can be expected to resolve over time as they are reabsorbed. Large hematomas may need to be drained; the patient should be referred back to the provider who performed the procedure.

■ Scrotal Mass

A scrotal mass can cause great concern for patient and clinician alike and may be detected by self-examination or during a routine physical. The key to diagnosing the mass is a thorough examination of the scrotal contents in an attempt to localize the mass and identify any associated structures.

History

The patient presents with complaints of a painful or nonpainful mass in the scrotum. He may provide a long history of its presence in the scrotum or a history of recently increasing size. There may also be discomfort associated with the mass, and it may worsen with activities such as running, weight lifting, or the Valsalva maneuver.

Physical Examination

A routine genital examination is required, with additional special maneuvers based on findings and the suspected cause.

INGUINAL HERNIA

See Table 12.2 and discussions in Chapter 12.

HYDROCELE

See pp. 439–440.

VARICOCELE

See pp. 440–441.

SPERM GRANULOMA

After a vasectomy, sperm can leak from the testicular end of the vas, causing an inflammatory reaction and granuloma formation. This granuloma helps to vent the pressure that can build up in the epididymis after a vasectomy, as sperm production does not cease. It is commonly apparent on physical examination and can be mistaken for other scrotal pathology. It may also indicate that the patient has formed antibodies against his own sperm, which can potentially complicate attempts at pregnancy after a vasectomy reversal.

Signs and Symptoms

Usually no signs or symptoms are evident other than a nontender, firm mass at the end of the proximal vas deferens that can range in diameter up to 1 cm. In some cases, the granuloma may be tender on palpation.

Diagnostic Studies

Diagnosis is based partly on the physical examination; a scrotal ultrasound is not necessary or indicated based on the history of a vasectomy, but it will definitively confirm a granuloma at the proximal end of the vas and rule out any other pathology.

SPERMATOCELE

See p. 441.

■ Penile or Genital Lesions

Complaints of lesions on the genitals are a common presentation of otherwise healthy male patients. These lesions may be the result of a communicable disease or other skin condition. Any sort of genital lesion is often a cause of significant anxiety to the patient. There are many additional, albeit less common, lesions that are not discussed in this section. If there is any uncertainty about the identification of a lesion, a referral to a urology specialist or dermatologist is appropriate.

History

The male patient may give a history of transient, recurrent, or nonhealing lesions to the penis or scrotum; there may also be a urethral discharge. The lesions may be described as small or moderately sized or as blisters or papules. The patient may describe progressively worsening and increasingly painful lesions. There may be complaints of dysuria, urethral itching, or malaise. A history of prior STIs and other skin changes is important, as is medical history, including conditions such as diabetes.

Physical Examination

A thorough inspection is mandatory, including examination of the scrotal contents, distal urethra, and inguinal regions for adenopathy. Note characteristics of the lesion(s). The examination may also reveal scars that indicate previous lesions from STIs. Examination and culture of lesions or discharge is necessary but also may cause additional pain to the patient.

Penile Cancer

Relatively rare in the United States, cancer of the penis is usually a squamous cell lesion that presents on the prepuce, glans, shaft, or base of the penis. If the lesion involves the glans, prepuce, or penile shaft, it is called *erythroplasia of Queyrat*; if it presents on the other aspects of the male genitalia or perineal region, it is called *Bowen's disease*. Risk factors include not being circumcised; a history of STIs, particularly condyloma acuminatum; or a history of balanitis xerotica obliterans (BXO), which is discussed later in the chapter.

Signs and Symptoms

Patients may complain of a nonhealing ulcer, erythema that does not resolve, induration of the skin, or a lesion with a warty appearance. Patients may also report a history of difficulty with foreskin retraction—the lesion being concealed by the foreskin.

There may be associated itching and/or burning with the lesion, and there may be visible ulceration of the penile tissue. Lesions are most common on the glans. On physical examination, the presentation of a lesion has a variety of appearances, including flat and erythematous or papillary, but is typically a well-marginated lesion. The tissue surrounding the lesion may feel less pliable than unaffected areas, and the foreskin of an uncircumcised male may be difficult to retract. The entire penis must be palpated to assess the possible extent of the lesion into the corpora and deeper tissues. There may be palpable inguinal adenopathy, and the lesion may show evidence of a secondary bacterial infection. A DRE is necessary to evaluate for prostatic or urethral involvement.

Diagnostic Studies

Definitive diagnosis is via biopsy. The patient should be referred urgently to a urologist for diagnosis and management (emergently if he has difficulty voiding due to the location of the lesion). If inguinal adenopathy is present, the patient can be started on an antibiotic in advance of the urology appointment to attempt to treat any superimposed bacterial infection. A CT scan may be required to assess the extent of any inguinal adenopathy.

SEXUALLY TRANSMITTED INFECTION–RELATED LESIONS

An STI can present in many ways in the male patient. Any complaint of lesions on the genitals should be thoroughly evaluated, including questioning the patient regarding his sexual activity and frequency of new partners.

Signs and Symptoms

Some STIs may be accompanied by complaints of constitutional symptoms or malaise. Refer to Table 13.3 for details of the lesion presentation on physical examination.

Table 13.3

Sexually Transmitted Infections and Their Presentation in the Male Patient

Sexually Transmitted Infection	Clinical Presentation in the Male Patient
Chancroid	Tender ulcer with deep, undermined border may be soft or indurated; friable base with ragged edges; purulent exudate possible; painful lymphadenopathy.
Chlamydia	Scant mucoid or mucopurulent urethral discharge; may be accompanied by mild dysuria and urethral itching.
Genital *herpes simplex*	*First episode:* Fluid-filled painful vesicles that may coalesce, with erythema to surrounding skin, and that eventually rupture, resulting in painful ulcerative lesions with erythematous edges; tender adenopathy, fever; dysuria also common. Lesions typically last 2 to 3 weeks, possibly up to 6 weeks.
Genital warts (human papillomavirus)	*Recurrences:* Prodromal pain, burning, tingling at site where vesicles will erupt with shorter course of constitutional symptoms; lesions usually resolve after 7 to 10 days.
Gonorrhea	Soft, fleshy, exophytic lesions with raised granular surfaces; commonly seen on glans and prepuce; also present as small papular lesions on the skin or nonhealing penile lesion(s). The majority of lesions are subclinical and can be detected by using 3% to 5% acetic acid.
Nongonococcal urethritis	Urethral discharge may be yellowish or gray-brown, purulent, and accompanied by itching and dysuria; may be accompanied by epididymal or testicular pain; asymptomatic in 5% to 10% of cases; rare superficial lesions to the penile shaft.
Pediculosis pubis	Mild to moderate clear or white urethral discharge or thin mucoid urethral discharge; accompanied by mild dysuria and urethral itching.
Scabies	Severe pruritus; observation of ectoparasites on hair and/or skin in the genital area. Papular or linear burrow-like lesions.
Syphilis	*Primary:* Solitary, painless, nontender, and rubbery ulcer (chancre), superficial or deep, with indurated edge and no exudate. *Secondary:* Papulosquamous or maculopapular rash indicative of systemic infection.
Trichomoniasis	Usually asymptomatic, may cause urethritis.

Diagnostic Studies

STIs can be diagnosed with the appropriate cultures, Gram stains, swabs, and serological studies. Unless a patient appears ill and a white blood cell count seems indicated, no additional laboratory work or imaging studies are indicated. Many STIs must be reported to the local health department. For complex, extensive, or refractory cases of genital warts, the patient can be referred to a urologist or dermatologist. Consult the most recent CDC guidelines for details of evaluation and treatment.

BALANITIS

Generally seen in uncircumcised males or very obese males with a retracted penis, balanitis is an inflammation of the glans, commonly caused by a *Candida albicans* infection. Men with poorly controlled or newly diagnosed diabetes mellitus are at particular risk for balanitis, as are morbidly obese patients who demonstrate a retractile penis as a result of their body habitus.

Signs and Symptoms

The patient may present with a combination of symptoms that include edema, erythema, and pain of the glans; dysuria; urethral discharge; and a history of a discharge from between the foreskin and the glans. Physical examination will confirm the edema, erythema, and exudates; there may be a cracked appearance to the prepuce. Palpation should always be done to the affected area to evaluate for changes in the consistency of the tissue. The patient should also be examined for any inguinal adenopathy.

Diagnostic Studies

Any exudates should be cultured for STIs and for other viral and fungal organisms; KOH (potassium hydroxide) and Tzanck preparations should also be included.

BALANOPOSTHITIS

This condition is generally seen only in uncircumcised males and is an inflammation that involves both the glans and foreskin.

Signs and Symptoms

The presentation and physical examination are similar to those for balanitis but can include an edematous and painful foreskin that may not retract.

Diagnostic Studies

Diagnostic studies are the same as for balanitis.

BALANITIS XEROTICA OBLITERANS

BXO is a variation of lichen sclerosus et atrophicus, which is common in middle-aged men and is a painful condition associated with patches of white, thinned skin. Uncircumcised and diabetic males have an increased risk, and the patient with long-standing BXO has a higher risk for squamous cell carcinoma of the penis.

Signs and Symptoms

Patients may complain of localized penile discomfort, painful erections, or urinary obstruction. On physical examination, there can be a whitish patch or patches on the prepuce or glans, and the meatus may become involved. The meatus itself may become edematous and indurated. As the condition progresses, there can be erosions, fissures, or meatal stenosis, and the foreskin may adhere to the glans.

Diagnostic Studies

Diagnosis can be made only via biopsy. If BXO is suspected, a referral to a urologist is mandatory, particularly because meatal stenosis or urinary obstruction can occur over time.

TRAUMA

The patient may present with a history of some manner of trauma to the genitalia (including robust sexual activity or the use of an unlubricated condom), with some resulting lesions. In the case of bruising to the genitals, the causative trauma may have happened a few days earlier. The patient may also admit to the use of some kind of penile enlargement or enhancement device with resulting trauma to the penis. Trauma may also result during BDSM practices.

Signs and Symptoms

Examination of the genitalia reveals ecchymotic areas on the penile shaft, scrotum, or glans. There may also be abraded areas on the genitalia.

Diagnostic Studies

No laboratory work or imaging studies are indicated. If the resulting lesions are severe or there is evidence of infection, a referral to a urology specialist is recommended.

■ Inability to Retract or Advance the Foreskin

Complaints of difficulty manipulating the foreskin occur only in males who have not been circumcised. These complaints are often accompanied by a history of chronic irritation or poor personal hygiene.

History

The patient will report difficulty at retracting the foreskin, possibly complicated by a history of poor personal hygiene and/or a recent groin skin infection. Alternatively, there may be a history of pain and progressive difficulty with retraction. There may be complaints of the inability to advance the foreskin over the glans, possibly after a prolonged period of retraction. Pain may also be associated with any of these complaints. In addition to investigating personal hygiene, recent infections, and history of conditions such as diabetes and cardiovascular disease, explore whether similar episodes have been experienced previously.

Physical Examination

A thorough genital inspection is required along with a gentle attempt to retract or advance the foreskin.

PHIMOSIS

This condition is seen only in males who are uncircumcised. The patient will often present with a history of progressive difficulty at retracting the foreskin and, in some cases, urinary obstruction. This is commonly preceded by poor personal hygiene, chronic balanitis or balanoposthitis, or poor control of diabetes mellitus. Long-standing phimosis will create a risk for chronic inflammation and squamous cell cancer of the penis.

Signs and Symptoms

The patient may complain of pain when retracting or attempting to retract the foreskin and possibly a "ballooning" of the foreskin when voiding. If the patient reports a complete inability to retract the foreskin, physical examination may show that the opening of the foreskin has contracted to the point at which the actual opening is quite small. There may be evidence of balanitis or balanoposthitis.

Diagnostic Studies

History and presentation are usually sufficient to confirm the diagnosis. The patient should be referred to a urologist or urology specialist for further evaluation and management, as a dorsal slit or circumcision may be required.

PARAPHIMOSIS

Paraphimosis is a condition in which the foreskin has been retracted and cannot be advanced forward to its normal position over the glans. It results from chronic inflammation under the foreskin and is commonly preceded by poor personal hygiene, chronic balanitis or balanoposthitis, or poor control of diabetes mellitus. Over time, a tight ring of tissue forms when the foreskin is retracted, resulting in additional edema to the glans with retraction of the foreskin.

Signs and Symptoms

The patient may present with complaints of pain, swelling, and possible discoloration of the glans. Physical examination will reveal a foreskin that cannot be reduced or can be reduced with some difficulty; the shaft of the penis and glans may be tender or painful on palpation. There may be evidence of balanitis or balanoposthitis.

Diagnostic Studies

Although history and presentation are usually sufficient to confirm the diagnosis, paraphimosis is a urological emergency. The patient should be referred to a urology specialist for further evaluation and management because arterial occlusion and necrosis of the glans and distal urethra may result if the paraphimosis is not reduced. Any exudates should be cultured for STIs and for other viral and fungal organisms; KOH and Tzanck preparations may also be included.

BALANITIS

See p. 446.

BALANOPOSTHITIS

See p. 446.

GENERALIZED EDEMA

The patient who suffers from generalized edema, such as that seen in cardiovascular or congestive heart failure patients, may also experience difficulty with advancing or retracting the foreskin.

Signs and Symptoms

The complaints are similar to those for phimosis or paraphimosis. Physical examination shows a swollen glans, discolored skin if this condition has persisted, and the glans, penile shaft, and foreskin may be painful to palpation. Generalized scrotal edema may be noted. Physical examination should also yield evidence of edema of the feet, legs, and possibly trunk, along with findings consistent with the causative condition(s).

Diagnostic Studies

History and presentation are usually sufficient to confirm the diagnosis. The patient should be urgently referred to a urology specialist for management if paraphimosis is noted. Otherwise, a routine referral to a urology specialist is recommended for consideration of dorsal slit or circumcision in the case of phimosis, if personal hygiene becomes an issue (although any elective surgical intervention will be delayed by persistent edema).

■ Absence of One or Both Testes in the Scrotum

The patient may present at any age with the complaint of the absence of one or both testes in the scrotum. Evaluation of the testes is a required physical assessment point in male infants, but it is not uncommon for adolescent or adult males to present with this complaint in the absence of a surgical history that indicates a testicle was removed.

History

The patient (or possibly a parent if the patient is a minor) will complain of the absence of one or both testicles in the scrotum. If the patient is an adult, he may provide a history of difficulty conceiving with his female partner or a history of semen analysis abnormalities. If there is a failure of both testicles to descend, the patient may report late, or failure of, puberty onset. There may also be a history of inguinal or lower abdominal pain.

Physical Examination

Physical examination involves a genital examination that notes the absence of one or both testicles in the scrotum. It is vital to note the stage of development of secondary male characteristics. The patient may have a testicle that is palpable in the inguinal canal that can be tender on examination. There may be age-appropriate secondary sexual characteristics, particularly with one descended testicle.

Congenital Cryptorchidism or Ectopic Testicle(s)

This is the condition in which one or both testes have failed to descend normally into the scrotum. Descent may have stopped at any point between the renal and scrotal areas, but most commonly the undescended testes are found in the inguinal canal. In male infants with undescended testes, more than half will descend into the scrotum during the first month after birth. There are no genetic abnormalities associated with this condition, and many males with a unilaterally undescended testicle do not have trouble initiating a pregnancy, despite decreased sperm counts. There is an increased risk of infertility and for testicular cancer owing to damage to the seminiferous tubules, depending on the length of time after birth the testes were brought down into the scrotal sac. The majority of patients with bilateral cryptorchidism become appropriately androgenized as adults but are at increased risk for inguinal hernias.

Signs and Symptoms

There can be complaints of pain, as the testes may be in an uncomfortable position. The patient may complain of infertility. On physical examination, the scrotum on the affected side will be atrophic. The testes may be felt in the inguinal canal or may not be palpable at all. If the testicle is palpable, it cannot be manipulated into the scrotum. An inguinal hernia may also be present on the affected side. The stage of development of secondary sexual characteristics should be noted in postpubertal males.

Diagnostic Studies

Ultrasound is usually successful if the suspected testis is in the groin; a CT scan or magnetic resonance imaging (MRI) will detect an intra-abdominal testis in a postpubertal male. Laboratory work can include testosterone, follicle-stimulating hormone (FSH), and luteinizing hormone (LH); FSH and LH may help differentiate intra-abdominal from bilateral anorchia because both are significantly elevated in this condition. A routine referral to a urology specialist for further evaluation and management should also be made.

Severe Atrophy of One or Both Testicles

Severe atrophy can result from a mumps infection in the prepubertal male, although it is rare in this era of a successful mumps vaccine. The patient will give a history of mumps before puberty and will often relate a history of profound swelling of one of the testicles. Orchitis will result in approximately 30% of males who contract mumps, with approximately one-third of those developing testicular atrophy.

It is also possible to encounter severe atrophy of a testicle as the result of a varicocele that has been present for many years (see earlier section on varicoceles for details).

Signs and Symptoms

Possible signs include complaints of size differential between the testicles or altered semen analysis. On physical examination, pronounced testicular atrophy compared with the unaffected side is apparent. The affected testicle is nontender on examination and has a softer consistency.

Diagnostic Studies

History and examination are usually sufficient. A scrotal ultrasound is not necessary but will definitively confirm the size differences and rule out any additional pathology.

KLINEFELTER SYNDROME

Klinefelter syndrome is the most common abnormality of sexual differentiation. It occurs in approximately 1 in 500 live births, is one of the most common causes of primary hypogonadism, and is the most common sex chromosome abnormality seen in infertile men. Patients present with the typical triad of small, firm testes; gynecomastia; and elevated urine gonadotropins. Variants of Klinefelter syndrome may also result in increased height, diabetes mellitus, obesity, and decreased intelligence. Although testicles are not absent, their small size may lead to lack of recognition as the testes.

Signs and Symptoms

Patients complain of delayed completion of puberty and delayed virilization. There are usually few physical complaints associated with Klinefelter disease other than possible concern regarding testicle size. Physical examination reveals a lack of development of secondary sexual characteristics (small [less than 3 cm] atrophic testes, small phallus, diminished body hair, diminished muscle bulk) and truncal fat distribution that often includes gynecomastia. Patients will be tall due to a delay in the fusion of the epiphyseal plates in the long bones.

Diagnostic Studies

Karyotype analysis will show 47, XXY or a mosaic 46, XY/47, XXY. Hormone studies will demonstrate decreased or normal testosterone, decreased free testosterone, elevated estradiol, normal or elevated LH, and elevated FSH. A scrotal ultrasound is unnecessary but can confirm the presence and small size of the testes. If fertility is an issue, the patient should be routinely referred to a urologist specializing in male infertility, as semen analysis will show azoospermia.

The rare male patient may present with a history of one or both of his testicles "climbing into his belly" or inguinal canal. This is a normal variant due to a hyperactive cremasteric reflex. Usually it can be demonstrated in children and into puberty, at which point it resolves. Occasionally, it can persist into adulthood. The patient will demonstrate normal male physiological development.

Signs and Symptoms

The patient will report that one or both testicles retract to the point that they are no longer palpable or visible in the scrotum. The important point of the physical examination is to locate the testicle and gently manipulate it into its usual anatomical position. This does not usually cause the patient pain. The scrotum will also be normally developed with no sign of atrophy.

Diagnostic Studies

The history and examination is typically sufficient. A scrotal ultrasound will aid in the diagnosis. If there is any doubt or trouble locating a testicle, the patient may be referred to a urology specialist.

ETIOLOGY OF ERECTILE FUNCTION COMPLAINTS

■ Erectile Dysfunction

Male erectile dysfunction (ED) is a common clinical complaint that may have far-reaching effects on the self-esteem and relationships of those involved. Some estimates project that 150 million men worldwide suffer from some degree of ED, and the incidence can be as high as 80% in men older than age 70 (Kessler et al., 2019). The actual incidence is likely to be greater because ED is an underreported condition, and questions regarding sexual function may not be asked during routine clinic visits.

Several underlying causes contribute to ED: arteriogenic, venogenic, endocrinological, neurological, psychological, and medicinal. Vascular disease is one of the most common causes of organic ED. Many epidemiological studies have shown that ED coexists with hypertension and that as the severity of hypertension increases, so do reports of ED severity from patients. Many men will complain of erectile problems in the absence of any other currently diagnosed pathologies, and ED may provide a clue to the subtle onset of many systemic diseases. This is particularly true in patients who proceed to formal diagnoses of hypercholesterolemia, hypertension, or diabetes mellitus. However, a complete discussion of ED is beyond the scope of this chapter. ED can be successfully treated without knowing the precise nature of its cause.

History

The patient will often give a history of declining erectile function, usually insidious and progressive, that may span several years. Alternatively, he may provide a history of relatively rapid or recent onset of decline in erectile function, perhaps associated with the history of recently starting new medication. Some degree of ED is a frequent complaint after prostate, bladder, rectal, or other retroperitoneal surgery.

The history should include several points specific to the patient's sexual functioning: the precise nature of the dysfunction (i.e., whether the problem is attaining or sustaining an erection, insufficient rigidity, penetration, absence of climax or anejaculation); whether ED occurs with all sexual partners or only specific partners; psychosocial factors, including the nature of current relationship(s); the presence or absence of nocturnal and morning erections and their quality; and any treatments (pharmacological and nonpharmacological) the patient has tried.

An assessment of the degree to which this condition has impacted the patient's quality of life is also important. This can be assessed using the Sexual Health Inventory for Men (Cappelleri & Rosen, 2005) or the International Index of Erectile Function (Rosen et al., 2002); both are short questionnaires validated for the assessment of ED.

Physical Examination

If ED is a complaint in a man with no other recognized medical conditions, a full physical examination is necessary. In the patient with recognized chronic conditions, the focus should be on the routine genital examination along with a cardiovascular examination for cardiovascular risk assessment (Nehra et al., 2012).

Diagnostic Studies

Based on the clinical suspicion for undiagnosed underlying disease, screening begins with a testosterone level, urinalysis, complete blood count, glucose or HgbA1c, blood urea nitrogen, serum creatinine, and cholesterol profile. A bioavailable testosterone may be considered, particularly if hypogonadism is suspected. If these tests are inconclusive, the patient can be referred to a urology specialist for further evaluation with specialized diagnostic testing as well as management if first-line pharmacological management is not sufficient. If the history and physical examination appear to suggest a stronger psychological than organic component to the ED, a referral to a sexual counselor or therapist is helpful.

Categories of Erectile Dysfunction

See Table 13.4, which is representative and is not all inclusive. Systemic disease–induced causes for ED are usually a combination of other etiological categories (Box 13.2). Medications that contribute to ED are listed in Table 13.5.

■ Prolonged Erection/Priapism

Priapism is the presence of a prolonged erection that occurs in the absence of sexual stimulation or that remains after orgasm. This condition usually affects only the corpora cavernosa of the penis. It is uncommon, and although it can occur in any age group, it is more common from ages 20 to 50. Priapism is usually painful, and it is a urological emergency. Failure to reverse the erection can result in scarring of the penile corpora and permanent ED owing to tissue

Table 13.4

Categories of Erectile Dysfunction and Selected Examples

Category of Erectile Dysfunction	Examples of Causes
Arteriogenic	Atherosclerosis, hypertension, hyperlipidemia, smoking, pelvic trauma, diabetes mellitus
Cavernosal (venogenic)	Vascular disease, diabetes mellitus, Peyronie's disease, insufficient trabecular smooth muscle contraction, age
Endocrinological	Hypogonadism, hyperprolactinemia, hyperthyroidism, hypothyroidism, diabetes mellitus, orchiectomy
Medication-induced	Antihypertensives, antidepressants, antipsychotics, alcohol abuse, smoking, antiandrogens, alpha adrenergic blockers, beta blockers, tranquilizers, thiazide diuretics, centrally acting sympatholytics, cimetidine, estrogens, polypharmacy, marijuana use, chemotherapy
Neurological	Retroperitoneal surgery, bowel resection, SCI, MS, diabetes mellitus, pelvic trauma, spina bifida, CNS tumors, alcohol abuse, Parkinson's disease, Alzheimer's disease, CVA, pelvic irradiation
Psychological	Performance anxiety, depression, psychological stress, relationship issues, psychotic disorders, misinformation or ignorance of normal anatomy/function
Systemic disease—induced	CRF, coronary heart disease, COPD (fear of inducing exacerbation), CHF, hepatic failure, recent MI, cirrhosis

CHF = congestive heart failure; CNS = central nervous system; COPD = chronic obstructive pulmonary disease; CRF = chronic renal failure; CVA = cardiovascular accident; MI = myocardial infarction; MS = multiple sclerosis; SCI = spinal cord injury.

Box 13.2

Decision Rule: Erectile Dysfunction

ED is a well-established risk marker for the presence of treatable underlying medical conditions, such as undiagnosed diabetes, lipid disease, or hypertension, that reduce quality and length of life when left untreated. The degree of ED strongly correlates with the severity of cardiovascular disease (CVD), and ED may be considered a sentinel marker that identifies men with occult CVD. In younger men, ED predicts up to a 50-fold increase in CVD events. The Princeton III criteria provide guidance for providers when considering if further cardiac evaluation is warranted prior to treating ED by designating patients as low, intermediate, or high risk. Men presenting with ED complaints give providers an opportunity to offer evaluation and assessment of global cardiovascular risk factors (AUA, 2018; Nehra et al., 2012).

Table 13.5

Selected Medications Reported to Contribute to Erectile Dysfunction

Medication Class	Selected Examples
Antiandrogenic	α-5 reductase inhibitors, luteinizing hormone-releasing medications, hormone analogs, antiandrogens
Anticholinergics	Diphenhydramine
Antihypertensives	Diuretics (thiazides), vasodilators, central sympatholytics (methyldopa, clonidine), beta blockers, calcium channel blockers, angiotensin-converting enzyme inhibitors
Benzodiazepines	Diazepam, clonazepam
Lipid-lowering agents	Lovastatin, pravastatin sodium
Miscellaneous medications	Cimetidine, lithium, baclofen, narcotics
Monoamine oxidase	Phenelzine, procarbazine inhibitors
Recreational drugs	Alcohol, marijuana, barbiturates, opiates, nicotine
Tranquilizers	Haldol
Tricyclic antidepressants	Nortriptyline hydrochloride, amitriptyline hydrochloride

ischemia. Unfortunately, there can be a significant time delay between the onset of priapism and the patient's presentation for evaluation and treatment.

History

The patient will complain of a persistent erection that did not resolve with cessation of sexual activity or after climax. There does not have to be 100% erection to be considered priapism. The erection may have occurred spontaneously. The patient may complain of pain, depending on length of time the penis has remained erect (pain does not usually occur until after 6 to 8 hours) and the specific mechanisms of the blood flow. He may also provide a history of use of injectable erectogenic agents, sickle cell disease, or similar episodes that resolved painlessly after a couple of hours. It is vital to establish as accurately as possible the duration of the erection.

Physical Examination

A routine genital examination will establish the presence of an erection; the corpora will be partially to fully rigid, depending on the etiology of the priapism. The penis may be tender on examination. The penis feels somewhat tense and congested, but the corpus spongiosum and glans are of normal consistency. There may be skin discoloration. A DRE, abdominal examination, and neurological examination should also be performed.

Table 13.6

Selected Causes of Priapism

Causes of Priapism	Explanation
Idiopathic (primary) priapism	Accounts for up to 60% of cases
Medication-induced priapism	Resulting after penile injection treatment for erectile dysfunction, some recreational or psychotropic drugs (e.g., cocaine, alcohol)
Priapism caused by other medical condition	Sickle cell disease, leukemia, pelvic tumor, spinal cord trauma, thromboembolic event, neoplastic causes due to metastases
Priapism due to trauma	Perineal or penile trauma can lead to high-flow (arterial) priapism

Selected Causes

See Table 13.6.

Diagnostic Studies

None are necessary. Priapism requires immediate referral to the nearest emergency department and often requires evaluation by a urology specialist.

■ Curvature of the Penis

Male patients of any age may present with curvature of the penis, which is usually noticeable only when the penis is erect. As men present at older ages, the likelihood that the curvature is congenital decreases, especially if they report that the erection was previously straight. The proper course of care for these patients is referral to a urologist for further examination and treatment, particularly in a case such as congenital penile corporal disproportion. Most complaints of curvature (in the absence of a clinically apparent plaque) are amenable to some type of surgical correction.

History

The patient will report a progressive curvature of the shaft of the penis with erection; the curve can occur at any site along the shaft of the penis. There may be a concurrent history of a decline in erectile function with the onset of curvature as well as pain with erections. Some patients report a history of some sort of trauma to the shaft of the penis with resulting bruising and pain that preceded the onset of the curvature. Alternatively, the patient may give a history that curvature has "always" been present, with no pain associated with erections, no impact to erectile function, and merely cosmetic concerns.

Physical Examination

A routine genital examination is necessary, and a palpable plaque may be felt anywhere along the shaft of the penis. Plaque can also be absent, particularly if the history indicates that the curvature may be congenital.

PEYRONIE'S DISEASE

Although the precise cause of Peyronie's disease is not known, current belief regarding its etiology is that the plaque formation results after disordered wound healing, often with calcium deposition in the plaque (AUA, 2015). During regular sexual activity, susceptible patients may suffer nonpainful minor trauma to the penis that leads to a decrease in the elasticity of the tissue and fibroblast formation, eventually resulting in plaque. The plaque is present in the tunica albuginea of the corpora cavernosa, which leads to shortening and curvature of the shaft of the penis. The resulting curvature can be in any direction: lateral, ventral, or dorsal. Often the quality of erection distal to the plaque is poor and prevents adequate penetration during sexual activity. Peyronie's disease is most commonly seen between the ages of 45 and 60, and complaints of ED may predate the curvature. There is a 30% association with Dupuytren's contracture of the tendons of the hand (AUA, 2015).

Signs and Symptoms

The patient complains of curvature of the penis, noticeable with erections. The curve may be progressive or may have stopped curving. If it is painful, it is only while the penis is erect. Physical examination may yield evidence of a palpable plaque that involves the tunica albuginea; the plaque is commonly located at or near the dorsal midline of the shaft.

Diagnostic Studies

History and physical examination are usually sufficient to confirm the diagnosis. A routine referral to a urologist can be considered for further treatment and possible surgical intervention.

PENILE CORPORAL DISPROPORTION

This is a relatively rare congenital condition in which the corpora cavernosa of the penis are not of identical length. This leads to painless curvature with erection; there are no associated erectile function complaints. The curvature will cause some distress to the patient, and he will seek evaluation to correct the curvature. The patient may have also (incorrectly) self-diagnosed Peyronie's disease.

Signs and Symptoms

The patient will describe curved erections without a history of having previously had straight erections. On physical examination, the difference between the corpora may be palpable. The patient will demonstrate age-appropriate development of secondary sexual characteristics.

Diagnostic Studies

Diagnosis is typically through history and physical examination. Routine referral to a urology specialist is recommended; this condition can be corrected with injected medication or surgery.

PENILE FRACTURE

Penile fracture results in an acquired curvature of the penis and is the result of trauma during intercourse that causes a rupture to the tunica albuginea of one of the corpora cavernosa of the penis. The patient will present with a history of a lateral buckling of the penis and a "snap" heard during intercourse, typically when the woman is in the superior position. This is followed by possible bleeding from the urethra, loss of penile rigidity, and eventual ecchymosis of the penis. The trauma may also be less severe and result in a gradual curvature over time. Often there is an accompanying loss of rigidity or pain with subsequent erections. There may also be some disruption of the urethra. This can occur in milder forms, without profound pain, bleeding, or ecchymosis.

Signs and Symptoms

The patient will complain of decreased and/or painful erections. On physical examination (including GU, rectal, and lower abdominal examinations), there may be a palpable indentation or scar at the site of the corporal rupture and possibly ecchymosis of the scrotum if the presentation is shortly after injury. If the patient presents acutely, there may be blood at the meatus. Physical findings depend on the length of time since the injury and its severity.

Diagnostic Studies

History and physical examination are usually sufficient to confirm the diagnosis. An urgent consult to a urologist should be made if the patient presents acutely. A routine referral to a urology specialist can be considered for further evaluation, treatment, and possible surgical intervention if the patient presents after the acute period.

■ Low Testosterone

Low testosterone is less a direct patient complaint than being representative of a combination of symptoms. There may be moodiness, loss of interest in usual activities, loss of libido, fatigue, and even diminished muscle bulk. The key in its evaluation is establishing the cause of the low level of testosterone. There is strengthening evidence regarding the role of testosterone in cardiovascular health, although no evidence supports testosterone replacement as a method to reduce cardiovascular disease.

History

There is likely to be an insidious onset of some degree of ED, loss of libido, depressed mood, and fatigue. If this has been progressing over a significant length of time, decreased muscle mass and strength and loss of facial and body hair may occur. A thorough history is essential, including past and current conditions, prescribed treatments and other agents taken, and a broad review of systems. Explore emotional status as well.

Physical Examination

A complete physical is necessary, including routine genital examination and DRE. Attention should focus on secondary sexual characteristics and testicular size. The physical examination is unrevealing in the majority of cases.

HYPOGONADISM

Hypogonadism is failure of the testes to produce normal levels of testosterone (and/or sperm). It primarily results from testicular failure; secondarily, it results from pituitary or hypothalamic causes. Combined hypogonadism is due to the decreased pulsatility of gonadotropins plus decreased testicular Leydig cell response. Hypogonadism is estimated to affect 4 to 5 million men in the United States alone; in aging males, the causes are more likely to be secondary. As males age, there is both decreased production of testosterone and decreased clearance beginning at age 40; however, it is not analogous to menopause in women because men retain reproductive capacity, and not all men decline below the normal limits for serum testosterone. Hypogonadism represents the only cause of male infertility that can successfully be treated with hormone therapy, although the response is largely dependent on the length of time of the hypogonadism. A complete discussion is beyond the scope of this chapter. Table 13.7 summarizes several causes of hypogonadism.

Signs and Symptoms

The patient may have a variety of complaints, including fatigue, truncal obesity, atrophic testes, loss of facial and pubic hair, and decreased muscle bulk. In the adult male, hypogonadism is manifested by changes in sexual function, behavior, and muscle mass and some loss of secondary sexual characteristics. The patient may report mood and behavioral symptoms (e.g., depression, irritability, loss of

Table 13.7		
Selected Causes of Hypogonadism		
Primary Hypogonadism	**Secondary Hypogonadism**	**Combined Hypogonadism**
• Aging	• Aging	• Aging
• Chemotherapy/irradiation	• Hemochromatosis	• Cirrhosis
• Cryptorchidism	• Hypertrophic hypogonadism, Kallmann syndrome	• Sickle cell disease
• Chromosome abnormalities (e.g., Klinefelter syndrome)	• Medication-induced (e.g., antiestrogens for treatment of prostate cancer)	
• Myotonic dystrophy	• Obesity	
• Orchitis (e.g., mumps)	• Pituitary mass lesions	
• Testicular loss from trauma, tumor	• Prolactinoma	
	• Psychological stress	
	• Uremia	

motivation) in addition to lethargy or loss of energy. Physical examination may demonstrate some regression of secondary sexual characteristics such as hair loss and possible loss of muscle bulk. There is no change to penis or prostate size.

Diagnostic Studies

Hypogonadism can be confirmed by checking a testosterone level; morning values are superior to afternoon blood samples because testosterone is secreted in the morning. If the patient is not available for morning laboratory draws, at least three afternoon values at close to the same time of day can provide an average testosterone value. If the total testosterone is low, obtain a free testosterone level, which is the most accurate measurement of a significant deficiency. Additional hormones can also be evaluated (e.g., LH, FSH, estradiol, prolactin, thyroid profile) if secondary causes are suspected. An MRI is necessary if pituitary lesions are suspected. A semen analysis will show oligospermia or azoospermia in the patient with hypogonadism.

CONGENITAL HYPOGONADISM

The most common variant of congenital hypogonadism is Klinefelter syndrome. See p. 451.

OBESITY

Obesity can lead to the aromatization of testosterone in fatty tissue to estradiol, leaving lowered amounts of testosterone available for maintenance and virilization functions.

Signs and Symptoms

The patient is a clinically obese male, with possible evidence of feminization or regression of secondary male sex characteristics found on physical examination.

Diagnostic Studies

Testosterone and free testosterone levels, along with estradiol, LH, and FSH levels, should be done. Routine referral to an endocrinologist or urology specialist, preferably one with expertise in male infertility (if this is an issue) and andrology, is recommended.

COMPLAINTS RELATED TO MALE FERTILITY AND SEXUAL FUNCTION

■ Infertility

In 30% of all heterosexual couples being evaluated for infertility, there is a clear, significant male factor alone involved; both male and female factors are present in approximately 20% of couples seeking an infertility evaluation (AUA, 2020). Many of these male factors can be sufficiently corrected or improved so that the couple can conceive naturally or can take advantage of less-expensive assisted reproductive technologies. An infertility evaluation is usually initiated after a 1-year history of unprotected intercourse that fails to achieve a pregnancy, although this length of time can be shortened as the female partner's age increases. Ideally, both partners should be evaluated.

History

The patient may give a history of trying to achieve pregnancy for a lengthy period of time. It is vital to carefully detail the duration of the couple's infertility, previous pregnancies for either partner, the regularity of the female partner's menstrual cycle, the timing of intercourse in relation to ovulation, and the use of lubricants. Inquire about any established abnormal semen analysis that may have been ordered by the female partner's clinician. There may also be a history of male or female siblings (or members of the extended family) who have had trouble conceiving. Several aspects of the male's medical history are particularly important: any specific childhood illnesses (e.g., mumps, orchitis), a history of cryptorchidism, the timing of puberty, and any GU or abdominal surgeries as an infant or child.

It is possible for a couple to present with a history of little difficulty achieving a first pregnancy and yet be unsuccessful in establishing a second pregnancy (secondary infertility).

Physical Examination

A complete physical examination may demonstrate that the male has failed to attain secondary male sex characteristics, lacks the vas deferens, or is obese. A careful GU examination is required. The physical examination may be completely normal. A semen analysis should be performed, with attention to sperm concentration, morphology, and motility.

VARICOCELE

See pp. 440–441.

HYPOGONADISM

See p. 459. See also sections on cryptorchidism, testicular atrophy, and Klinefelter syndrome.

CONGENITAL BILATERAL ABSENCE OF THE VAS DEFERENS

Congenital bilateral absence of the vas deferens is a genetic abnormality seen with cystic fibrosis (CF) and its variants. If not previously diagnosed with CF, the patient may present with a history of chronic bronchitis requiring hospitalization, recurrent respiratory infections as a child and adolescent, or asthma or an asthma-like condition. There are usually no other physical complaints. There may be a family history of infertility or persistent respiratory illnesses.

Male patients with CF frequently demonstrate malformation of the epididymis; the vas deferens, seminal vesicles, and ejaculatory ducts are atrophic or absent. However, spermatogenesis is usually normal. It is possible that the patient has a much more rare unilateral absence of the vas deferens.

Signs and Symptoms

Usually there are no signs and symptoms other than infertility if the patient has not been previously diagnosed with CF. Physical examination may show complete absence of the vas deferens unilaterally or bilaterally or show a palpable gap in the vas deferens. Testes are usually of normal size and consistency, and the patient will demonstrate normal libido and age-appropriate secondary sexual characteristics.

Diagnostic Studies

Physical examination is usually sufficient to confirm the absence of the vas deferens. Testosterone levels will be normal. Because this is a genetic abnormality, referrals to a urology specialist with expertise in male infertility, a reproductive endocrinologist, and a medical geneticist to discuss genetic analysis of the couple should be encouraged, as establishing a pregnancy will require high-level assisted reproductive technologies.

EXOGENOUS TESTOSTERONE SUPPLEMENTATION OR ANABOLIC STEROID USE

Supplementation with testosterone or with testosterone-like substances can result in decreased endogenous testosterone and LH, hypogonadotropic hypogonadism, and suppressed spermatogenesis. Hypogonadism induced by exogenous steroid use is usually temporary, and endogenous hormone production and spermatogenesis rebound approximately 4 months after discontinuation of supplements.

Signs and Symptoms

The patient may complain of increased or decreased libido and possible ED. Patients using anabolic steroids may also have skeletal muscle hypertrophy, acne, gynecomastia, and striae. There may be some noticeable testicular atrophy on examination.

Diagnostic Studies

Semen analysis will show oligospermia or azoospermia, and total testosterone will be above the normal range (or supraphysiological with anabolic use). Levels of LH and FSH will be decreased. Routine referral to a urologist, preferably one with expertise in male infertility and andrology, is recommended.

◾ Ejaculatory Dysfunction

In some cases of ejaculatory dysfunction, the cause is idiopathic and may be due to a failure of bladder neck closure. Men with diabetes can develop retrograde ejaculation. Neurological disease, such as multiple sclerosis and spinal cord injury, can lead to retrograde ejaculation or anejaculation. GU infections can also contribute to ejaculatory dysfunction, commonly owing to obstruction of the vas deferens or ejaculatory ducts.

History

The patient may present with complaints of cloudy urine after ejaculation, hematospermia, possible recent-onset anejaculation, oligospermia or azoospermia with a low-volume ejaculate on semen analysis, and a history of retroperitoneal or bladder neck surgery or neurological disease. There may also be complaints related to a decreased amount of ejaculate, a decreased volume of ejaculate, or the inability to ejaculate. It is possible that ejaculatory dysfunction will present during a male infertility evaluation.

Physical Examination

A routine GU examination, which is usually benign, is needed, as is a careful inspection of the abdomen to examine for surgical scars.

Selected Causes

Refer to Table 13.8.

Diagnostic Studies

Order a semen analysis—an antegrade and retrograde semen analysis if retrograde ejaculation is suspected. The evaluation of the semen sample will show a fructose-negative, acidic pH, azoospermic sample if obstructed. Routine referral to a urology specialist for further evaluation and treatment is necessary.

■ Painful Ejaculation

Male patients may occasionally complain that they experience pain with or following ejaculation, intermittently or with each climax. This can be distressing and, over time, may cause avoidance of sexual activity, which in turn can affect the quality of the relationship with a partner.

Table 13.8	
Selected Causes of Ejaculatory Dysfunction	
Selected Causes	**Example**
Anatomical	Congenital bilateral absence of the vas deferens, obstruction of seminal vesicles, bladder neck abnormalities, retrograde ejaculation
Functional	Premature ejaculation
Medical	Selective serotonin reuptake inhibitors, monoamine oxidase inhibitors, beta blockers, antipsychotics, benzodiazepines, alcohol, methadone
Neurological	Diabetes mellitus, spinal cord injury, multiple sclerosis
Surgical	Bladder reconstructive surgery, retroperitoneal lymph node dissection, radical prostatectomy, transurethral resection of the prostate, cystoprostatectomy, bowel resection

History

The patient will describe pain on ejaculation, usually of relatively recent onset. The pain may localize to a specific scrotal structure or radiate into the testes. There also may be decreased volume of ejaculate, hematospermia, or difficulty with bowel movements.

Physical Examination

The examination will include a careful inspection and palpation of the scrotal contents and a DRE.

EJACULATORY DUCT OBSTRUCTION

In this condition, one or both of the ducts leading from the seminal vesicles into the prostate become partially or completely blocked. This causes only prostatic fluids to contribute to the ejaculate volume, resulting in decreased volume, possible hematospermia, and possible azoospermia if both ducts are blocked. An increased risk of obstruction is associated with recent GU instrumentation or repeated urinary tract infections.

Signs and Symptoms

Testes are usually normally sized. If the obstruction is long-standing, there may be evidence of epididymal induration on physical examination. A DRE may demonstrate distended seminal vesicles, but this condition is often difficult to distinguish.

Diagnostic Studies

The ejaculate will be of low volume, acidic, and with no sperm, fructose, or coagulation factors on a semen analysis. Routine referral to a urology specialist is indicated, particularly if fertility is an issue.

EPIDIDYMITIS/ORCHITIS

See pp. 438–439.

PROSTATITIS

See Chapter 12.

■ Hematospermia

Blood in the ejaculate, or hematospermia, like other changes to the ejaculate, can cause concern for the male patient. Although this is a relatively uncommon complaint, it does have some common causes.

History

If the patient or patient's partner complains of blood in the ejaculate, it may have been present intermittently for several months preceding the patient's presentation. The ejaculate will be pink, reddish (new blood), or brownish (old blood). The presence of blood may be intermittent or occur with each ejaculate, there may be a history of recent GU instrumentation, or the patient may describe some sense of pressure with ejaculation.

Physical Examination

A routine GU examination is necessary, including DRE.

EJACULATORY DUCT OBSTRUCTION

See p. 464.

PROSTATITIS

See Chapter 12.

BENIGN PROSTATIC HYPERPLASIA

See Chapter 12.

RECENT GENITOURINARY PROCEDURE

It is possible to have several episodes of hematospermia after a prostate biopsy, resection of the prostate, incision, or other procedure that involves trauma to the prostate. In this case, the hematospermia will be transient and self-limited and is usually not associated with pain.

Signs and Symptoms

The patient will complain of blood in the ejaculate and provide history of prior procedure.

Diagnostic Studies

A history of recent procedure involving the prostate will confirm the diagnosis.

REFERENCES

American Urological Association (AUA) Guideline. (2015). Peyronie's Disease: AUA Guideline. AUA Board of Directors. https://www.auanet.org/guidelines/guidelines/peyronies-disease-guideline

American Urological Association. (2020). Diagnosis and Treatment of Infertility in Men: AUA/ASRM Guideline. https://www.auanet.org/guidelines/male-infertility

Burnett, A. L., Nehra, A, Breau, R. H., Culkin, D. J., Faraday, M. M., Hakim, L. S., Heidelbaugh, J., Khera, M., McVary, K. T., Miner, M. M., Nelson, C. J., Sadeghi-Nejad, H., Seftel, A. D., & Shindel, A. D. (2018). Erectile dysfunction: AUA guideline. *Journal of Urology, 200*, 633.

Cappelleri, J., & Rosen, R. (2005). The Sexual Health Inventory for Men (SHIM): A 5-year review of research and clinical experience. *Int J Impot Res, 17*, 307–319. https://doi.org/10.1038/sj.ijir.3901327

Kessler, A., Sollie, S., Challacombe, B., Briggs, K., & Van Hemelrijck, M. (2019). The global prevalence of erectile dysfunction: a review. *BJU International, 124*, 587–599.

Nehra, A., Jackson, G., Miner, M., Billups, K. L., Burnett, A. L., Buvat, J., Carson, C. C., Cunningham, G. R., Ganz, P., Goldstein, I., Guay, A. T., Hackett, G., Kloner, R. A., Kostis, J., Montorsi, P., Ramsey, M., Rosen, R., Sadovsky, R., Seftel, A. D., . . . Wux, F. C. W. (2012). The Princeton III Consensus recommendations for the management of erectile dysfunction and cardiovascular disease. *Mayo Clinic Proceedings, 87*(8), 766–778.

Rosen, R. Cappelleri, J., & Gendrano, N. (2002). The international index of erectile function. *Int J Impot Res, 14*(4), 226–44. doi: 10.1038/sj.ijir.3900857

Scanlon, V. C., & Sanders, T. (2015). *Essentials of anatomy and physiology* (7th ed.). F.A. Davis.

Waldert, M., Klatte, T., Schmidbauer, J., Remzi, M., Lackner, J., & Marberger, M. (2010). Color Doppler sonography reliably identifies testicular torsion in boys. *Urology*, 75:1170–1174.

Chapter 14

Female Reproductive System

Aimee Holland ·
Ashton Strachan ·

Anatomy and Physiology

Figures 14.1 and 14.2 show the major structures of the female reproductive system. The hormones involved in the pathway that controls the female reproductive system are as follows: (a) gonadotropin-releasing hormone, which is produced in the hypothalamus and released to the pituitary gland; (b) follicle-stimulating hormone, which is produced in the pituitary and released to the ovaries for the development and maturation of the ovarian follicle and the control of ovum production; (c) luteinizing hormone, also produced in the pituitary, stimulates the ovaries to produce estrogen and progesterone resulting in ovulation, the development of the corpus luteum. Progesterone also thickens the endometrium in preparation for a fertilized ovum. If fertilization does not take place, the endometrium is shed during menses.

■ Reproductive Hormones

- **Estrogen**—A group of estrogenic hormones, termed the *female hormones*, produced by the ovary. Estrogens are responsible for the development of secondary sexual characteristics in the female patient and for cyclic changes in the vaginal epithelium and uterine endometrium.
- **Progesterone**—A steroid hormone secreted by the corpus luteum and placenta that is responsible for changes in the endometrium in the luteal phase of the menstrual cycle, making implantation possible. It is used in combination with estrogen in oral contraceptives.
- **Follicle-stimulating hormone (FSH)**—A hormone produced by the anterior pituitary that stimulates the Graafian follicles of the ovary for follicular maturation and secretion of estradiol.
- **Luteinizing hormone (LH)**—A hormone produced by the anterior pituitary that stimulates ovulation, which involves rupture of the mature ovarian follicle, transformation of the follicle into the corpus luteum, and secretion of progesterone and estrogen by the corpus luteum.

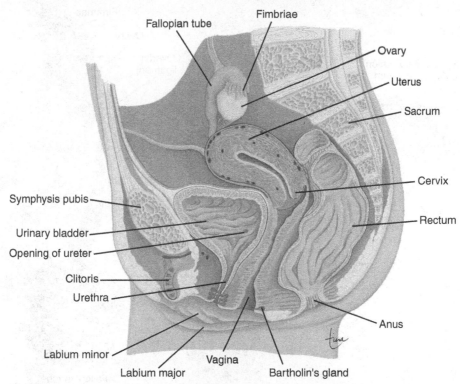

Figure 14.1 Internal female genitalia. (From Scanlon, V. C., & Sanders, T. [2015]. *Essentials of anatomy and physiology* [7th ed.]. Philadelphia, PA: F. A. Davis. Reprinted with permission.)

- **Prolactin level**—A hormone produced by the pituitary gland that stimulates breast development and lactation during pregnancy, in conjunction with estrogen and progesterone. In the postpartum period, sucking by the infant stimulates prolactin so milk continues to be produced. Elevations in prolactin in the female patient can cause amenorrhea, galactorrhea, and infertility, and in the male patient, erectile dysfunction. These symptoms in a patient should alert the examiner to the possibility of a pituitary tumor.
- **Estradiol**—A steroid produced by the ovary that is a component of estrogen. It is found in large quantities in pregnant patients. In the body, it is converted to estrone, another of the estrogenic hormones.
- **Testosterone**—An androgen and principal hormone produced by the testicle. Some testosterone is also produced by the adrenal cortex in both male and female patients. It is responsible for the development of secondary sexual characteristics and for sexual function in male patients. It also accounts for the larger muscle mass in men compared with women and for distribution of fat in male patients. It affects blood flow and other metabolic activities.
- **Thyroid-stimulating hormone (TSH)**—A hormone produced by the anterior pituitary that stimulates the thyroid gland to secrete thyroxine and triiodothyronine.

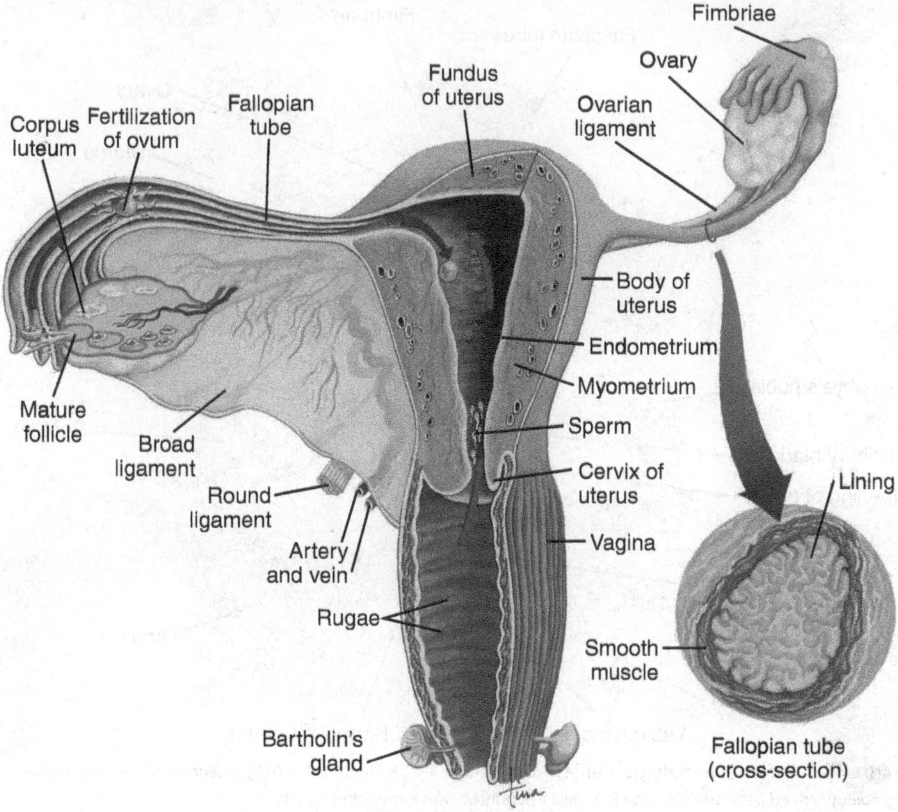

Figure 14.2 Internal structures of adnexa. (From Scanlon, V. C., & Sanders, T. [2015]. *Essentials of anatomy and physiology* [7th ed.]. Philadelphia, PA: F. A. Davis. Reprinted with permission.)

History

■ General Female Reproductive History

The gynecological history is complex, and complaints should not be treated lightly. Gynecological cancers may present with vague, nonspecific complaints, and an index of suspicion is necessary for early diagnosis and treatment. The last menstrual period is one of the most important questions to ask, particularly when prescribing medications, because many are contraindicated in pregnancy. If menstrual cycles are not regular, pregnancy should be ruled out first, and then other diagnoses can be considered. The menstrual history includes any episodes of amenorrhea (absence of menstrual bleeding), menorrhagia (excessive bleeding at the time of the menstrual cycle), metrorrhagia (bleeding at irregular noncyclic intervals), dysmenorrhea (pain/cramping with menstruation), and postmenopausal bleeding. Amenorrhea has many causes, including pregnancy; anorexia nervosa; excessive exercise; low body fat; and disorders or tumors of the

The Menstrual Cycle

The menstrual cycle is regulated by complex interactions between LH, FSH, and the sex hormones estrogen and progesterone (Fig. 14.3). The menstrual cycle has three phases:

- **Follicular Phase** (before release of the egg) begins with the onset of the menstrual cycle. Estrogen and progesterone are low at this time, causing shedding of the top layers of the uterine lining (endometrium). Small amounts of follicle-stimulating hormone (FSH) are released for production of several follicles in the ovaries. Each follicle contains an egg. This phase lasts 13 to 14 days.
- **Ovulatory Phase** (egg release) begins with a surge of LH and FSH, which stimulates egg release (ovulation). Estrogen levels surge during this time, and progesterone begins to increase. This phase last 16 to 32 hours.
- **Luteal Phase** (after egg release) begins with a drop in LH and FSH. The ruptured follicle closes after releasing the egg and forms a corpus luteum, which produces progesterone. Estrogen and progesterone remain elevated, causing the lining of the uterus to thicken, preparing for possible fertilization. If fertilization does not occur, the corpus luteum degenerates, progesterone and estrogen decrease, and the endometrium sheds, leading to menstruation. This phase lasts about 14 days unless fertilization occurs.

hypothalamus, pituitary gland, ovary, uterus, and thyroid gland. Menorrhagia is most commonly caused by uterine fibroids, but hematologic disorders should be considered. Metrorrhagia can be caused by anovulation, intrauterine devices (IUDs), and ovarian and uterine tumors. Primary dysmenorrhea is common and generally does not indicate pathology, particularly in the young population. It is most severe in the first few days of the menstrual cycle. Secondary amenorrhea can occur with fibroids, IUDs, cervical stenosis, and pelvic inflammatory disease (PID). The pain is more persistent with menstrual flow, and nausea, vomiting, or fever occasionally accompanies the pain. Bleeding that occurs after menopause has been established is cause for concern. It may indicate endometrial cancer, and referral for endometrial biopsy or dilation and curettage (D&C) is warranted. If the patient is menopausal, ask about age of menopause, symptoms of menopause, and past or current use of hormone replacement therapy.

Ask the patient about the type of birth control being used, if any. If the patient is not in a monogamous relationship, ask about condom use. Be sure to inquire as to the consistency with which the patient uses birth control methods. Often patients deny the use of birth control, deny the desire for pregnancy, and yet admit to being sexually active. This definitely indicates the need for health teaching and counseling.

Inquire about any masses or lesions that the patient may feel on the external genitalia, which could indicate infection, sexually transmitted infection (STI),

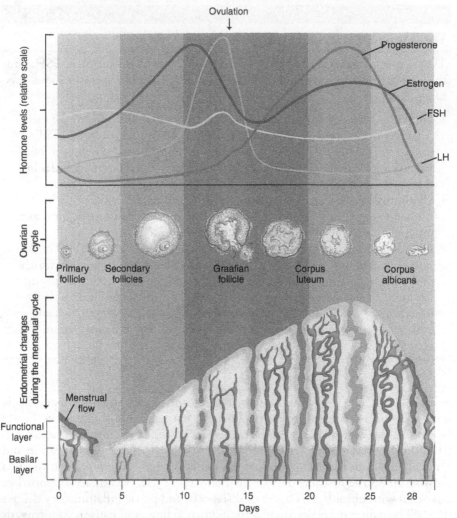

Figure 14.3 The menstrual cycle. (From Scanlon, V. C., & Sanders, T. [2015]. *Essentials of anatomy and physiology* [7th ed.]. Philadelphia, PA: F. A. Davis. Reprinted with permission.)

vulvar malignancy, Bartholin's or Skene's gland infection/inflammation, uterine prolapse, cystocele, or rectocele.

If the patient complains about vaginal discharge, inquire as to the amount, color, consistency, odor, itching, burning, inflammation, or lesions, and history of STIs.

Dyspareunia is one symptom that patients may be reluctant to mention or discuss, so specific inquiries should be made by the practitioner. Dyspareunia may accompany infections caused by inflammation of the vaginal mucosa, uterus, or pelvic structures; vaginal dryness or atrophy usually seen in postmenopausal patients; fibroids; endometriosis; sexual difficulties; or psychosomatic illnesses.

Infertility may be caused by anovulation, decreased function of the corpus luteum, or blocked or scarred fallopian tubes. Any of these can occur even though the patient may be having menstrual cycles. A history of menstrual irregularities may suggest anovulation or thyroid disease, either of which can cause infertility. A history of STIs could lead to scarring of the tubes. If the patient has not already done so, ask her to chart her menstrual cycles and basal body temperatures for 3 months to determine whether and when ovulation is occurring.

■ Past Medical History

Past medical history includes age at menarche, menstrual irregularities, gynecological surgeries or procedures, history of ovarian cysts or uterine fibroids, endometriosis, infertility, STIs, and chronic diseases that might impact hormonal or menstrual function—the most common one being thyroid disease. Ask the patient about past or present use of medications, such as oral contraceptives, hormone replacement therapy, fertility drugs, or thyroid medicine. An obstetrical history should include pregnancies, live births, miscarriages, and abortions.

■ Family History

Family history includes gynecological malignancies in the patient's mother or female siblings or the use of diethylstilbestrol (DES) by the patient's mother during pregnancy. Before the 1970s, the drug DES was widely used in pregnant patients with threatened abortion. Subsequently, it was found to cause abnormalities and malignancies of the reproductive tract in the children of those patients. Its use was banned in the United States in 1971 and in Europe in 1978.

■ Gynecological Cancer History

When inquiring about an individual's family history, it is important to ask about gynecological cancers. Types of cancer that originate in the reproductive organs are referred to as gynecological cancers. Gynecological cancers include ovarian, endometrial/uterine, cervical, vaginal, and vulvar. Endometrial cancer is the most common gynecological cancer. Ovarian cancer has the highest incidence in postmenopausal women. Cervical cancer is the only gynecological cancer with reliable screening tests. The human papillomavirus (HPV) vaccine protects against types of HPV that commonly cause cervical, vaginal, and vulvar cancer.

■ Lifestyle Impacts

The matter of sexual activity and sexual partners is one of the more important areas to inquire about, especially with the high risk of HIV and other STIs. Multiple sexual partners, even in the absence of STIs, puts women at risk for infection with HPV. Smoking may also contribute to the development of HPV infection. Exercise habits, if extremely rigorous or excessive, can contribute to menstrual irregularities. Stress, if significant and prolonged, can cause menstrual irregularities. The use of drugs or alcohol may put patients at risk for unsafe sexual practices or date rape.

Physical Examination

■ Order of the Examination

The United States Preventive Services Task Force (USPSTF) updated cervical cancer screening guidelines were published in 2014 to assist providers with decisions for safe, cost-effective screening practices (Table 14.1).

Patients are often uncomfortable with the gynecological examination, so it is important to spend a sufficient amount of time taking the history and establishing a rapport before beginning the examination. A thorough explanation of the examination both before and as you perform it will help allay the patient's fears. Be sure to have the patient empty the bladder before beginning. The examination should start with an abdominal examination, proceed to external genitalia examination, and end with the speculum and bimanual examination.

Inspection

Inspect the abdomen for any signs of masses, visible pulsations, peristaltic waves, or swelling, which might indicate ascites. Inspect the lower extremities for edema, which can be attributed to many things, one of which is lymphedema secondary to a malignancy. Inspect the external genitalia for lesions, ulcerations, inflammation, warts, swelling, discharge, or nodules. Inspect the perineum and anal areas for fissures, hemorrhoids, inflammation, lesions, ulcers, warts, or nodules. Assess the support of the vaginal outlet by asking the patient to bear down while you look for bulging at the introitus, suggesting a cystocele, rectocele, or prolapsed uterus. Observe the Bartholin's and Skene's glands for inflammation or swelling.

Table 14.1	
USPSTF Cancer Screening Guidelines	
Population	**Recommendation**
Women ages 21–65	Screen with cytology (Pap test) every 3 years. Grade: A
Women ages 30–65	Screen with cytology every 3 years, or hrHPV testing every 5 years, or cotesting (cytology/HPV testing) every 5 years. Grade: A
Women younger than age 21	Do not screen. Grade: D
Women older than age 65 who have had adequate prior screening and are not high risk	Do not screen. Grade: D
Women after hysterectomy with removal of the cervix and with no history of high-grade precancer or cervical cancer	Do not screen. Grade: D

hrHPV = high-risk human papillomavirus.
    USPSTF Cancer Screening Recommendations (2018).

Auscultation

Auscultate the abdomen before beginning the gynecological examination. Listen for bowel sounds and bruits. Note any abnormalities in the bowel sounds. Gynecological malignancies can cause abnormalities of bowel sounds owing to peritoneal inflammation, infection, ascites, or gastrointestinal obstruction.

Percussion

Percuss the abdomen, paying particular attention to the suprapubic area and the right and left lower quadrants. An enlarged uterus will percuss dull in the suprapubic region. Inflammation, causing peritoneal irritation, may cause discomfort with percussion. Percuss for shifting dullness in the abdomen, indicating ascites, which may be the first sign of ovarian cancer.

Palpation

Palpate the abdomen for rebound tenderness, ascites, or masses. Palpate the inguinal lymph nodes for swelling or tenderness. STIs often cause inguinal lymphadenopathy with tenderness. Ovarian cancer that has metastasized to the lymph system will cause inflammation and swelling of the lymph nodes in the inguinal area.

Speculum Examination

A speculum examination is recommended during an annual wellness examination when indicated by an individual's medical history or current symptoms (ACOG, 2020). If a speculum examination is needed to perform cervical cancer screening, to screen for an STI, or to examine symptoms present, the provider should follow current evidence-based guidelines. A pelvic examination is not a requirement before initiating or prescribing contraception, except when placing an IUD (ACOG, 2020).

When performing a speculum examination, the provider should observe the cervix for inflammation, lesions, growths, nodules, discharge, or bleeding. Observe the vaginal walls for inflammation, discharge, color changes, or ulcers. Infection can cause discharge and redness of the vaginal walls. Infection is also associated with vaginal bleeding from the cervix. Menopause causes the vaginal walls to be pale and smooth as opposed to the normal pink and rugose. Varicose veins may be seen on the sides of the vaginal walls mostly in pregnant and obese patients. A parous cervix will be more open and may show healed lacerations. The cervix of a pregnant patient will be purplish in color. Cervical polyps are nonmalignant growths that appear as pedunculated, teardrop growths from the cervical os.

Bimanual Examination

The bimanual examination is performed to determine the position, size, shape, consistency, and mobility of the uterus and ovaries. It is also used to assess tenderness that might be associated with inflammation, infection, or cysts.

The uterus should be pear-shaped, smooth, mobile, nontender, and firm but not hard. Malignancies may occur, causing the uterus to be hard and fixed. Fibroids present as firm, nodular growths. Ultrasound or a computed tomography (CT) scan is needed to determine whether the growths are benign fibroids or malignant growths. Tenderness with movement of the cervix and uterus occurs in PID, termed *cervical motion tenderness*.

Variations in the position of the uterus are not considered abnormal, but significant variations may be related to back pain, especially during menses or childbirth, and occasionally to infertility. Figure 14.4 shows the common

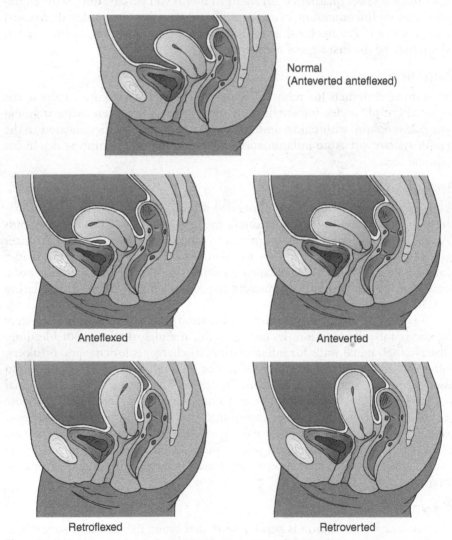

Normal
(Anteverted anteflexed)

Anteflexed

Anteverted

Retroflexed

Retroverted

Figure 14.4 Common uterine positions. (From Swartz, M. [1998]. *Textbook of physical diagnosis* [3rd ed.]. Philadelphia, PA: W. B. Saunders, p. 442. Reprinted with permission.)

uterine positions (i.e., normal, retroverted, retroflexed, anteverted, anteflexed). The uterus can be situated in the midline, posteriorly toward the sacrum, or anteriorly toward the abdominal wall, termed *normal, retroverted,* or *anteverted,* respectively. The long axis of the uterus can also be bent over on itself either backward or forward, termed *retroflexed* or *anteflexed.* A digital rectal examination is useful for indirect palpation of the uterus and is particularly helpful if the uterus is retroverted or retroflexed.

The ovaries are small and almond-shaped, smooth, mobile, nontender, and firm. Ovaries are more difficult to palpate because of their small size and anatomical location. Ovarian cysts or inflammation cause a significant increase in tenderness that is easy to diagnose. Unilateral adnexal pain and tenderness in a patient in the first trimester of pregnancy should alert you to the possibility of a tubal pregnancy, considered a surgical emergency. Malignancies may result in nodular, enlarged, hard, and fixed ovaries, but the cancer may have been present for some time before the physical examination signs are detected. Any masses or abnormalities found on palpation of the uterus or ovaries warrant prompt ultrasound or CT.

Differential Diagnosis of Chief Complaints

■ Mass and Swelling at the Introitus

Vaginal infections or malignancies may lead to irritation and swelling of the external genitalia. Swelling and/or infection of a Bartholin's gland presents as a very painful, inflamed, tender cyst on either side of the introitus. Nontender masses include uterine prolapse, cystocele, and rectocele. Occasionally, pregnant patients develop painful varicose veins in the vagina that appear swollen and purplish in color. Inspection and palpation are most helpful in the diagnosis. Laboratory tests and diagnostics are usually not necessary for initial diagnosis. Referrals to the surgeon or gynecology specialist are necessary for treatment in most cases.

History

A childbirth history is important in patients with this complaint because difficult or numerous childbirths may lead to problems with the pelvic support structures or damage to the bladder or rectal wall. Any change in elimination patterns is one of the most important questions to ask this group of patients. Ask about urinary incontinence or more frequent urinary tract infections. Uterine prolapse and cystocele can cause frequency, incontinence, and residual urine, thus increasing the risk for urinary tract infections. Ask about changes in bowel movements, such as constipation, difficulty with evacuation, and rectal fullness, which could be symptoms of a rectocele.

Physical Examination

A thorough pelvic examination, including a speculum and bimanual examination, is necessary. Assess for support of the vaginal outlet. It may be possible to visualize a mass or swelling in the vaginal area on inspection. If not, ask the

---

| RED FLAG | Red Flags for Examination of the Female Reproductive System |

- *Significant unilateral adnexal pain in an early pregnant patient*
- *Frank uterine bleeding in a pregnant patient*
- *Frank uterine bleeding in a postpartum or postabortion patient for more than 7 days*
- *Fever or significant abdominal pain in a postpartum or postabortion patient*
- *Free fluid in the peritoneal cavity (ascites)*
- *Uterine bleeding in a postmenopausal patient*
- *A uterus or ovaries that are fixed, hard, or nodular on palpation*

---

patient to strain down while you insert your finger into the vaginal opening. Feel for the mass to come to meet your finger when the patient bears down. Palpate superiorly, inferiorly, and on the sides over the Bartholin's glands for swelling and tenderness.

UTERINE PROLAPSE

Uterine prolapse is a downward placement of the uterus into the vaginal canal. It occurs more in older, multiparous patients as a result of injury, weakening, and stretching of the pelvic musculature and ligaments. Prolapse can be due to traumatic vaginal delivery, multiple births, chronic straining, pelvic tumors, and obesity. It may take years for the prolapse to develop, which partly explains why it is seen more often in older patients. Prolapse of the uterus is often accompanied by cystocele and rectocele. Risk factors for pelvic organ prolapse include age, parity, obesity, chronic constipation, hormone status, previous gynecological surgery, smoking, high-impact activity, and genetic predisposition.

Signs and Symptoms

Early on, the patient may complain of a full feeling in the vaginal area or may be unaware that the uterus is prolapsed until it is discovered on physical examination. As the uterus prolapses further, the patient will feel a mass at the introitus or even protruding from the vagina. The patient may also have complaints of urinary frequency or incontinence owing to pressure on the bladder from the uterus. Kegel exercises and estrogen therapy, either oral or vaginal, can be used as prevention or treatment of mild prolapse. The use of a pessary will hold the uterus in place and lessen symptoms. Surgical intervention may be required, particularly when cystocele and rectocele are present.

Diagnostic Studies

The diagnosis is made by physical examination, although pelvic ultrasound may help to rule out other conditions. The degree of prolapse depends on the degree of weakness of pelvic support:

- In first-degree uterine prolapse, the uterus partially descends into the vagina.
- In second-degree uterine prolapse, the uterus descends into the introitus.
- In third-degree uterine prolapse, the uterus can be visualized outside of the vagina, and often the vagina becomes inverted.

CYSTOCELE

A cystocele occurs when a portion of the bladder herniates into the vagina. Similar to uterine prolapse, it is the result of weakness of the supporting muscles and ligaments, and cystocele often accompanies uterine prolapse.

Signs and Symptoms

Although a cystocele can contribute to urinary frequency, urgency, and infection, it is not the only cause of stress incontinence. The bimanual examination reveals a smooth, soft bulge of the anterior vaginal wall that is more pronounced with straining.

Diagnostic Studies

The most beneficial diagnostic test is a voiding cystourethrogram (VCUG), which is an x-ray taken while the patient is voiding. It is helpful in determining the size and shape of the bladder and the presence of an obstruction to urine flow in the ureter, bladder, or urethra. It can also be helpful in determining whether reflux is present. If VCUG is inconclusive, an ultrasound, CT scan, or magnetic resonance imaging (MRI) of the abdomen and pelvis are useful to determine the etiology of the patient's complaint. Surgical repair of the cystocele, including hysterectomy, may be necessary in order to avoid recurrence.

RECTOCELE

A rectocele occurs when a portion of the connective tissue of the rectal wall herniates into the vagina. As in uterine prolapse and cystocele, rectocele occurs more often in multiparous patients as they age. Breech deliveries and episiotomies also may contribute to the development of a rectocele.

Signs and Symptoms

Patients are often asymptomatic but may complain of difficult or painful defecation, constipation, sensation of incomplete evacuation, or a feeling of rectal fullness. Rectovaginal examination reveals a soft bulge in the posterior vaginal wall.

Diagnostic Studies

Rectoceles are commonly found by an evacuation proctogram (defecography), a barium x-ray that looks at pelvic organs while the patient is straining. It gives information about the size of the rectal bulge and how efficiently the rectum empties.

Rectoceles are considered abnormal if barium trapping (the rectocele does not completely empty upon evacuation) is noted. Colonoscopy may be necessary to rule out malignancies, which often give rise to symptoms similar to those of rectocele. Surgical repair may be indicated if the rectocele obstructs and impairs fecal evacuation.

Bartholin's Cysts

The two Bartholin's glands are mucus-secreting glands, one located in each lateral wall of the vagina at the introitus. They can become abscessed in acute or chronic inflammatory processes, usually as a result of bacteria that are prevalent in the vaginal and perineal area, but also by thickened mucus or congenital narrowing of the duct. In postmenopausal patients, a malignant cause should be considered in the differential diagnosis.

Signs and Symptoms

Acutely, Bartholin's abscesses are extremely painful, in part due to their anatomical location, which makes sitting difficult. The area becomes swollen with the presence of a tender, inflamed, fluctuant cyst that is easily visualized. Systemic symptoms are usually absent. The cysts often become chronically inflamed, in which case a marsupialization procedure may be indicated. Occasionally, solid malignant tumors can occur in the Bartholin's glands and will need prompt referral. Other considerations include vaginal wall cysts (Gartner's duct cysts), Skene's gland cysts, or urethral diverticulum, although the latter two are located superiorly to the Bartholin's gland. As previously mentioned, malignancy should always be considered in postmenopausal patients.

Diagnostic Studies

The diagnosis is made by physical examination. Antibiotics are necessary only when infection is present. If malignancy is suspected, prompt referral and biopsy are necessary.

■ Vaginal Discharge

Vaginal discharge is one of the more common complaints in both primary care and gynecological health. The history and physical examination are often sufficient to give a diagnosis, but in some cases, further laboratory testing may be necessary for a definitive diagnosis. If the history, physical examination, and vaginal cultures lead to a diagnosis of an STI, further serology is indicated, and patient education is of utmost importance in treatment and future prevention. When a patient presents with a complaint of vaginal discharge, several diagnoses should be considered, including yeast, trichomoniasis, chlamydia, gonorrhea, bacterial vaginosis, cervicitis, gynecological cancer, PID, and pregnancy.

History

The history includes the length of time the patient has had the discharge, the color and consistency of the discharge, presence of itching or odor, unusual bleeding, abdominal pain, or fever. Abdominal pain or fever suggests inflammation in the

Box 14.1

How To Be Reasonably Certain That a Patient Is Not Pregnant

A health-care provider can be reasonably certain that a patient is not pregnant if there are no signs or symptoms of pregnancy and any one of the following criteria is met:

- is 7 days or less after the beginning of the last normal menses
- has not had sexual intercourse since the last menses
- has been correctly and consistently using a reliable method of contraception
- is ≤7 days or less after spontaneous or induced abortion
- is within 4 weeks postpartum
- is fully or almost fully breastfeeding, amenorrheic, and less than 6 months postpartum

CDC (2017).

fallopian tubes and ovaries rather than being confined to the vaginal area. It is imperative to obtain a menstrual and sexual history as well as method of birth control and history of STIs. Before prescribing medications, it is necessary to confirm and document that a patient is not pregnant. A health-care provider can be reasonably certain that a patient is not pregnant by performing a pregnancy test or by using the Centers for Disease Control and Prevention's (CDC's) "reasonable certainty" method (Box 14.1) (CDC, 2017b).

Physical Examination

A thorough gynecological examination is necessary, including a speculum examination to observe the discharge and presence of inflammation of the vaginal mucosa or cervix, a wet prep to examine the discharge microscopically, cervical cultures if necessary to rule out STIs, and a bimanual examination to rule out tenderness or enlargement of the uterus or ovaries. See Table 14.2 for differentiation of vaginal discharge.

YEAST VAGINITIS (CANDIDIASIS)

Yeast vaginitis is one of the more common vaginal infections in young patients and is caused by the fungus *Candida albicans*. It is not considered an STI, and transmission to or from sexual partners is unlikely. Since the advent of over-the-counter (OTC) preparations to treat yeast vaginitis, it is not seen in office practice as frequently. There should be a high index of suspicion in patients who complain of failure with OTC preparations because they have most likely misdiagnosed their problem or perhaps have more than one infection occurring. Patients who have documented recurrent yeast vaginitis should be screened for diabetes because this type of infection is common in the diabetic population. The high concentration of glucose in the blood offers a favorable medium for yeast to flourish. In addition, HIV is a concern because yeast is more prevalent

Table 14.2

Differentiation of Vaginal Discharge

Characteristic	Yeast	Trichomoniasis	Bacterial vaginosis	Chlamydia	Gonorrhea
Color	White	Grayish	White/yellow	Yellowish	Yellowish
Odor	Absent	Foul	Fishy	Absent	Absent
Consistency	Thick, curdy	Frothy	Creamy	Purulent	Purulent
Location	Adheres to vagina, walls	Pooled in vagina	Introitus, vagina	Introitus, vagina, cervical os	Introitus, vagina, cervical os
Vulva	Erythematous and pruritic	Edematous	Normal	Normal	Normal
Vaginal	Erythematous	"Strawberry spots"	Normal	Normal	Normal mucosa
Cervix	No discharge	"Strawberry spots"	Normal	Purulent discharge	Purulent discharge
Wet Prep	Hyphae, yeast buds	Motile protozoa	Clue cells and whiff test	Numerous white cells	Numerous white cells

in immunocompromised individuals. Other causes include medications, particularly antibiotics but also oral contraceptives and corticosteroids.

Signs and Symptoms

The discharge associated with yeast vaginitis can be differentiated from other infections by symptomatology and wet prep examination. The discharge is very thick and curdlike and adheres to the vaginal walls. Intense vulvar itching accompanies the discharge. Because the discharge is thick, patients often give a history of itching but no discharge since it adheres to the vaginal walls and may not be seen by the patient. In most cases, inflammation and swelling around the labia and introitus occur. This inflammation causes dyspareunia and burning of the labia with urination. Partners generally do not have any related complaints.

Diagnostic Studies

A high suspicion of yeast can be made on physical examination with a wet prep to confirm the diagnosis of *C. albicans*. A 10% KOH (potassium hydroxide) wet prep is most helpful for visualizing budding yeast and hyphae microscopically. A saline wet prep should also be done in looking for alternative causes of the discharge. The presence of *C. albicans* may be reported on a Pap test.

BACTERIAL VAGINOSIS

Although it is believed that the *Gardnerella vaginalis* bacteria can be transmitted through sexual contact, it is not strictly considered an STI. A change in the vaginal pH to a value greater than 4.5 and a change in the bacterial flora with a decrease in lactobacilli give rise to increases in aerobic and anaerobic bacteria. *G. vaginalis* is the most prevalent vaginal infection, although many of the patients with this infection are asymptomatic. It is considered a risk factor for preterm labor, and pregnant patients should always be treated aggressively. Also, patients who are undergoing pelvic surgery are believed to benefit from treatment before surgery.

Signs and Symptoms

Of those patients who are symptomatic, the overwhelming complaint is of a malodorous discharge. *G. vaginalis* has a distinct fishy odor. The odor is usually noticeable during the pelvic examination, but a few drops of 10% KOH solution on the wet prep slide augment the odor. The discharge is fairly thick and white. Patients do not complain of itching, and, generally, there is no inflammation of the vaginal mucosa. Male partners do not complain of discharge, odor, or dysuria, although it is believed they may harbor the bacteria without being symptomatic. The higher pH of semen may be related to the higher vaginal pH that triggers the overgrowth of anaerobes and aerobes.

Diagnostic Studies

The diagnosis is made on symptomatology and KOH wet prep. Microscopically, the wet prep shows the characteristic clue cells (epithelial cells embedded with bacteria), and the odor of *G. vaginalis* is unmistakable.

TRICHOMONIASIS

The STI *Trichomonas vaginalis* is a unicellular, flagellate protozoan. It is associated with an increased incidence in the transmission of HIV; therefore, women with trichomoniasis should be screened for other STIs, including HIV, gonorrhea, chlamydia, and syphilis. *T. vaginalis* has also been associated with perinatal complications.

Signs and Symptoms

The presenting complaints with trichomoniasis are discharge and itching. It can be differentiated from yeast by the discharge, which is thin and frothy rather than the thick, curdlike discharge of yeast. It can also be differentiated from *G. vaginalis* by the presence of vulvar itching and inflammation but no complaint of odor. Inflammation with petechiae of the vaginal walls, known as *strawberry spots*, is diagnostic of *T. vaginalis*. Male partners are usually asymptomatic but harbor the organism, and they must be treated along with the patient; intercourse should be avoided or condoms used until treatment is completed by each partner.

Diagnostic Studies

T. vaginalis is easily seen on a wet prep as a flagellate protozoan in the majority of cases. If they are present, it is diagnostic. If protozoa are not seen on wet prep and trichomoniasis is suspected, a culture is recommended. A Pap test may also show the presence of *T. vaginalis* but is only 60% to 70% accurate for diagnosis.

CHLAMYDIA

Chlamydia is an STI caused by the bacteria *Chlamydia trachomatis*. In addition to cervical or higher reproductive organ infection, *C. trachomatis* can affect the urethra, rectum, or throat. It is thought to be the main cause of salpingitis and scarring of the fallopian tubes, thus leading to ectopic pregnancy or infertility. It can also cause conjunctivitis in the neonate if present during delivery.

Signs and Symptoms

Patients are often asymptomatic with chlamydia infections but may present with mucopurulent discharge, dysuria, abdominal pain, fever, and abnormal vaginal bleeding. Cervicitis and cervical motion tenderness on physical examination indicate PID. It is the causative organism in the majority of nongonococcal urethritis in both women and men and in most cases of cervicitis. Reiter's syndrome, a serious systemic complication of chlamydia infection that occurs more commonly in men, is characterized by urethritis, arthritis, and conjunctivitis or uveitis.

Diagnostic Studies

A nucleic acid amplification test (NAAT) from a urine sample or from the endocervix or vagina offers increased sensitivity and specificity, and it is recommended by the CDC (2021) for detection of both gonorrhea and chlamydia. A Gen-Probe cervical culture may still be used depending on cost and the patient's insurance coverage. Because chlamydia is an STI, both the patient and any partners should be screened and treated. Patients should abstain from intercourse during treatment. Test of cure follow-up is not advised for individuals treated with the recommended regimen, unless therapeutic adherence is uncertain, symptoms continue, or reinfection is suspected (CDC, 2021).

GONORRHEA

Gonorrhea is an STI caused by *Neisseria gonorrhoeae* that can present in any degree, ranging from asymptomatic to severe infection. In addition to cervical or higher reproductive organ infection, *N. gonorrhoeae* can affect the urethra, rectum, or throat. In spite of ongoing public education on STIs, the incidence of gonorrhea has continued to increase.

Signs and Symptoms

Patients may be asymptomatic or present with complaints of mucopurulent discharge, fever, abdominal pain, lymphadenopathy, and joint pain. Be suspicious of infection with *N. gonorrhoeae* in a young patient who complains of abrupt onset of polyarthritis. *N. gonorrhoeae* can persist, leading to salpingitis, abscess, and peritonitis. As with chlamydia, long-term complications include scarring of the fallopian tubes, ectopic pregnancy, and infertility. In addition, *N. gonorrhoeae* can cause conjunctivitis in newborns of infected patients.

Two more serious complications of gonorrhea are disseminated gonococcal infection (DGI) with bacteremia and gonococcal arthritis. In DGI, symptoms of genital infection may be absent. The patient presents instead with systemic complaints, such as fever, malaise, migratory polyarthralgias, and pustular skin lesions on the limbs. The bacteremia occasionally can lead to pericarditis, endocarditis, and meningitis; therefore, prompt diagnosis and treatment are necessary. Gonococcal arthritis presents with more severe and localized joint symptoms. The patient is usually febrile with severe joint pain, limited range of motion, redness, tenderness, and effusion of a few joints rather than disseminated as seen in DGI. Prompt treatment is required to avoid articular destruction.

Diagnostic Studies

As with chlamydia, a NAAT can be performed and is more accurate for diagnosis of both *N. gonorrhoeae* and *C. trachomatis*; however, it is also more expensive. A Gen-Probe cervical culture can still be used to detect gonorrhea and chlamydia if cost is an issue. A test of cure is not recommended for individuals who received a diagnosis of uncomplicated urogenital or rectal gonorrhea if treated with one of the recommended regimens; however, individuals diagnosed with pharyngeal gonorrhea should return within 7 to 14 days after treatment for a test of cure (CDC, 2021). If DGI is suspected, blood cultures or synovial fluid cultures should be drawn. In gonococcal arthritis, a joint aspirate will show pus and the presence of gonococci.

PELVIC INFLAMMATORY DISEASE AND SALPINGITIS

PID is defined as an infection of the uterus, fallopian tubes, and adjacent pelvic structures. It is often secondary to an STI or other infection of the lower reproductive tract that migrates upward into the uterus and tubes. *N. gonorrhea* and *C. trachomatis* are two of the commonly offending organisms. Pelvic infections can also occur postsurgery, postpartum, or postabortion but are generally caused by other organisms, such as staphylococcus or streptococcus.

Signs and Symptoms

Abdominal pain, mucopurulent cervical discharge, and often fever are the more common presenting symptoms. Rebound tenderness indicates peritoneal irritation. Dysuria, nausea, and vomiting may also be present. The abdominal pain is midline and often accompanied by right and left lower quadrant pain, particularly when accompanied by salpingitis. During the pelvic examination, there is pain with cervical motion and with palpation of the uterus and ovaries. Risk factors include a history of PID or STIs, multiple sexual partners, douching, and IUDs. Infertility may occur as a complication owing to scarring and occlusion of the fallopian tubes.

Diagnostic Studies

The diagnosis is based mostly on history and physical examination. A positive culture of the cervical discharge identifying a bacterial organism is helpful. An elevated white blood cell count will be present. If suspected, surgical emergencies such as ectopic pregnancy or appendicitis must be ruled out by ultrasound or abdominal CT scan. Culdocentesis, endometrial biopsy, and laparoscopy can be performed if the diagnosis is unclear or to isolate the causative organism.

GENITOURINARY SYNDROME OF MENOPAUSE

Genitourinary syndrome of menopause, formerly known as atrophic vaginitis, is not an infection and does not cause a discharge. Signs and symptoms can mimic the *C. albicans* yeast vaginitis. It occurs in postmenopausal patients owing to a lack of estrogen. It can occur with surgical or natural menopause and occasionally in lactating patients.

Signs and Symptoms

The vaginal mucosa thins and becomes smooth and pale. The complaint most often heard from patients is itching owing to dryness and atrophy of the vaginal tissue. It is often mistaken for *C. albicans* by patients because of the pruritus, but the physical examination shows no similarity.

Diagnostic Studies

The diagnosis is dependent on the history and physical examination. Common symptoms reported include vaginal and vulvar dryness and irritation, dyspareunia, and urinary frequency, dysuria, nocturia, or incontinence. A wet prep may show the presence of leukocytes and a lack of lactobacillus.

■ Labial Lesions

Common causes of labial lesions include the herpes simplex virus (HSV), condyloma acuminatum, cancer of the vulva, syphilitic chancre, and, just inferior to the labia, a Bartholin's cyst. Although HSV is the most common cause of this complaint, it depends somewhat on the age and sexual history of the patient.

History

As with most gynecological complaints, a thorough sexual history is imperative: the number of partners, type of birth control, condom use, history of STIs, length of time in current relationship, perceived monogamy of the relationship, last Pap test, and history of abnormal Pap test. Ask the patient to describe the location and characteristics of the lesion and whether it is a single lesion or multiple lesions. Inquire about accompanying symptoms, such as pain, tenderness, burning, itching, excoriation, redness, swelling, or discharge. Herpetic lesions usually burn or itch in the prodromal stage and then become painful and tender; condyloma often itch but are not painful; syphilitic chancres are usually not tender; cancerous labial lesions usually are neither tender nor pruritic; and Bartholin's cysts present with severe discomfort and tenderness, especially with sitting. The age of the patient can play a part in prioritizing differential diagnosis because labial cancer rarely occurs in patients younger than 50 years.

Physical Examination

The physical examination includes a thorough visualization of the skin over the entire body to look for other lesions or skin changes, particularly in the anal area, mouth, palms, and soles. Labial lesions caused by STIs may also be present in the mouth or anus, depending on sexual practices. Syphilis may manifest itself with pigmented or light-red macules or papules on the soles or palms.

Examine the abdomen for tenderness, and check the lymph nodes, especially in the inguinal area. A thorough gynecological examination is necessary, including a speculum examination, wet prep, viral and/or bacterial cultures, and Pap test. A scraping or biopsy of the lesion may be necessary if cancer is suspected. A blood sample for the Venereal Disease Research Laboratory (VDRL) is needed if syphilis is suspected.

HERPES SIMPLEX VIRUS

There are two types of HSV: HSV1 and HSV2. The majority of genital herpes infections are due to HSV2 that has been transferred to the labial area by either genital or oral contact. Although blood tests can be done to determine the presence or absence of antibodies to HSV1 and HSV2, it is mostly academic as the symptoms, transmission, and treatment are the same regardless of type.

Signs and Symptoms

Although antibodies to the herpes virus can be found in the majority of patients 3 weeks after exposure, the symptoms may be absent or mild enough to go unnoticed by the patient. Approximately 10% to 15% of persons who carry the virus are asymptomatic, but they can still shed the virus—referred to as *asymptomatic viral shedding*. This, among other things, contributes to the spread of the herpes virus. The lesions begin with a slightly reddened area on the labia that is pruritic and tingling. There may be systemic symptoms, such as fever, headache, malaise, lymphadenopathy, and urinary frequency/dysuria. After a few days, a patchy lesion appears, containing several small vesicles. The vesicles then rupture, and a painful, tender ulcerated area remains for 10 to 14 days. Lesions may be single or multiple. They may also occur on the cervix, perianal area, and mouth, depending on contact area. Lesions can reoccur as frequently as once a month, often with menstruation, or as infrequently as once a year or longer. The virus may remain dormant for years until a stress or illness causes a recurrence. Treatment with antiviral medication can lessen and sometimes prevent recurrence. Suppressive therapy is encouraged to help reduce recurrent infections.

Diagnostic Studies

A viral culture of the active lesion will yield positive results in the acute phase. Additionally, about 85% of patients will develop antibodies within 21 days of exposure, and a blood test will be positive for immunoglobulin M (IgM) antibodies. Type-specific assay tests are available to distinguish HSV1 from HSV2.

CONDYLOMA ACUMINATUM

Condylomas are one of the manifestations of HPV, which is the most common STI. There are over 100 types of HPV, 40 of which commonly affect the anogenital region. Most HPV infections are self-limiting and asymptomatic. The virus is categorized by DNA pattern (genotype) rather than by host antibodies to the virus (serotype). Types 6 and 11 are most commonly associated with condylomas. There is an increased incidence of cervical cancer in patients infected with HPV, with neoplasias being associated with types 16 and 18. HPV is highly contagious and can be transmitted through intercourse or oral/anal sex and from pregnant patient to infant. HPV can affect the respiratory or reproductive tract of newborns, termed *respiratory papillomatosis*. Condylomas grow more rapidly in pregnancy. However, the presence of lesions during delivery is not always a contraindication to a vaginal delivery. Those who are immunocompromised are also at greater risk for infection or proliferation of condylomas. HPV vaccination can prevent genital warts.

Signs and Symptoms

Lesions are white with a rough, granular appearance with fingerlike projections often containing capillaries or a mosaic pattern. Condylomas may be single or multiple and can occur on the vagina, cervix, vulva, perineum, and perianal areas. Symptoms are rarely associated with condyloma but may include itching or irritation.

Diagnostic Studies

Diagnosing condyloma through physical examination can be a challenge. Lesions are often very small, even microscopic, and the rugae of the vaginal mucosa may mask the lesion. Applying white vinegar to a suspected lesion helps to distinguish it from normal tissue. Condyloma will turn white against the surrounding tissue when the vinegar is applied. Many of the small lesions can be seen only on colposcopy. If dysplasia is seen on the Pap test, biopsies should be taken to rule out intraepithelial neoplasia because more than 90% of the cervical neoplasias are caused by HPV. Unfortunately, barrier contraceptives offer only limited protection against the spread of HPV infection.

SYPHILIS

Syphilis is an STI caused by the spirochete *Treponema pallidum*. It is transmitted through intact or abraded mucous membranes and rapidly spreads to the lymph nodes and throughout the body. The incidence of syphilis has risen dramatically in the last 30 years with the increase in HIV and other STIs. The latest data, from 2017 to 2018, shows an increase of nearly 13.3% in all stages. Syphilis cases have steadily been on the rise for men who have sex with men, but an increase in cases is also evident in men who have sex with women. This is particularly concerning in untreated female patients of childbearing age. Congenital syphilis cases have increased by nearly 40%. Untreated syphilis in pregnant patients can lead to infection of the fetus in up to 80% of cases and may result in stillbirth or infant death in up to 40% of cases (CDC, 2017a).

Signs and Symptoms

The primary chancre lesion occurs anywhere from 10 to 90 days after exposure. It appears as a firm, indurated, painless papule that erodes into an ulcer with raised or reddened borders. Chancres are usually single lesions and can occur on any mucous membrane or skin area. Nontender lymphadenopathy is present in the regional nodes. Genital lesions are most commonly seen in women on the external genitalia. Symptoms may be mild enough to go unnoticed, especially when they are in areas other than the genitalia, and they heal without treatment in 4 to 8 weeks.

If the primary infection is not treated, secondary syphilis develops and is characterized by more systemic symptoms, such as diffuse lymphadenopathy, malaise, fever, headache, anorexia, joint pain, and rash, which appears most commonly on the soles and palms but can also be present on the trunk. The rash can be macular, papular, or pustular, making the differential diagnosis variable. Erosion of the mucous membranes occurs, mostly in the mouth, forming grayish-white patches. Alopecia also may occur in patches. In secondary syphilis, anemia, jaundice, albuminuria, neck stiffness, and syphilitic meningitis may develop, causing cranial nerve lesions and deafness. If secondary syphilis is untreated, a latent stage develops. Approximately one-third of those infected go on to develop tertiary syphilis, although it may not manifest for many years. Tertiary syphilis affects the skin, bones, and cardiovascular and neurological systems.

Diagnostic Studies

Serum for VDRL/rapid plasma reagin (RPR) is the necessary laboratory test for diagnosis, and it will generally convert to positive 3 to 6 weeks after infection or 3 to 4 weeks after appearance of the primary lesion. False-positive serological reactions are common, transient, and usually with a low titer. Confirmatory testing is necessary. Although there are several confirmatory choices—including the fluorescent treponemal antibody absorption test (FTA-ABS), microhemagglutination assay (MHA-TP), *T. pallidum* particle agglutination assay (TPPA), *T. pallidum* enzyme immunoassay (TP-EIA), and chemiluminescence immunoassays (CIA)—the CDC's *Morbidity and Mortality Weekly Report* (2011) recommends the TPPA, which has a high predictive value. With treatment, a positive VDRL/RPR syphilis test result usually becomes negative. Treponemal tests (FTA-ABS, MHA-TP, TPPA, TP-EIA, and CIA) stay positive for life, regardless of treatment (CDC, 2011). *T. pallidum* also can be detected by dark-field examination of specimens from skin and mucous membrane lesions, but serological testing is more reliable. Polymerase chain reaction is specific for detecting *T. pallidum* in serum, spinal fluid, and amniotic fluid.

CANCER OF THE VULVA

Vulvar carcinoma accounts for less than 6% of gynecological cancers (American Cancer Society, 2022). It occurs more commonly in patients older than 50 years. The majority of these cancers are squamous cell carcinomas; the remaining are basal cell, melanomas, Paget's disease, and Bartholin's adenocarcinoma.

Signs and Symptoms

The lesions of vulvar carcinoma are easily seen and palpated by the patient but are not recognized as serious and often do not bring the patient into the office for many months. They are often pruritic, white, macerated lesions initially on the vulva that may extend to the vagina, urethra, and anal area. They begin superficially but can become quite extensive in depth and breadth if left untreated. They may become infected, ulcerated, and necrotic.

Diagnostic Studies

Biopsy is the definitive diagnostic procedure, and for squamous cell carcinoma, radical vulvectomy with inguinal and femoral lymph node dissection is the definitive treatment. Patients should be followed closely for at least 5 years for early detection of recurrences. Prognosis depends on the depth of the lesion.

■ Abnormal Pap Test

The Pap test is designed to detect cancer cells in the cervix and vagina. It was developed in the 1940s, and since then, the incidence of cervical cancer has declined more than 70%. The technology for the interpretation of Pap tests has improved greatly over the years, with computer-generated procedures now being used. In 2018 and 2019, updated screening guidelines were released by the USPSTF and the American Cancer Society (ACS), respectively. The American Society for Colposcopy and Cervical Pathology (ASCCP) updated risk-based management guidelines for abnormal cervical cancer screening tests in 2019. The USPSTF guidelines recommend a Pap test beginning at age 21 and a Pap test every 3 years for patients ages 21 to 29. For patients ages 30 to 65 years, the USPSTF recommends screening every 3 years with cervical cytology alone, every 5 years with high-risk human papillomavirus (hrHPV) testing alone, or every 5 years with hrHPV testing in combination with cytology (cotesting). The ACS recommends cervical cancer screening beginning at age 25. The recommendation for first-line screening is an hrHPV test. If this cannot be performed, a Pap test performed every 3 years or a Pap and HPV test every 5 years is acceptable. Recommendations for patients with a history of abnormal Pap tests should be managed following the ASCCP guidelines.

Patients who are immunocompromised, have been exposed to DES before birth, have been treated for a precancerous cervical lesion or cervical cancer, or who have HIV need more frequent screening and may need to continue screening beyond age 65. Women who have had a hysterectomy do not need cervical screening, unless the hysterectomy was done to treat a precancerous cervical lesion or cervical cancer. Patients older than 65 years may need a pelvic and bimanual examination if the patient is having vaginal bleeding or symptoms that might indicate ovarian cancer, such as pelvic/abdominal pain, bloating, fullness, urinary frequency and fatigue.

History

Ask the patient about a history of abnormal Pap tests, cryosurgery, colposcopy, or cervical/endometrial biopsy. Ask about any history of STIs, especially HSV and HPV, both of which can be a reason for an abnormal Pap test. Ask about the use of DES by the patient's mother during pregnancy since it can cause abnormalities and malignancies of the reproductive tract in the children of those women. Ask about family gynecological malignancies.

Physical Examination

While obtaining the Pap test, a thorough gynecological examination should be performed and notations made of any cervical inflammation (cervicitis), discharge, STIs, or other reproductive abnormalities. It is important to continue Pap tests in postmenopausal patients for cervical and endometrial cancer screening. Surprisingly, 25% of cervical cancers occur in patients older than 65 years. It has been suggested that the increased risk for cervical cancer among older patients stems from nonadherence to screening at younger ages. The peak incidence of endometrial cancer occurs in postmenopausal patients between 50 and 60 years (American Cancer Society, 2021). In patients who have had hysterectomies, a smear of the vaginal cuff is still suggested as well as inspection of the vaginal mucosa and external genitalia looking for signs of malignancy.

Signs and Symptoms

Patients rarely exhibit symptoms of an abnormal Pap test unless it is due to infection or inflammation, in which case vaginal discharge is commonly present.

Diagnostic Studies

Diagnosis is made solely through the Pap test cytology report from the sample taken of the endocervix, cervix, and vaginal pool, or the vaginal cuff in the case of hysterectomy. The Bethesda system is the standard for reporting cervical cytology (National Cancer Institute, 2001). See Table 14.3 for an outline of the Bethesda

Table 14.3

Bethesda 2014 Classification System for Cervical Cytology

Negative for Intraepithelial Lesion or Malignancy Organisms	Epithelial Cell Abnormalities Squamous Cell	Other
• Trichomoniasis • Fungal • Bacterial vaginosis • HSV • Cytomegalovirus	• ASC-US; ASC-H • LSIL • HSIL • Squamous cell cancer	• Endometrial cells in patients older than 45 years
Non-neoplastic Findings	Glandular cell	
• Reactive cellular changes, such as inflammation, radiation IUD • Glandular cells status—posthysterectomy • Non-neoplastic cellular variations including atrophy, squamous metaplasia, keratotic changes, tubal metaplasia, or pregnancy-associated changes	• Atypical endocervical cells (not otherwise specified or favor neoplastic) • Atypical endometrial cells (not otherwise specified) • Atypical glandular cells (not otherwise specified or favor neoplastic) • Endocervical adenocarcinoma in situ • Adenocarcinoma; includes endocervical endometrial, extrauterine, not otherwise specified	

ASC-H = ASC cannot exclude high-grade squamous intraepithelial lesion; ASC-US = atypical squamous cells of undetermined significance; herpes simplex virus (HSV); HSIL = high-grade squamous intraepithelial lesion; IUD = intrauterine device; LSIL = low-grade squamous intraepithelial lesion system. For other abnormalities, referral should be made to a specialist for colposcopy and/or biopsy.

■ Abnormal Uterine Bleeding

Abnormal uterine bleeding is much more common in the younger population, especially during the teen years when menstrual patterns are becoming established. Also, during the early reproductive years, malignancies are much less likely to be the cause. Most cases of abnormal uterine bleeding are due to organic causes and to dysfunction of the hypothalamic-pituitary-ovarian axis. Bleeding after menopause has been established as cause for concern, and referral for endometrial biopsy is a must.

History

Start with the date of the last menstrual period and reconstruct as much of the menstrual history as possible, including age at menarche, menstrual patterns, and episodes of amenorrhea or abnormal bleeding in the past. Ask for a complete description of the current problem with abnormal bleeding. Important things to know include the time of onset; the pattern of bleeding (intermittent or constant); the amount and frequency of bleeding; the color of the blood (bright red or dark); and any history of trauma, vaginal discharge, recent STIs, abdominal pain, fever, or missed periods. Inquire about type of birth control and sexual activity. Determine whether there is a history of abnormal Pap tests. In postmenopausal patients, ask about the use of unopposed estrogen replacement, which is a risk factor for endometrial cancer. Bleeding disorders can arise, so it is important to ask the patient about easy bruising or any recent gum bleeding or nosebleeds.

Physical Examination

Both an abdominal and a pelvic examination should be done to assess for masses or tenderness and the size, consistency, and mobility of the uterus and ovaries. During the pelvic examination, a Pap test should be obtained to rule out cervical cancer. An endometrial biopsy might be needed to rule out endometrial cancer, especially in middle-aged and older patients, but it is wise to wait for the results of the Pap test before proceeding with a biopsy. A pelvic ultrasound or MRI should be considered to rule out pelvic mass. A human chorionic gonadotropin (hCG) measurement should be performed to rule out pregnancy, and a complete blood count (CBC) and platelet count should be done to rule out hematologic causes.

ENDOMETRIAL CARCINOMA

Endometrial cancer can follow atypical hyperplasia or can originate on its own. It occurs more often in white patients, but black patients are more likely to die from it. The peak incidence is between 60 and 70 years but has been reported in patients as young as 20 years. Although it is the most common pelvic genital cancer in women, a complaint of abnormal uterine bleeding assists in early detection. Patients with hyperestrogenism that is due to either altered estrogen metabolism or the use of unopposed estrogen are at increased risk. Patients taking tamoxifen for breast cancer are also at increased risk.

Signs and Symptoms

Abnormal bleeding occurs in the majority of patients with endometrial cancers. Spotting or bleeding of any kind in a postmenopausal patient is a red flag, and endometrial biopsy is warranted. A small number of patients complain of lower abdominal pain or cramping. Physical examination is usually not helpful in the early stages but in later stages may reveal an enlarged, fixed uterus. It is necessary to refer the patient to a gynecological surgeon for hysterectomy.

Diagnostic Studies

A Pap test should be part of the routine examination and may show abnormal cytology indicative of endometrial carcinoma. For definitive diagnosis and histological typing, an endometrial biopsy or D&C is necessary. Serum CA-125, a tumor marker for ovarian cancer, is also elevated in endometrial cancer, with the advanced stages more likely to have elevations. A complete metabolic profile, CBC, urinalysis, and chest x-ray should be performed at the time of diagnosis to identify or rule out metastases.

HORMONAL IMBALANCES

Irregular bleeding occurs more frequently early in menarche, before the body establishes a regular pattern, as well as during the perimenopausal period, when hormones are changing. Other causes of hormonal imbalances are discussed throughout this chapter.

ORAL CONTRACEPTIVES

If the progesterone component of the pill is not sufficient to maintain the lining of the uterus, metrorrhagia may occur in the luteal phase of the cycle. If a patient complains of spotting or bleeding during this time, a different pill with a stronger or different type of progesterone should be prescribed. If the bleeding continues, consider stopping the pill temporarily to determine whether that is the aggravating factor. There are enough choices of pills available to find one that the patient can take without unwanted side effects.

FIBROIDS

Uterine leiomyomas, more commonly known as uterine fibroids, are benign growths consisting mostly of smooth muscle. The etiology is unknown, but their growth is hormone dependent; therefore, they are seen in approximately 25% of patients during their reproductive years. They generally do not originate after menopause and, if present, will decrease in size after menopause. A tumor that arises in a postmenopausal patient should always have a high suspicion for malignancy rather than benign leiomyoma. Leiomyomas are more common in black patients, occurring in as many as 50%. They can be single or multiple, usually measuring less than 15 cm. A very small percentage (0.1% to 0.5%)

may undergo malignant transformation to become a leiomyosarcoma, requiring prompt surgical intervention.

Signs and Symptoms

Heavy menstrual bleeding (menorrhagia) and irregular bleeding (metrorrhagia) are the most common presenting symptoms, although a large percentage of patients are asymptomatic. Other symptoms include heaviness or fullness in the lower abdomen, pelvic pain, backache, dysmenorrhea, and urinary complaints. The pain can be severe if caused by torsion of a pedunculated fibroid. Fibroids are thought to contribute to infertility, spontaneous abortion, preterm labor, and problems with labor and delivery. Most leiomyomas can be palpated on bimanual examination, and some larger fibroids can be palpated through the abdomen. The uterus may feel enlarged, irregular, or nodular; pedunculated fibroids can be difficult to differentiate from other pelvic or abdominal masses. A retroverted uterus may obscure palpation.

Diagnostic Studies

A pregnancy test should be performed to rule pregnancy out as a cause of the symptoms. A CBC is needed in cases of heavy bleeding to determine whether anemia or platelet disorder is present. Pelvic ultrasound or MRI should be performed if symptoms of leiomyoma are present or for any palpable pelvic mass detected on physical examination. Imaging assists in differentiating ovarian cancer, leiomyosarcoma, endometrial cancer, or other neoplasms. An endometrial biopsy, D&C, or laparoscopy may be necessary to rule out malignancies.

VON WILLEBRAND DISEASE

Von Willebrand disease (VWD) is an inherited bleeding disorder. VWD is caused by a deficiency in or dysfunction of von Willebrand factor (VWF) and affects nearly 3.2 million people in the United States. VWF is further affected by factors such as race, blood type, inflammatory mediators, and hormonal status. While the condition affects both male and female patients and may be diagnosed at any age, it is often identified during evaluation of menstrual bleeding disorder. Bleeding can be life-threatening.

Signs and Symptoms

The severity of signs and symptoms depends on the severity of the condition. The patient often has experienced easy bruising, nosebleeds, and abnormal bleeding following dental procedures, surgeries, or other procedures, in addition to heavy or prolonged menses. If the patient has given birth, there is often a history of prolonged bleeding following delivery. There may be a positive family history of bleeding disorders or of abnormal bleeding. Physical findings may not be present at the time of evaluation.

Diagnostic Studies

CBC, partial thromboplastin time (PTT), prothrombin time (PT), and a fibrinogen level of a thrombin time (TT) should be ordered to guide subsequent evaluation. These studies will not provide definitive diagnosis of VWD or rule the condition out, but they will provide an indication of a coagulation disorder. If VWD or another bleeding disorder is suspected, the patient should be referred to a hematology specialist.

ANOVULATION

The causes of chronic anovulation are numerous, with some resulting in abnormal uterine bleeding and some resulting in amenorrhea. The main categories for causes are as follows:

- Inappropriate feedback, including polycystic ovary syndrome (PCOS); neoplasms that produce excess androgens, estrogens, or hCG; and excess estrogen production associated with obesity or liver disease
- Pituitary dysfunction related to tumors or hypopituitarism
- Hypothalamic dysfunction associated with stress, exercise, malnutrition, or anorexia nervosa
- Endocrine or metabolic dysfunction, including thyroid disease, adrenal hyperfunction as seen in Cushing's disease, and prolactin or growth hormone excess

Signs and Symptoms

Anovulation may present with amenorrhea but also may present with abnormal uterine bleeding, polymenorrhea, or menorrhagia. The symptoms vary with the cause. Overweight may be seen with several of the causes, including hypothyroidism, PCOS, and pituitary and adrenal dysfunction. Underweight is seen in anorexia nervosa, excessive exercise, hyperthyroidism, or stress-induced anovulation. Hirsutism, acne, and other skin changes can be seen with imbalances in LH, FSH, and androgens, as seen in polycystic ovary disease. Delayed puberty or regression of sexual characteristics is seen in hypopituitarism; galactorrhea can be the presenting symptom in pituitary tumors.

Diagnostic Studies

Appropriate laboratory and diagnostic testing depends on the history and physical examination and on the preliminary differential diagnosis. TSH, LH, FSH, estradiol, and testosterone levels will give information about sex and thyroid hormone levels as well as ovarian function. If polycystic ovary disease is suspected, a pelvic ultrasound is necessary, although it may be normal even with the disease. If pituitary or adrenal dysfunction is suspected, tests include glucose, cortisol, growth hormone, TSH, adrenocorticotropic hormone (ACTH), prolactin, LH, and FSH. Abnormalities in any of these studies may warrant MRI or CT scanning of the head.

PERIMENOPAUSE

Generally, there is no objective way to determine when the perimenopausal period begins, but from subjective data gathered from patients, menstrual changes begin to take place in the fourth decade of life.

Signs and Symptoms

FSH and LH remain normal, but patients who had regular menstrual cycles all of their lives begin to complain of more frequent periods with more dysmenorrhea or, conversely, missed periods. Patients may also begin to have sleep disturbances, decreased energy, increased weight, urinary frequency, and other complaints that are usually associated with menopause.

Diagnostic Studies

Pregnancy and pathology must be ruled out. The following laboratory tests and diagnostics are recommended: hCG; urinalysis; Pap test with bimanual examination to rule out fibroids or a malignancy; CBC to rule out anemia, which can cause menorrhagia; and FSH and LH tests to ensure that the patient is not menopausal. A pelvic ultrasound is indicated if fibroids or malignancy is suspected. If the symptoms are established to be benign perimenopausal symptoms, then no treatment is really necessary as the symptoms are bothersome but not dangerous. However, they can be managed with low-strength birth control pills if there are no contraindications.

■ Amenorrhea

The four main causes of primary amenorrhea are disorders of the outflow tract, disorders of the ovary, disorders of the anterior pituitary, and disorders of the hypothalamus. Secondary amenorrhea can occur for many reasons: pregnancy, oral contraceptives, high prolactin due to a pituitary microadenoma, stress, rapid weight change, anorexia nervosa, menopause, vigorous exercise, hypothyroidism, chronic disease, and polycystic ovary disease.

History

It is necessary to determine whether the amenorrhea is primary or secondary. Primary amenorrhea is defined as the absence of menarche by age 16. Secondary amenorrhea is the absence of menstruation for more than 3 months in a patient with past menses. If there is no history of menses, consider the age and Tanner stage of the patient. Constitutional delay occurs in teenagers whose family has a history of late growth. These teens can experience late but normal sexual maturation. In the case of no menstrual cycle, consider also the disorders of the outflow tract and hypoestrogenic amenorrhea. If the patient has had menstrual cycles in the past, inquire as to age of onset, duration, amount of flow, regularity, and date of last menstrual period.

Irregular menses is very common in adolescents and does not necessarily indicate pathology. Ask the patient about lifestyle, exercise and eating habits, and weight gain or loss that might indicate thyroid disease, polycystic ovary disease, or an eating disorder. It is necessary to know about prescription or OTC medications; use of oral contraceptives; birth control method, if any; and sexual activity that might indicate pregnancy or oral contraceptive–induced amenorrhea. Major stresses or life-changing events and/or chronic illness that can cause physical and emotional stress have been shown to cause amenorrhea.

Ask the patient about the presence of galactorrhea, indicating the possibility of a pituitary tumor.

Physical Examination

A height and weight are a good start and give you an idea about several possible explanations for the amenorrhea. Short stature, obesity, or underweight are associated with both primary and secondary causes of amenorrhea. Inspect for webbing of the hands and neck that accompany the short stature of Turner's syndrome. Assess the skin for dryness and the hair for signs of dryness, thinning, or brittleness, indicating hypothyroidism or altered nutritional state. Inspect the patient for hirsutism, which can occur in pituitary and hormonal abnormalities. The gynecological examination includes inspection for patency of the introitus and cervix; inspection of the vaginal mucosa for dryness or atrophy, which accompanies a lack of estrogen; a bimanual examination to determine uterine size, which can be enlarged in pregnancy or tumors; and palpation of the ovaries for cysts.

Diagnostic testing is necessary in most cases because a cessation of menses may be the only symptom and physical examination findings may be absent. The initial step should be to rule out pregnancy with a urine or serum hCG analysis. If negative, a TSH and prolactin level should be drawn to rule out thyroid disease or pituitary tumor. A decreased TSH, indicating hyperthyroidism, can result in hypomenorrhea or amenorrhea. Hyperprolactinemia can lead to lower FSH and LH levels and hypogonadism. If the prolactin is normal and galactorrhea is absent, a pituitary tumor can be ruled out; likewise, a normal TSH rules out thyroid disease. Before ordering other expensive or extensive laboratory studies, a progesterone challenge should be given. If the patient experiences menstrual bleeding after 7 days of oral progesterone, it can be assumed that the endometrium is sufficiently prepared by endogenous estrogen and that there is at least minimal function of the ovary, pituitary, and central nervous system. This rules out primary ovarian failure and tells you that the patient has some circulating estrogen. In this case, the patient is likely not ovulating and therefore is not getting the postovulatory rise in progesterone needed for menses. Polycystic ovary disease is the most common cause of anovulation, and an increase in LH, estrogen, and androgen levels along with a decreased FSH can help to confirm this. Although in PCOS the ovaries are not always enlarged or cystic, a pelvic ultrasound may assist in the diagnosis. Adrenal dysfunction plays a part in ovarian and menstrual function, although in the case of adrenal dysfunction, menstrual irregularities are only one of many other more serious symptoms related to the action of adrenocortical hormones.

If bleeding does not occur with the progesterone challenge, estrogen should be added to the progesterone challenge to differentiate a disorder of the outflow tract from hypoestrogenic amenorrhea. An ultrasound will also assist in the diagnosis of an outflow tract disorder. In the case of no menses with the combination estrogen and progesterone challenge, an FSH and LH test as well as an MRI of the sella turcica are needed to determine gonadal failure versus hypothalamic amenorrhea caused by pituitary adenoma or other hypothalamic/

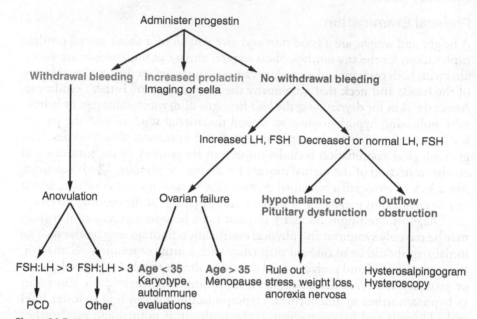

Figure 14.5 Evaluation of amenorrhea. (From Kiningham, R. B., Apgar, B. S., & Schwenk, T. L. Evaluation of amenorrhea. *American Family Physician*, 53, 4, 1185–1194, 1996. Reprinted with permission.)

pituitary abnormalities. Figure 14.5 provides a flowchart for the evaluation of amenorrhea.

POLYCYSTIC OVARY SYNDROME

Formerly called Stein-Leventhal syndrome, PCOS is a hypothalamic-pituitary-ovarian axis disorder resulting in high levels of LH, low levels of FSH, a high nonfluctuating level of estrogen, and an overproduction of androgens. It occurs in 4% to 12% of the female population.

Signs and Symptoms

PCOS is characterized by anovulation, amenorrhea, and hirsutism, although some patients with PCOS have menorrhagia or abnormal uterine bleeding rather than amenorrhea. It also has been associated with infertility, insulin resistance, truncal obesity, and dyslipidemia. Enlarged ovaries are usually present but are not required for diagnosis. Other physical findings associated with PCOS include acne, alopecia, and acanthosis nigricans.

Diagnostic Studies

No single test can give a definitive diagnosis of PCOS. There are several tests that assist in the diagnosis. Elevated androgen values (free testosterone, dehydroepiandrosterone sulfate, total testosterone) are seen in many patients, most commonly free testosterone. If elevated androgen levels are present, adrenal tumors need to be ruled out. Elevated levels of LH and an elevated LH-to-FSH ratio may be present, although results vary widely, depending on the timing of the laboratory testing. Prolactin and TSH levels are normal but will assist in ruling out pituitary tumors or thyroid disease as a cause of the amenorrhea. Cushing's disease should be ruled out because PCOS has many similar signs and symptoms. Ultrasound of the ovaries may assist in the diagnosis, but many women who have cystic ovaries do not have PCOS. If PCOS is suspected, a glucose tolerance test, insulin levels, and a lipid profile should be done to monitor other health problems associated with PCOS. Management includes hormone therapy, insulin-sensitizing drugs, and weight loss. Weight loss will help to prevent diabetes, dyslipidemia, and cardiovascular disease and will also reduce circulating testosterone.

MENOPAUSE

Menopause is the absence of menses without a pathological cause for at least 12 months. See Box 14.2 for physiological changes that occur with menopause.

Signs and Symptoms

In addition to inquiring about the typical menopausal symptoms as mentioned above, ask the patient about recent major life changes, as stress has been shown to affect menstrual regularity. Age of menopause varies greatly, although age 50 to 55 years is the typical range of onset.

Diagnostic Studies

During transition to menopause, hormone levels are erratic and variable. Measuring hormone levels to confirm menopause is often inaccurate and no longer recommended by the North American Menopause Society (NAMS) or the American Congress of Obstetricians and Gynecologists (ACOG). Absence of menses in a patient around age 50 years without a pathologic cause is presumed to be menopause. The history is most helpful in determining the length of time menses has been absent.

Box 14.2

Physiological Changes With Menopause

- Hot flashes, fatigue, insomnia, urinary frequency and incontinence, nervousness, decreased libido, and depression
- Increased bone resorption, especially in the first 5 years of menopause, leading to osteopenia and osteoporosis
- Increased incidence of atherosclerosis
- Vaginal and urethral dryness and decreased integrity
- Decreased skin turgor

■ Dysmenorrhea

Dysmenorrhea is the most common gynecological complaint, particularly in the adolescent and young adult population. Primary dysmenorrhea is due to a rise in prostaglandins that occurs at the onset of menses; it has been found that prostaglandins are higher in patients with dysmenorrhea. Recently, it has been found that increased leukotriene levels contribute to dysmenorrhea. Other psychosocial variables may contribute, such as response to pain, anxiety, stress, and attitudes about menstruation.

Secondary dysmenorrhea is most often caused by endometriosis. Other causes include chronic PID, adhesions, IUDs, cervical stenosis, and uterine fibroids.

History

Take a menstrual history, including age at menarche, menstrual patterns, and the qualitative and quantitative factors of the dysmenorrhea. Important things to know include the time of onset in the menstrual cycle, pattern (intermittent or constant), regularity of the cycles, severity and duration of the pain, amount of lost work or school time, and medications taken for relief. Also ask about any history of trauma, vaginal discharge, recent STIs, fever, history of endometriosis, infertility, or missed periods. Inquire about the type of birth control and sexual activity. Determine whether there is a history of abnormal Pap tests.

Physical Examination

Both an abdominal and a pelvic examination should be done to assess for masses or tenderness. During the pelvic examination, a Pap test should be obtained along with cultures for chlamydia and gonorrhea. Assess for size, consistency, mobility, and tenderness of the uterus and ovaries.

PRIMARY DYSMENORRHEA

Primary dysmenorrhea is often used to describe menstrual cramping, but strictly speaking, the term should be used only to describe pain with menses that interferes with normal daily living and requires pain medicine, either opioid or nonopioid.

Signs and Symptoms

The pain is in the pelvic area and begins with the onset of menses or shortly thereafter. The pain can be so severe as to be accompanied by nausea, vomiting, and diarrhea. It is short in duration, usually lasting only the first day or two of the menstrual cycle. If pain worsens over time or occurs between cycles, secondary causes should be suspected.

Diagnostic Studies

In primary dysmenorrhea, diagnosis is by history because menstrual pain is a subjective complaint and cannot be measured objectively. However, if a secondary cause is suspected, an examination should be done to inspect for vaginal discharge that might indicate infection, and a NAAT is needed to test for gonorrhea and chlamydia. A bimanual examination should be done to palpate for tenderness that might indicate infection or fibroids. Laboratory tests and diagnostics to consider include a serum hCG for pregnancy, a pelvic ultrasound to rule out fibroids or endometriosis, an endometrial biopsy, and possibly laparoscopy if endometriosis is suspected in order to determine the extent of disease. Oral contraceptives will diminish the severity of the dysmenorrhea along with NSAIDs or other pain medication.

ENDOMETRIOSIS

Endometriosis is characterized by a proliferation of endometrial tissue in sites other than the lining of the uterus. It typically grows on the outside of the uterus, tubes and ovaries, broad ligament, uterosacral ligaments, large and small bowel, bladder, ureters, vagina, and cul-de-sac. It is almost exclusively found in premenopausal women and is estimated to cause as much as 50% of infertility in women. Several theories exist, but the exact cause is unknown. Theories include retrograde menstruation with transport of endometrial cells, lymphatic transport of endometrial cells, metaplasia of coelomic epithelium, or immune response resulting in endometrial hyperplasia. In addition, there seems to be a genetic predisposition, with a 6% to 10% increase in patients with first-degree relatives who have endometriosis.

Signs and Symptoms

The main symptom of endometriosis is dysmenorrhea, which sometimes makes it difficult to differentiate from primary dysmenorrhea. Other presenting symptoms include dyspareunia, infertility, and constant pelvic and low back pain that occurs before menses. Adhesions may cause chronic pelvic pain unrelated to the menstrual cycle. The physical examination may reveal a fixed uterus as a result of adhesions, causing pain on uterine movement; nodules on the posterior vaginal fornix; and tenderness in the adnexal area. In many patients, the physical examination is unremarkable.

Diagnostic Studies

The history and physical examination generally lead you to suspect endometriosis, but the definitive diagnosis is made through laparoscopic surgery and biopsy. The lesions seen in endometriosis, termed *endometrial implants*, are dark red to dark brown and give the appearance of a powder burn from a gunshot. They appear on the peritoneal, bladder, uterine, and ovarian surfaces. Over time they become thickened and produce scar tissue. Ultrasound may give information about the extent of the disease but should not be used as the sole diagnostic tool. Various hormonal treatments are helpful, as are laparoscopic ablation of extrauterine endometrial tissue and lysing of adhesions with the goal of restoring pelvic anatomy.

UTERINE FIBROIDS

Along with abnormal uterine bleeding, leiomyomas can cause dysmenorrhea, which is often one of the presenting complaints. See the section on fibroids under "Abnormal Uterine Bleeding" (pp. 490–494).

■ Ovarian Cancer

Although patients do not come in with a chief complaint of ovarian cancer, the symptoms and physical findings are usually vague or nonexistent, thereby making it a differential diagnosis or a diagnosis of suspicion rather than one based on history or physical. Ovarian cancer has the highest mortality of the gynecological malignancies because as much as 85% of cases have metastases outside the ovaries at the time of diagnosis and the cancer is usually widespread before the patient has signs or symptoms. It occurs most often in postmenopausal patients, in those with a positive family history, and in those with *BRCA1* and *BRCA2* gene mutations. Use of oral contraceptives may decrease a woman's risk of developing ovarian cancer (American Cancer Society, 2018).

History

The history should include both abdominal and gynecological complaints, as many patients with ovarian cancer present with vague gastrointestinal complaints. A menstrual history is necessary because some of the patients have abnormal uterine bleeding. A positive family history of ovarian cancer is a red flag, as is a patient's history of other gynecological or breast malignancies.

Physical Examination

In the premenopausal patient, 95% of ovarian masses are small (less than 8 cm), cystic, and benign, although ovarian malignancies do occur in this population. In the postmenopausal patient, there should be a high index of suspicion for ovarian cancer. Early symptoms are vague and include mild lower abdominal discomfort, feelings of fullness, bloating, distension, nausea, dyspepsia, constipation, and urinary frequency if the tumor is large. Abnormal uterine bleeding is uncommon. Pelvic pain, anemia, ascites, and cachexia are seen in late disease.

The characteristics typical of a malignant ovarian mass include solid, fixed, nodular, nontender, and bilateral. The abdominal examination is essential, looking for distension, changes in percussion, or ascites. As the cancer metastasizes, lymphadenopathy occurs, especially in the inguinal and supraclavicular areas. The cancer spreads by direct extension to the abdominal and pelvic peritoneum and through lymph nodes. Laboratory tests and other diagnostics are needed for a definitive diagnosis.

Pelvic examination has been shown to have a low sensitivity and specificity for ovarian cancer, with many tumors smaller than 10 cm being missed. Several diagnostic studies are useful for detecting ovarian cancer. The CA-125 blood test by immunoassay is used as a tumor marker for treatment decisions but can also be used as a diagnostic tool. Patients at high risk due to family history and *BRCA* gene mutations should begin screening at age 35 years. False-positive elevations in CA-125 do occur with endometriosis and PID; therefore, tests should be interpreted with caution and followed up with transvaginal ultrasound. Transvaginal ultrasound will show a solid, irregular mass that may be adhered to adjoining structures. A Pap test may contain malignant cells. X-rays may show metastatic lung or bone lesions. Prognosis is poor, but recent advances in cancer treatment have helped prolong survival, depending on stage at diagnosis and whether there is local spread or distant metastasis. Surgery is necessary for staging and also as the mainstay of treatment, along with chemotherapy and possibly radiation.

OVARIAN CYSTS

Several differentiating factors separate ovarian cysts from ovarian cancer. The primary factor is that cysts are fluid-filled sacs and cancer is a solid tumor. Ovarian cancer is much more prevalent in patients older than 50 years, although it can occur in younger patients. Ovarian cysts are common in the younger population and tend to occur in the latter half of the menstrual cycle. Many spontaneously resolve. Others may need surgical intervention if they cause the ovary to become twisted, owing to the risk of gangrene.

Signs and Symptoms

Right or left lower quadrant pain is usually the presenting complaint. Pelvic examination reveals significant tenderness in the affected adnexal area. Rebound tenderness may be present. Follicular cysts are most common, and the pain typically occurs in the second half of the menstrual cycle. These cysts usually resolve with menses and require no further treatment. Other cysts—including corpus luteum cysts, inflammatory cysts occurring with tubo-ovarian abscess, and endometriotic cysts—may require surgical intervention.

Diagnostic Studies

Tubal pregnancy must be ruled out immediately with a urine or serum hCG. Transvaginal ultrasound will give the best information for differentiating a blood- or fluid-filled cyst from a solid mass.

HYDATIDIFORM MOLE AND CHORIOCARCINOMA

These solid tumors are part of a category of gestational trophoblastic neoplasia. In the United States, the incidence is 1 in 1,500 pregnancies. Risk factors include low socioeconomic status, previous history of mole, and age younger than 18 or older than 40 years. Hydatidiform mole is generally benign, but a small percentage may develop into choriocarcinoma (Ghassemzadeh & Kang, 2020).

Signs and Symptoms

Clinical signs are those of a missed abortion: uterine bleeding, nausea, vomiting, and enlarged and/or tender uterus and ovaries. Collapsed vesicles from the mole may pass through the vagina.

Diagnostic Studies

A quantitative hCG should be done, as these values may differ from those of a normal pregnancy. Grapelike clusters within an enlarged uterus in the absence of a fetus and placenta are diagnostic for hydatidiform mole. In partial hydatidiform mole, pelvic ultrasound may show an embryo or gestational sac. These partial moles are slow growing but are more likely to become choriocarcinomas.

A solid mass on ultrasound is suspicious for choriocarcinoma and requires biopsy for diagnosis. Choriocarcinoma responds well to chemotherapy, and the prognosis is favorable.

UTERINE FIBROIDS

See "Abnormal Uterine Bleeding," pp. 491–492.

GASTROINTESTINAL, LIVER, PANCREATIC CANCERS

See Chapter 11.

IRRITABLE BOWEL SYNDROME

See Chapter 11.

■ Sexual Dysfunction

There are many causes of sexual dysfunction that may have a physical or psychological origin or a combination of both. Dysfunction generally stems from decreased desire, decreased arousal, orgasmic dysfunction, and physical discomfort.

History

A sexual history should be part of the gynecological review of systems, although it is often omitted as a result of examiner discomfort or a failure to view it as an integral part of the examination. If problems exist, the examiner should explore the patient's relationships, life circumstances and changes, medical conditions, surgeries, sexual activity and behaviors, sexual development, and fertility issues.

Physical Examination

There are no special examinations to be done for sexual dysfunction, although hormonal assessment may be helpful. A thorough gynecological examination is adequate to determine whether there is a physical cause for the problem. If dyspareunia is part of the complaint, a pelvic ultrasound may assist in the diagnosis of structural pathology.

LOSS OF LIBIDO AND DECREASED SEXUAL RESPONSE

Decreases in libido and sexual response are not uncommon with aging, although it is an erroneous stereotype to assume that sexual desire or functioning automatically declines with age. Inhibited or decreased sexual desire has many causes, including aging, marital discord, drug or alcohol abuse, pregnancy, physical illness or discomfort, depression, medications, including contraceptives, history of sexual abuse, sexual phobias, and anxiety.

Signs and Symptoms

The diagnosis of inhibited sexual desire is primarily a subjective one based on patient history. If organic causes such as illness and physical discomfort are ruled out, a thorough psychological evaluation is recommended. As previously mentioned, desire and response may slow with aging, but a good history should be able to discern when a psychological evaluation is warranted. In the older patient, lubricating agents may be helpful to deal with decreased or uncomfortable stimulation due to loss of lubrication.

Diagnostic Studies

Although a thorough history is most helpful, serum free testosterone will show an androgen deficiency, which has been blamed for decreased libido, particularly in the postmenopausal patient.

DYSPAREUNIA

The causes of dyspareunia are numerous and include vaginal infection or irritation, PID, endometriosis, pregnancy, atrophic vaginitis, decreased lubrication, episiotomy, labial lesions, Bartholin's cysts, adhesions from previous gynecological or abdominal surgeries, and psychological causes.

Signs and Symptoms

The age of the client should be considered because decreased estrogen can cause atrophic vaginitis and thus decreased lubrication leading to dyspareunia. The history can give information about pregnancy or delivery difficulties, past surgeries, and the possibility of adhesions. A thorough sexual history should be done to uncover any psychological issues. A pelvic examination should be done, looking for vaginal discharge, inflammation, or lesions.

Diagnostic Studies

Structural abnormalities should be ruled out, and transvaginal ultrasound may be helpful. If vaginal discharge is present, wet prep and cultures should be obtained to rule out infection. Blood samples for hormonal testing may be necessary, particularly if mucosal atrophy is evident on physical examination.

VAGINISMUS

Vaginismus is defined as a painful contraction of the lower vaginal and thigh adductor muscles that occurs unconsciously in a patient who does not desire penetration. It most often occurs in young women who have been molested, sexually abused, or raped, or it is secondary to gynecological trauma or medical procedures.

Signs and Symptoms

The physical or psychological causes can be uncovered during history and physical examination. A good history, inquiring specifically about sexual abuse, is necessary. Involuntary vaginal spasm can be observed during the pelvic examination, and the patient often exhibits avoidance behavior in response to the examiner and the pelvic examination.

Diagnostic Studies

Once structural and other physical causes have been eliminated, vaginismus can be treated with gradual dilation techniques. In many instances, psychotherapy is necessary.

■ Infertility

The workup for infertility is complex and will need to be referred to a gynecologist specializing in infertility. The causes are numerous but generally fall into the categories of anovulation, implantation failure, hormonal failure, chromosomal abnormalities, or low sperm count in the male partner. Preliminary tests that can be initiated by the nurse practitioner include the following:

- Pelvic examination to ensure that the cervix is open and that there are no uterine abnormalities
- Basal body temperature charts to plot monthly ovulation and menstrual patterns
- Laboratory testing, including TSH, FSH, LH, and estradiol
- Ultrasound, which shows the position of the uterus, the presence of fibroids or other growths, and the thickening of the endometrium that may occur in endometriosis, all of which can affect fertility
- Hysterosalpingography, a radiography of the uterus and fallopian tubes to assess patency and the presence of any structural abnormalities
- Sperm count for the male partner (one of the first things that should be done in an infertility workup)

REFERENCES

American Cancer Society. (2018). Can ovarian cancer be prevented? https://www.cancer.org/cancer/ovarian-cancer/causes-risks-prevention/prevention.html.

American Cancer Society. (2021). Key statistics for endometrial cancer. https://www.cancer.org/cancer/endometrial-cancer/about/key-statistics.html

American Cancer Society. (2022). Cancer facts & figures 2022: Key statistics for vulvar cancer. Atlanta, GA: American Cancer Society. https://www.cancer.org/cancer/vulvar-cancer/about/key-statistics.html

American College of Obstetricians and Gynecologists (ACOG). (2020). The utility of and indications for routine pelvic examination. https://www.acog.org/clinical/clinical-guidance/committee-opinion/articles/2018/10/the-utility-of-and-indications-for-routine-pelvic-examination

Centers for Disease Control and Prevention. (2017a). 2017 STD surveillance report. https://www.cdc.gov/nchhstp/newsroom/2018/2017-STD-surveillance-report.html

Centers for Disease Control and Prevention. (2017b). *National ambulatory medical care survey: 2017 summary.* National Center for Health Statistics. April 12, 2017, from https://www.cdc.gov/nchs/ahcd/

Centers for Disease Control and Prevention. (2018). Sexually Transmitted Disease Surveillance 2018: Syphilis. Retrieved March 24, 2021, from https://www.cdc.gov/std/stats18/syphilis.htm

Centers for Disease Control and Prevention. (2019). Basic information about gynecological cancers. www.cdc.gov/cancer/gynecologic/basic_info/index.htm

Centers for Disease Control and Prevention. (2021). 2015 sexually transmitted diseases treatment guidelines. Retrieved March 31, 2021, from https://www.cdc.gov/std/tg2015/

Ghassemzadeh, S., & Kang, M. (2020). Hydatidiform mole. StatPearls Publishing. ncbi.nlm.nih.gov/books/NBK459155

Havrilesky, L. J., Gierisch, J. M., Moorman, P. G., Coeytaux, R. R., Peragallo Urrutia, R., Lowery, W. J., Dinan, M., McBroom, A. J., Wing, L., Musty, D. D., Lallinger, K. R., Hasselblad, V., Sanders, G. D., & Myers, E. R. (2013). *Oral contraceptive use for the primary prevention of ovarian cancer.* Agency for Healthcare Research and Quality. https://www.ncbi.nlm.nih.gov/books/NBK148769/

National Cancer Institute. (2001). The Bethesda System for reporting cervical cytology. http://fosp.saude.sp.gov.br:443/docs/The+Bethesda+System+for+Reporting+Cervic.pdf

U.S. Preventive Services Task Force. (2018). Cervical cancer: Screening. Retrieved March 25, 2021 from https://www.uspreventiveservicestaskforce.org/uspstf/recommendation/cervical-cancer-screening

Chapter 15

Musculoskeletal System

Michael E. Zychowicz •

The bones and muscles provide the structure for stability and movement of the body. Individual abilities and limitations in strength, movement, ease, and grace are defined by the abilities of this system to respond to input and stimuli. Limitations are a result of disease, injury, metabolic disorders, and lack of conditioning, which can lead to temporary or permanent disability. Over 100 rheumatologic problems can cause musculoskeletal pain, swelling, and/or stiffness, with arthritis being the leading cause of disability in the United States. Complaints related to the musculoskeletal system are common across the life span. The types of problems vary among age groups.

As with all systems in the body, the musculoskeletal system is closely linked with other systems. The neurological and circulatory systems and the skin are most often associated with problems that also affect the musculoskeletal system. Problems affecting one system often produce associated problems in others. Problems with the musculoskeletal system can affect the joints, tendons, ligaments, muscle, nerve, bone, and surrounding soft tissues. A thorough examination of the affected body part must be performed to obtain a complete picture of the problem.

Assessment of Musculoskeletal Complaints

Patients who have musculoskeletal problems usually present with pain, deformity, and/or weakness. Joint pain, in general, is the most common problem, and backache, specifically, is the most common disorder for which patients seek health care. The examination is often centered on the joint(s) where the pain is focused, but frequently muscles and nerves are also a focal point of the examination. Conditions associated with joint pain can be categorized into four major groups: mechanical problems, soft tissue conditions, inflammatory diseases, and noninflammatory diseases. Conditions frequently associated with joint pain include osteoarthritis (OA), tendonitis, infection, gout/pseudogout, rheumatoid arthritis (RA), and systemic lupus erythematosus (SLE). A number of presentations are indications of urgent problems, requiring immediate recognition and

> **RED FLAG** ◀   **Red Flags in the Assessment of the Musculoskeletal System**
>
> - *History of major trauma*
> - *History of cancer*
> - *Hot and/or swollen joints*
> - *Systemic/constitutional symptoms*
> - *Focal or diffuse weakness*
> - *Neurogenic pain*
> - *Claudication*
> - *Unrelenting nighttime pain*
> - *Poorly localized pain*
> - *Recent joint surgery or procedure*
> - *Unexplained or unexpected weight loss*
> - *Pain at rest*

definitive treatment. It is essential that the history and physical examination be directed to identify any of the symptoms or signs noted in the Red Flag box.

History

■ General Musculoskeletal History

It is important to complete a thorough symptom analysis for any musculoskeletal complaint. When a musculoskeletal disorder is suspected, the review of that system should include a history of associated pain, discomfort, swelling, redness, stiffness, crepitus, limited motion, and weakness. Numbness and tingling can accompany musculoskeletal conditions with a neurological compromise. The clinician should have a clear understanding of the specific location and pattern or distribution of the patient's pain. Any locking, buckling, or giving way of a joint could be due to a tear of the cartilage, tendon, or ligament and should be noted. The onset and progression of symptoms are important to help differentiate among traumatic or acute problems and chronic conditions. The musculoskeletal history should be appropriate to the patient's age because many problems occur among certain age groups more often than others. The clinician should inquire about any deformity the patient has noted. While some deformity may be acute in origin due to an injury, chronic musculoskeletal conditions such as RA or OA may be accompanied by deformity that develops and progresses slowly over time. Ask about the use of adaptive and assistive devices, supports, and braces such as crutches, cane, walker, splint, or sling.

▪ Past Medical History

Identify any history of musculoskeletal disorders and procedures. The history of both remote and recent trauma and/or other injuries, and how they occurred, should be determined. Disorders to ask about include recent infections, which could explain symptoms such as polyarthritis, monoarthritis, or generalized aches, as well as a history of RA, OA, osteoporosis, gout, or other chronic musculoskeletal problems. The treatment and response related to any identified musculoskeletal problem(s) should be noted, with specific attention to prior joint procedures or surgeries. Obtain a list of all current or recently prescribed and over-the-counter medications or supplements. The medication list may shed light on disorders previously omitted from the overall medical history and may also provide clues to the etiology of complaints. Table 15.1 lists some medications that are commonly associated with musculoskeletal effects. Ask about previous treatments from physical therapists, chiropractors, massage therapists, acupuncturists, and practitioners of other disciplines relative to musculoskeletal complaints.

In addition to specific musculoskeletal disorders, determine whether the patient has a history of other disorders that might suggest a cause for the musculoskeletal complaint, such as gonococcal arthritis, Lyme disease, or SLE. Several endocrine disorders may result in musculoskeletal symptoms, including hyperparathyroidism, hyper- and hypothyroidism, and diabetes. The history of any neurological problems should be established.

▪ Family History

Identify the family history of various types of arthritis, osteoporosis, gout, SLE, and other musculoskeletal disorders. Also determine the history of related systems.

Table 15.1	
Medications With Musculoskeletal Effects	
Medications	Possible Musculoskeletal Side Effects
Diuretics	Secondary hyperuricemia
Chemotherapies for malignancies	May increase hyperuricemia
Hydralazine, procainamide, chlorpromazine, methyldopa, isoniazid, and oral contraceptives	Triggers for systemic lupus erythematosus
Anti-inflammatories, statins, fibrates, and erythromycins	May cause rhabdomyolysis
Quinilones	Black box warning for tendinitis/tendon rupture during and after treatment

■ Social History

Obtain a history of normal daily activity, including exercise, and any limitations realized since the presenting complaint was first noticed. Have the patient identify all occupational, social, and recreational physical activities, particularly those that require repetitive motions and/or stressors to the musculoskeletal system. Inquire if the current musculoskeletal complaint interferes with those activities. Environmental issues associated with where the patient works, lives, and spends recreational time should be explored. Identify and quantify all drug, alcohol, and tobacco products used.

Physical Examination

■ Order of the Examination

The general musculoskeletal examination includes inspection, palpation, range of motion (ROM), and assessment of strength, in addition to relevant "special maneuvers." After an initial observation of the patient's general appearance, gait, and gross ROM, the remainder of the general musculoskeletal examination is usually performed in a head-to-toe sequence. However, depending on the presentation, the general survey may be followed by a more focused examination of the affected area, with comparison to the opposite side/structures. Although assessment involves both inspection and palpation, there are "special maneuvers" or specific procedures used to assess individual joints that combine inspection with palpation to determine muscle tone, muscle strength, ROM, and joint stability. As specific complaints are assessed, the problem can be further identified by having the patient point to the specific region or site that is most painful and by more carefully assessing that area. A neurovascular examination of the body part may be needed to thoroughly evaluate a complaint.

General Survey

Observe the patient's general appearance, including body build, posture, obvious deformities, general gait, movement, and any assistive aids used (e.g., crutches, walker, cane, bracing). A limp, guarding, or obvious weakness can provide a valuable indication of a musculoskeletal or neurological problem and how the patient is compensating. Notice whether the patient appears comfortable in the current position or guards a particular extremity or region during the history and physical examination. Observe the patient's general skin condition. Note the vital signs.

Inspection

The focused musculoskeletal examination begins with inspection. For overall assessment, it is essential that patients disrobe, usually to their underwear or shorts. When examination is limited to a specific region, it is essential that the region be completely free of clothing to allow adequate observation. Once the patient is disrobed, the general posture should again be noted as well as any deformities, limited motion, and asymmetry of bony pairs or muscle groups. Identify any skin lesions, discoloration, scars, skin atrophy, bulges, nodules or masses, and areas of erythema or edema. Direct the patient through a variety of maneuvers intended to demonstrate ROM and general ability to control movement. These include a variety of gaits (normal, heel-toe, on toes, on heels, etc.) as well as full ROM of all joints without resistance. In addition to general inspection, more focused attention should be paid to any area of complaint. If an effusion, bulging, or redness is detected, the cause is more likely an inflammatory condition.

Palpation

For a complete musculoskeletal examination, palpation involves assessment of each joint as well as the major muscle groups and accessory structures, such as ligaments and tendons. For a focused musculoskeletal examination, the clinician will focus on examining a singular joint or just a few joints affected by a complaint. Joint assessments can be complex but can be performed in a systematic manner, with the examiner palpating with a purpose and considering the underlying anatomy during the examination. While palpating a body part, place attention on palpation of specific anatomical locations of the part to be examined. During palpation, note any palpable deformities, nodularities, tenderness, swelling, or warmth. Palpate muscles for tone, size, and tenderness. Note any palpable crepitus, which can be present with conditions such as a fracture or arthritis. Areas of warmth may suggest an inflammatory or infectious cause of pain, while cool areas may suggest vascular compromise. Point tenderness is important as a potential indicator of injury, inflammation, or infection.

■ Range of Motion

Active motion of a joint is performed prior to assessing passive and assisted motion. In each case, note any limitations or complaints while the joint is moving through the ROM in the applicable motion planes for that joint. The patient's response to active motion provides clues to how the examiner should best support the limb through passive motion. If a patient demonstrates full active ROM for a joint, passive or assisted ROM may not be necessary. A goniometer is a tool that assists the examiner to measure degrees of motion for a joint and provides an objective measure of ROM. A loss of motion occurs to some degree with age; it can be minimal but does vary from person to person. Substantial and asymmetric loss are abnormal findings. An injured or diseased joint will likely be painful on motion, and active ROM may be limited to a greater degree than passive ROM due to pain inhibition of motion. Motion in an abnormal plane may indicate laxity in ligaments. Crepitus and grating on movement often indicate cartilage degeneration of the articular surfaces. Clicks can occur from previous injuries to the joints, abnormalities of a meniscus, or merely from soft tissue sliding over bone. When performing a focused examination of a specific body part, be sure to assess for symmetry of ROM by assessing the same joint on the opposite side of the body.

■ Ligamentous Tests

When a patient complains of pain or injury to a joint, the stability of the joint should be determined. Ligamentous tests involve applying stress (i.e., stretch) to the ligaments by a variety of maneuvers, with the examiner flexing or extending the joint while applying pressure in a particular direction and determining the "feel" of the resulting movement and evaluating for any laxity, crepitus, or pain. Ligamentous stressing of a joint should start with only gentle pressure and then be repeated with increasing amounts of pressure/stress so that the test remains within the patient's pain tolerance yet provides information on the degree of laxity in a joint with any particular amount of stress. Symmetry of joint laxity should be assessed with the clinician examining the same joint on the opposite side of the body. Some patients may have lax joints as a component of their normal anatomical makeup without injury, and this will be demonstrated as symmetric bilateral laxity. Conversely, people who have had a ligamentous injury can have varying degrees of laxity, which can demonstrate as asymmetry in joint laxity when comparing the injured joint with the contralateral uninjured joint. The degree of laxity correlates to the degree of injury to a ligament.

■ Muscle Strength and Tone

Muscle strength is determined by asking the patient to attempt to move a particular body part in the specific planes of motion for the joint against the examiner's manual resistance. This is sometimes referred to as manual muscle testing. Muscle strength is graded on a scale of 0 (no evidence of muscle contraction or strength) to 5 (complete or full strength against resistance). Pain, contracture, and disease can all affect muscle strength. Table 15.2 depicts a rating scheme for muscle strength. As with many parts of the musculoskeletal examination, assessment for symmetry of strength is important, and the examiner should assess strength bilaterally.

Table 15.2

Muscle Strength Assessment

Muscle Strength Assessment	Grade Notation	% Normal
No muscle contraction noted when resistance applied	M0	0
A slight muscle contraction seen or palpated but insufficient for joint movement	M1	10
Weak contraction when the joint is held in position; full passive range of motion	M2	25
Contraction weak but there is full active movement against resistance	M3	50
Some muscle strength against resistance	M4	75
Normal strength is present	M5	100

Joint, tendon, and muscle pain typically increase when the muscle or tendon is stretched, and the joint is mobilized. For instance, an injured hamstring muscle is more painful when the leg is extended and the muscle pulled tight. Joint and tendon pain also increase when the area of injury is stressed.

Assessment of the muscle tone helps to assess innervation. A relaxed muscle should retain a slight residual tension, or tone. To assess muscle tone, passively stretch the muscle, ask the patient to relax, and then palpate the muscle, comparing side to side. It takes practice on the part of the examiner to develop a smooth motion when performing passive stretching. Alternatively, assessment of muscle tone can be combined with a determination of the patient's resistance to passive movement. Tense patients or those with increased muscle tone will have increased resistance to passive movements. Flaccid or hypotonic muscles may indicate peripheral nervous system disease, cerebellar disease, or spinal cord problems. A spastic muscle has increased resistance, which may vary as the limb is moved, as in "cogwheeling," such as seen in patients with parkinsonism. Resistance with both flexion and extension is called *lead-pipe rigidity*, as is sometimes seen in parkinsonism.

■ Special Maneuvers

A variety of special maneuvers are indicated during the assessment of specific muscle, ligament, and joint groups. Some of the major maneuvers are described in subsequent sections on specific complaints.

Diagnostic Studies

The diagnostic studies relevant to musculoskeletal assessment are numerous. Plain radiographs provide the appropriate initial imaging for many musculoskeletal complaints. However, a number of other imaging studies are available, depending on the presentation and differential diagnoses. These include computed tomography (CT) scans, magnetic resonance imaging (MRI), myelograms, ultrasound, nuclear scans, and others. Arthroscopic procedures provide an invasive means to visualize the internal joint structures and look for pathology or injury. Arthrocentesis allows for aspiration of fluid to assess for pathology, including septic arthritis or gouty arthritis. Doppler studies may be helpful in determining problems with blood flow, clotting, and inflammation in the veins. Blood work to determine the presence of infectious, metabolic, rheumatic, or other disorders may also be needed.

Differential Diagnosis of Chief Complaints

Pain is a common complaint associated with musculoskeletal disorders. Any complaint of musculoskeletal pain requires further symptom analysis. The analysis is very similar regardless of the specific joint or region involved. Box 15.1 identifies the basic symptom analysis for musculoskeletal pain. The subsequent sections of this chapter refer to this box.

Box 15.1

Musculoskeletal Symptom Analysis

Questions to determine what causes and/or relieves the pain:
- What, if anything, has been done to relieve the pain, and what was the response?
- Is there any situation or activity that relieves or diminishes the pain?
- Does anything seem to trigger the pain or make it worse?
- Is the pain worse or better at any particular time of day?

Questions to identify the type or quality of the pain:
- How can the pain be described?
- Is it burning, cramping, aching, sharp?
- Is it constant, throbbing, shooting?
- How bad is the pain on a scale?

Questions to determine the location and radiation of the pain:
- Where exactly does it hurt the most? (Ask the patient to point to the area where the pain is the worst.)
- Where does the pain radiate? Where else has there been pain?

Questions about associated symptoms:
- What other symptoms have been noticed since the pain first occurred?
- Have any other sensations, such as tingling or numbness, been noticed?
- Has there been any weakness, swelling, redness, limited motion, or popping?
- Have there been any other generalized symptoms, such as fever, malaise, or decreased energy?

Questions about the temporal sequence of the symptoms:
- When was the pain first noticed? What was the patient doing at the time?
- Since the pain was noticed, has it been persistent or intermittent?
- Since its onset, has the pain gotten worse or stayed the same?

■ Polyarthralgia

Polyarthralgia usually refers to arthralgia, or pain, in five or more joints, as opposed to monoarthralgia, which involves only one joint, or oligoarthralgia, which involves two to four joints. Arthralgia is differentiated from arthritis in that arthralgia simply indicates joint pain/discomfort, whereas arthritis indicates associated joint inflammation and/or degeneration. Therefore, one can have arthralgia with or without accompanying signs of arthritis.

The differential diagnosis for polyarthralgia is broad and includes infections, rheumatic conditions, noninflammatory degenerative disorders, malignancies, and endocrine disorders. For this reason, it is critical that the history and physical examination obtain the necessary information to narrow the differential diagnosis.

History

Essential components of the history include a description of the nature and characteristics of symptom onset and progression as well as the presence of extra-articular symptoms. Establish whether the pain and any other symptoms have been constant, progressive, or intermittent and whether the same joints are consistently involved or whether the pain migrates among differing joints. Family history is important, particularly for autoimmune disorders, RA, and OA. Ask about risks for developing a sexually transmitted infection and about history of tick bite as a potential causative factor for joint pain.

Physical Examination

A thorough musculoskeletal examination should be performed. When examining a patient who complains of pain in multiple joints, it is important to determine the distribution of the involved joints, noting the degree of symmetry and the types of joints (large weight-bearing versus small joints) affected. The clinician should attempt to discern if the discomfort is truly articular or if the pain is from the periarticular soft tissue structures. ROM and strength should be assessed and compared bilaterally. The presence of inflammatory signs helps to differentiate arthritic conditions from noninflammatory arthralgias. Other important signs include the presence or absence of nonarticular signs, including abnormalities of the ear-nose-throat, integumentary, cardiopulmonary, gastro-intestinal, genitourinary, neurological, or lymphatic systems. Be sure to evaluate for red flags of joint infection such as warmth, edema, erythema, fever, and joint pain with passive motion.

Diagnostic Studies

Many diagnostic studies can be used to evaluate musculoskeletal complaints. Imaging studies are commonly used to evaluate the structure and integrity of affected joints. The range of relevant imaging studies is broad, although plain films are generally the first images indicated. Depending on the presentation, appropriate laboratory studies include a complete blood count, a metabolic profile, a urinalysis, and a variety of rheumatologic tests. Analysis of synovial fluid is often warranted to differentiate among potential etiologies, including gout and joint infection.

RHEUMATOID ARTHRITIS

RA is a progressive, inflammatory, and erosive condition that usually affects multiple joints. Women are affected by RA at a greater rate than men. In addition to the articular changes associated with RA, there is a range of systemic effects. RA is an autoimmune condition with onset of the disease most commonly between age 30 and 50 years.

Signs and Symptoms

RA typically affects the joints symmetrically. Symptoms may wax and wane, but the effects are cumulative and progressive. Although RA can affect any joint, it commonly affects the small joints of the hands and feet, with the characteristic deformity often helpful in making the diagnosis. There is often history of prolonged morning stiffness for longer than an hour and fatigue. Affected joints are often tender, swollen with effusions, warm, and inflamed. Nodules and deformities are common to RA. The disease most commonly affects metacarpophalangeal and proximal interphalangeal joints. Over time, a variety of typical RA deformities develop, including subluxation of the metacarpophalangeal joints and ulnar deviation and hyperextensions of the proximal interphalangeal (swan neck) joints. Deformities of the feet will include claw toes and hallux valgus (bunion). RA is also associated with nonarticular findings, including changes in the eye consistent with scleritis and episcleritis, interstitial lung disease, and pericardial disease.

Diagnostic Studies

A variety of laboratory tests are used to diagnose RA, including the rheumatoid factor, which is positive in up to 80% of persons with RA but not specific to this disorder. It is often falsely positive in patients with other diseases, including lupus, sarcoidosis, and syphilis. RA is often associated with normocytic, hypochromic anemia as well as elevations in sedimentation rate and C-reactive protein. Other laboratory tests that may be positive at diagnosis include antinuclear antibody (ANA) and anticyclic citrullinated peptide (anti-CCP) antibodies. The anti-CCP antibodies are more specific to RA than the rheumatoid factor. Radiological images show loss of joint space, periarticular osteopenia, and bony erosion.

OSTEOARTHRITIS

OA is another common cause of polyarthralgia. It is the most prevalent form of arthritis, affecting over 30 million Americans. This progressive disorder is associated with age and with wear and tear. OA causes a loss of cartilage and progressive erosion of bone.

Signs and Symptoms

Compared with RA, OA has a higher likelihood of affecting larger joints, such as the hips and knees. Like RA, OA also frequently involves the small joints of the hands, although it tends to occur at the distal interphalangeal joints (Heberden's nodes) and proximal interphalangeal joints (Bouchard's nodes). Most frequently, the second or third digits and the base of the thumb at the carpometacarpal joint are involved. The distribution is asymmetrical. Patients may complain of pain, stiffness, loss of motion, or deformity and swelling. The pain and stiffness associated with OA often improve with moderate use and are worse after extended periods of rest. If three or more metacarpophalangeal joints are swollen, the differential should include RA.

Diagnostic Studies

Plain films reveal characteristic and progressive changes to the joints, including diminishing joint space due to loss of articular cartilage, subchondral sclerosis, subchondral cyst formation, and osteophyte formation. Serum laboratory studies are typically not necessary for patients with OA. Inflammatory markers, such as C-reactive protein and erythrocyte sedimentation rate, as well as rheumatoid factor, will be negative.

FIBROMYALGIA

The etiology of fibromyalgia is not known. This complex, chronic, multifactorial disorder affects approximately 2% of the population and occurs primarily in women between age 20 and 60 years. Although patients may present with complaints of multiple joint pain, the disorder does not actually involve joints. Instead, it is a noninflammatory soft tissue disorder.

Signs and Symptoms

The most common symptoms are generalized pain, fatigue, stiffness, and decreased ROM, with multiple-point tenderness. The diagnostic criteria currently rest on a patient reporting point tenderness/pain in at least 11 of 18 specified sites (Fig. 15.1) and the presence of widespread pain for at least 3 months. The most common painful/tender sites are in the neck, shoulders, spine, and hips. Other common symptoms include morning stiffness, paresthesias of the feet and/or hands, anxiety, depression, sleep disturbances, "brain fog," headache, chest pain, and irritable bowel syndrome.

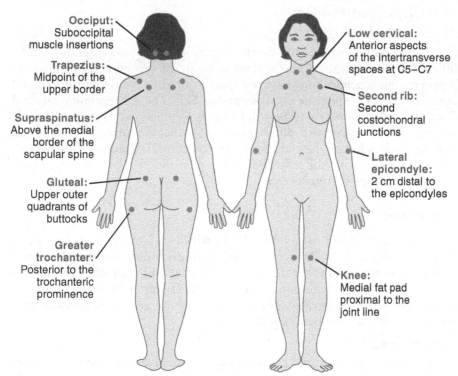

Figure 15.1 The 18 pressure points must be accurately located and tested by applying just enough pressure with one finger to barely blanch the nailbed.

Diagnostic Studies

There are no definitive diagnostic biomarker studies for fibromyalgia. If the clinician is suspicious for underlying pathology or comorbidities, appropriate laboratory studies or diagnostic imaging may be ordered to evaluate for or rule out disorders.

SYSTEMIC LUPUS ERYTHEMATOSUS

SLE is a chronic autoimmune disorder that has widespread effects. A majority of patients with SLE will have joints affected by this disease. The prevalence is much higher in women, particularly in the childbearing years, than in men.

Signs and Symptoms

SLE has many potential symptoms. The classic findings include a malar rash. Patients often have arthralgias, myalgias, fever, fatigue, Raynaud's syndrome, and neuropathy. SLE effects depend on the organs involved. Involvement of cardiovascular, renal, pulmonary, hematological, neurological, ophthalmic, gastrointestinal, dermatological, and musculoskeletal symptoms is possible. Patients can exhibit large joint involvement including pain, swelling, and synovitis. Hand and wrist synovitis, swelling, and ligament laxity are common. Patients taking oral steroids for SLE treatment can develop osteonecrosis of the hip and subsequent hip pain and disability.

Diagnostic Studies

The diagnostic findings depend on the organs involved, and diagnosis can be difficult. A positive ANA occurs at some point in the condition in the majority of patients but is neither consistent nor specific for SLE. Positive anti-DNA and lupus erythematosus prep are also common to SLE. The sedimentation rate and C-reactive protein level are increased. Other helpful laboratory studies include complete blood count with differential, creatinine, albumin, and urinalysis. Imaging study selection depends on the presentation. Imaging studies are necessary for patients with SLE who develop hip pain and have been managed with steroids to evaluate for osteonecrosis.

SARCOIDOSIS

Sarcoidosis is an inflammatory disorder in which patients develop noncaseating granulomas and a wide range of symptoms, including arthritis. It is most commonly diagnosed in persons between ages 20 and 40 years. Exposure to environmental antigens can initiate a cell-mediated immune response in people who are genetically susceptible. The inflammatory immune response of sarcoidosis leads to the development of granulomas.

Signs and Symptoms

Although the disorder may be asymptomatic and resolve spontaneously, it often is accompanied by multiple symptoms, including joint pain and chronic illness. Arthralgias occur in approximately 3% of patients with sarcoidosis, and the most commonly affected joints include the ankles, feet, and hands. The patient may complain of constitutional symptoms, including fatigue, malaise, weakness, fever, weight loss, and altered appetite. Respiratory symptoms, including cough, wheezing, and shortness of breath, are primary symptoms. Others include lymphadenopathy, rash, eye changes, and palpitations.

Diagnostic Studies

Appropriate diagnostic studies depend on the symptoms and the involved organs. However, definitive diagnosis involves biopsy of the affected organs. Other laboratory abnormalities depend on involved organs and degree of pathology. There is often an elevated sedimentation rate and normocytic, normochromic anemia. Chest films should be ordered when sarcoidosis is suspected.

REACTIVE ARTHRITIS

Reactive arthritis is a type of seronegative spondyloarthropathy that is typically acute in onset. Presentation of reactive arthritis occurs most commonly in men younger than 40 years. The complex of symptoms develops after a gastrointestinal or genitourinary infection. *Chlamydia, Shigella, Salmonella, Yersinia, Campylobacter,* and *Clostridium difficile* are infections commonly associated with onset of reactive arthritis.

Signs and Symptoms

Multiple joints are usually involved, primarily affecting the knee, ankle, and sacroiliac joint, which may develop within a few weeks of an infection. The distribution of affected joints is asymmetrical, and the arthritis is migratory. In addition to the arthritis pain, often present are urethritis, dactylitis, enthesitis, conjunctivitis, or iritis as well as diarrhea and fever.

Diagnostic Studies

There are no studies specific to Reiter's syndrome, and this is frequently a clinical diagnosis. Erythrocyte sedimentation rate and C-reactive protein are often elevated. Studies may identify the offending infectious agent. Signs of infection may be present in urinalysis if a genitourinary infection is present. Serum HLA-B27 antigen is positive in most patients.

GONOCOCCAL ARTHRITIS

This infectious or septic arthritis is more common in young sexually active men and follows infection with gonorrhea. Gonococcal arthritis occurs as part of disseminated infection and frequently presents with polyarthralgia, but it may also be isolated to a single infected joint.

Signs and Symptoms

This septic arthritis can be migratory and affect lower extremities and the hands or may involve a singular infected joint. In addition to the arthritis, the syndrome usually includes a nonpruritic dermatitis and tenosynovitis. Generalized muscle aches and fever are also common. An infected joint will often be warm, erythematous, edematous, and painful to touch. The patient may have pain with ROM and have an inability to bear weight.

Diagnostic Studies

The sedimentation rate and C-reactive protein are often elevated. Plain films will reveal joint distension, which can later progress to joint destruction. Synovial fluid aspiration with increased polymorphonuclear leukocytes and positive culture occur in fewer than 50% of patients.

GOUTY ARTHRITIS

Gout is a form of acute inflammatory arthritis that results from the deposition/collection of monosodium urate crystals in joint tissue. The condition usually occurs after middle age and is associated with an elevated serum uric acid level. Patients will experience intermittent flares of pain with asymptomatic periods. The frequency of how often a patient develops a painful flare varies widely.

Signs and Symptoms

Gout is a classic cause of acute monoarthritis but more rarely affects multiple joints. It should be considered when polyarthritis recurs over a long period of time. Even though most cases involve a joint in the lower extremities, other joints may be affected. Approximately 50% of gout flares will involve the great toe. Acute pain usually develops in one joint, with swelling, redness, and warmth, and the severity of the pain increases rapidly; this is frequently referred to as a gouty flare. Patients may experience a fever during an attack. ROM of the affected joints is limited by pain, and there is significant tenderness to the site. Patients who have had gout for an extended time often have gouty tophi, which are soft tissue nodules containing urate crystals. The olecranon bursa is a common site for tophi development, which can be painful.

Diagnostic Studies

Plain films are generally negative unless the condition has persisted for a long time. In this case, films may reveal bone spurs and subchondral erosions of the bone. The serum uric acid level may be elevated; however, during a gouty pain flare, the serum levels can reduce to normal. Joint fluid aspiration and evaluation of the fluid using polarized light microscopy is considered by many to be the gold standard for diagnosing gout. The aspirate will reveal characteristic urate crystals. There may be a mild increase in white blood cells, and sedimentation rate is increased on examination of serum.

LYME DISEASE

In the United States, Lyme disease is one of the most frequent causes for vector-borne illness. Lyme is caused by the bacterium *Borrelia burgdorferi* and is transmitted by a bite from a deer tick. Whereas the incubation period ranges from 3 to 30 days, the onset of symptoms typically appears in 7 to 14 days. Lyme infections primarily occur in the upper Midwest and Northeast regions of the United States.

Decision Rule

While microscopic assessment of joint aspirate for urate crystals is believed to be the gold standard, not all clinicians are trained to aspirate joints. In particular, the small joints (e.g., the great toe) can be difficult to aspirate. As an alternative to aspirating a joint, a clinical diagnosis algorithm can be used to come to a diagnosis of gout. The sensitivity and specificity of the Clinical Gout Diagnosis tool (AHRQ, 2017) are 97% and 96%, respectively. This clinical decision tool proposes a diagnosis of gout when any 4 of the following 8 specified findings are present:

History of more than one attack of acute arthritis
Development of maximum inflammation within 1 day
Monoarthritis or oligoarthritis
Redness over joints
Painful or swollen first metatarsophalangeal joint (podagra)
Unilateral tarsal joint attack
Tophi
Risk factors such as hyperuricemia

Signs and Symptoms

Early disease will demonstrate a classic solitary bulls-eye–appearing lesion (erythema migrans) that may be followed by multiple lesions. A patient can develop arthralgias, myalgia, headache and neck stiffness, and fatigue, and fever can occur early in the disease. The patient can develop meningitis, neuropathy, Bell's palsy, radiculopathy, heart block, and pericarditis. Lyme arthritis is a common late finding with this disease, typically affecting large joints. Late disease may also be accompanied by encephalopathy, radicular pain, and paresthesia, as well as cognitive deficit.

Diagnostic Studies

The diagnosis of early Lyme is often based on the physical findings. Definitive diagnosis is based on laboratory studies. Initially, an enzyme-linked immunosorbent assay (ELISA) or indirect immunoglobulin G and M (IgG, IgM) antibody is obtained; if the initial test is positive, it is followed by Western blot.

ACUTE RHEUMATIC FEVER

Acute rheumatic fever (ARF) is becoming more rare in the United States. However, this disease should be considered when children and young adults develop polyarthralgia. This complex of symptoms occurs following an infection with streptococci, typically streptococcal pharyngitis. For those people who have had a prior episode of ARF, they have nearly a 50% risk of developing another episode of ARF with another untreated streptococcal pharyngitis infection.

> RED FLAG ◄ **Red Flags in the Assessment of the Patient With Neck Pain**
>
> - *History of injury/trauma preceding onset of pain*
> - *Associated neck stiffness (nuchal rigidity) with fever*
> - *Neck pain in a child*
> - *Pain that is unrelenting and/or worsening in patients who have tried and failed conservative treatment*
> - *Acute, severe pain, with or without radicular symptoms, upon awakening in the morning*
> - *Pain relieved by elevating the arm above the head on the side of the pain*
> - *Severe pain, with or without radicular symptoms, on flexion or extension of the neck*
> - *Chronic neck pain with weakness of upper or lower extremities, stumbling, muscle atrophy, bowel or bladder incontinence*
> - *Pain with a history of malignancies*

Signs and Symptoms

There is typically a history of recent sore throat preceding development of pain in the larger joints. Symptoms frequently begin approximately 2 to 3 weeks following a streptococcal pharyngitis infection. The joint pain is often migratory and can be accompanied by edema and warmth over the joint. Joint pain most commonly affects the elbow, wrist, knee, and ankles. Cardiac symptoms may be present, including heart failure, murmur, or pericarditis. Other signs include fever, rash, and subcutaneous nodules. The rash is usually a faint pink and nonpruritic.

Diagnostic Studies

There may be elevations of sedimentation rate and C-reactive protein as well as a prolonged PR interval on electrocardiogram. Throat culture is positive in approximately 25% of patients.

■ Neck Pain

Neck pain is a common complaint and may originate from the neck structures or radiate to the neck from another region of the body. Many of the potential causes are benign and self-limiting. Neck pain may also be an indication of a rheumatologic disorder, traumatic injury, or neurological disorder. Signs and symptoms associated with neck pain are listed in the Red Flag box.

History

When a patient presents with neck pain, it is important to obtain a thorough history of the complaint and any associated symptoms. An analysis of the pain should be completed (see Box 15.1). Determine whether the pain is isolated to just the neck or if there is any associated pain in other areas, including the head, shoulders, back, and upper extremities. Ask about stiffness or decreased ROM as well as whether certain motions or positions increase or decrease the discomfort. Identify the patient's normal occupational and recreational activities and any unusual exertion/activities. Always determine whether a recent injury or a trauma has occurred and the mechanisms involved in the injury/trauma.

Physical Examination

The neck examination should be thorough and performed with the patient undressed from the waist up. It can be helpful to observe the patient undressing, noting movement and any apparent discomfort or weakness. Observe the patient's general posture, head placement, cervical curve, and symmetry of movement. The neck structures should be observed and palpated, noting any deformity, tenderness, muscle spasms, or other abnormalities. Active ROM of the neck should be performed in all planes (flexion, extension, rotation, lateral flexion) within the patient's tolerance, followed by passive movement if any limitations are identified. Neck or arm pain associated with neck movement should be noted. Assess the ROM, sensation, and reflexes of the upper extremities to assess cervical nerve compromise. The strength and tone of the neck and upper extremities should be determined as well. The examination of neck pain may vary depending on the presentation. For patients with recent trauma, such as a motor vehicle accident, a brief initial examination to determine stability may be performed and then radiographs obtained before proceeding with a more comprehensive examination.

Diagnostic Studies

In orthopedics generally, the history and clinical findings should help guide the determination of when to order diagnostic studies and what studies to order. Selecting the appropriate imaging study can also be guided by evidence and appropriateness criteria such as those available through the American College of Radiology (ACR). Patients with a recent onset of neck pain but no neurological symptoms, such as weakness or loss of reflexes, and no history of trauma do not necessarily require imaging. A CT scan is superior for looking at bony architecture and should be obtained for patients who have potential for a fracture due to a history of high-risk trauma or who present with neurological signs, altered sensorium, or abnormal radiographic findings. Box 15.2 depicts indications of high-risk trauma. MRI is superior in imaging soft tissues such as intervertebral disk, spinal cord, or nerve roots. When patients have neurological symptoms along with neck pain, an MRI can be ordered to assess for nerve or spinal cord compromise. When the patient cannot tolerate or has other contraindications to the use of an MRI, a CT scan can be obtained and followed by a myelogram as necessary. Electromyography (EMG) and nerve conduction studies (NCS) are helpful in identifying level and distribution of nerve involvement.

Box 15.2

High-Risk Trauma

- Fall from 3 or more feet
- Fall from five or more stairs
- Fall involving axial load (e.g., diving accident)
- Vehicular accident at high speed (more than 100 km/hr), with rollover and/or ejection
- Accident involving recreational vehicle or bicycle

ACR (2021).

CERVICAL DISK HERNIATION/ RADICULOPATHY

Cervical disk herniation can occur when the central portion of an interverte-bral disk (nucleus pulposus) herniates through the outer fibrous covering of a disk (annulus fibrosis), resulting in neck pain and/or radiculopathy. When the disk herniates, it can compress upon or irritate a cervical nerve root leading to the characteristic radicular pain along the distribution of the affected cervical nerve(s). In the neck, the nerves most affected are the C6 and C7 cervical nerves. Cervical disk herniation can result from an increased intradiscal pressure follow-ing a trauma or injury. With aging and the degenerative process, intervertebral disks can develop fissures or tears in the annulus, which increases the potential for a herniation.

Signs and Symptoms

Patients with a cervical disk herniation with radiculopathy will primarily com-plain of unilateral arm pain with or without neck pain. Some patients can have a disk herniation without nerve irritation and no neck or arm symptoms. There may be complaints of muscle spasm with the neck pain. Coughing and straining can increase the pain, which may radiate to the shoulder and arm. Elevating the arm and placing the hand on top of the head may provide relief (positive relief sign). The distribution of radiating symptoms of pain, numbness, and tingling depends on the affected nerve root. Neurological findings can include altered upper extremity deep tendon reflexes, weakness, and loss of sensation. If disk rupture is due to injury or trauma, the onset of symptoms will typically be acute. The patient should be assessed for signs of cervical myelopathy such as bowel and bladder dysfunction or disturbance in gait. This can occur with a large cervical disk herniation that compresses upon the spinal cord.

A positive Spurling's sign is noted if this maneuver reproduces neck and radicular pain, suggesting herniated disk. Spurling's sign is tested for by lightly pressing downward on the top of the patient's head while tilting head and neck back and toward the side of pain. The Lhermitte's sign, a hallmark finding in patients with multiple sclerosis, also may support suspicion of a herniated disk.

This test is conducted by having the patient flex the neck in a chin-to-chest motion and is positive if an electric shock–like sensation down the spine results. The sign may also be positive in a number of other conditions, including spondylosis, radiation myelopathy, and Chiari I malformation.

Diagnostic Studies

When patients are alert, not intoxicated, able to allow assessment of the neck, and demonstrating rotation of 45 degrees in both directions, cervical images are typically not indicated. The ACR (2021) cites the Canadian C-Spine Rule as an indicator that images should be considered. These criteria include being older than 65, paresthesia of extremities, history of rigid spinal disease (e.g., ankylosing spondylitis), and the considerations listed in Box 15.2. Plain films often identify the diminished disk space and should include anteroposterior (AP), lateral, open-mouth, and both oblique views. An MRI is indicated for chronic neck pain with diminished disk space and/or neurological findings.

CERVICAL SPONDYLOSIS/STENOSIS

Cervical spondylosis is a degenerative process involving the cervical spine. It is characterized by degeneration and arthritis of the joints of the cervical spine, degeneration of the intervertebral discs, and thickening of the spinal ligaments. The term *cervical stenosis* is used when the degenerative changes lead to the spinal canal or the neuroforamen becoming smaller than normal. The stenosis can result in compression of the spinal cord or the nerve roots, potentially resulting in either motor or sensory neurological symptoms. Patients in whom symptomatic cervical spondylosis is identified should be referred to specialty evaluation and treatment.

Signs and Symptoms

Neck discomfort and headache are common findings of cervical spondylosis. The neurological symptoms and clinical findings are specific to the affected nerve root or level of the spinal cord. These can include radicular pain and dysesthesias, abnormal deep tendon reflexes, and weakness. Patients may exhibit symptoms of radiculopathy or myelopathy.

Diagnostic Studies

Plain radiographs identify degenerative changes of the spine, osteophyte formation, and narrowing of the intervertebral disc spaces. An MRI will identify the sites and degree of stenosis and nerve tissue compression. Alternatively, a CT with myelogram can be a useful tool to image the anatomy of the cervical spine.

NECK STRAIN

Neck strain is a common problem, which can be caused by chronic strain from positioning and posture or overuse and repetitive use of the neck and related structures. An acceleration/deceleration injury, or whiplash, is a form of neck strain typically seen following a motor vehicle crash.

Signs and Symptoms

The most common symptom of neck strain, regardless of the cause, is neck pain. However, there is often associated radiating occipital, shoulder, and/or upper back pain. The history usually identifies the source of the strain. With more severe strain, such as is seen with whiplash injuries, other common complaints such as paresthesias of the upper extremities can be noted. The strength and reflexes of the upper extremities are typically within normal limits, and the patient should be neurologically intact. The patient with a neurological deficit should be considered for a referral for further evaluation.

Diagnostic Studies

Radiographs of the cervical spine should be obtained to assess for cervical fractures and subluxation if a trauma has occurred or any neurological findings are present. If spasm is present, the only radiological finding may be loss of the lordotic curve. In the absence of injury or neurological symptoms, most patients will not require imaging.

SYRINGOMYELIA (SYRINX, HYDROSYRINGOMYELIA)

Syringomyelia is a fluid cavity in the spinal cord that can occur in the cervical and/or thoracic areas. The most common cause of syringomyelia is Chiari malformation (see "Chiari Malformation" in the "Headache" or "Cephalalgia" section of Chapter 16). Less common causes include spinal tumor, arachnoiditis, or trauma. These fluid cavities can lead to neurological deficit as they gradually expand.

Signs and Symptoms

The patient often describes burning pain in the neck or thoracic area and paresthesias or numbness in the neck or thoracic areas as well as in the extremities. Progressive weakness of the extremities and limited ROM of the neck and/or back may occur. Other possible symptoms include bladder retention or incontinence and diminished sensation, strength, and reflexes. The gait may be altered.

Diagnostic Studies

The test of choice for diagnosis of syringomyelia is an MRI of the cervical, thoracic, and lumbar spine with and without contrast. The area of the spine that is imaged is determined by the area of symptoms reported by the patient.

PATHOLOGICAL FRACTURE AND METASTATIC TUMOR

Any spontaneous fracture should be explored for possible relation to carcinoma, either metastatic or multiple myeloma, in an older adult. Other noncancerous causes for pathologic fracture can be due to collapse of the bone from osteonecrosis, osteomyelitis, or benign bone tumor.

FIBROMYALGIA

See pp. 515–516.

■ Low Back Pain

Low back pain (LBP) is extremely common. Nearly three-fourths of the world's population will have at least one disabling episode of LBP in their lives. It is the most common cause of limited activity and most common reason for office visits for patients younger than 45 years in the United States. Most episodes are self-limited and resolve in less than 3 weeks. The cause of LBP can be difficult to differentiate/diagnose, and the condition may be poorly treated. Many patients forgo traditional medical assessment and treatment in favor of chiropractic care, massage, or acupuncture. Many factors can affect how fast or soon a person returns to work after a work-related back injury. For example, the longer an employee is absent from work owing to LBP, the lower the chance the employee has of returning to the workplace.

History

As with all pain syndromes, it is important to obtain a detailed history of the onset and progression of the pain. A thorough pain history should be completed, noting its quality, location, radiation, and intensity as well as any exacerbating and relieving factors. A thorough review of systems is necessary to identify any associated symptoms that may indicate an urgent problem. These include altered bowel and/or bladder function, fever, weight loss, and/or weakness. The medical history should identify previous episodes of back pain and other musculoskeletal disorders and should include the treatment and responses for them. Specifically ask about a history of malignancy, arthritis, recent infection, and neurological disorders. Identify any history of recent trauma, including the mechanisms involved. Family history should be obtained. The patient's recreational and

---

RED FLAG ◀ **Red Flags in the Assessment of the Patient With Low Back Pain**

- *Pain associated with neurological deficits (weakness, altered sensation, bowel/bladder changes)*
- *Pain in a child*
- *Pain associated with fever and/or stiff neck*
- *Pain associated with unexplained weight loss with or without a previous history of malignancy*
- *Pain worse at rest*
- *Pain associated with radiation to the abdomen or stomach area or lower extremities*
- *Pain related to history of urinary tract infections, drug use, or other infections (including AIDS)*
- *Pain increases with coughing/sneezing or straining*

occupational activity patterns should be determined. A history of all medications, both over the counter and prescription, should be identified. See the Red Flag box for signs and symptoms associated with LBP.

Physical Examination

The physical examination should begin by noting the patient's posture and apparent level of discomfort. The standing patient should be directed through a series of maneuvers to assess the back motion, including flexion, hyperextension, lateral flexion, and rotation, as the smoothness of motion, ROM, and any obvious signs of discomfort are noted. Next, palpate along the spinal column with the patient standing and then bending forward. Note the presence or absence of the natural curvature and any focal, midline tenderness. Observe the patient walking on heels and on toes, noting any signs of weakness.

Next, with the patient resting supine on the examination table, perform the straight leg maneuver. As the patient rests supine with both legs extended, the examiner should passively elevate one leg at a time. A positive test is indicated if the patient experiences pain in the leg with elevation. Note how far down the leg the pain extends. Note whether any pain is experienced on the side of the raised leg or contralaterally. Consider the results of the straight leg test in combination with the rest of the physical examination, including neurosensory and reflex testing. If the results indicate nerve impingement or disk injury, further radiographic testing is then indicated.

Throughout the assessment, be attentive for signs of serious diseases associated with LBP, including malignancy, abdominal aortic aneurysm, fracture, and bone infection.

Diagnostic Studies

The following diagnostic tests should be considered on the basis of history and presentation:

- Lumbar x-rays with AP/lateral and flexion/extension views provide information about bony abnormalities. Acute fractures and subluxation are often discernable on plain x-rays.
- An MRI of the lumbar spine with and without contrast is the test of choice for prolonged symptoms and/or diagnosis of herniated disks, intra- or extradural mass lesions, spina bifida occulta, and cauda equina syndrome or with history of recent trauma or advanced age.
- For blunt trauma history associated with back pain, a CT scan without contrast or a multidetector CT should be considered.

MECHANICAL LOW BACK PAIN

Mechanical LBP is extremely common, and most individuals experience some type of mechanical back pain at least once in their lives. This is a frequent cause for LBP. The causes are varied.

Signs and Symptoms

Pain in the back, buttocks, and thighs may be severe. The onset can occur after new or unusual exertion. There is usually no history of major trauma, systemic infection, or malignancy. Pain relief is frequently achieved when lying down. Physical examination can reveal paravertebral tenderness/spasm, scoliosis, or loss of natural lumbar lordosis with no neurological signs or radiculopathy.

Diagnostic Studies

None are needed unless the patient fails to improve with conservative treatment, the symptoms progressively worsen, or the patient exhibits red flag symptoms.

LUMBAR HERNIATED INTERVERTEBRAL DISK

Herniated disks are most common after age 30 and occur more frequently in men than in women. A herniation occurs when the inner portion of the intervertebral disk (nucleus pulposus) herniates through the outer portion of the disk (annulus fibrosis). Symptoms depend on the degree of disk herniation. The herniated portion may push against the spinal ligaments, spinal cord, or nerve roots. Most herniations will occur at the L4/5 and L5/S1 level. The symptoms for a majority of patients will improve with conservative care within 3 months. A flexion injury or trauma may precede the onset of symptoms.

Signs and Symptoms

The acute phase is often associated with symptoms of radicular irritation such as pain, numbness, and tingling into the lower extremities. Other symptoms include diminished reflexes and strength. A major prolapse may be associated with bilateral weakness and bowel and bladder dysfunction. Pain associated with chronic nerve irritation is usually dull and unilateral. Lying with hips flexed may provide pain relief. Associated paravertebral tenderness and muscle spasm often result in awkward posture. Patients with a disk herniation will often show a positive straight leg raise on examination.

Diagnostic Studies

Patients with a disk herniation, without an injury and with symptoms of only pain, numbness, and tingling, typically do not require imaging until they have had unimproved symptoms for 6 to 8 weeks. Patients who have a loss of strength or reflexes require imaging x-ray and MRI. A CT or myelogram may be indicated if the patient is unable to obtain an MRI. An EMG may give supporting documentation regarding the level of nerve damage.

SPINAL STENOSIS

Caused by progressive degenerative spine changes, spinal stenosis is most common at middle age or later. Spinal stenosis results in narrowing of the central spinal canal or the neuroforamen. A majority of patients will have spinal stenosis at the L4/5 level, and it is the leading cause of surgery for people older than 65 years.

Signs and Symptoms

Patients with spinal stenosis will experience back, buttock, and/or leg pain. Spinal stenosis pain is usually worse during the day. It is aggravated by standing and walking but relieved by rest, sitting, and leaning forward. The pain varies from severe to mild. The level of neurological findings varies and can include weakness and bowel or bladder dysfunction. OA signs may be present.

Diagnostic Studies

Radiological findings may indicate extensive vertebral osteophytes and degenerative disk disease. An MRI or CT scan can be helpful if initial x-rays are inconclusive.

OSTEOARTHRITIS

See pp. 514–515.

MALIGNANCY

When assessing back pain, it is important to consider that the complaints and findings may suggest a malignancy. Back pain in a patient with cancer is an indication of metastasis. The most common primary sources of metastatic cancer affecting the spine include lung, breast, and prostate cancer.

Signs and Symptoms

The patient is often older than 50 years and presents with dull pain that has gradually increased in intensity. Patients may have symptoms such as an unexplained weight loss, pain that wakes the patient up from sleep, pain at rest, or more severe neurological symptoms including bowel and bladder dysfunction, extremity pain, weakness, or numbness of the extremities. Tumors of the vertebral bodies may lead to collapse and fracture of the vertebral body. Neurological findings vary by the level of involvement. The potential increases with a history of another malignancy.

Diagnostic Studies

When malignancy is suspected, plain films should be ordered, followed by CT, MRI, and/or bone scan.

SPINAL INFECTION

Vertebral osteomyelitis is rare, but it should be considered, particularly with at-risk patients. These include persons with advancing age, history of intravenous drug use, and compromised immune systems. Most vertebral infections will occur in the thoracic or lumbar vertebrae with only 10% occurring in the cervical spine.

Signs and Symptoms

The history includes fever and chills with possible weight loss. There may be a recent history of an infection such as pneumonia, urinary tract infection, or dermatological infection. The pain can be severe and insidious in onset and is often worse at night or with activities. There is point tenderness with percussion over the infected vertebrae along with elevated skin temperature. There are usually no neurological complaints; however, this depends on the degree and level of involvement and can present with radiculopathy or myelopathy.

Diagnostic Studies

In advanced infections, plain films reveal vertebral and intervertebral disk destruction. An MRI with contrast is highly useful in making this diagnosis. While bone scans could be used for patients who cannot tolerate MRI, they are not specific. Blood cultures should be obtained. The sedimentation rate and C-reactive protein are elevated.

COMPRESSION FRACTURE

Compression fractures are most commonly associated with osteoporosis and have a higher incidence with age. Nearly half of adults older than 80 will be affected by a compression fracture.

Signs and Symptoms

The patient complains of back pain that may range from mild to severe. Palpation on the spinous process of the affected vertebrae can cause pain. Onset can be gradual or acute. With acute onset, the patient can often describe a precipitating injury. There is a loss of height. Kyphosis results from thoracic fracture and lordosis from lumbar fracture. Depending on the degree of deformity associated with the fracture(s), pulmonary symptoms may be present. A patient may exhibit symptoms of spinal nerve compression, while spinal cord compression is rare.

Diagnostic Studies

Plain films reveal compression deformity with loss of vertebral height and/or wedge deformity.

ANKYLOSING SPONDYLITIS

Ankylosing spondylitis is one of the chronic autoimmune spondyloarthropathies, which have genetic predispositions and are inflammatory disorders. The incidence is higher in men than in women, and onset is generally in young adulthood. Patients will experience inflammation of the tendon and ligament attachments to bone. Inflammation will lead to erosion of the bone and ossification of the adjacent soft tissue, which will lead to ankylosis, or fusion, of affected joints. The axial skeleton (spine and pelvis) is primarily affected.

Signs and Symptoms

Early symptoms include LBP and stiffness, which gradually become persistent and increase in severity. Later, the pain may again become intermittent. Neck pain is a late symptom and often occurs some time after the development of LBP. Other symptoms can include bony tenderness, malaise, loss of appetite, fever, and fatigue. There is loss of spine mobility, and posture gradually changes, with fixed flexion of the neck, increased kyphosis of the thoracic region, and loss of the lumbar curve. Although chest expansion is affected, respiratory function usually remains intact.

Diagnostic Studies

The *HLA-B27* gene is present in most patients. Most have elevations of erythrocyte sedimentation rate and C-reactive protein as well as some degree of anemia. Radiographs show abnormality of the sacroiliac joint with progressive erosion. Spinal x-rays will show bone bridging between vertebrae due to ligament ossification. A CT scan is useful to identify sacroiliitis.

■ Shoulder Pain

Shoulder pain arises both from disorders affecting the shoulder structures and conditions involving other structures, such as the neck. The shoulder includes complex structures, and many of the conditions have very similar symptoms and physical findings. Shoulder pain in patients younger than 45 years is often related to trauma. Shoulder pain in patients older than 45 years is more often related to degenerative disease. Biomechanical trauma to the shoulder accentuates degenerative changes and symptoms. Shoulder syndromes frequently arise from inflammation. Most frequently, the capsule of the glenohumeral joint, the supraspinatus tendon, and the subacromial bursa are involved. When patients present with shoulder pain, always consider the possibility of a cardiac, cervical spine, or gastrointestinal cause.

The history should be directed to identify any potential injuries from trauma or overuse as well as any previous experience of shoulder pain. Determine whether the onset was acute or gradual. Ask about any activities or positions that are associated with diminished or increased pain. Details of self-treatment and response are important to elicit. Personal and family history of autoimmune and inflammatory disorders should be investigated.

The physical examination for shoulder pain starts with observations of the patient's posture and how the arm is "carried." General ROM, palpation, and testing of strength and sensation are important. A number of maneuvers are helpful in differentiating the source of shoulder pain; they are depicted in Figures 15.2 through 15.6, which appear in the following sections. In general, if images are considered, the best choice for initial study for shoulder pain is plain radiographic images. If the x-ray does not aid in making a diagnosis and there is persistent or significant pain, the ACR (2017) recommends an MRI without contrast as the next step.

TRAUMA

Trauma to the shoulder can result in a range of injuries, including brachial plexus injury, acute rotator cuff tear, acromioclavicular injury, and fractured humerus or clavicle.

Signs and Symptoms

The history includes the description of the traumatic event, such as direct blow, fall on the shoulder, or twisting injury. Physical findings are typically consistent

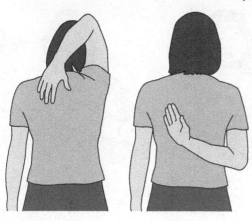

Figure 15.2 Apley's test involves range of motion as the patient reaches overhead and behind the lower back to touch the scapula.

with the degree of trauma and involvement of the shoulder and other surrounding structures. Rotator cuff injuries (see next subsection) can result from acute trauma as well as chronic impingement and degeneration. A fall or blow to the shoulder area may result in a fractured clavicle, which is often associated with an obvious deformity at the site of the fracture and significant pain when pressure is applied over the fracture site. Acromioclavicular separation or strain typically results in an obvious deformity as well as pain that increases as the arm is elevated. The presence of deformity after a shoulder injury depends on the severity of fracture, edema, separation, or displacement. A brachial plexus injury with trauma and stretch to C5–T1 nerves is indicated by paresthesia and/or sharp pain that radiates to the arm, paired with significant weakness and decreased sensation.

Diagnostic Studies

An x-ray should be ordered for any complaint of shoulder pain following an acute trauma. If the patient is younger than 35 years, a magnetic resonance angiogram should be considered. Patients with a brachial plexus injury may require chest and neck x-rays to rule out a fracture. EMG/NCS can assess injury and location of the cervical nerves with a brachial plexus injury.

ROTATOR CUFF SYNDROME AND IMPINGEMENT SYNDROME

The rotator cuff consists of the supraspinatus, infraspinatus, subscapularis, and teres minor. Injury to the rotator cuff is frequently due to chronic impingement with degenerative changes over time. It is most common in persons older than 40 years. Impingement results in rotator cuff tendinitis or bursitis of the subacromial bursa. As the structures thicken, increased mechanical injury occurs, which can eventually lead to partial- or full-thickness rotator cuff tears.

Signs and Symptoms

The patient typically complains of anterior and lateral shoulder pain that increases with arm elevation and reaching overhead. The pain is usually progressive and may be associated with repetitive activities. Pain at night or with side lying may

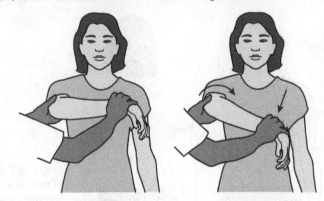

Figure 15.3 Hawkins' test involves internally rotating the patient's arm as it is elevated to 90 degrees.

cause sleep disturbance. ROM is typically preserved. Apley's (see Fig. 15.2) and Hawkins' (Fig. 15.3) impingement tests may reproduce the pain, depending on the component of the rotator cuff involved. There may be point of diffuse tenderness to the shoulder area. Crepitus or arm weakness can accompany significant weakness of the rotator cuff muscles or a possible acute tear.

Diagnostic Studies

Plain films are often normal but may show subacromial spurs. MRI will show soft tissue inflammation and injury; however, it is typically not indicated unless suspicious for a tear or if the patient is failing to improve with usual management.

ROTATOR CUFF TEAR

Tear to the rotator cuff usually follows chronic impingement and degenerative changes over time. A tear to the structures may also result from acute trauma. Degenerative cuff tears occur more frequently in older patients, while acute tears occur more frequently in younger patients. Tears range in size and severity. They may be complete full-thickness tears to the tendon or minor partial tears.

Signs and Symptoms

Pain associated with an acute tear of the rotator cuff is sudden in onset and may be worse at night and with movement. Atrophy of surrounding structures can be due to long-standing tears with disuse. Associated weakness and limited ROM may be present. The limitation is sometimes connected with the pain, as it is painful for the patient to lift the arm; however, injury of the periarticular structures also contributes to weakness. With a large full-thickness tear, the patient may only be able to shrug the shoulder but not lift the arm. Tenderness is frequently greatest at the supraspinatus insertion, since this is the most common site for injury, and pain may radiate to the deltoid region. Crepitus is often noted between 60 to 120 degrees of abduction, as this maneuver compresses the injured tissue. Additionally, an injured rotator cuff allows the head of the humerus to migrate upward and rub against the acromion during motion, leading to a

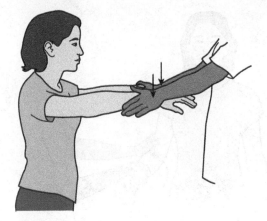

Figure 15.4 The empty can test involves the patient's arms held anteriorly with thumbs down (as if emptying a can) while resisting downward pressure applied by the examiner.

sound of crepitus. To compensate, the patient may rotate the palm up (supination) during abduction, which rotates the shoulder, widens the rotator cuff, and changes the muscles engaged in shoulder movement, decreasing the pain on movement. Apley's (see Fig. 15.2), Hawkins' (see Fig. 15.3), and the empty can (Fig. 15.4) tests may be positive, depending on the location of the tear. A drop arm test will be positive for patients with a full-thickness tear of the supraspinatus.

Diagnostic Studies

Shoulder x-rays may demonstrate underlying degenerative joint disease and arthritic spurring, which may correlate with long-standing degenerative cuff disease. With an acute injury, x-rays may be beneficial to screen for an associated fracture. Full rotator cuff tears may allow the head of the humerus to migrate up toward the acromion, decreasing the space between the two on x-ray. MRI should be considered if shoulder pain persists, the onset of pain was preceded by trauma, or the patient has an acute loss of shoulder motion with a suspected full tear.

BICEPS TENOSYNOVITIS

Inflammation of the biceps tendon is another common cause of anterior shoulder pain. The patient is usually middle-aged or is an athlete with repeated injuries related to the throwing motion. This can also be associated with rotator cuff

Decision Rule

The sensitivity and specificity of the empty can test for full rotator cuff tears are 75% to 98% and 58% to 88%, respectively. The full can test is 71% to 89% sensitive and 68% to 81% specific for full tears. These findings can be used to guide further diagnostic workup (Dinnes et al., 2003).

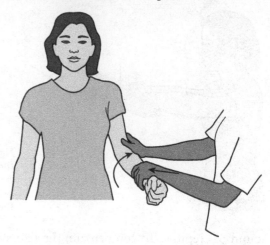

Figure 15.5 Yergason's test involves the patient holding the arm with elbow flexed 90 degrees, in thumb-up position, and then attempting to further flex and supinate the arm as the examiner offers resistance.

injury or impingement syndrome. In cases of constant wear and tear with heavy lifting, the biceps tendon can fray and eventually tear. Biceps tendon rupture, while uncommon, can occur typically when an unexpected force is applied to a flexed arm (e.g., catching a heavy falling object). It can rupture proximally or distally.

Signs and Symptoms

Anterior shoulder tenderness is noted with active and passive motion and with palpation of the tendon sheath. The tendon becomes inflamed in the bicipital groove, which can be felt on palpation. Discomfort can radiate down the biceps. A positive Yergason's test (Fig. 15.5) suggests biceps tendon instability or tendonitis. The test is positive if pain is produced at the bicipital groove. A Speed's test may also indicate biceps tendonitis if pain is reproduced during the examination. In a tendon rupture, a pop may be felt initially, followed by the appearance of a "Popeye arm."

Diagnostic Studies

No radiological testing is indicated for tenosynovitis. For suspected rupture, radiographs may be done to rule out an associated avulsion fracture. An MRI can be performed to assess the amount of damage. Surgical repair is necessary.

ADHESIVE CAPSULITIS ("FROZEN SHOULDER")

Frozen shoulder, or adhesive capsulitis, is a condition that, as the name implies, results in loss of shoulder motion. Adhesive capsulitis is more common among women and adults between ages 40 and 60 years. It is typically a self-limited disorder that has a greater incidence among patients with thyroid disease or diabetes. The disorder may be idiopathic or can develop following a trauma or surgery of the shoulder.

Signs and Symptoms

A period of pain without limited motion often precedes the loss of motion. Then, progressive stiffness (freezing) associated with the pain may occur until the patient recognizes inability to perform certain tasks requiring elevation of the arm or reaching behind the head/back. At the point that passive and active ROM are affected, there is generally diffuse pain and tenderness. The patient is unable to abduct the affected arm beyond 90 degrees with the scapula on that side stabilized/immobilized.

Diagnostic Studies

Plain films may be helpful in identifying other disorders that cause secondary adhesive capsulitis, such as OA, fracture, avascular necrosis, and calcific tendinitis. Laboratory studies may be useful to evaluate for or control diabetes or thyroid disease.

GLENOHUMERAL INSTABILITY

Unlike the other conditions affecting the shoulder, glenohumeral instability is most common in young patients who are physically active. A patient may have had a previous injury leading to shoulder instability, or the patient may have inherently lax joints. The instability can result in displacement of the humeral head in various directions.

Signs and Symptoms

The patient will experience sudden onset of pain and be unwilling to move the arm. The displacement may follow an acute injury/trauma or may be associated with specific movements or overuse. A positive apprehension test, in which the patient feels as if the shoulder will dislocate, suggests anterior glenohumeral instability (Fig. 15.6). This can be somewhat validated by performing the relocation test, in which the movement of the apprehension test is reversed, and the sense of impending dislocation is eliminated. Inferior instability can be assessed

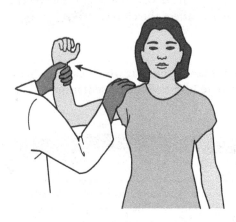

Figure 15.6 The apprehension test involves the patient holding the arm in a neutral position, elevated to 90 degrees. Then the examiner places mild pressure on the anterior aspect of the arm while externally rotating it.

with a sulcus sign examination of the shoulder, while a posterior jerk test can assess for posterior instability.

Diagnostic Studies

Plain x-ray image may help to identify the direction of instability and may show a defect of the humeral head that is associated with the instability. If the humerus is dislocated due to instability, this will clearly be noted on x-ray. An MRI may provide clear imaging of joint capsule and ligamentous laxity and possible tears or other pathology.

CARDIAC PAIN

When patients present with complaints of exertional pain in the left shoulder region, it is important to maintain a level of suspicion for referred cardiac pain. The presentation would likely include pain relieved with rest, and the patient would likely have a history of cardiac risk factors. See Chapter 8.

PULMONARY PAIN

Pulmonary disorders can be associated with pain that is referred to the shoulder region. See Chapter 9.

REFERRED ABDOMINAL PAIN

Certain abdominal conditions, such as gallbladder disease, may result in pain that refers to the right shoulder. See Chapter 11.

■ Elbow Pain

Pain related to the elbow is commonly mechanical in origin. The elbow is a very complex joint, with articulations between the humerus and radius, the humerus and ulna, and the ulna and radius. The innervation is also complex, with risk for entrapment between the various soft tissues and bony structures. Overuse and repetitive movement are responsible for many causes of elbow pain. However, rheumatoid, gouty, and septic arthritis can also affect the elbow.

TRAUMA

As with other joints, the elbow is at risk for acute trauma, which can result in fracture or dislocation or can trigger reactive tendinitis. The presentation will be specific to the trauma experienced.

Decision Rule

For adult patients, the extension test has been demonstrated to be 98% sensitive and 48% specific to elbow fracture following a trauma. This point can be used to guide the decision on obtaining images (Appelboam et al., 2008).

EPICONDYLITIS

Epicondylitis involves inflammation of the tendon/tendon insertion of the forearm. This tendinitis results in either lateral or medial elbow pain associated with overuse of the wrist extensors (tennis elbow) or wrist flexors and rotation (golfer's elbow) respectively. It is common for the overuse to be associated with microtears of the affected tendons.

Signs and Symptoms

Point tenderness is noted at the medial or lateral epicondyle. The onset and severity of pain is usually gradual and progressive but may have relatively acute onset following an activity involving significant repetitive use. The pain may be referred to the forearm and is increased by the offending motion (e.g., wrist flexion, extension, or rotation). Pain is usually greater when the motion is made against resistance or with stretching the affected muscle and tendon groups. There may be a locking sensation with motion, and the area of point tenderness may be swollen. Patients may have pain and weakness with gripping activities.

Diagnostic Studies

Plain films are often normal but may reveal spurs, loose bodies, or loss of joint space. Imaging is typically not necessary; however, it may be indicated, particularly if there is a history of trauma.

OLECRANON BURSITIS

The olecranon bursa is superficial and at risk for repeated trauma. Olecranon bursitis can result from repetitive overuse, trauma, and infection.

Signs and Symptoms

The patient will complain of swelling and tenderness at the "tip" of the elbow over the olecranon. Point tenderness is common, although it is found most frequently in patients with septic bursitis. Typically, there is no loss of elbow motion. Septic bursitis is also often associated with a skin lesion either over the bursa or distal to the elbow. There may be an elevated body temperature as well as redness and warmth over the infected bursa.

Diagnostic Studies

Plain x-rays of the elbow will typically be negative. An aspiration of the bursa should be performed for culture (septic bursitis) as well as determination of whether there is a collection of crystals (gouty bursitis) or elevated white cell count (greatest in septic bursitis). Following a direct trauma, there may be blood present in the aspirated fluid.

NURSEMAID'S ELBOW

Also known as *pulled elbow* or *toddler's elbow*, nursemaid's elbow involves the head of the radius slipping under the annular ligament in children, usually between 1 and 4 years of age. The condition occurs when traction is applied to the young child's hand or wrist.

Signs and Symptoms

There is a history of sudden onset of pain associated with sudden immobility of the affected arm as the child protects the elbow. The parent may be able to identify a situation in which the child's hand was held and traction applied. The child may have moved in an opposite direction, or injury could have occurred while pulling the arm through clothing. There is no associated swelling or inflammation. Examination is otherwise normal with the exception of resistance to attempts to move the arm, elbow, and possibly the wrist. There may be tenderness along the upper margin of the radius.

Diagnostic Studies

None are usually indicated unless history suggests the need to rule out fracture. Some clinicians perform x-rays to confirm a dislocation and then follow-up x-rays after a reduction of the dislocation to confirm.

GOUT

Although gout typically involves a lower extremity joint, it is a frequent cause of elbow inflammation.

RHEUMATOID ARTHRITIS

RA is a systemic condition but may affect individual joints. See pp. 513–514.

OSTEOARTHRITIS

See pp. 514–515.

■ Wrist and Hand Pain

Pain and numbness of the hand and wrist may be unilateral or bilateral, and they are usually associated with injuries or overuse. The hands are common sites of both OA and RA.

The history should include a thorough description of the pain and its impact on activities, as well as personal and family history of inflammatory or autoimmune conditions. Ask about occupational and recreational routines to identify potential overuse or ergonomic and traumatic etiologies. The potential impacts of trauma to the fingers, hands, and wrists are numerous and not specifically addressed. However, the nature and mechanisms of any trauma or injury should be specifically evaluated.

The examination includes careful inspection and palpation of the structures of the wrists, hands, and fingers with side-to-side comparisons. ROM and strength are tested. For trauma, plain x-ray images should be ordered. If these are inconclusive or there are persistent findings or pain, repeat radiographs, CT, or MRI should be obtained.

CARPAL TUNNEL SYNDROME

The carpal tunnel is a space located at the wrist formed by the carpal bones and the transverse carpal ligamentous forming the roof of the tunnel. The median nerve and several flexor tendons traverse through the carpal tunnel. With overuse and repetitive movements, the tissues of the carpal tunnel may undergo hypertrophy, causing a loss of space and impingement on the median nerve. The types of activities associated with carpal tunnel syndrome include computer use and painting. Space-occupying lesions (e.g., cysts) located within the carpal tunnel can lead to compression of the medial nerve as well.

Signs and Symptoms

Carpal tunnel syndrome causes a range of neurological symptoms, including pain, paresthesia, clumsiness of the hands, and weakness. Frequently, nighttime pain that wakes a person from sleep is an early symptom. There may be a swelling at the wrist related to inactivity or flexion at night. The pain and paresthesias typically involve the anterior aspects of wrist, radial side of the palm, and first three digits on the affected hand. However, pain may radiate up the forearm to the shoulder with numbness and tingling along the median nerve. Over time, hand weakness with atrophy of the thenal eminence often develops with untreated carpal tunnel syndrome. Pain and paresthesia are often relieved by the patient "shaking" the affected hand in a downward fashion; this is called the flicking sign. A positive Tinel's sign is elicited by tapping on the median nerve at the carpal tunnel, causing pain and tingling along the median nerve distribution. Phalen's maneuver reproduces the pain after 1 minute of wrist flexion against resistance. A Durkan's test, which involves compressing the carpal tunnel with the examiner's thumbs for 30 seconds, will also reproduce the symptoms if positive for carpal tunnel.

Diagnostic Studies

This is typically a clinical diagnosis with no diagnostic studies. Nerve testing, including EMG/NCS, may be indicated to determine the location and extent of the compression, if the patient is not improving with conservative management or if the clinician is unsure of the diagnosis. An ultrasound may depict synovitis. Imaging with x-ray or MRI may provide evidence for secondary causes for carpal tunnel such as wrist arthritis or a cyst.

DE QUERVAIN'S TENDONITIS/TENOSYNOVITIS

De Quervain's tenosynovitis involves irritation of two tendons (extensor pollicis brevis and abductor pollicis longus) located within the first dorsal compartment on the radial side of the wrist, near the thumb. With overuse, the tissues surrounding the tendon sheath hypertrophy, causing pressure on the tendon, and making it difficult to move. This condition occurs more frequently in women than in men, most typically between ages 30 and 50 years.

Signs and Symptoms

The pain is usually limited to the radial aspect of the wrist and the area immediately around the base of the thumb. Pain increases with use of the hand, such as with gripping maneuvers. Other symptoms include swelling, decreased sensation, and limited ROM with a locking sensation with thumb motion. The Finkelstein's maneuver (Fig. 15.7) is used to diagnose De Quervain's disease. A positive test results in pain, which is often severe. Patients who can repeatedly

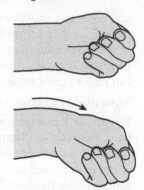

Figure 15.7 Finkelstein's maneuver involves the patient making a fist with the fingers flexed over the thumb, which is flexed against the palm of the hand, and then holding the fist closed while deviating the wrist toward the ulnar surface.

open and close the fist with smooth thumb motion are unlikely to have De Quervain's disease.

Diagnostic Studies

Plain x-rays of the wrist are normal.

GANGLION CYSTS

Ganglion cysts are common soft tissue abnormalities involving the wrist and/or hand. The fluid-filled synovial cysts typically develop adjacent to a tendon sheath. The etiology is not clear, but ganglia are believed to be associated with some degenerative or traumatic damage to tendon sheaths or joints.

Signs and Symptoms

Ganglion cysts are frequently asymptomatic and typically pose only cosmetic concern due to a bump that may be present. There may be an obvious swollen defect over the fluid-filled ganglion cyst, and the area can become inflamed and painful if the cyst is distended. The presence and severity of discomfort is variable and may be mild and/or limiting to hand motion. The size of the ganglion cyst may vary over time. The cyst should transilluminate. Ganglion cysts at the wrist have the potential to compress on the medial nerve or the radial/ulnar artery, leading to associated symptoms.

Diagnostic Studies

Plain films will be negative and are typically not necessary. Ultrasound will reveal the cystic structure and can be useful at times in differentiating a cystic mass from a vascular aneurysm.

OSTEOARTHRITIS

See pp. 514–515.

RHEUMATOID ARTHRITIS

See pp. 513–514.

■ Hip Pain

There are many potential causes of hip pain. Among adults, the most common cause is OA with degenerative changes. In younger patients, the cause is often strain of the muscles or tendons. In comparison to other joints, the hip can be difficult to assess, in part because much of the joint and its periarticular structures lie deeper than those of other joints.

As with other joint-specific pain, it is critical to obtain a history of the pain's onset, progression, and nature, starting with the questions in Box 15.1. Previous history of hip pain as well as inflammatory or degenerative conditions must be explored. A history of recent activities (overuse) and trauma is important.

The examination begins by noting the patient's posture and apparent limitations or discomfort with walking, sitting, rising, and so forth. The ROM should be thoroughly tested, actively, passively, and against resistance. Note pain, crepitus, clicking, and limitations. When images are indicated, plain films of the pelvis and/or hip should be done initially. Strength, sensation, and reflexes should be noted.

OSTEOARTHRITIS

OA causes degenerative hip changes and is a frequent cause of hip pain in adults, becoming more prevalent after age 50. In younger patients, it may be secondary to trauma or congenital problems, such as a congenital hip dislocation or slipped capital femoral epiphysis. See pp. 514–515.

TROCHANTERIC BURSITIS

Trochanteric bursitis involves a presumed inflammation or irritation of the trochanteric bursa, which lies laterally over greater trochanter. Overuse is a common cause and may be seen in runners and other contact sport athletes. A tight iliotibial band repetitively sliding back and forth over the trochanteric bursa at the lateral hip with activities such as running can cause irritation and inflammation. Lateral hip surgery may also be associated with trochanteric bursitis. Other problems that result in changes in the patient's gait tend to increase the stress on the joint.

Signs and Symptoms
The patient presents with pain at the lateral hip and thigh to the knee or numbness. Pain is precipitated by walking, climbing, or prolonged standing. There is point tenderness at the greater trochanter, with increased pain on resisted abduction and external rotation.

Diagnostic Studies
X-rays are usually not helpful and may show no abnormalities.

OSTEONECROSIS/AVASCULAR NECROSIS OF THE FEMORAL HEAD

This condition involves bone deterioration associated with diminished circulation stemming from trauma or other disorders such as malignancy, sickle cell disease, lupus, infections, or Legg-Calvé-Perthes disease. It is also associated with the use of corticosteroids or protease inhibitors, alcoholism, and radiation treatment. Avascular necrosis can also affect other structures, such as the humeral head and knee. This occurs more frequently in males. The diminished blood flow of avascular necrosis will eventually lead to fracture and collapse of the affected bone.

Signs and Symptoms

The patient presents with complaints of hip pain and difficulty bearing weight. There is a history of an offending medication, trauma, or condition. The actual onset of pain can be very sudden or gradually recognized. In addition to weight-bearing activities, other actions such as coughing and other non-weight-bearing movements often increase pain, and the pain often persists at rest and occurs at night. ROM is significantly limited. Pain is often located anteriorly at the hip and radiates down the anterior thigh.

Diagnostic Studies

Early in the progression, plain x-rays may be normal or reveal increased bone density (sclerosis). As collapse of the affected bone occurs, the density increases. However, these changes may not be evident until the disorder is very advanced. For this reason, definitive diagnosis is made with MRI, which is more sensitive than plain x-rays. A bone scan will show increased uptake in the region surrounding the necrotic bone.

TENDONITIS

This inflammation in a hip tendon typically follows overuse activities, with strain and/or inflammatory changes. Injury and inflammation of the iliopsoas tendon, a hip flexor, is common and can result in anterior hip and groin discomfort. The condition can be acute or chronic.

Signs and Symptoms

The patient usually can identify recent activities that included repetitive motions and/or risk for straining tendon structures related to the hip. The onset of pain is delayed until some time following the repetitive activity. The pain is localized and increases with further activity. There is often a snapping or catching sensation. Point tenderness and swelling may be present.

Diagnostic Studies

The diagnosis is typically made on physical findings and history alone. X-rays will be normal. Although an MRI or ultrasound may reveal the injury to the tendon, these studies are not usually indicated or ordered.

INFLAMMATORY ARTHRITIS

RA and other forms of inflammatory arthritis, such as gout and Reiter's syndrome, should be considered in assessment of hip pain. See section under Polyarthralgias in this chapter.

Slipped Capital Femoral Epiphysis

This condition involving growth plate disruption causes hip pain in adolescents. Slipped capital femoral epiphysis involves slippage of the femoral epiphysis in relation to the metaphysis at the growth plate of the femoral neck. It is more common in overweight male adolescents during a time of rapid growth. Because the patient often presents with referred pain to the groin, thigh, or knee, diagnosis and treatment are frequently delayed.

Signs and Symptoms

The progression of symptoms is usually gradual, with stiffness and decreasing ROM progressing to pain and subsequent development of a limp. There is usually no history of preceding activity or trauma. Pain often involves the buttocks and/or groin and can radiate to the medial knee. The presentation may be knee pain, with normal knee examination. Comfort is increased with external rotation of the hip; passive internal rotation of the flexed hip increases pain. If advanced, avascular necrosis may occur, resulting in collapse of the femoral head. The condition is bilateral in approximately 25% of cases, although the complaint may be limited to one hip.

Diagnostic Studies

X-rays with AP and lateral frog leg views reveal widening of the epiphyseal line and/or femoral displacement.

▪ Knee Pain

The knee is vulnerable to injury from recreational or occupational activities and a variety of pathologic conditions. Assessment of the knee requires skill and practice in performing special maneuvers such as McMurray's test and tests of ligament integrity, including the drawer test and Lachman's test.

This section does not address knee fractures. However, the Ottawa knee rules provide a set of evidence-based criteria by which to determine when radiographs of the knee are warranted following trauma.

Decision Rule

The Ottawa knee criteria have been shown to have 100% sensitivity and 49% specificity for fracture of the knee. According to the findings, x-rays should be ordered following a traumatic injury to the knee only if at least one of the following criteria are met: The patient is at least 55 years of age, tenderness is present at the tibial head, isolated tenderness is present at the patella (i.e., no other knee tenderness), the patient cannot flex the knee to 90 degrees, or the patient cannot bear weight for four steps (i.e., two steps on each foot) even with limping (ACR, 2021).

A number of special maneuvers are useful in differentiating the cause of knee pain. These are shown in Figures 15.8, 15.9, and 15.10, which appear in subsequent sections.

MENISCUS (LATERAL, MEDIAL) TEAR

The medial and lateral menisci are C-shaped fibrocartilage that sit on the proximal articular surface of the tibia. The meniscus provides for some stability and shock absorption at the knee. Tears or disruptions of the meniscus are associated with OA in older persons and with athletic activities in younger persons. Injury to the medial meniscus is more common than injury to the lateral. Patients who have anterior cruciate ligament (ACL) laxity or tears are at greater risk for meniscus injury.

Signs and Symptoms

There is typically a sudden onset of pain and swelling over the lateral or medial joint line as well as locking or clicking and painful popping. Onset often follows a twisting injury. Point tenderness is present over the joint line, with mild effusion. A positive McMurray's test is often present (Fig. 15.8).

Diagnostic Studies

If meniscal tear is suspected, radiographs are usually of little use to visualize this soft tissue condition, and they are usually negative. An MRI will reveal the defect in most cases. Arthroscopy can be performed alternatively or as a follow-up to the MRI.

LIGAMENTOUS INJURIES

The cruciate and collateral knee ligaments are vulnerable to injury in athletic activities. The mechanism through which the ACL is typically injured involves deceleration combined with sudden turning or pivoting. The posterior cruciate ligament (PCL) can be torn due to a hyperextension injury or in a motor vehicle crash if the flexed knee impacts the dashboard. The medial collateral ligament (MCL) is most prone to injury through motions that place valgus stress on the knee. Compared with ACL and MCL injury, damage to the lateral collateral

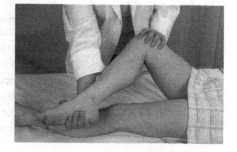

Figure 15.8 McMurray's test assesses the menisci. The medial meniscus is tested with the hip flexed and externally rotated as the examiner moves the knee from full flexion to extension and applies gentle varus pressure to the knee. To test the lateral meniscus, the hip is flexed and internally rotated during the procedure with gentle valgus pressure applied to the knee while it is being extended. A snap heard or felt during this maneuver suggests a tear of the tested meniscus.

ligament (LCL) is much less frequent but typically occurs when sudden varus stress is placed on the knee.

Signs and Symptoms

The patient often relates a history of an acute trauma followed by onset of pain, swelling, and limited mobility. Often patients recall hearing or feeling a "pop" at the moment of injury and/or a "give-away" sense. ACL injury is identified through a positive anterior drawer (Fig. 15.9) or Lachman's test (Fig. 15.10). Conversely, the PCL will be assessed using the posterior drawer test or sag sign. Laxity of the MCL and LCL is assessed by placing valgus and varus stress on the knee with the leg both extended and flexed.

Diagnostic Studies

Radiographs may be indicated, and clinicians are encouraged to use imaging decision tools such as the Ottawa rules. If a fracture is suspected, an x-ray will be useful to visualize it. If there is an ACL injury, plain film may reveal the presence of a tibial avulsion fracture. Ligament tears will best be visualized with MRI.

Decision Rule

Among patients with ACL tears, the combination of effusion, popping sensation, and giving-away is associated with 71% sensitivity and 71% specificity. When the anterior drawer test was added, sensitivity was 63% and specificity increased to 85% (Wagemakers et al., 2010).

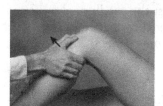

Figure 15.9 The drawer sign is elicited by the examiner holding the patient's leg at the level of the tibial tubercle and firmly pulling anteriorly on the lower leg as the patient's knee is flexed at 90 degrees. The test is positive for anterior cruciate ligament injury when there is laxity and forward motion and positive for posterior cruciate ligament injury when there is laxity in posterior movement.

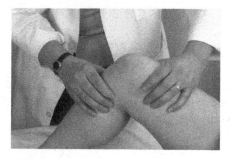

Figure 15.10 Lachman's test is performed with the patient's knee flexed to 30 degrees, noting laxity in anterior and posterior movement of the lower leg with the maneuver. Laxity of the medial collateral ligament is assessed by placing valgus stress on the knee first with the leg extended and next with it flexed at 30 degrees.

Decision Rule

Among patients with MCL, history of pain, trauma, and laxity (with valgus stress at 30 degrees flexion) were associated with 56% sensitivity and 91% specificity (Kastelein et al., 2008).

CHONDROMALACIA PATELLA

Chondromalacia patella is seen in young active persons, with women having a greater incidence than men. The condition is also commonly called *patella-femoral syndrome* or *runner's knee and leads to anterior knee pain with pathologic changes and damage to the articular undersurface of the patella*. This is often idiopathic; however, in some cases it is associated with other conditions, such as poor tracking of the patella in the trochlear groove, muscle weakness, and limb malalignment.

Signs and Symptoms

The pain involves the anterior knee, often develops gradually, and is moderate in intensity. For some, there is a sudden onset of patellar pain. The pain is often noticed when rising to stand after sitting for a prolonged time, when walking up and down stairs, or with squatting. Runners sometimes indicate that their discomfort was first noticed when running downhill. The pain is relieved during rest. Pain can be reproduced by pressing the patella against the femoral condyles, and there is tenderness on palpation around the patella. Other maneuvers that reproduce the pain include applying pressure against the patella as the patient extends the lower leg, flexing the quadriceps, and moving the patella from side to side. Crepitus and effusion are often present. In some patients, there may be weakness or atrophy of the quadriceps.

Diagnostic Studies

Diagnostic studies are not necessarily warranted. However, sunrise view x-rays may reveal an irregular undersurface of the patella.

Decision Rule

Two or more of the following symptoms are associated with 60% sensitivity and 85% specificity for patellofemoral pain syndrome: pain reported on muscle contraction, squatting, or kneeling. The one maneuver with the greatest diagnostic strength is pain on resisted contraction (Cook et al., 2010).

PATELLAR TENDONITIS

Tendonitis can develop in any of the knee tendons but is common with the patellar tendon. It most commonly affects boys during their teens and those engaged in jumping athletic activities. This is also referred to as *jumper's knee*. Diminished flexibility of the hamstrings and/or quadriceps is a risk factor in developing patella tendonitis. Initially, patients will have pain only after activities, but tendonitis can progress to pain during and after activities or even be continuous with persistent pain.

Signs and Symptoms

The patient complains of pain inferior to the patella at the site of the patellar tendon. The pain is often vague and increases with walking, climbing stairs, or jumping. There is point tenderness over the tendon, and pain can be reproduced by having the patient extend the knee against resistance. There is usually no effusion or crepitus; however, edema may be present.

Diagnostic Studies

No studies are indicated unless the patient fails to improve with several weeks of conservative management.

PREPATELLAR BURSITIS

Bursitis often accompanies tendinitis and can be associated with mild trauma. Prepatellar bursitis is also called *housemaid's knee*, which is common to persons whose occupation requires extended periods of kneeling, such as plumbers and carpet layers. This is the most common type of bursitis affecting the knee, but bursitis can also be caused by an infection.

Signs and Symptoms

There is often a history of prolonged kneeling prior to the onset of pain and inflammation. The patient complains of pain in the area inferior to and over the patella, and there is swelling and inflammation of the bursa. The swelling and pain can occur suddenly, and there is point tenderness over the affected area. The pain is worse with activity and does not bother the patient at night. The problem can become chronic. The clinician should assess for warmth and erythema of the skin over the bursitis, which may be associated with septic bursitis.

Diagnostic Studies

No diagnostic imaging studies are generally performed. However, aspiration of the bursa can be performed to assess for crystalline deposits (gout) or evidence of infection with Gram stain and culture of the fluid.

OSGOOD-SCHLATTER DISEASE

This self-limited condition is a cause for anterior knee pain, which occurs in adolescents. Inflammation and pain occur at the site where the patellar tendon inserts on the tibial tubercle. Traction and stress from the patella tendon cause enlargement, irregularity, and fragmentation of the tibial tubercle. This can occur bilaterally in 20% to 30% of adolescents. While this condition occurs more frequently in boys, if a girl has this condition, it typically occurs earlier in adolescence than in boys.

Signs and Symptoms

The patient complains of pain centered 2 to 3 inches inferior to the patella at the tibial tubercle that usually corresponds with an enlarged raised area of the anterior tibia. The pain ranges from mild to severe. Pain may occur only with extensive activity or persist regardless of activity level. Point tenderness and swelling are often present, with the pain worsened with kneeling. Resisted extension of the affected knee will also exacerbate the discomfort.

Diagnostic Studies

Images are typically not necessary, as the diagnosis can be made on history and physical findings. However, if plain x-rays are ordered, they often reveal an area of fragmentation and bony irregularity over the tibial tubercle.

BAKER'S CYST

This is a popliteal cyst that often arises secondary to some other knee condition (e.g., degenerative joint disease) or injury (e.g., meniscus tear). This synovial cyst develops from fluid of the gastrocnemius-semimembranosus bursa or a defect in the synovial lining of the knee joint.

Signs and Symptoms

Baker's cysts can cause mild to moderate discomfort in the posterior knee/popliteal fossa. The cyst is palpable as an area of fullness. Other physical findings depend on associated knee pathology or injury, such as meniscal tear. Cysts have the potential to enlarge significantly to inhibit venous blood flow or entrap/compress nerves. This can lead to physical examination findings of calf edema and numbness, tingling, or weakness of the lower leg.

Diagnostic Studies

Diagnosis is typically based on physical findings of the palpable cyst. However, an ultrasound of the popliteal space or MRI can provide definitive diagnosis.

OSTEOARTHRITIS

See pp. 514–515.

INFLAMMATORY ARTHRITIS

See pp. 513–518.

■ Ankle and Foot Pain

Although this section does not address fractures, the Ottawa ankle and Ottawa foot rules provide evidence-based criteria to determine when, following acute trauma/injury, radiographs are warranted. These are summarized in Table 15.3.

Table 15.3	
Ottawa Ankle and Foot Rules	
Ankle Rule: Order X-Ray if One of the Following Is Met	**Foot Rule: Order X-Ray if One of the Following Is Met**
Inability to bear weight for four steps (both immediately and in emergency department)	Inability to bear weight for four steps (both immediately and in emergency department)
Bone tenderness at posterior edge or tip of either malleolus	Bone tenderness at navicular or base of fifth metatarsal
Sensitivity = 100%	Sensitivity = 100%
Specificity = 79%	Specificity = 79%

(ACR, 2021)

The identified specificity and sensitivity are based on adequate training in application of the rules.

SPRAINS

Sprains are the most common of all ankle injuries and a leading cause for missing athletic participation. Most ankle sprains involve the lateral ligament complex and are caused by forceful inversion and plantar flexion.

Signs and Symptoms

The patient relates a history of an ankle injury followed by sudden onset of pain. Pain is noted in the region of the strained muscles/tendons or sprained ligaments with local tenderness on palpation. There can be a varying degree of edema and ecchymosis. The clinician should be deliberate when determining where the pain is located and attempt to differentiate pain from injured soft tissue from pain on palpation of injured bone. Ankle stability is assessed in a manner like that used to test the ligaments of the knee. By immobilizing the lower leg, grasping the foot while applying anterior and posterior stress, a drawer test is achieved. Valgus and varus pressure can also be applied, with inversion and eversion of the foot. Assess if the patient can bear weight. Sprains can be classified using the Ottawa guidelines to provide information concerning the degree of disability and requirements for treatment. Table 15.4 lists the classifications for strains.

Diagnostic Studies

The Ottawa foot and ankle rules can assist the clinician to determine if imaging is needed.

PLANTAR FASCIITIS

Plantar fasciitis is often incorrectly referred to as heel spur pain. In fact, this condition can occur in the absence of a calcaneal heel spur. It involves inflammation of the plantar fascia associated with biomechanical tension on the fascia and microtears of the tissue, most commonly involving the site of insertion at the

Table 15.4	

Classification of Strains

Grade	Degree of Injury
I	Partial tear but no instability or opening of the joint on stress maneuvers
II	Partial tear with some instability indicated by partial opening of joint on stress maneuvers
III	Complete tear with complete opening of joint on stress

calcaneal tubercle. It can be caused by prolonged standing, walking, or running in poorly designed shoes with no arch support. Obesity is a risk factor for development. This occurs in men and women with a similar frequency.

Signs and Symptoms

The history includes pain on the undersurface of the heel. This can be worse upon weight bearing after periods of rest, first step out of bed in the morning, or dorsiflexion of the toes. Walking generally helps to reduce the discomfort. It can be present in one or both feet, but bilateral problems may represent an early symptom of gout, RA, or ankylosing spondylitis. There is point tenderness at the fascia insertion site. Some patients may have an associated tight Achilles tendon and limited dorsiflexion.

Diagnostic Studies

Images are typically not warranted. The absence of a calcaneal spur does not rule out the condition. However, plain x-rays can rule out stress fracture. If further indicated by prolonged pain and/or disability, an MRI would be the next image to consider.

MORTON'S NEUROMA/INTERDIGITAL NEUROMA

Interdigital neuroma is not actually neuroma but rather a perineural fibrous tissue thickening and entrapment of the interdigital nerves, typically in the space between the second and third or third and fourth metatarsal heads. They occur most frequently in women and may be associated with footwear, such as high heels or shoes with a narrow toe box.

Signs and Symptoms

Most common is localized pain that is increased with walking and decreased with rest and/or removal of shoes. Paresthesia may be present on the plantar surface of the foot at the webspace between the affected toes. Palpation of the space between the affected metatarsals often reproduces the sharp pain. Pain can also be reproduced by squeezing the forefoot and compressing the metatarsal heads together.

Diagnostic Studies

No diagnostic studies are indicated. X-rays can be used to rule out other causes.

ACHILLES TENDINITIS

Chronic overuse of the muscles of the calf or extreme stress on the Achilles tendon from activities such as jumping can lead to inflammation. Tendon ruptures may occur with untreated or prolonged tendinitis.

Signs and Symptoms

Passive stretching of the tendon by dorsiflexion of the ankle reproduces this pain. The patient may not be able to stand on the ball of the foot due to tenderness. Edema may be present. The ankle ROM is usually diminished. Progressive enlargement of the Achilles insertion site at the calcaneus can occur with prolonged inflammation. Thompson's test is positive if a full thickness rupture of the tendon has occurred. Thompson's test involves squeezing the calf, a maneuver that causes plantar flexion of the foot with an intact Achilles tendon. With Achilles tendon rupture, there is a loss of movement in the foot when the calf is squeezed. There is often inability to bear weight, edema, ecchymosis, and significant pain. The patient will frequently report hearing an audible pop when the tendon ruptured.

Diagnostic Studies

X-ray can be helpful to rule out fracture. Ultrasound identifies the degree of tendon thickening. If an Achilles rupture is suspected, an MRI is indicated.

HALLUX VALGUS/BUNION

Hallux valgus deformity results from medial displacement of the first metatarsal head with a valgus deformity and angulation at the first metatarsal phalangeal (MTP) joint. This condition is more common in women. Some risk factors include flat feet, rheumatoid arthritis, family history, and wearing narrow-toed shoes.

Signs and Symptoms

Pain and valgus deformity are the initial complaints with tenderness and redness over the affected MTP joint. Shoe wear can be painful and difficult due to the deformity.

Diagnostic Studies

X-rays will help rule out degenerative changes and differentiate soft tissue injuries from valgus deformity of the MTP joint.

GOUT

The great toe is the most common site of gouty arthritis, which can also affect other areas of the foot or ankle. See p. 518.

OSTEOARTHRITIS

See pp. 514–515.

RHEUMATOID ARTHRITIS AND OTHER FORMS OF INFLAMMATORY ARTHRITIS

See pp. 513–518.

■ Myalgia

Myalgia, or muscle pain, is a nonspecific complaint accompanying many conditions. The history and physical examination are essential in arriving at a definitive diagnosis. Whereas myalgia is a finding in many conditions, it is the central complaint in others, which are described in the following sections.

FIBROMYALGIA

Myalgia is often the primary complaint in fibromyalgia. See pp. 515–516.

POLYMYALGIA RHEUMATICA

Polymyalgia rheumatica is usually identified in adults age 50 or older and is more common in women. While the actual etiology of this condition is unknown, it is generally believed to be an inflammatory condition. Giant cell arteritis occurs in about 15% of those with polymyalgia rheumatica, and the two conditions may be different expressions of the same etiology.

Signs and Symptoms

The patient typically complains of sudden onset of widespread pain. Commonly affected sites include the neck, shoulders, and pelvis. Pain is accompanied by fatigue and stiffness. The stiffness is most profound in the morning or after resting. There is no actual muscle weakness. Unlike RA, there is no small joint inflammation or effusion.

Diagnostic Studies

The C-reactive protein and sedimentation rate are often elevated. Biopsy and EMG are normal.

RHEUMATOID ARTHRITIS

Although RA typically affects multiple joints, it is not unusual for patients to present with complaints of muscle aches. See pp. 513–514.

INFECTION

A variety of infections cause varying degrees of myalgia. Myalgia is a common component of viral syndrome.

Signs and Symptoms

The patient describes an acute onset of symptoms, which often includes complaints more specific to the infectious agent. There is often an elevated temperature and signs of viral infection.

DRUG-INDUCED MYALGIA

Myalgia is associated with several medications, including diuretics, anticonvulsants, lipid-lowering agents, hydralazine, chloroquine, and procainamide.

Signs and Symptoms

The signs and symptoms are dependent on the specific medication and dosage taken. If the myalgia is related to rhabdomyolysis, the urine is often reddish brown.

Diagnostic Studies

In general, no diagnostic studies are ordered. However, when drug-induced myalgia is present, there is often eosinophilia. For drug-induced SLE, ANA is positive. For rhabdomyolysis myalgia, the serum creatine kinase is significantly elevated.

REFERENCES

Agency for Healthcare Research & Quality. (2017). Clinician summary. Diagnosis and management of gout: Current state of the evidence. https://effectivehealthcare.ahrq.gov/topics/gout/clinician/

American College of Radiology. (2017). ACR Appropriateness Criteria® shoulder pain–atraumatic. Retrieved April 8, 2022, from https://acsearch.acr.org/docs/3101482/narrative/

American College of Radiology. (2021). ACR Appropriateness Criteria. Retrieved June 18, 2021, from https://www.acr.org/Clinical-Resources/ACR-Appropriateness-Criteria

Appelboam, A., Reuben, A. D., Benger, J. R., Beech, F., Dutson, J., Haig, S., Higginson, I., Klein, J. A., Le Roux, S., Saranga, S. S. M.,Taylor, R., Vickery, J., Powell, R. J., & Lloyd, G. (2008). Elbow extension test to rule out elbow fracture: Multicentre, prospective validation and observational study of diagnostic accuracy in adults and children. *British Medical Journal, 337*, a2428. www.bmj.com/content/337/bmj .a2428.pdf%2Bhtml

Cook, C., Hegedus, E., Hawkins, R., Scovell, F., & Wyland, D. (2010). Diagnostic accuracy and association to disability of clinical test findings associated with patellofemoral pain syndrome. *Physiotherapy Canada, 62*(1), 17–24.

Dinnes, J., Loveman, E., McIntyre, L., & Waugh, N. (2003). The effectiveness of diagnostic tests for the assessment of shoulder pain due to soft tissue disorders: A systematic review. *Health Technology Assessment, 7*(29), 1–166.

Grelsamer, R. (2017). Physical examination of the knee: Meniscus, cartilage, and patellofemoral conditions. *The Journal of the American Academy of Orthopaedic Surgeons, 25*(10), e243. https://doi.org/10.5435 /JAAOS-D-17-00331

Kastelein, M., Wagemakers, H. P., Luijsterburg, P. A., Verhaar, J. A., Koes, B. W., & Bierma-Zeinstra, S. M. (2008). Assessing medial collateral ligament knee lesions in general practice. *American Journal of Medicine, 121*(11), 982–988.

Wagemakers, H. P., Luijsterburg, P. A., Boks, S. S., Heintjes, E. M., Berger, M. Y., Verhaar, J. A., Koes, B. W., & Bierma-Zeinstra, S. M. (2010). Diagnostic accuracy of history taking and physical examination for assessing anterior cruciate ligament lesions of the knee in primary care. *Archives of Physical Medicine and Rehabilitation, 91*(9), 1452–1559.

Zwerus, E. L., Somford, M. P., Maissan, F., Heisen, J., Eygendaal, D., & van den Bekerom, M. P. (2018). Physical examination of the elbow, what is the evidence? A systematic literature review. *British Journal of Sports Medicine, 52*(19), 1253–1260. https://doi.org/10.1136/bjsports-2016-096712

Chapter 16

Neurological System

• Michael Zychowicz

N eurological conditions are commonly encountered in primary care settings. Often neurological problems result in nonspecific symptoms that require careful investigation for timely diagnosis. Some of the content described in this chapter overlaps that in others. For instance, dementia and delirium are described here in detail but are also addressed in the chapters addressing mental health (Chapter 18) and older patients (Chapter 21). Sensory vision and hearing changes are addressed in Chapters 6 and 7, respectively.

History

■ Chief Complaint and the History of Present Illness

The history of present illness should include the primary symptom or constellation of symptoms, the associated factors, and the onset and duration of the symptoms. Ask patients to describe the chief complaint in their own words. Ask whether the primary symptom began acutely or gradually and whether an injury or traumatic event precipitated the onset of symptoms. If an injury was involved, explore the mechanism of injury, any associated loss of consciousness, and emergent treatments at the time of injury. Ask whether there has been any change in the character, severity, location, or duration of the symptoms. Identify measures that make the symptom better or worse (e.g., lying down, movements, Valsalva maneuver, medications).

■ General History and the Review of Systems

The general history should include a review of all body systems because symptoms of neurological diseases often overlap with other systems. For example, endocrine disorders may manifest themselves with symptoms of lethargy, fatigue, dizziness, or paresthesias; musculoskeletal disorders may manifest as weakness, muscle atrophy, and balance or gait problems; and psychiatric disorders may mimic signs of neurological dysfunction. Therefore, a thorough review of systems is recommended. Specific to the neurological system, the review should include questions to determine whether the patient has experienced headaches or other pain, sensory changes, motor disturbances, confusion or other altered thought processes, dizziness, syncope, or altered speech.

Past Medical and Surgical History

The medical history should include all disorders for which the patient has been treated in the past. This includes both recent and remote history. If the patient is a child or adolescent, inquire about common childhood illnesses and immunizations. Ask whether the patient has ever been treated for the same or a similar complaint. If so, identify what diagnosis was made at that time, what treatments were rendered, and what was the response. The history should include conditions that have potential neurological effects, including cardiovascular disorders, such as atherosclerosis or hypertension; endocrine disorders, such as diabetes or hypothyroidism; and malignancies. Include any history of blood transfusions and allergy or adverse reaction to medications or treatments. Explore the history of surgery or interventional procedures and experience with anesthesia. Identify the history of any serious injuries. Document all medications, including over-the-counter (OTC) and herbal agents, as well as the patient's understanding of their indication.

The specific neurological history should include any past neurological disorders, excluding the presenting chief complaint. This includes stroke, carotid artery disease, aneurysm, head or spine trauma, altered level of consciousness, exposure to toxins or infectious diseases (e.g., tick bites, spider bites, mononucleosis, insecticides), seizures, or psychiatric disorders. Also inquire about the history of melanoma or malignancies of the lung, breast, colon, or kidney.

Social History

Ask about current and past use of tobacco (cigarette, cigar, pipe, or smokeless), alcohol, or drugs, including the quantity and duration of each. Document the amount of caffeine the patient consumes per day (include coffee, tea, other caffeinated beverages, and chocolate). Identify the type and frequency of activity performed and any recreational risks. Document the patient's highest level of education and current and former occupations, including any possible occupational hazards.

Family History

Inquire about the immediate family history, including parents, siblings, and children. Family history of neurological diseases, including familial tremor, stroke, cerebrovascular disease, and neuromuscular disorders, is particularly important. Establish whether there is a family history of cardiovascular, endocrine, or other conditions with neurological effects. Also include any family history of substance abuse or mental illness.

Physical Examination

The neurological examination should start with a review of the patient's vital signs and a general survey. The breadth of the actual examination will depend on the patient's presentation. However, familiarity with each aspect is important, and these are described next.

General Appearance and Affect

Observe the patient when entering the room and during the interview. Note general appearance as it relates to nutrition, body habitus, cleanliness, attention to grooming, and affect. Observe the physical appearance of the skull, identifying any asymmetry or gross lesions. Note fluidity of movements, gait, and facial expressions. Abnormalities that may be detected during the assessment of general appearance include obesity, cachexia, poor grooming, sullen or flat affect, involuntary movements, hyperactivity, jocularity, and obvious craniofacial deformities.

Mental Status

A good screening tool for use in the outpatient setting is the Mini-Mental Status Exam, described in detail in Chapter 21. Ask the family or significant other whether the patient's behavior patterns have changed. If the patient does not speak or write English, have an interpreter available during the examination. Box 16.1 describes the components of the mental status examination. Mental status abnormalities include confusion, inability to recall recent or remote events,

---

Box 16.1

Mental Status Components

Orientation—The patient should normally be aware of person, date, and place. Ask patients their full name, current date, and place in which the examination is being done.

Memory—Recent and remote memory should normally be intact. Ask what the patient had for lunch yesterday (recent) and where the patient graduated from elementary school (remote).

Fund of knowledge (take into consideration the patient's level of education)— Ask about any recent news events or significant upcoming or past holiday.

Attention span—Ability to focus on the interviewer without being easily distracted. Ask the patient to repeat a short list of numbers (e.g., 7-8-9-3-0-2). Inability to repeat six or more numbers indicates attention deficit.

Concentration—Ability to concentrate on a question or task. Ask the patient to remember three unrelated words (e.g., *red, happy,* and *five*) and then to repeat them in 5 minutes, or ask the patient to count backward from 100 by 7.

Language—Use and understanding of language. Ask the patient to write a full sentence or to spell *world* backward. Distinguish between dysphonias and dysarthrias, as these indicate mechanical disturbances often due to CN dysfunction. Assess fluency of speech by asking the patient to repeat "no ifs, ands, or buts about it." Dysfluent speech is Broca's aphasia. Speech that is devoid of content indicates Wernicke's aphasia.

Abstract thoughts—Ask the patient to interpret a common proverb (e.g., a stitch in time saves nine), or ask the patient to answer an abstract question (e.g., "Is my sister's brother a man or a woman?").

inability to concentrate on conversation or examination, confabulation, inappropriate crying or laughter, slurred speech, word-finding difficulty, jocularity, or difficulty with calculations or abstract reasoning.

Cranial Nerve Examination

Examination of the cranial nerves (CNs) offers information about localization of the abnormality. Table 16.1 summarizes the CN examination.

Table 16.1	

Cranial Nerve Examination

Cranial Nerve (CN)	Technique
CN I, olfactory	After establishing patency of nostrils, assess ability to recognize smell, such as alcohol swab, soap, or coffee (never ammonia); test one side at a time. (Abnormalities: inability to discriminate between odors, asymmetric sense of smell)
CN II, optic	Check visual acuity, visual fields; observe optic disk. (Abnormalities: diminished vision, optic disk pallor, papilledema; see Chapter 6)
CN II, oculomotor	Test pupil responses to light and accommodation. (Abnormalities: asymmetry of pupil size or reaction to light; inability to accommodate with near/far vision test) Check lid position for ptosis; see Chapter 6. Also check for eye position with test for extraocular movement (CNs III, IV, and VI).
CN III, oculomotor	Observe relative position of each eye and eye movements.
CN IV, trochlear	(Abnormalities: asymmetrical gaze, nystagmus, limited movement of either eye or both eyes)
CN VI, abducens	
CN V, trigeminal	Assess facial and corneal sensation and masseter muscles' tone/strength. (Abnormalities: asymmetric facial sensation, inability to blink upon threat, inability to clench jaw, jaw pain)
CN VII, facial	Observe facial symmetry during conversation, at rest, during exaggerated expressions; assess strength of eyelids, taste on the anterior two-thirds of the tongue, sensation, and elevation of the palate. (Abnormalities: decreased or absent taste, palate numbness, facial asymmetry or droop, asymmetric facial sensation)
CN VIII, vestibulocochlear	Assess hearing and balance. (Abnormalities: positive Romberg, poor balance, altered acuity of hearing, tinnitus)
CN IX, glossopharyngeal CN X, vagus	Assess swallowing, gag reflex, and quality of voice; observe palate elevation, taste, and sensation. (Abnormalities: absent gag reflex, dysphagia, asymmetry or deviation of uvula, asymmetric decreased/absent taste or numbness of the tongue, hoarseness/altered voice quality)
CN XI, spinal accessory	Assess head movement, strength of sternocleidomastoid (SCM) and trapezius muscles. (Abnormalities: asymmetric movements or weakness) *Note:* Both central and peripheral lesions cause ipsilateral SCM weakness: Central lesions cause ipsilateral trapezius weakness, whereas peripheral lesions cause contralateral trapezius weakness.
CN XII, hypoglossal	Observe tongue position and movement. (Abnormalities: fasciculations, atrophy, tongue, or palate deviation) The tongue will deviate *toward* the side of the lesion.

Motor Function

If possible, the assessment of motor function should begin when the patient walks into the room and is seated. Note the strength of handshake. Observe posture, resting movements of limbs, blinking frequency, and facial movements. More detailed assessment involves attention to isolated muscle groups, noting strength, tone, bulk, and contour of muscles. Abnormalities include a lack of muscle tone, rigidity, cogwheel rigidity, atrophy, asymmetric strength, spasticity, flaccidity, fasciculations, and tremor.

■ Reflexes

Test deep tendon reflexes in all extremities. Some patients will have diminished or absent reflexes, which is a normal variant if the finding is symmetrical. If necessary, reinforcement can be accomplished by having the patient clench the jaws or tighten muscles of extremities not being tested. The grading scale for reflexes is provided in Box 16.2. The nerves related to each of the reflexes are listed in Box 16.3. Special reflex maneuvers include the Babinski reflex, assessing for upper motor neuron lesions of the lower extremities, assessing for upper motor lesions of the upper extremities, and the Hoffman response. Abnormalities of the deep tendon reflexes include hyperreflexive responses, with clonus. Diminished or absent reflexes are particularly important if they are unilateral or limited to specific sites while others remain intact.

Box 16.2

Reflex Grades

0 = absent
1+ = hyporeflexia
2+ = normal
3+ = hyperreflexia
4+ and 5+ = abnormally strong contractions with clonus

Box 16.3

Deep Tendon Reflexes

Biceps: C5, C6
Brachioradialis: C5, C6
Triceps: C6, C7
Patellar: L3, L4
Achilles: S1

Box 16.4

Coordination Tests

Finger-to-nose testing—Ask patients to touch your index finger with their index finger, then touch their nose repeatedly. Poor coordination of movement indicates dysmetria.

Rapid alternating movements—Ask patients to perform rapid pronation and supination of the hand on their thigh or on the examining table.

Heel-to-shin testing—Ask patients to take the heel of one side and repeatedly move up and down the shin of the opposite leg.

Romberg—Ask patients to stand with feet together, arms abducted outward with palms up, and eyes closed. Positive Romberg is observed as a swaying motion, or inability to maintain balance, and indicates cerebellar dysfunction.

■ Coordination

Test fluidity of movements. Inability to coordinate volitional movements suggests cerebellar dysfunction. Also note any involuntary movements, such as tremors or an inability to perform tests. Box 16.4 lists coordination tests.

■ Cerebrovascular

Auscultation of the carotid arteries is an important portion of the neurological examination, particularly for older patients or those with a history of tobacco abuse. Patients should be asked to hold their breath during auscultation. A bruit in the carotid artery may be an indicator of potential stroke or carotid artery stenosis and should be followed by further tests, such as carotid duplex and carotid ultrasound.

■ Funduscopic Examination

The funduscopic examination is fully described in Chapter 6.

■ Sensory Examination

The sensory examination should be the final portion of the neurological examination. The sensory examination indicates the patient's ability to interpret cutaneous sensory information. The test is performed with a clean, unused safety pin, the end of a cotton swab, and a tuning fork. Test each dermatome individually for ability to feel light touch, sharp/dull discrimination, and vibratory sense. Asymmetry of sensation implies impaired sensory distribution to the particular dermatome being tested.

Differential Diagnosis of Chief Complaints

■ Headache or Cephalalgia

Headache is one of the most prevalent presenting complaints in the outpatient clinical setting as well as a leading cause of missed days of work. The occasional headache sufferer accounts for the expenditure of billions of dollars annually for

OTC symptom remedies. Those who suffer one or fewer headaches per month are unlikely to seek professional advice; however, those who suffer chronic pain of two or more episodes per month are more likely to consult their health-care provider.

The considerable frequency of headache in the general population has led to the development of the International Headache Society (IHS) classification of headaches (IHS, 2018). This classification is useful for appropriate diagnosis and treatment of headaches. Headaches are broadly categorized as primary (e.g., migraine, tension, cluster) and secondary (associated with space-occupying masses, infection, trauma, or substances).

History

The patient history is critical to head pain assessment and is often more telling than the physical examination. The headache history should follow the basic history format, with an emphasis on the head pain episodes. Key elements of the history should include full symptom analysis. Have patients describe the pain in their own words (e.g., throbbing, aching, pressure, sharp, stabbing), rate the severity on a scale of 1 to 10, and point to the area of pain. An account of activities preceding the onset of the headache may help to identify potential triggers, such as straining, exertion, coitus, foods, substances, and the like—although the relationship may be coincidental rather than causative. Determine whether the onset of pain was acute or gradual and its duration. If similar headaches have been experienced previously, ask about prior treatments and response. Identify any associated symptoms, such as fever, nausea, vomiting, confusion, stiff neck, or vision changes, as well as the history of any prodromal symptoms or aura. Determine whether the patient has recently altered any habits, such as caffeine intake. Identify all recently used OTC or prescribed medication, illicit/recreational drugs, tobacco, and alcohol. Determine whether the patient has recently experienced or been exposed to a viral or bacterial infection, traveled out of the country, or been exposed to any environmental toxins. Inquire about a history of lung disease or obstructive sleep apnea (OSA) since cerebral hypoxia can cause headache. Ask about any recent trauma, specifically a fall or blow to the head. Explore with patients their occupation, habits, family stressors, marital relationship, sexual factors, social relationships, hobbies, and coping strategies. A thorough psychosocial investigation should precede additional testing. See the Red Flag box for headache presentations.

For recurrent headaches, a headache diary is helpful in arriving at a definitive diagnosis. Although details can be simply recorded on a calendar, a number of headache diaries are available and downloadable on the internet. Regardless of the format used, the diary should provide a space for the patient to identify daily whether a headache was experienced. When headache is experienced, the form should allow the patient to identify the type, severity, and duration of pain experienced; accompanying symptoms; treatment and response; and any suspected triggers.

> **RED FLAG** ◄ **Red Flags in the Assessment of Patients With Headaches**
>
> - *Acute onset, severe headaches described as "the worst headache of my life" in a patient who has no history of headache*
> - *Unrelenting headaches, unrelieved with conservative treatments or with pain that steadily worsens*
> - *New-onset headaches in patients older than 50 years without previous history of headache*
> - *Lancinating, "ice pick" head pain*
> - *Severe headaches associated with a stiff neck and/or fever*
> - *Headache accompanied by a change in mentation or level of consciousness*
> - *Persistent headaches following trauma to the head or neck*
> - *Headaches that are significantly different in pattern or severity in a patient with a long-standing chronic headache history*

Physical Examination

The neurological examination for headache should include all of the basic elements with an emphasis on the CNs. Vital signs should be recorded, noting blood pressure and heart rate to assist in determining possible vascular components of the headache and any fever, which may indicate an inflammatory or infectious process. The physical examination should include examination of the eyes/fundi, neck, throat, sinuses, and nose. Pay particular attention to the funduscopic examination, which can provide information about increased intracranial pressure. Palpate the head and temporal arteries for any gross abnormalities. The remainder of the neurological examination should be conducted to detect any sensory or motor dysfunction, difficulty with coordination, diminished reflexes, or altered mental status. Lesions or tumors of the brain, in particular, may cause subtle or insidious symptoms, requiring a thorough examination and strict attention to detail.

Patients exhibiting any of the red flags noted previously require immediate definitive diagnosis. For example, any patient with an acute, severe headache, described as "the worst headache of my life," with or without associated symptoms, should be referred immediately to the emergency department because this type of complaint may indicate an intracranial bleed. Any patient with headache associated with fever and stiff neck should be referred to the emergency department for evaluation of possible meningitis. Any patient older than 50 years with new onset of headache that is unrelieved by medication and without a previous history of headache should trigger suspicion of a space-occupying lesion, and imaging studies should be obtained to further assess the complaint.

Box 16.5

Diagnostic Studies for Headache

Magnetic resonance imaging (MRI) with and without contrast is the test of choice for diagnosis of occult lesions and organic disorders unless contrast is otherwise contraindicated. The MRI should be performed in the sagittal, axial, and coronal planes.

Computed tomography (CT) scan is a useful screening tool for emergent detection of expanding mass lesions such as subdural or epidural hematoma, hemorrhagic stroke, or large mass lesions. CT with contrast will help to visualize mass lesions, although it is less sensitive than MRI. CT of the brain also helps to determine evidence of hydrocephalus.

Magnetic resonance angiography (MRA) of the head is used for imaging arteries (and less commonly veins) in order to evaluate for stenosis, occlusions, aneurysms, or other vascular abnormalities.

Plain skull films are helpful in identifying bony, extracranial abnormalities, such as skull fractures or lesions. However, they lack the sensitivity to diagnose intracranial abnormalities.

Lumbar puncture (LP) is an invasive test to be performed only when symptoms warrant and if no expanding mass lesion is found on contrast MRI of the brain. Patient must be fully informed of the risks and benefits of the procedure.

Select laboratory studies such as CBC, ESR, and basic metabolic profile are used to detect infectious processes, anemia, and metabolic abnormalities. Thyroid function tests identify hypothyroidism.

Diagnostic Studies

Depending on the presentation and findings, further studies may be warranted. Box 16.5 provides a brief discussion of diagnostic studies relevant to the assessment of headache.

MIGRAINE HEADACHE

Migraine is one of the most common vascular headache types and accounts for a significant percentage of clinic and emergency department visits each year. They occur more frequently in women, with the typical onset at approximately age 6 years through adolescence. Black people and those of Hispanic descent are more likely to experience migraine compared with white people and those of Asian descent. The majority of patients report a family history of migraine. Onset of migraine is uncommon after age 40 years. Thus, patients with an onset of headache beyond this age should be evaluated for other head pain etiologies. Migraines often subside or completely resolve during pregnancy and menopause. The IHS defines migraine as a recurring, idiopathic headache that generally lasts 4 to 76 hours. They generally do not occur daily and are often associated with the menstrual cycle. The frequency of episodes can be one to four times per month or only several times per year. Migraines can occur with or without aura.

Signs and Symptoms

Typical migraine pain begins unilaterally but may become generalized and may lateralize to the opposite side and/or radiate to the face or neck. The pain ranges from a dull ache to a throbbing or pulsatile pain. The pain is often severe and/or incapacitating and is often aggravated by movement, light, and noise. Accompanying symptoms may include nausea, vomiting, photophobia, phonophobia, osmophobia, dizziness, chills, and/or ataxia. There may be tenderness to palpation of the temporal arteries. Auras, if experienced, may include blurred vision and scotoma and/or other prodromal symptoms such as anorexia, irritability, restlessness, or paresthesias lasting from 30 minutes to 3 hours before the onset of migraine pain. The patient may be able to identify headache triggers; common migraine triggers are listed in Table 16.2.

Diagnostic Studies

Although not usually indicated, further diagnostic studies may be desired to rule out other conditions, based on the history and physical examination. These tests can include complete blood count (CBC), erythrocyte sedimentation rate (ESR), metabolic profile, computed tomography (CT) scan with contrast, and magnetic resonance imaging (MRI) of the brain with and without contrast to rule out conditions such as hemorrhage or intracerebral lesions. It is often helpful to ask the patient to keep a headache diary and record any factors precipitating the headache.

CLUSTER HEADACHE

One of the most severe and incapacitating forms of headache is the cluster headache, so named because the pain occurs in episodic clusters of attacks. The pain of cluster headache can be so intense as to precipitate suicidal thoughts or

Table 16.2

Headache Triggers: Migraine, Cluster, Tension

Migraine	Cluster	Tension
• Stress	• Smoking	• Stress
• Caffeine	• Alcohol	• Fatigue/lack of sleep
• Altered sleep and fatigue	• Vasodilators	• Anxiety/depression
• Specific foods, missed meals	• Seasonal changes	• Caffeine/tobacco overuse
• Menses	• Altitude changes	• Latent hostility
• Alcohol		
• Hormone supplements		
• Dehydration		

actions in order to find relief. Cluster headaches are more common in men, with onset in the second to third decades of life. Rare cases have been reported in children. The pain is believed to emanate from a hypersensitized ophthalmic nerve.

Signs and Symptoms

There is usually complaint of headaches that are episodic and unpredictable in nature and that may be cyclic. Episodes often occur more frequently in spring and autumn. Cluster periods last, on average, 2 to 3 months and may remit for months to years. Remissions are typically shorter than 2 years. The pain is not preceded by aura. Cluster headaches have rapid crescendo patterns, peaking in approximately 10 to 15 minutes and often lasting 30 to 60 minutes per episode (rarely lasting over 2 hours each). Attacks occur as frequently as two to three times per day. The pain is generally in the area of the trigeminal nerve and is described as unilateral, penetrating, sharp, excruciating, and unrelenting in nature. There may be associated unilateral lacrimation, nasal congestion or rhinorrhea, pallor, flushing, conjunctival redness, ptosis—all on the *same side* as the pain. Some people may experience bradycardia during the episode. During an episode, the patient is restless, may hold the head, and is often anxious and unable to sit still. Cluster headache triggers are listed in Table 16.2.

Diagnostic Studies

Diagnostic studies and workup are not definitive but should be selected if needed to rule out other disorders. These include an MRI or CT scan of the brain with contrast to rule out life-threatening differential diagnoses such as tumor or hemorrhage. Imaging can also assist in ruling out abnormalities of the eye, sinuses, and cervical vasculature. An ophthalmological examination with dilation may help to rule out ocular causes of the pain. CBC, ESR, and C-reactive protein may be helpful, particularly if giant cell arteritis is part of the differential.

TENSION HEADACHE

Tension headaches are quite common. Whereas many people with episodic tension headaches do not seek treatment, those who suffer from frequent or chronic tension headaches may enlist the help of their provider. Other terms to describe tension headache include *stress headache, essential headache, idiopathic headache,* and *muscle contraction headache.* Tension headaches can occur with greater frequency in women (as compared with men), in white people, and in those with a higher education level.

Signs and Symptoms

Typical symptoms of tension headache include mild to moderate nonthrobbing pressure or squeezing pain that can occur anywhere in the head or neck. The pain often starts slowly as a dull and aching discomfort that progresses to holocranial pain and pressure. The pain can recur intermittently, lasting from minutes to hours and usually remitting with rest or removal of the stressful trigger. There is usually no associated nausea and vomiting. Although patients may report photophobia and phonophobia, it is less severe than that associated with migraines.

Tension headaches are not aggravated by movement or activity. The neck muscles are often tight to palpation. Tension headache triggers are listed in Table 16.2.

Diagnostic Studies

Diagnostics and further workup should be ordered only if necessary to rule out other conditions.

SUBDURAL HEMATOMA

Subdural hematomas can be either acute or chronic. Acute subdural hematomas are usually associated with an acute head injury and can cause a range of symptoms, including headache and loss of consciousness. A chronic subdural hematoma in an older person may enlarge significantly before the patient begins to notice head pain.

Signs and Symptoms

The headache associated with subdural hematoma is generally dull and aching in nature and may be transient. The history often includes a blow to the head, fall, or other injury, which preceded the pain. The pain is progressive and will gradually worsen over days to weeks. The pain may wake a patient from sleep or worsen with changes in patient posture. In older adults, the history of head trauma may be more remote than in younger patients. A change in mentation may precede pain in older patients. The physical findings vary depending on the severity of the trauma. There may be progressive neurological deterioration, including personality change, sleepiness, or sensory changes, which may advance to include loss of consciousness or coma. Patients may experience seizures, weakness, nausea, and vomiting.

Diagnostic Studies

A CT scan of the brain is the test of choice in the acute setting and will show both acute and chronic subdural hematoma. An MRI of the brain with and without contrast will demonstrate any associated abnormalities.

SUBARACHNOID HEMORRHAGE

Head trauma is a common cause of subarachnoid hemorrhage (SAH). However, an SAH can be spontaneous, stemming from vascular malformations, uncontrolled hypertension, or hemorrhagic disease. SAH most commonly occurs due to a ruptured arterial aneurysm, which is frequently located where arteries branch (e.g., circle of Willis). SAH most typically occurs in adults age 50 to 60 years, and persons who smoke have a significantly higher risk of SAH. This type of headache represents a true medical emergency and necessitates immediate referral or transfer to a local emergency department for triage and treatment.

Signs and Symptoms

The pain associated with SAH is generally described as severe and acute in onset. The headache onset is often described as being like a "thunderbolt" or "thunderclap." The severity is described as "the worst headache of my life." It is generally made worse by lying down. There is often associated nausea and/or vomiting and possible rapid deterioration in neurological function and diminished level of consciousness.

Diagnostic Studies

A noncontrast CT scan followed by CT angiography (CTA) of the brain can rule out SAH with greater than 99% sensitivity (McCormack & Hutson, 2010). If SAH is included in the differential diagnosis, a lumbar puncture (LP) is generally not recommended in the acute phase because it may result in increased bleeding or herniation. If an LP is performed, the cerebrospinal fluid (CSF) may have a yellowish appearance because of bilirubin from the hemorrhage that has mixed with the CSF. If a vascular abnormality is found, magnetic resonance angiography (MRA) may be helpful to determine the exact etiology.

VIRAL OR BACTERIAL MENINGITIS

Meningitis is an inflammatory central nervous system (CNS) disease generally caused by either viral or bacterial infection. The etiology of meningitis includes community-acquired, posttraumatic, aseptic, carcinomatous, or transferred from another bodily source. The most common organisms belong to such genera as *Streptococcus, Neisseria (meningitides), Haemophilus (influenzae), Listeria, Staphylococcus (aureus)*, and gram-negative bacilli and gram-positive cocci. Meningitis can affect persons of all ages; however, infants, adolescents, and young adults have a greater risk. Risk is also increased for those living in close quarters or crowded spaces such as college dormitories. When obtaining the history, inquire about any travel or exposure, which may be a causative factor. The patient may have had a recent infection or may have an underlying immunocompromised state that increased the risk for developing meningitis. Patients with meningitis represent a medical emergency and should be referred to an emergency department for treatment.

Signs and Symptoms

The headache associated with meningitis is described as diffuse and throbbing and is often severe or intense in nature. There is usually associated fever, photophobia, phonophobia, nausea, vomiting, and nuchal rigidity. Tachycardia and rapid respiratory rate can accompany meningitis. Patients can rapidly decline to delirium, seizures, and, if untreated, coma. On neurological examination, the patient may be lethargic and febrile and have altered mentation along with nuchal rigidity and/or guarding, contracted and sluggish pupils, and a generally "toxic" appearance. Brudzinski's and Kernig's signs are helpful in assessing potential meningeal conditions (Box 16.6). Delirium or acute confusion necessitates immediate transfer to an emergency department for treatment, as the patient can rapidly deteriorate to coma.

Diagnostics Studies

Diagnostic tests should include CBC, ESR, C-reactive protein, and a CT scan or MRI to rule out a space-occupying lesion. An LP to obtain CSF for cell count,

Box 16.6

Meningeal Tests

Brudzinski's test—With patient lying on examination table, gently flex the patient's neck to a chin-to-chest position. The test is positive if the patient attempts to lift legs and flex hips to relieve pain caused by the maneuver.

Kernig's test—With patient resting on examination table, hold leg with hip and knee flexed. Without moving the upper leg, slowly extend the knee, straightening the leg. The test is positive if the maneuver results in pain, with the patient flexing the neck in attempt to relieve the pain.

protein, glucose, cultures, and possible polymerase chain reaction (PCR) is generally performed only after ruling out a mass through imaging.

CHIARI MALFORMATION

Chiari malformations are brainstem and cerebellar malformations where a portion of the cerebellum extends through the foramen magnum at the base of the skull and into the spinal canal. CSF flow as well as cerebellar function may be impaired. There are three types of Chiari malformation. Chiari type 1 occurs when the lowest portion of the cerebellum is pushed through the foramen magnum and is most often associated with occipital headaches; it is generally seen in the adult population but can be diagnosed at any age. Type 1 symptoms may be very vague and transient, and it is often misdiagnosed as another neurological disease. Type 2 is generally diagnosed in infants or children, associated with myelomeningocele or other open neural tube defects, or in adults with undiagnosed spina bifida occulta or tethered cord. Type 2 is characterized by both the brainstem and the cerebellum passing through the foramen magnum. Type 3 malformation is rare, diagnosed in infants, and associated with cervical myelomeningocele or pseudomeningocele; it carries a very poor prognosis.

Signs and Symptoms

The typical presentation of Chiari malformation includes a persistent headache that occurs most often in the occipital area and may radiate diffusely or behind the eyes. The headache is triggered or worsened by the Valsalva maneuver or by flexion/extension of the neck. There is often complaint of neck or skull base pain as well as dizziness or disequilibrium, also worsened by movement or flexion/extension of the neck. Other complaints may include tinnitus and decreased hearing; weakness, numbness, paresthesias, and extremity pain; extreme fatigue, difficulty sleeping, and generalized body weakness; difficulty swallowing and voice hoarseness (often with diminished or absent gag reflex); and altered memory or concentration.

Diagnostic Studies

The test of choice for the diagnosis of Chiari malformation is an MRI of the brain and brainstem with and without contrast.

Brain Abscess

Brain abscess can be caused by an extension of an existing extracranial infection, extension of a blood-borne infection, intracranial procedures, or penetrating head injury. Infections of the lung, heart, ear, or sinus are the most common sources of abscess transference. The cause is idiopathic in approximately 15% to 25% of the cases. Inquire about recent visits to developing countries because abscess is more common and easily spread in these geographic areas. Also inquire about recent or remote consumption of poorly cooked meats or unwashed vegetables. The most common vectors are Streptococcus and Staphylococcus.

The abscess generally causes head pain only after the lesion has enlarged enough to result in mass effect on the brain tissue, so timely treatment for brain abscess requires immediate transfer to an emergency department for neurosurgical and infectious disease consultation.

Signs and Symptoms

If the condition represents an extension of a preexisting problem, the history will be consistent with that condition and with the symptoms specifically related to the abscess. The history usually includes a gradual onset of symptoms that progress as the inflammatory process increases. These symptoms include headache, nausea (with or without vomiting), lethargy, and fever. Over time, if the lesion expands, the symptoms progress to include seizures, lethargy, nuchal rigidity, hemiparesis, and altered mental status. If left untreated, the patient can rapidly decline to seizures and coma.

Diagnostic Studies

Diagnostic tests for patients suspected of brain abscess include CBC (may be normal in the early stage or in older patients), ESR, C-reactive protein, and blood cultures (may be negative). An MRI of the brain with and without contrast will show enhancing lesions, and this is the test of choice for localization. Magnetic resonance spectroscopy may also help in determining the activity of the abscess. LP is not recommended in the initial workup for intracranial abscess. The abscess can be aspirated during surgery or with stereotactic CT for culture, Gram stain, acid fast stain, and fungal stain.

Tumor

An intracranial malignancy can result in a wide range of complaints and findings depending on the size and location of the mass, as they commonly stem from increased pressure on tissues, obstruction of the circulation, or increased intracranial pressure. Because the brain tissue does not feel pain, most patients do not present with headache until the lesion is large enough to significantly increase intracranial pressure. A majority of brain tumors will include acoustic neuroma, meningioma, glioma, pituitary adenoma, or metastasis. Meningioma is the most likely tumor to cause headache. Brain tumors include benign, primary malignant, and metastatic lesions.

Signs and Symptoms

Progressive neurological deterioration is one of the most common symptoms of an intracranial mass lesion. Many older patients may show slow, progressive mental decline over months to years and may be misdiagnosed as experiencing depression or dementia. Head pain generally overlies the area of the mass lesion. Tumors of the sella generally refer pain to the vertex. The pain associated with tumors is often described as dull, aching, and transitory. New-onset seizures in the adult population should be considered the result of a mass lesion until proven otherwise. Vomiting without nausea implies increased intracranial pressure. Some persons report improvement in their symptoms for a brief time after vomiting. Unilateral extremity numbness or paresthesias and weakness may be either slowly or rapidly progressive. Mass lesions of the cerebellum may cause disequilibrium or gait disturbance. Acute unilateral hearing loss or tinnitus may imply a lesion of the acoustic nerve, and unilateral visual disturbances may imply a lesion or compression on the optic nerve. The physical examination may reveal alterations in vital signs, particularly new-onset hypertension. The neurological examination may be normal until the lesion exerts enough mass effect to increase intracranial pressure or obstruct the flow of CSF. Focal neurological findings may include anisocoria, unilateral hearing loss, nystagmus, visual field defects, extremity weakness, numbness or paresthesia of the extremities, tongue deviation, and papilledema.

Diagnostic Studies

An MRI of the brain with and without contrast is the imaging study of choice for assessment of intracranial lesions. Magnetic resonance spectroscopy will help to assess cell activity within the tumor. If suspicious for metastasis, imaging of the suspected area may aid in evaluation of the tumor type. If a lesion is found in the cerebellum, an MRI of the cervical spine will help to assess for any drop lesions. Surgical biopsy of the intracranial tumor is the test of choice for definitive diagnosis of tumor type.

TEMPORAL ARTERITIS

Temporal arteritis is also referred to as *giant cell arteritis* or *cranial arteritis*. It is characterized by chronic inflammation and the presence of giant cells in large arteries, usually the temporal artery, but it can occur in the cranial arteries, the aorta, and the coronary or peripheral arteries. It affects the arteries containing elastic tissue, resulting in narrowing and eventual occlusion of the lumen. It occurs more among persons older than 50 years and is slightly more common in females than in males. The cause is unknown, but there seems to be a genetic predisposition. If left untreated, arteritis can rapidly lead to blindness that is often irreversible.

Signs and Symptoms

The most common chief complaint is bitemporal, frontal, or vertex head pain that is lancinating, sharp, or "ice pick" in nature. The pain can be quite severe and debilitating. Patients often complain of visual changes, including amaurosis, diplopia, blurred vision, visual field cuts, eye pain, periorbital edema, and intermittent unilateral blindness. Other common presenting symptoms include scalp and/or jaw tenderness, facial pain, and tenderness to palpation as well as potential pulselessness of the affected artery. The pain is generally hemicranial but can be bilateral or diffuse. There may be eye pain, which is usually bilateral; periorbital edema may be present. Other potential associated symptoms include an intermittent fever (generally low grade), chills, nausea, and/or weight loss. Patients can experience polymyalgia rheumatica at the same time as temporal arteritis.

Diagnostic Studies

In temporal arteritis, the white blood cell count may be elevated, although often it is normal in older patients. The ESR and C-reactive protein may be elevated. Definitive diagnosis of arteritis is determined by temporal artery biopsy. An MRI of the brain with and without contrast will help to rule out other structural causes; however, its use is not definitive for the diagnosis of arteritis. Patients with acute visual change should be referred immediately to a neurologist or neuro-ophthalmologist to prevent blindness from ischemic optic neuropathy, which occurs in approximately 20% of patients; treatment with corticosteroids should be started immediately while diagnostic studies are completed.

MEDICATION-OVERUSE HEADACHE, OR ANALGESIC REBOUND HEADACHE

Susceptible patients who take analgesic or abortive medications on a frequent basis for recurrent headaches may develop medication-overuse headaches. In addition to the susceptibility of the individual patient, the regularity with which the particular agent is taken is an important variable. Overuse or rebound headache should be considered in patients who develop chronic, daily headaches during therapy for primary headaches. Although this discussion is specific to the development of chronic headaches following overuse of headache agents, chronic headaches can also be associated with overuse of or withdrawal from a variety of other agents or may be an adverse effect of a wide range of substances. Withdrawal of medication or substances may require detoxification.

Signs and Symptoms

The headache is usually described as migraine-like. History reveals frequent use of analgesic or abortive agents (e.g., acetaminophen, aspirin, compounds, codeine, triptans) taken, for example, 15 or more times a month, usually for a period of 3 or more months. The chronic daily headaches resolve or revert to the earlier pattern of frequency when the patient is successfully withdrawn from the associated drug for a period of 2 months.

Diagnostic Studies

None are typically warranted; however, they may be necessary to rule out other potential causes. Urine or serum toxicology screens may aid in determining the levels of certain medications.

TRAUMA

Blunt trauma to the head can result in acute or chronic headache, regardless of whether there was loss of consciousness or traumatic brain injury (TBI). Generally, the severity of the trauma is correlated with the duration of the headache, but that is not always the case. Depending on the severity of the head trauma, within the skull there may be injury to the blood vessels, hemorrhage, contusion, nerve axon injury, meningeal irritation, edema, and hypoxia. Falls, motor vehicle crashes, and being hit by an object are leading causes of head trauma, contributing to significant morbidity and mortality in the United States.

Signs and Symptoms

The headache related to trauma is highly variable in frequency, intensity, and duration and can be difficult to manage. The pain may be localized to the site of the injury or generalized. The patient may be irritable or may complain of dizziness, difficulty with concentration, and difficulty sleeping owing to the pain. There may be an apparent motor deficit, loss of consciousness, and behavioral changes, as well as auditory or verbal deficit. Stress and/or depression may play a role. Severity of the head trauma will determine the severity of the signs and symptoms. The specific signs and symptoms the patient experiences may correlate to specific areas of the brain injured with a head trauma. The clinician should conduct a thorough neurological examination and assess the patient for signs and symptoms of increased intracranial pressure.

Diagnostic Studies

An acute head injury with complaint of severe headache warrants an emergency CT scan, MRI, or skull x-ray to rule out a cerebral contusion, subdural or intracerebral hematoma or hemorrhage, or skull fracture.

CEREBRAL HYPOXIA/EDEMA

Cerebral hypoxia results in edema and can occur in TBI, chronic obstructive pulmonary disease (COPD), congestive heart failure (CHF), and sleep disorders, specifically OSA.

Signs and Symptoms

In TBI, the hypoxia can be severe and the neurological injury significant, ranging from temporary loss of consciousness to a vegetative state. In chronic, low-level hypoxia—as seen in COPD, CHF, and OSA—the headache is dull and persistent. Hypertension can accompany COPD and OSA; hypotension may be present in individuals with CHF.

Diagnostic Studies

The diagnosis for TBI is usually obvious from the history of trauma. For chronic hypoxemia, arterial blood gases, oxygen saturation readings, pulmonary function tests, echocardiography, CBC results, and sleep studies can help in determining the cause.

■ Altered Mental Status

Alteration in mental status is generally a chief complaint of the older population. However, some unusual forms of dementia can be diagnosed as early as the second decade of life. The causes of mental status changes include, but are not limited to, Alzheimer's disease, multi-infarct dementia, stroke, CNS infections, neurodegenerative disorders, head injury, mass lesions, metabolic disorders, and hydrocephalus. It is estimated that approximately 10% to 20% of mental status changes are due to treatable causes, such as vitamin B deficiency, polypharmacy, intoxication or drug abuse, and infectious processes. Chapters 18 and 21 include additional content on altered thought processes. It is important to consider psychiatric conditions in the differential diagnosis for altered mental status.

History

A thorough history of the chief complaint should emphasize the mental status baseline and changes that have occurred. It is best if a family member or significant other can be present when taking the history because the patient may not have full awareness of the mental status changes. Identify when the mental status change was first noted by the patient or others. Determine whether onset was an acute change or developed over time; ask whether the changes are most notable at any particular time of day. Identify the baseline level of function and cognition. Determine the highest level of education, current or previous occupation, and daily routine, including whether the ability to perform activities of daily living independently has been affected. Determine whether the patient is aware of any functional change, as patients in the early stages of dementia often have insight into their functional capacity changes. Note whether the patient is easily frustrated with the level of abilities or cognition. Ask whether the patient's interpersonal relationships have been altered. Identify any history of excessive use of alcohol or drugs, any exposures to environmental toxins (e.g., lead, ammonia, carbon monoxide, heavy metals), or recent trauma. Review all current medications because polypharmacy, especially in the older population, can cause states of confusion. Review recent or remote exposure to any infectious disease, such as AIDS, herpes, meningitis, mononucleosis, or syphilis. Explore psychosocial factors, such as depression, anxiety, or the loss of a loved one. See the following box for red flags associated with mental status changes.

Physical Examination

The neurological examination should focus on assessment of cognition and mental status by using the Mental State Examination or another validated screening instrument. Observation is a key element in the neurological examination for the patient with mental status changes and should include the patient's dress and personal grooming, affect, any obvious agitation or frustration, and reliance on a significant other for assistance during the history or examination. Note the fluidity of speech and speech content. Also note whether the speech reveals a flight of ideas, confabulation, or echolalia (repeating vocalizations of others), as well as whether hallucinations are potentially present. Assess orientation to person, place, and time by asking patients to recite their full name, current location/place (e.g., clinic, hospital, home), and the date (day of the week, month, and year). Knowledge of time is generally impaired first, followed by place. The inability to recite or recognize one's name implies a significant deficit in mental status. All of the areas addressed in Box 16.1 should be considered during the mental status examination.

Diagnostic Studies

The range of potential diagnostic studies for a complaint of mental status change is immense, and studies should be selected on the basis of history and physical findings as well as differential diagnoses. A basic metabolic profile should be considered to determine metabolic abnormalities with particular attention to electrolytes, blood urea nitrogen, creatinine, calcium, and liver functions. Other common studies include serum B_{12} and folic acid levels. For older patients, consider urinalysis to rule out urinary tract infection and chest x-ray and pulse oximetry for respiratory compromise. A CBC with differential can determine evidence of infectious process or anemia. HIV testing, fluorescent treponemal antibody absorption test (FTA-ABS) for tertiary syphilis, and Lyme serology are important to establish the specific infectious condition. An ESR can be used to assess an inflammatory process. Thyroid function tests should be considered to evaluate thyroid status. An electrocardiogram or diagnostic imaging may be appropriate depending on the patient condition.

A 24-hour urine collection for heavy metals and/or toxicology screen should be considered. An electroencephalogram can determine the presence of subtle seizure activity or localized slow wave activity. An LP for CSF studies should be ordered if CNS infection is suspected.

DELIRIUM

Delirium can be observed in both older and younger patients and is generally defined as an *acute* confusional state, affecting all aspects of cognition and mentation, and is often related to a treatable disorder. These include an

---

RED FLAG ◀ Red Flags in the Assessment of Patients With Mental Status Changes
• *Acute changes associated with fever, stiff neck, or headache*
• *Acute changes in the older person (patient should be worked up for a possible infectious process, particularly urinary tract infections)*
• *Acute changes associated with any type of head trauma*
• *Progressive changes associated with gait disorder or incontinence*
• *Gradual but significant changes*

Table 16.3

Select Treatable Causes of Symptoms Associated With Delirium/Confusion

Condition	Findings
Vitamin B deficiencies	Depending on the particular deficiency, peripheral neuropathy, skin or mucous membrane changes, fatigue, constipation
Hypothyroidism	Fatigue, depression, skin/hair changes, cold intolerance, constipation, anemia
Infections	Highly dependent on the condition; for meningitis, nuchal rigidity, and fever
Nutritional deficit	Weight loss, nausea/vomiting, anorexia, weakness, electrolyte imbalances

almost endless list of potential causes, such as, but not limited to, intoxication, substance abuse, medication overdose, polypharmacy, infectious processes, mass lesion, intracranial bleed, thyroid imbalance, metabolic disturbances, encephalopathy, anemia, hypoxia, acute obstructive hydrocephalus, vitamin B deficiency, nutritional deficiency, and environmental exposures.

Signs and Symptoms

The signs and symptoms of delirium generally have a more acute or rapidly progressive onset as opposed to the slow, gradual decline noted in the organic dementias. The acute mental status change is often associated with other signs or symptoms—such as agitation, hallucinations, illusions, incoherent speech, inattention, memory difficulty, and constant aimless activity—that help to narrow the differential diagnosis. Table 16.3 describes some of the associated findings for several of the causes of treatable delirium or confusion. The history may reveal trauma, exposure to toxins, or medications if these are responsible for the mental status changes. In spite of the confusion, the patient's sensorium is usually intact, although some conditions (such as intoxication and severe metabolic derangements) result in altered level of consciousness as well.

STROKE

Stroke, or cerebrovascular accident, is one of the leading causes of death in the United States. Patients with stroke often have a history of hypertension, diabetes, cardiac disease, hyperlipidemia, smoking, drug or alcohol abuse, and family history of stroke. Strokes are divided into two main categories: ischemic (absence of blood flow) and hemorrhagic (bleeding); however, the two can be difficult to differentiate using clinical signs and symptoms. A majority of people experiencing a stroke will experience an ischemic stroke. Black Americans are at greater risk than white Americans for experiencing and dying from a stroke. Women have a greater risk than men of dying from a stroke, as well. While strokes can lead to permanent disability or death, a patient may alternatively experience temporary ischemia to a specific portion of the brain without permanent disability, known as a transient ischemic attack.

Signs and Symptoms

The onset is usually an abrupt altered level of consciousness accompanied by hemiparesis or hemiplegia. Patients may experience confusion, memory impairment, aphasia, ataxia, or visual disturbance. Signs and symptoms vary with the location and severity of the stroke. Mentation and cognitive changes may be temporary or permanent, depending on the extent of injury. Communication alterations stemming from fluent or receptive aphasia may be mistaken for dementia.

Diagnostic Studies

A CT scan, without contrast, is the preferred imaging study in early stroke because hemorrhage may be difficult to determine on an MRI in the first 48 hours. Although many hospitals recommend plain CT for diagnosis, CTA gives a more comprehensive and detailed picture of the stroke etiology. In studies of ischemic stroke patients, researchers have shown the reversibility of abnormalities on CT or MRI through the use of thrombolytic therapy within a 3-hour window.

PARKINSON'S DISEASE

Parkinson's disease (PD) is a common neurodegenerative disease affecting middle-aged to older adults. Although altered mental status is usually not the first manifestation of PD, mild cognitive dysfunction is often seen. Because of the flat affect and facies that patients with PD exhibit, these symptoms may be mistaken for psychosis, depression, or dementia, which can often coexist. PD occurs in all ethnic groups, with approximately equal sex distribution, and usually begins between ages 45 and 65 years. Another form of PD, known as *posttraumatic parkinsonism* or *dementia pugilistica*, is a combination of dementia and parkinsonism that develops in boxers or persons sustaining repeated blows to the head. Parkinsonian symptoms may also occur secondary to a number of other causes, including medications, infections, and toxins. The following discussion is not inclusive of the range of secondary parkinsonism.

Signs and Symptoms

Unilateral pill-rolling tremor at rest is often the first symptom. The tremor is maximal at rest but absent during sleep and can be differentiated from essential tremor, which is absent at rest and worsens with voluntary movement. The bradykinesia of PD affects gross and fine motor movement, speech volume, swallowing, and blinking. While the patient will have rigidity, there is generally no muscle weakness, and deep tendon reflexes are normal. Although Alzheimer's disease can also manifest with rigidity, bradykinesia, and gait disorders, no resting tremor is seen with Alzheimer's. Nonspecific secondary manifestations include cognitive dysfunction, sleep disturbances, constipation, dysphagia, blurred or double vision, nocturia, frequency, urgency, autonomic dysfunction (e.g., erectile dysfunction), dizziness, and drooling.

Diagnostic Studies

No diagnostic studies are specific to PD, and the patient should be referred to a neurologist for definitive diagnosis. If secondary parkinsonism is suspected, laboratory studies such as a metabolic profile or toxicology screens may be warranted.

Due to a lack of definitive diagnostics, there is a high rate of missed diagnosis of PD. MRI can be used to rule out masses or structural pathology of the brain, if warranted. A U.S. Food and Drug Administration (FDA)–approved specialized imaging technique called DaTscan captures detailed pictures of the dopamine system in the brain. Although DaTscan is not definitive, it can be used as a tool to assist in the diagnosis of parkinsonian syndrome.

NORMAL PRESSURE HYDROCEPHALUS

The etiology of normal pressure hydrocephalus is not fully understood. It is seen primarily in persons older than 60 years and involves enlargement of the ventricles with excess CSF, often without increased CSF pressure. Intraventricular pressures may be high or normal. Blockages of CSF circulation from tumor, trauma, hemorrhage, or infection can result in the development of normal pressure hydrocephalus. Another theorized cause includes intermittent pressure increases. This is slightly more common in men than in women.

Signs and Symptoms

The patient often first notices some degree of gait disorder, followed by the onset of a "clouding" of thought processes, which gradually progresses. The typical picture is a patient who has a triad of gait disturbance, altered thought processes, and urinary incontinence. Strength and sensation are usually within normal limits. However, focal neurological findings are present and include increased deep tendon reflexes, the inability to tandem walk, positive Babinski, and/or positive Romberg. This condition can worsen over time and requires surgical intervention.

Diagnostic Studies

Imaging with MRI or CT can provide for a definitive diagnosis.

TUMOR

See p. 568.

BRAIN ABSCESS AND CNS INFECTION

See pp. 566 and 568.

ORGANIC, PROGRESSIVE DEMENTIAS

Dementia generally affects persons older than 60 years; however, people in the fourth and fifth decades of life can show mental status changes as a result of some other offending cause. Approximately 15% of people older than 70 years will experience dementia, which involves a substantial cognitive loss and decrease in mental ability. Alzheimer's dementia is a frequent cause of progressive organic dementia. Other causes with similar findings include Pick's disease, alcoholism-related dementia, PD, and the causes discussed separately in previous entries. Chapters 18 and 21 also include brief discussions of progressive dementia of this type.

Signs and Symptoms

Unlike delirium, most organic dementias develop over months to years. There are typically no physical motor or sensory alterations until the condition is advanced. Memory impairment is the predominant symptom; however, cognition, personality, and language are affected. There may be impairment in another area of cognitive functioning, such as with aphasia (producing language and understanding it), agnosia (perceptual impairments not due to dysfunction of the primary sensory organ), apraxia (inability to perform complex motor acts), and impairment in executive functioning (inability to plan, organize, sequence, and think abstractly). Progressive mental status changes associated with focal motor or sensory findings should not be attributed to Alzheimer's or Pick's diseases.

Diagnostic Studies

The studies are based on patient history and presentation. It is crucial to rule out any correctible cause of confusion or altered mental status, such as drug toxicity or other medical condition, in a timely manner.

■ Dizziness and Vertigo

Patients interpret the subjective complaint of dizziness and vertigo differently, and clinicians at times use the words interchangeably. With vertigo, the patient experiences a spinning sensation or a sensation that their surroundings are rotating or spinning; however, with dizziness, the patient experiences light-headedness or unsteadiness. Table 16.4 differentiates between light-headedness and dizziness or vertigo.

History

The dimensions of the symptom are important to understand, particularly onset and duration, because many cases of dizziness are paroxysmal, short, and self-limiting. Dizziness that is not vertigo is often associated with quick movement or bending over and is often worse upon first arising in the morning or when

Table 16.4	
Causes of Vertigo and Light-headedness	
Symptom	Causes
Light-headedness/presyncope (sense of faintness)	Dehydration Hypotension Hypoglycemia/hyperglycemia Heart block Infection Cardiovascular and cerebellar perfusion
Vertigo/disequilibrium (sense of motion/spinning)	Vestibular disturbances Middle ear disturbance Cerebellar

rising from a recumbent position. Vertigo, by contrast, describes the sense of spinning. It can occur at any time of the day or night. Many people report vertigo associated with listing to one side while walking, often running into walls or doorjambs while walking. Nystagmus is often associated with vertigo but rarely with dizziness. Nausea and vomiting can be associated with both dizziness and vertigo.

Dizziness that becomes frequent or lasts extended periods of time deserves closer investigation. Sustained periods of dizziness with near fainting can be a precursor to syncope or stroke and may have a neurovascular or cardiac etiology. Neurocardiogenic syncope, also called *vasovagal syncope*, is a common cause of dizziness and fainting and is caused by a sudden decrease in blood pressure and heart rate after prolonged standing, by stress, or by dehydration. It is a result of sympathetic sensitivity causing a reflexive response that suddenly causes bradycardia and venous dilation. Hypotension and dizziness result.

Dizziness can also be a precursor (or aura) of seizures. Dizziness that leads to disequilibrium can result in inability to drive, falls, and injuries, and can be quite disabling for some persons. Light-headedness in older persons or in persons with vascular insufficiency is not uncommon. It is crucial to identify any associated symptoms, specifically nausea, vomiting, fevers, vision changes, speech disturbances, and numbness or weakness of the face or extremities.

The history of head or ear trauma as well as exposure to infections should be determined. A thorough review of the patient's current medications must be included because polypharmacy can cause dizziness in many patients. Social and recreational history is important. Activities such as scuba diving, high-elevation hiking, or air travel can contribute to the development of dizziness, as can dehydration related to exercising in the heat. Other potential causes include vestibular dysfunction, causing transient dizziness and balance difficulties, and alcohol or substance abuse. Because dizziness can be associated with hyperventilation or anxiety, ask about a history of anxiety or panic attacks. Review the family history of stroke, seizures, Ménière's disease, or other conditions associated with dizziness or vertigo. Refer to the following Red Flag box that lists red flag presentations of dizziness.

Physical Examination

The neurological examination should focus on vital signs, gait, station, and CN function. Blood pressure should be taken both lying and standing, looking for orthostatic changes. Measure the rate and regularity of the pulse and obtain an electrocardiogram if necessary. Note fever, which might indicate infection. The examination should include an assessment of gait, including tandem walking. Gait ataxia is noted when patients are so uncoordinated that they cannot walk a straight line without stumbling. The Romberg test should be performed; a positive Romberg test is noted when the patient is unable to maintain an upright posture with feet together and arms extended and sways or falls to the side. The finger-to-nose test should be performed, observing for dysmetria, and rapid alternating movement is tested, observing the smoothness of motion.

RED FLAG	Red Flags in the Assessment of Patients With Dizziness/Vertigo

- *Near fainting or fainting*
- *Slurred speech, numbness of the face or limbs, or loss of limb movement*
- *Visual changes, particularly diplopia*
- *Acute onset, associated with nausea/vomiting*

CN testing is important, particularly CNs II, III, IV, and VI. The eye nerves are particularly sensitive to increases in intracranial pressure. Note any vision or pupillary changes; decreases in visual fields; and nystagmus on upward, downward, or lateral gaze with extraocular movements. Assess any asymmetry in facial sensation or movements (CN VII), which could indicate a transient ischemic attack or cerebrovascular accident or pressure on the nerve from a tumor. CN VIII is the most sensitive to test for vestibulocochlear abnormalities. Always perform the Rinne and Weber tests to localize hearing loss or tinnitus.

Diagnostic Studies

The studies useful in assessing dizziness are identified in Box 16.7.

Box 16.7

Diagnostic Studies for Dizziness

MRI of the brain with and without contrast will help to rule out evidence of a mass lesion or demyelinating process.

MRA of the head is used for imaging arteries (and less commonly veins) in order to evaluate for stenosis, occlusions, aneurysms, or other vascular abnormalities.

MRI of the internal auditory canal is sensitive for mass lesions on the inner ear and acoustic nerve.

Audiogram is useful for assessing inner ear and hearing damage. This can also be helpful in assessing inflammatory disorders.

Electronystagmogram is useful for determining eye movements in relation to a stimulus and helps with localizing the lesion to the nerve.

Carotid ultrasound or duplex will determine vascular insufficiency.

Brainstem and auditory evoked potentials help with determining whether the defect lies with the nerve or within the inner ear.

Tilt table test can be performed to rule out neurocardiogenic syncope.

Home blood pressure monitoring may be helpful for those patients with hypo- or hypertension-induced dizziness.

CENTRAL NERVOUS SYSTEM LESIONS

The causes of CNS vertigo include brainstem vascular disease or tumor, arteriovenous malformations, cerebellar tumor, multiple sclerosis (MS), and vertebrobasilar migraine (Douglas & Aminoff, 2021).

Signs and Symptoms

The findings depend on the location and progression of the lesion. Most patients present with disequilibrium or dizziness. Children may present with gait disorders.

Vertigo from central lesions is constant and causes difficulties with the activities of daily living. Other symptoms may be present, such as CN dysfunction, diplopia, dysarthria, motor and sensory dysfunction, nausea and vomiting, and cerebellar dysfunction.

Diagnostic Studies

An MRI of the brain with and without contrast is the test of choice for diagnosis of central lesions. An MRI of the internal auditory canal is sensitive for mass lesions on the inner ear and acoustic nerve.

MÉNIÈRE'S DISEASE

The exact cause of Ménière's disease is unknown; however, the symptoms are associated with increased fluid and pressure in the labyrinth. This affects men and women with an equal distribution and typically occurs in adults between ages 30 and 60 years. Allergies, alcohol, caffeine, and hormonal fluctuation are believed to be risk factors in the development of Ménière's disease.

Signs and Symptoms

Ménière's disease commonly involves a triad of symptoms: severe vertigo, tinnitus, and sensorineural hearing loss. The vertigo is transient but recurrent. The tinnitus and hearing loss may also be intermittent or recurrent but often become worse over time. A sensation of ear fullness may precede an episode. During the episode, vertigo is often debilitating and is associated with nausea and vomiting. Although the tinnitus and hearing loss are usually unilateral, some patients experience bilateral symptoms. Vestibular maneuvers, including the Nylen-Barany test, are often positive, reproducing the patient's complaint. An otoscopic examination should be performed to evaluate for associated pathology such as otitis media or cholesteatoma.

Diagnostic Studies

Although not specific to Ménière's disease, an audiogram is helpful to confirm hearing loss. Rinne and Weber tests should be performed to assess for sensorineural hearing loss. The patient will exhibit laterization of sound to the unaffected ear due to the sensorineural hearing loss. Because the symptoms and findings of Ménière's disease and acoustic neuroma are so similar, an MRI is helpful to exclude tumor. A number of other studies, including auditory evoked potentials, are typically performed by specialists.

CENTRAL AUDITORY AND VESTIBULAR SYSTEM DYSFUNCTION

Diseases in this category include acoustic neuroma, vascular compromise, and MS. Acoustic neuromas are benign and are one of the most common intracranial tumors. Due to their location, they can compress CN VIII and cause hearing loss and difficulty with speech discrimination. While they are benign, acoustic neuromas can grow large enough to be life threatening.

Vertebrobasilar insufficiency is seen mostly in older persons and is exacerbated by extension of the neck or changes in head position. Migraines and vascular loops may cause vascular compromise and vertigo. MS can also cause chronic imbalance and unilateral hearing loss. See under "Weakness" in Chapter 17.

Signs and Symptoms

The vertigo from central lesions is more likely to be persistent and chronic rather than intermittent, as is seen with other causes of vertigo. The dizziness may be described as a constant sense of disequilibrium rather than a true vertigo. Unlike benign positional vertigo, central and vestibular nystagmus is "often nonfatigable, vertical rather than horizontal in orientation, without latency, and unsuppressed by visual fixation" (Lui et al., 2021). Unilateral hearing loss should be suspect for acoustic neuroma or MS. A history of migraines may suggest vascular compromise.

Diagnostic Studies

An MRI with and without contrast of the internal auditory canal is necessary for a definitive diagnosis of acoustic neuroma. An MRA or a cerebral angiogram is used to diagnose vascular abnormalities. An LP and an MRI with and without contrast are necessary for a diagnosis of MS.

VIRAL (SEROUS) OR BACTERIAL (SUPPURATIVE) LABYRINTHITIS

Labyrinthitis is caused by the invasion of the ear by bacteria or a virus leading to inflammation of the vestibulocochlear nerve. Bacterial labyrinthitis is more serious because it may lead to meningitis. Prompt treatment with antibiotics is necessary.

Signs and Symptoms

Labyrinthitis is characterized by severe vertigo, nystagmus, and sensorineural hearing loss. Suppurative labyrinthitis may be secondary to bacterial otitis media or other bacterial infection. Serous labyrinthitis can be secondary to a variety of viral illnesses, including measles, mumps, chickenpox, influenza, mononucleosis, and adenovirus. Some patients complain of nausea, vomiting, diaphoresis, and visual disturbances. A comprehensive neurological examination to include CN assessment and otoscopic examination should be performed.

Diagnostic Studies

The diagnosis is mainly made by history and physical examination. A CBC or mono spot can assist in the diagnosis, and a culture of the fluid from the middle ear will differentiate a bacterial from a viral cause. Rinne and Weber tests should be performed to assess for sensorineural hearing loss. The patient will exhibit laterization of sound to the unaffected ear due to the sensorineural hearing loss.

CHOLESTEATOMA

See Chapter 7.

HEAD TRAUMA/PERILYMPHATIC FISTULA

A fistula may form from a blow to the head or from barotrauma significant enough to cause a rupture of or fissures in the round or the oval window. Other causes include whiplash, inability to equalize the ears during scuba diving, or ear/ear drum trauma. Perilymphatic fluid from the inner ear escapes to the middle ear through fistula.

Signs and Symptoms

Vertigo, ataxia, nausea, vomiting, and hearing loss can result from this fistula. A patient may complain of fullness of the ear and dizziness. A medical history provides the necessary information for an index of suspicion for this cause of dizziness. Sneezing, coughing, lifting heavy objects, or changes in altitude can all potentially worsen a patient's symptoms.

Diagnostic Studies

In addition to a good history, a CT scan or MRI of the head can assist in the diagnosis. Surgical repair is necessary.

BENIGN PAROXYSMAL POSITIONAL VERTIGO/ CUPULOLITHIASIS

Benign paroxysmal positional vertigo, or cupulolithiasis, is the most common vestibular disorder, resulting from otolithic crystals/particles detaching from the utricle membrane and migrating to the semicircular canal. It can occur spontaneously with motion or position change or as a result of vascular or labyrinth trauma.

Signs and Symptoms

Characterized by sudden-onset dizziness lasting 30 to 60 seconds and following a head position change, cupulolithiasis may be accompanied by nystagmus. A patient may also experience nausea, vomiting, or difficulty with balance. It usually subsides but may recur at any time. Three characteristics that differentiate benign positional vertigo from vertigo caused by a central lesion include a latency period of several seconds from head movement to vertigo, symptoms that subside in 10 to 60 seconds, and repetition of the positional change leading to habituation (decreased responsiveness to repeated stimulus). In central lesions, there is no latency, no fatigability, and no habituation.

Diagnostic Studies

In addition to the history, a provocative test for positional nystagmus can be performed (Hallpike maneuver), although it is not always positive. The provocative test involves moving the patient quickly from a sitting position to a lying position with the head turned to the side and the head dependent over the side of the examination table. After a few seconds, vertigo and nystagmus occur. This response fatigues with immediate repetition of the test. A CT scan or MRI may be necessary to rule out CNS lesions; however, the vertigo associated with CNS lesions is not as severe, does not have a latency period, and does not fatigue. The Epley repositioning maneuver, also called *vestibular exercises*, can assist in alleviating the problem.

■ Tremors

Tremors make up the largest category of movement disorders. The etiology is vast, with a recent consensus statement classifying etiologies as acquired, genetically defined, or idiopathic. A tremor is "an involuntary, rhythmic, oscillatory movement of a body part" due to muscle groups cycling between contraction and relaxation (Bhatia et al., 2018).

History

History should include details surrounding the onset of the tremors, including the approximate date or age of onset, any perceived precipitating factors (e.g., stress, illness, medications), and progression since onset. A past medical history and family history should explore conditions such as essential tremor, neurodegenerative diseases (e.g., PD, MS), epilepsy, and thyroid disease. Past medical history should further include history of brain injury, stroke, and infectious diseases. Ask about substance use; obtain a history of all prescribed and OTC drugs/agents. Symptoms related to the tremor, and underlying pathology, may be revealed through a thorough review of systems. Ask the patient to describe the actual tremor. If necessary, ask about fine, pill-rolling, dystonic, jerky, and other movements, demonstrating what is meant by these terms, if necessary. Ask whether the tremors are associated with action or rest, as well as any actions that stimulate or alleviate the tremor. Determine which body parts are involved, as well as any accompanying symptoms (e.g., altered balance, gait, voice change, mental status). Many presentations may be confused with tremors, including tics, asterixis, epilepsy, clonus, and myoclonus. Inquire if, and how, the tremor affects the patient's activities of daily living.

Physical Examination

Physical examination should include a general observation of the patient during the history, noting fluidity of speech, any abnormal movement, signs of illness, and so on. A thorough neurological examination should be completed, noting the presence or absence of any tremors during this period. It is critical to conduct a focused assessment of the abnormal movement or tremor, recognizing that physiological tremors (very fine tremors occurring when a position is held against gravity and do not cause difficulties) are normal.

Tremors are generally categorized as positional, resting, or intentional. Resting tremors are commonly associated with PD or parkinsonian disorders. Causes of intentional tremors include conditions such as essential tremor and cerebellar disease. When assessing for tremor, face the patient so that the affected and contralateral sides are visible. As you inspect and the patient is instructed to assume different positions, spend up to 30 seconds assessing each position; a tremor may initiate or cease only after a brief period when a new position is assumed.

When assessing for tremor at rest, the associated body part must be placed in a fully relaxed and supported position. For a tremor of the neck, head, upper arms, or lower limbs, this generally requires reclining. For hands and forearms, an armchair can usually provide adequate support for the patient during assessment for a resting tremor. Cognitive and motor distraction techniques can optimize resting tremor assessment by either increasing or decreasing the amplitude of the tremor. Cognitive distraction methods include having the patient perform a serial sevens test or list types of objects (e.g., vegetables, car models) during the examination; motor distraction methods include actions such as tapping the contralateral hand or foot and forming then releasing contralateral fist. Postural tremor should be assessed with the affected body part held against gravity—for example, arms elevated with hands both supinated and pronated. Intentional tremors can be assessed by having the patient perform simple movements (finger-to-nose test) and more intentional movements (writing or drawing) (van der Wardt et al., 2020). Document presence or absence of tremor in varied positions, noting amplitude and general description of any involuntary movement detected. The literature often differentiates between tremors based on the frequency or "speed" of tremor repetitions per second, using the term *hertz* (Hz). These measures require equipment such as an accelerometer. Recent research supports the potential for tremor assessment using smartphones and other mobile health devices (Fuchs et al., 2021). These descriptions of frequency help clinicians understand the variations common among different tremors.

Diagnostic Studies

The need for diagnostic studies is dependent on the suspected cause. For essential, physiological, or psychogenic tremors, no additional studies may be warranted. Studies that may be considered include electromyography to better document characteristics of a tremor, imaging if neurological lesions are suspected, and laboratory studies if a metabolic disease, infection, or genetic condition is suspected (Bhatia et al., 2018). However, referral to a neurologist or movement specialist will expedite definitive diagnosis of other conditions.

RED FLAG	Red Flags in the Assessment of Patients With Tremors

- *Sudden onset and progression*
- *Mental status change*
- *Focal neurological signs*
- *Metabolic symptoms*

ESSENTIAL TREMOR

An essential tremor may affect almost any body part, although the hands, head, and voice are commonly involved. Onset is gradual, usually after age 40 years. Risk increases with age and among those with a family history. Progression is usually slow, and the tremors are generally benign. However, the tremors can impact ability to perform daily and recreational activities as the tremors typically occur with intentional movement. The term "ET Plus" is used when the primary symptom of tremor is accompanied by other findings, such as resting tremor or ataxia.

Signs and Symptoms

Patient has history of slow progression of an intentional tremor, commonly affecting upper limbs, head, and voice. Symptoms are usually bilateral, and the tremor frequency is faster than that of PD. The patient may describe improvement with alcohol intake and worsening with stress. When the head is involved, the tremor is often a side-to-side motion, as if saying "No." Voice involvement can be enhanced by having the patient hold a long syllable, such as "AAAA" or "EEEE."

Diagnostic Studies

Diagnostic studies are usually not required unless specific pathology needs to be ruled out. The diagnosis is typically based on history and clinical examination.

PARKINSON'S DISEASE/PARKINSONIAN TREMOR

PD and secondary parkinsonism have slow and progressive onsets. PD involves degeneration of basal ganglia cell groups resulting in decreased dopamine release and uptake. Although tremor is not always present, a unilateral resting tremor involving a hand (or foot) is often the first symptom noticed. The tremor of the hand or fingers is generally slow and rhythmic. PD tremor can affect other body parts. Bradykinesia, with slow and rigid movements, and postural instability, with altered gait and risk of fall, are common. PD is complex and difficult to diagnose; patients often have had symptoms of the condition for years before a definitive diagnosis is made.

Signs and Symptoms

Initial complaints may include history of resting tremor, postural instability with history of falls, and altered gait. Family members may report changes such as altered facial expression, softening of voice, diminished size of handwriting, and apathy. The resting tremor generally disappears with intentional action. The patient may have difficulty rising from a chair and initiating ambulation. Rigidity of the extremities can be accompanied by a ratchet-like or cogwheel type of movement. A flexed posture may be noticed as the disease progresses. Patients with PD often exhibit dysphagia, hyperhidrosis, dysarthria, a "mask-like" appearance of the face, and urinary urgency. Cognitive, personality, and behavioral changes are not uncommon with patients experiencing PD. Balance can be tested by pulling the patient's shoulders from behind to test ability to correct. Repetitive motions such as toe tapping or opening and closing a fist are often slower in the affected hand or in comparison to the norm. The Movement Disorders Society Unified Parkinson's Disease Rating Scale (MDS-UPDRS) is available online and provides a psychometrically tested means of analyzing a patient. However, it is time consuming to administer and requires knowledge of the maneuvers.

Diagnostic Studies

Diagnosis of PD is clinical and best made by movement disorder specialists. Referral to a movement disorder clinic is ideal.

MULTIPLE SCLEROSIS

MS is a disease associated with periods of relapse and remission with varied symptoms. The tremors associated with MS are intermittent, usually associated with intentional movement and involuntary muscle contractions. MS is also associated with nystagmus. See Chapter 17.

PSYCHOGENIC TREMOR

Psychogenic tremor is one of several psychogenic movement disorders. The cause is not well understood, as history of traumatic events is not universal among persons with this diagnosis. Psychogenic tremors most often affect the hand; they are more common among women. Completion of a thorough psychosocial history is important, in addition to the relevant past medical history, family history, review of systems, and symptom analysis. Close observation may reveal that a patient is able to complete certain movements when distracted, but not during the examination. Associated psychiatric diagnoses are common.

Signs and Symptoms

Psychogenic tremor has a sudden onset and may be associated with a precipitating situation. The tremor may be present with both rest and movement and have a spontaneous remission. Tremors are often inconsistent with any of the classified organic causes of tremors; often complex in nature; not limited to rest, posture, or intention; and/or involve unusual distribution patterns. Movements during the examination may reflect more effort or weakness than would be expected and are accompanied by facial expressions such as grimacing.

Diagnostic Studies

When psychogenic tremor is suspected, refer to a movement disorder specialist. In this way, neurophysiological studies can be conducted, often with added imaging and/or laboratory studies to evaluate potential organic causes.

DRUG-INDUCED TREMORS

Many medications can cause either resting or action tremors. Accurate diagnosis requires a thorough medication history. While some medications may cause tremors soon after they are initiated, others may have delayed onset of tremor, associated with elevated levels. Some antiseizure, asthma, antidepressant, or antihypertensive medications can cause tremor. Withdrawal of substances (alcohol and drugs) is also associated with tremors. The tremors may occur at rest or with movement.

METABOLICALLY INDUCED TREMORS

Tremors are associated with numerous metabolic derangements. These include hypoglycemia, hyperthyroidism, hepatic disorders, and many electrolyte disturbances. Serum laboratory studies will be directed toward identification of a metabolic cause for a tremor.

REFERENCES

Bhatia, K., Bain, P., Bajaj, N., Elbel, R., Hallett, M., Louis, E., Raethjen, J., Stamelou, M., Testa, C., Deuschl, G., & the Tremor Task Force of the International Parkinson and Movement Disorder Society. (2018). Consensus statement on the classification of tremors. From the task force on tremor of the International Parkinson and Movement Disorder Society. *Movement Disorders, 33*(1), 75–87.

Douglas, V. C., & Aminoff, M. J. (2021). Nervous system disorders. In M. A. Papadakis, S. J. McPhee, & M. W. Rabow (Eds.), *CURRENT: Medical diagnosis & treatment* (60th ed., pp. 1032–1037). McGraw Hill.

Fuchs, C., Nobile, M., Zamora, G., Degeneffe, A., Kubben, P., & Kaymak, U. (2021). Tremor assessment using smartphone sensor data and fuzzy reasoning. *BMC Bioinformatics, 22*(suppl. 2). https://dx.doi.org /10.1186%2Fs12859-021-03961-8

International Headache Society. (2018). Classification of headaches disorders. Accessed July 29, 2021, from https://ichd-3.org

Lui, F., Foris, L. A., Willner, K., & Tadi, P. (2021). Central vertigo. In: StatPearls [Internet]. Treasure Island (FL): StatPearls Publishing; 2022 Jan. Available from: https://www.ncbi.nlm.nih.gov/books/NBK441861/

McCormack, R. F., & Hutson, A. (2010). Can computed tomography angiography of the brain replace lumbar puncture in the evaluation of acute-onset headache after a negative noncontrast cranial computed tomography scan? *Academic Emergency Medicine, 17*(4), 444–451.

Van der Wardt, J., van der Stouwe, A., Dirkx, M., Eltin, J., Post, B., Tijssen, M., & Helmich, R. (2020). Systematic clinical approach for diagnosis upper limb tremor. *Journal of Neurology, Neurosurgery, and Psychiatry, 91*(8), 822–830.

Chapter 17

Nonspecific Complaints

• Laurie Grubbs

History and Physical Examination

Some of the more challenging chief complaints for any health-care practitioner are those "generic" complaints that have a multitude of causations, such as fatigue, weakness, dizziness, numbness/tingling, headache, and so on. Deciding on which system to start with is often difficult. Because there are so many possibilities for the origin of these complaints, all systems should be considered, although the neurological and cardiac systems are often a good place to start. Proceed with the history in the typical format because the complaint may be related to past health problems, medications, a familial or genetic predisposition, or simply a new-onset problem. Be sure to include in your review of systems the questions under the general assessment, such as weight loss, changes in appetite or nutritional patterns, fevers, chills, night sweats, lethargy, weakness, inability to perform the activities of daily life, and changes in mental status. Pay attention to the general appearance and behavior of the patient, including personal hygiene, dress, grooming, speech patterns, mood, and affect. Patients who are depressed or ill may show signs of poor hygiene and flat affect.

Differential Diagnosis of Chief Complaints

■ Fatigue

A complaint of fatigue has strong psychological overtones, making it extremely important to consider a psychological as well as a physical cause. There are a multitude of possible causes of clinically significant fatigue, including hyperthyroidism, hypothyroidism, infection, diabetes, heart disease, autoimmune disorders, renal disease, hematologic disorders, lung disease, cancer, sleep disturbances, medications, nonprescription drugs, alcohol, stress, anxiety, or depression.

History

Key symptoms to inquire about include generalized weakness, easy fatigability, and mental fatigue. A thorough medication history, including over-the-counter drugs, is imperative. Ask about tobacco, alcohol, and other drug use. Investigate a history or family history of cardiac, respiratory, endocrine, gastrointestinal (GI), or hematologic disease. A family history of type 2 diabetes mellitus (DM) presents a significant risk for the patient developing it as well. Thyroid disease seems to show a family predisposition. A history of anemia in a patient with fatigue should raise the index of suspicion for chronicity. Always ask the date of the last menstrual period for a young woman regardless of whether she is using oral contraceptives. Other common causes, particularly in older patients, include arrhythmias, congestive heart failure (CHF), infection, and malignancy. Two uncommon causes of fatigue could be adrenal dysfunction (e.g., Addison's and Cushing's diseases), but patients might describe weakness rather than fatigue, especially in the case of Cushing's disease, in which there is muscle wasting. It is important to take a thorough psychosocial history as part of the review of systems. Ask about living arrangements, relationships with family and significant others, environment, occupational history, economic status (including job satisfaction), daily profile (rest–activity patterns, exercise habits, social activities), and patterns of health care. In today's society, it is not uncommon for a person to be working, caring for children, and caring for older parents, possibly as a single parent and sole family support. People are often not aware of the physical toll that long-term stress can take on the body and immune system.

Physical Examination

The physical examination should follow most closely with the system suspected as causing the fatigue, although other systems should be included. The practitioner's index of suspicion involves many variables, including age of the patient, current health, past history, and presenting symptoms. As usual, vital signs are a good place to start. Hypotension, bradycardia, tachycardia, or fever could indicate a cardiac or infectious cause as well as Addison's disease. Unexplained weight loss might indicate a thyroid disease, DM, Addison's disease, malignancy, or depression. In the head, ears, eyes, nose, and throat examination, pay particular attention to the thyroid and lymph system. Significant findings in the cardiac examination include an arrhythmia or murmur, which might be compromising cardiac output, or ventricular hypertrophy, which might indicate heart failure. Electrocardiogram (EKG) changes may demonstrate the ventricular hypertrophy seen in heart failure or the conduction delays as seen in Addison's disease. Shortness of breath, tachypnea, or adventitious sounds may indicate a cardiac or respiratory cause of the fatigue. Masses in the abdomen might indicate a malignancy. Bruits, particularly over the renal arteries, could affect blood flow to the kidneys, giving rise to renal impairment and fatigue. Skin changes may be seen in thyroid disease, with dry skin seen in hypothyroidism and moist skin in hyperthyroidism, or in Addison's disease, which causes hyperpigmentation. A thorough neurological assessment is also in order, especially in older patients, because depression and dementia are more common and could present as fatigue or lethargy. The remainder of the assessment involves laboratory or other diagnostics, which are discussed under each differential diagnosis.

STRESS, ANXIETY, DEPRESSION, AND DYSTHYMIA

Psychiatric disorders may be responsible for complaints of fatigue in the primary care setting and may manifest as physical illness, injury, or drug and alcohol abuse. With the increased acceptance and recognition of depression as an illness, and with the treatment choices now available, patients are much more likely to seek help for depression. Often, they are not aware of being depressed, and they present with somatic symptoms such as fatigue.

Signs and Symptoms

Subjectively, patients admit to feelings of sadness, hopelessness, and worthlessness with diminished interest in both work and recreation. There may be cognitive complaints, such as difficulty thinking and concentrating, obsessive ruminations, and difficulty making decisions. There may be difficulty sleeping, appetite changes, loss of energy, and decreased libido. Often depression is accompanied by anxiety, agitation, or various somatic complaints, such as fatigue, headache, nausea, and irritability.

Diagnostic Studies

There are many diagnostic tools to evaluate depression and other psychiatric problems. The Beck Inventory of Depression I and II are widely used. In clinical family practice, abbreviated "bedside questionnaires" can be used to evaluate the patient for referral to a mental health counselor. A detailed discussion of stress, anxiety, depression, and dysthymia can be found in Chapter 18.

TYPE 2 DIABETES MELLITUS

The incidence of type 2 DM in the United States has risen dramatically in the last two decades, mainly owing to the rise in obesity. The Centers for Disease Control and Prevention (CDC) estimates that there are 34.2 million people in the United States with diabetes (1 in 10) and an additional 88 million with pre-diabetes (1 in 3) (CDC, 2020a). Patients who are overweight and sedentary, with a positive family history, are at high risk for developing type 2 DM.

Signs and Symptoms

Polydipsia, polyphagia, and polyuria are the hallmark signs of diabetes, but fatigue, unexplained weight loss, and blurred vision are often the symptoms that bring patients into the office.

Diagnostic Studies

According to the American Diabetes Association, a fasting glucose level higher than 126 mg/dL and/or a HgbA1c higher than 6.5% mmol/mol is considered diagnostic for diabetes. A glucose tolerance test (GTT) can also be done to look for fluctuations in glucose metabolism but is used infrequently. A test of the hemoglobin A1c level gives an estimation of blood glucose over the previous 3 months and is the gold standard for diagnosing, monitoring, and managing diabetes.

HYPOTHYROIDISM

Primary hypothyroidism is the most common form of hypothyroidism and is thought to be autoimmune in origin. Secondary hypothyroidism is due to a failure of the hypothalamic-pituitary axis. There are numerous causes of hypothyroidism, including Hashimoto's thyroiditis; iodine deficiency; genetic thyroid enzyme defects; medications (amiodarone, iodine-containing contrast media, lithium, methimazole, phenylbutazone, sulfonamides, aminoglutethimide, interferon-α); thyroid cancer; and infiltrative disorders, such as sarcoidosis, amyloidosis, scleroderma, cystinosis, and hemochromatosis. In general, the incidence of hypothyroidism is greater in women and more common in people older than 40 years.

Signs and Symptoms

Because the onset of hypothyroidism can be insidious, patients may not be aware that their thyroid levels have diminished. The severity of symptoms ranges from unrecognized states found only by thyroid-stimulating hormone (TSH) screening to striking myxedema. Symptoms include fatigue, cold intolerance, constipation, modest weight gain, depression, menorrhagia, hoarseness, dry skin and hair, cool skin with slow capillary refill, paresthesias of the hands and feet, bradycardia, cognitive dullness, delayed deep tendon reflexes (DTRs), periorbital edema, anemia, and hyponatremia. The thyroid may be of normal size or enlarged and nodular, depending on the cause. In rare and extreme cases, myxedematous coma may ensue, with severe hypothermia, hypoventilation, hyponatremia, hypoxia, hypercapnia, hypotension, and seizures. In older patients, the presenting symptom may be CHF. Also see the subsection on goiter in Chapter 5.

Diagnostic Studies

Whereas the physical examination may raise the index of suspicion, the measurement of TSH and free T_4 confirms the diagnosis. Because thyroid function requires a feedback loop between the pituitary gland and the thyroid gland, in hypothyroidism, the free T_4 levels are below normal and the TSH is above normal. A thyroid ultrasound and thyroid radionuclide scan are helpful for determining the size and differentiation of nodules.

MALIGNANCY

A malignancy any place in the body may cause the patient to feel fatigued. It is often an indirect cause of fatigue stemming from anemia, shortness of breath, decreased appetite, nausea and vomiting, decreased renal function, or a variety of other symptoms caused by the malignancy.

Signs and Symptoms

The signs and symptoms depend on the system where the malignancy exists. If a patient presents with a primary complaint of fatigue, an index of suspicion for a malignancy should alert you to ask about other signs or symptoms the patient might have noticed. If malignancy is advanced enough to cause fatigue, there are usually other symptoms present.

Diagnostic Studies

The diagnostics also depend on the system thought to be involved. A complete blood count (CBC), urinalysis, complete metabolic profile, liver function tests, and a chest x-ray are helpful. Depending on the age of the patient, a mammogram and/or colonoscopy may be warranted. New-onset anemia, especially in an older person, should be thoroughly investigated, as it may be secondary to blood loss as a result of colon cancer or decreased red blood cell (RBC) production due to a hematologic malignancy. Excessive use of anti-inflammatory medications may also cause new-onset anemia from an occult gastrointestinal bleed.

ANEMIA

The anemia may be primary or secondary to a hematologic disease or a malignancy. It is important to determine whether the anemia is due to decreased production or increased destruction of RBCs owing to diseases affecting the bone marrow, blood loss, or other hemolytic conditions. A patient with a history of anemia should alert the practitioner to start there with the differential diagnosis of fatigue. Ask about the cause or type of anemia and any past or current treatments.

Signs and Symptoms

Fatigue and decreased activity tolerance may be the symptoms that bring the patient to the clinic. The degree of fatigue is often proportional to the degree of anemia; however, patients with long-standing anemia compensate and may be asymptomatic, even with a significant anemia. Along with fatigue, the patient may appear pale with pale conjunctivae and mucous membranes. There may be neurological symptoms, such as paresthesias, or decreased proprioception, as is the case in B_{12} deficiency. Cardiac functioning may be affected with severe, long-standing anemia.

Diagnostic Studies

A CBC with differential is the first laboratory test to obtain. A reticulocyte count and red cell distribution width (RDW) assist in differentiating whether the anemia is due to increased destruction of RBCs, resulting in a high reticulocyte count and high RDW, or to decreased production of RBCs, resulting in a low reticulocyte count and low RDW. Bilirubin in the urine or an elevated serum bilirubin suggests RBC destruction. Serum iron, total iron-binding capacity, ferritin, and B_{12} tests give important information about the specific type of anemia. Positive hemoccult tests alert the practitioner to the need for a GI consultation to determine the source of bleeding. See Figures 17.1, 17.2, and 17.3 for anemia workups.

CHRONIC RENAL FAILURE

The main causes of chronic renal failure are diabetes and hypertension (greater than 50%). Polycystic kidney disease and glomerulonephritis account for another 12%, and the remaining causes are unknown (Dirkx & Woodell, 2021). The three stages of chronic renal failure are diminished renal reserve; renal

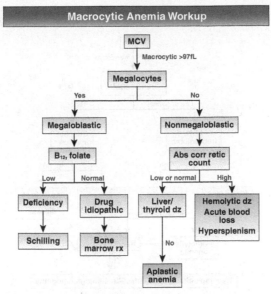

Figure 17.1 Macrocytic anemia workup. (From Lee, B. Y. [2009]. *Medical notes clinical medicine pocket guide.* Philadelphia, PA: F.A. Davis. Reprinted with permission.)

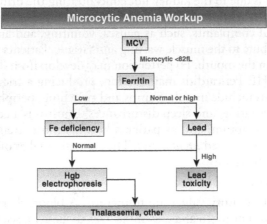

Figure 17.2 Microcytic anemia workup. (From Lee, B.Y. [2009]. *Medical notes clinical medicine pocket guide.* Philadelphia, PA: F.A. Davis. Reprinted with permission.)

insufficiency, in which azotemia develops and is reflected in elevations of plasma urea and creatinine; and uremia, which is accompanied by fluid and electrolyte imbalances.

Signs and Symptoms

Patients with mild renal dysfunction are generally asymptomatic, but as the disease progresses, vague symptoms appear. Fatigue and weakness are early signs, as are decreased cognitive functioning and irritability. Patients may complain of

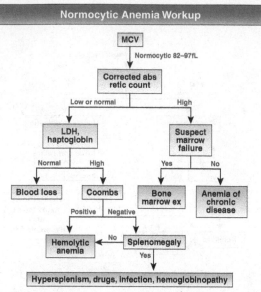

Figure 17.3 Normocytic anemia workup. (From Lee, B.Y. [2009]. *Medical notes clinical medicine pocket guide.* Philadelphia, PA: F.A. Davis. Reprinted with permission.)

nocturia, which is due to the kidney not concentrating the urine at night. Many of these early signs are nonspecific, and patients often pass them off as a normal part of aging. GI complaints, such as nausea, vomiting, and anorexia, are common and contribute to the muscle wasting and fatigue. Patients may complain of a metallic taste in the mouth. Hypertension may develop from fluid overload and can result in CHF. Pericarditis may develop, producing a friction rub. Neurological symptoms include muscle cramps and twitching, peripheral neuropathy, difficulty concentrating, and sleep disturbances. Pruritus is a common and very uncomfortable symptom, and as patients become more uremic, crystals may appear on the skin, termed *uremic frost.* The skin often takes on a yellow-brown tone with easy bruisability.

Diagnostic Studies

The abnormal laboratory values are numerous. A blood chemistry will reveal elevated blood urea nitrogen and creatinine. Metabolic acidosis, hyperphosphatemia, hypocalcemia, and hyperkalemia are present. A normocytic, normochromic anemia is present. Imaging studies of the kidney may be helpful if the chronic renal failure is due to a cystic or structural problem in the kidney. For additional information on renal failure, see Chapter 12.

ARRHYTHMIAS

Both atrial and ventricular arrhythmias may cause fatigue. They may be secondary to age, coronary artery disease, valvular heart disease, or endocrine diseases. Atrial fibrillation is very common in older patients, with an increased incidence due to the aging population. Other atrial and ventricular arrhythmias can occur at any age with or without the presence of other disorders. Supraventricular tachycardia is usually paroxysmal in nature and results from an abnormal pathway within or around the atrioventricular node. Intraventricular conduction delays may be seen in Addison's disease, in which fatigue is a common symptom. The only ventricular arrhythmias that might present with a complaint of fatigue are bigeminy or trigeminy. Ventricular tachycardia or ventricular fibrillation is life-threatening, and the patient generally does not remain conscious for any significant length of time after the onset of the arrhythmia.

Signs and Symptoms

In atrial fibrillation, the symptoms generally depend on the ventricular response rate. The patient may be very symptomatic, with shortness of breath, decreased exercise tolerance, and fatigue, or the patient may be completely asymptomatic. In supraventricular tachycardia, the rate is usually quite high, up to 200 beats per minute, and the patient is aware of palpitations. There may be accompanying complaints of shortness of breath and fatigue, particularly if the arrhythmia persists for any length of time. With bigeminy and trigeminy, patients are usually aware of palpitations or the sensation of missed beats. They may complain of shortness of breath and probably have more a complaint of weakness or lightheadedness than fatigue.

Diagnostic Studies

An EKG is a simple way to quickly and definitively diagnose an arrhythmia, as long as it is occurring when the patient presents to the office, clinic, or emergency department. A Holter monitor worn for 24 to 72 hours can detect a recurring arrhythmia not present at the time of the office or emergency department encounter. A detailed discussion of arrhythmias can be found in Chapter 8.

CONGESTIVE HEART FAILURE

CHF, commonly occurring in older patients or in patients with past myocardial infarctions or cardiomyopathy, can often present with complaints of fatigue, decreased activity tolerance, and/or shortness of breath. A detailed discussion of CHF can be found in Chapter 8.

CHRONIC OBSTRUCTIVE PULMONARY DISEASE

Chronic obstructive pulmonary disease such as chronic asthma/bronchitis, bronchiolitis, and emphysema may be associated with fatigue. These conditions are discussed in Chapter 9.

PREGNANCY

Females of child-bearing age should always be asked the date of their last menstrual period, and some index of suspicion should be present for any young female who presents with a complaint of fatigue.

Signs and Symptoms

A missed menstrual cycle, fatigue, breast tenderness, and nausea are the typical pregnancy signs and symptoms.

Diagnostic Studies

A urine or serum hCG is diagnostic.

MONONUCLEOSIS

Mononucleosis is a viral infection that typically occurs in adolescence and early adulthood and is caused by the Epstein-Barr virus. Mononucleosis is described in Chapter 7.

FIBROMYALGIA

Fatigue is a common finding in fibromyalgia and is described in detail in Chapter 15.

ADDISON'S DISEASE

Addison's disease is a chronic, progressive hypofunctioning of the adrenals caused by atrophy or destruction of the adrenal cortex, usually with an autoimmune origin. Other causes include medications, tuberculosis (TB), amyloidosis, malignancy, or inflammation. It affects everyone equally, regardless of gender, and can be seen in all ages. The main hormones produced by the adrenal gland are cortisol, aldosterone, and adrenal androgens. Addison's disease is characterized by electrolyte imbalance—there is an increase in Na^+ excretion and a decrease in K^+ excretion that leads to low blood levels of Na^+ and Cl^- and high levels of K^+. This produces volume depletion, dehydration, and hypotension. The cortisol deficiency causes alterations in carbohydrate, fat, and protein metabolism and in insulin sensitivity. The metabolic changes lead to hypoglycemia and decreased liver glycogen, causing fatigue and weakness. The decreased cortisol levels affect melanocyte-stimulating activities, thus producing the characteristic hyperpigmentation of the skin.

The acute form of the disease, termed *adrenal crisis*, is a more severe and life-threatening form, and it is characterized by profound weakness, severe abdominal and back pain, nausea, vomiting, diarrhea, confusion, renal shutdown, and circulatory collapse.

Signs and Symptoms

Weakness and fatigue are early signs of Addison's disease. The patient may complain of light-headedness owing to volume depletion, and orthostatic hypotension is found on examination. In most cases, the skin and mucous membranes are hyperpigmented, especially over creases, bony prominences, and nipples. The patient may complain of anorexia, nausea, vomiting, or diarrhea, and weight loss is evident. A complaint of light-headedness or syncope may lead the practitioner to do an EKG, which shows decreased voltage owing to a small heart and prolonged PR and QT intervals.

Diagnostic Studies

The blood chemistry findings suggestive of Addison's disease include low serum Ca^+, high K^+, elevated blood urea nitrogen, decrease in plasma bicarbonate, and low fasting glucose. The CBC may show an elevated hematocrit owing to volume depletion, a low white blood cell count, lymphocytosis, and increased eosinophils. Chest x-ray shows a small heart and possibly evidence of TB. Abdominal films may show calcifications in the adrenals and renal TB. More sophisticated tests can be performed using an adrenocorticotropic hormone (ACTH) challenge to determine its effect on plasma cortisol levels. Other tests can help to differentiate primary from secondary adrenal insufficiency, such as the insulin-induced hypoglycemia test, corticotropin-releasing hormone test, antibody screen, prolonged ACTH stimulation test, and imaging studies such as computed tomography (CT) and magnetic resonance imaging (MRI). Replacement of adrenal hormones results in a good prognosis for these patients.

■ Postacute COVID-19 Syndrome

Also known as "long COVID," postacute COVID-19 syndrome refers to patients who experience persistent symptoms of COVID-19 after the acute infection, which can last weeks to months. One study showed that for those patients who were hospitalized, over 75% had at least one symptom 6 months from acute infection. Women age 40 to 60 years are at greater risk of debilitating long-term symptoms (BMJ, 2021; Huang et al., 2021). Pediatric patients can also suffer from long COVID, but it may present differently than in adults and is not necessarily commensurate with the severity of the original illness (CDC, 2021).

Signs and Symptoms

Persistent symptoms vary but those most frequently reported include the following:

- Tiredness or fatigue
- Fever
- Difficulty thinking or concentrating (sometimes referred to as "brain fog")
- Vasomotor instability
- Headache
- Cognitive impairment, depression or anxiety
- Sleep disturbances
- Persistent loss of smell or taste
- Gastrointestinal dysmotility
- Dizziness on standing
- Tachycardia, palpitations, chest pain, postural tachycardia
- Difficulty breathing or shortness of breath, cough
- Joint or muscle pain
- Symptoms that get worse after physical or mental activities
- Multisystem inflammatory disorder

Diagnostic Studies

The etiology of the long-lasting effects of COVID-19 is still under investigation. Diagnostic tests and treatments are available based on the system(s) affected. Potential mechanisms for postacute COVID-19 syndrome include persistent cardiac or pulmonary injury, deconditioning, direct neuroinvasion of the brain or brainstem, damage of peripheral nerves, indirect neuronal injury and glial activation, persistent autoimmune inflammatory response, and mast cell activation.

Sleep Disorders

Sleep disorders can obviously contribute to fatigue and affect daily performance. Common disorders associated with sleep disturbances include insomnia; obstructive sleep apnea (OSA); restless leg syndrome; pain syndromes; substance abuse; CHF; asthma; stress, anxiety, depression, and dysthymia; and fibromyalgia.

History

The history should explore the type of sleep disturbance experienced. Determine how many hours the patient sleeps each night. Ask if the patient experiences trouble falling asleep, awakens through the night, or awakens early. Determine whether the patient feels rested upon awakening. A sleep diary may help to determine the type of disturbance experienced. A complete medical and mental health history are necessary to explore both physical and psychological etiology because there are numerous causes of sleep disturbances. Ask about chronic and acute conditions that could interfere with sleep, including those that affect the respiratory system, cause pain, or affect emotional state. A medication history may reveal that the patient is self-medicating in order to fall asleep or may identify medications that contribute to sleep alterations. A history of illegal drug or alcohol use is significant. A family history may help to uncover hereditary or psychosocial links. Living conditions and environmental exposures are important to explore, as are occupational and recreational activities. It is important to ask how, if at all, the altered sleep affects daily activities.

Physical Examination

Vital signs, body mass index (BMI), and oxygen saturation should be obtained. A thorough mental status and neurological examination is a good place to start. An examination of the mouth, throat, and respiratory system is necessary to assess for conditions that might cause OSA. Check for peripheral pulses, sensation, and edema in the lower extremities to assess for decreased circulation or neuropathy. Examine the thyroid for enlargement or nodularity and check for systemic signs and symptoms of thyroid disease.

PRIMARY INSOMNIA

Insomnia has a multitude of causes, including age, menopause, chronic illness, pain, stress, anxiety, depression, poor sleep habits, endocrine disorders, or medications. The *DSM-5* criteria for primary insomnia are as follows (American Psychiatric Association, 2013):

1. The sleep disturbance is defined as difficulty initiating or maintaining sleep, or nonrestorative sleep, for at least 1 month.
2. The sleep disturbance (or associated daytime fatigue) causes clinically significant distress or impairment in social, occupational, or other important areas of functioning.
3. The sleep disturbance does not occur exclusively during the course of narcolepsy, breathing-related sleep disorder, circadian rhythm sleep disorder, or a parasomnia.
4. The disturbance does not occur exclusively during the course of another mental disorder (e.g., major depressive disorder, generalized anxiety disorder, delirium).
5. The disturbance is not due to the direct physiological effects of a substance (e.g., drug or medication) or a general medical condition.

Signs and Symptoms

Daytime sleepiness, irritability, and cognitive impairment are the most common symptoms of insomnia. Patients may also complain of weight changes, anxiety, and depression.

Diagnostic Studies

A polysomnogram can be performed, but only to rule out physiological causes. It is important to ask the patient to keep a sleep diary for at least 1 week. A sleep history is important and should include estimated time to fall asleep, awakening time and total sleep time, number of times awakening during the night and amount of time staying awake, number and length of naps, amount and time of alcohol and caffeine intake, amount of stress during the day, amount of daily exercise, appetite during the day, level of fatigue and irritability during the day, and medication use. Treatment depends on the cause, and behavioral changes or pharmaceutical sleep agents may be necessary (Figure 17.4).

OBSTRUCTIVE SLEEP APNEA

The incidence of OSA has increased with increased obesity rates. Besides obesity, other predisposing and risk factors include narrowed upper airways, macroglossia, tonsillar hypertrophy, sleep medicines, alcohol, smoking, nasal obstruction, and hypothyroidism. It occurs more often in middle-aged men. A thorough medication history, respiratory history, neurological history, and mental health assessment should be performed.

Signs and Symptoms

One of the more common symptoms of OSA is snoring, usually reported by the spouse. The spouse may also report prolonged periods of apnea and restlessness. The patient may complain of frequent nighttime awakening, morning drowsiness, headache (caused by carbon dioxide buildup in the brain), cognitive impairment, erectile dysfunction, and weight gain, which can be both a cause

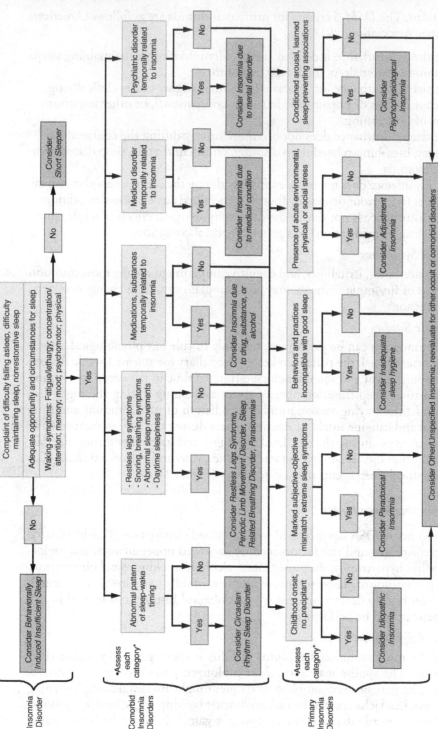

Figure 17.4 Algorithm for the evaluation of chronic insomnia. When using this diagram, the clinician should be aware that the presence of one diagnosis does not exclude other diagnoses in the same or another tier, as multiple diagnoses may coexist. Acute adjustment insomnia, not a chronic insomnia, is included in the chronic insomnia algorithm in order to highlight that the clinician should be aware that extrinsic stressors may trigger, perpetuate, or exacerbate the chronic insomnia. (From Schutte-Rodin, S., Broch, L., Buysse, D., Dorsey, C., & Sateia, M. (2017). Clinical guideline for the evaluation and management of chronic insomnia in adults. *Journal of Clinical Sleep Medicine, 4(I),* 495, Figure 1. Reprinted with permission.)

and an effect. Systemic hypertension is a complication of OSA but often resolves when the cause of the apnea is corrected.

Diagnostic Studies

An overnight sleep study (polysomnogram) is diagnostic for OSA. It records sleep wave activity, breathing patterns, heart rate and rhythm, and oxygen saturations. Oxygen saturations drop during periods of apnea, and brady- or tachyarrhythmias may occur. A CBC may show erythrocytosis to compensate for the hypoxemia. A continuous positive airway pressure (CPAP) machine is recommended, but if possible, the underlying cause should be corrected.

RESTLESS LEG SYNDROME

Although the exact cause of restless leg syndrome (RLS) is unknown, it has been associated with obesity, pregnancy, smoking, iron-deficiency anemia, peripheral neuropathy, heavy metal toxicity and other toxins, endocrine disorders, renal failure, caffeine and alcohol use, and certain medications, particularly H_2 blockers and some antidepressants. A hereditary basis has also been suggested.

Signs and Symptoms

RLS is characterized by an uncontrollable need to move the limbs, especially during times of rest and relaxation. Other symptoms attributed to RLS include tingling, itching, burning, or aching in the legs (and sometimes arms). Other conditions that may mimic RLS include Parkinson's disease, neuropathic or circulatory conditions, muscle diseases, or joint conditions. Eliminating tobacco and alcohol and adding exercise to the daily routine can help alleviate symptoms.

Diagnostic Studies

RLS is diagnosed primarily through the history. Laboratory tests include CBC to check for anemia, complete metabolic panel for endocrine and renal disorders, and tests for heavy metals.

PAIN SYNDROMES

Pain should be explored as a potential cause of sleep disturbance. Pain is described in general in the following sections, and specific types of pain are described in earlier chapters.

SUBSTANCE ABUSE

See Chapter 18.

CONGESTIVE HEART FAILURE

See Chapter 8.

ASTHMA

See Chapter 9.

STRESS, ANXIETY, DEPRESSION, AND DYSTHYMIA

See earlier in this chapter, p. 590.

FIBROMYALGIA

See Chapter 15.

■ Weakness

Although many of the previously discussed diagnoses for fatigue could also fit into a chief complaint of weakness, this complaint connotes a lack of strength rather than a feeling of lethargy, and it is manifested in many neurological diseases and in adrenal dysfunction, hyperthyroidism, and malignancy.

History

The history should include the type of weakness, whether it is proximal weakness, which might alert you to thyroid disease, malignancy, adrenal dysfunction, or distal weakness, which would raise an index of suspicion for a neurological cause, especially if it was accompanied by paresthesias. Ask the patient when and with what types of activities the weakness is most prominent and how much it interferes with activities of daily living. Inquire about changes in speech patterns or slurring that might indicate a neurological cause. Ask whether there are any cognitive or personality changes, which are often seen with adrenal dysfunction. The review of systems should include headache, cold or heat intolerance, change in appetite, weight gain or loss, nausea, vomiting or diarrhea, changes in balance or gait, numbness or paresthesia, diplopia or other vision changes, and difficulty with speech or swallowing.

Physical Examination

The physical examination should focus on the neurological and musculoskeletal examinations because both are very closely related and provide much information about the type, site, and severity of the weakness. Evaluate muscle mass, strength, and tone; the condition of the joints; and any fasciculations or spasticity. A complete neurological examination should be done, including cranial nerves, mental status, motor and sensory function, and DTRs. Assess the skin for any color or texture changes, as seen in adrenal or thyroid dysfunction. The head and neck should be assessed particularly for lymphadenopathy or enlarged or nodular thyroid.

MULTIPLE SCLEROSIS

Multiple sclerosis (MS) is a degenerative, demyelinating disease that is usually diagnosed in the second to fourth decades of life. It occurs more often in women than in men. The presentation of MS is often vague and transient, with episodic remission and exacerbation. Patients may have relapsing-remitting or primary/secondary progressive MS. The etiology is unknown, but it is thought to be autoimmune. A genetic susceptibility is suspected since it is seen more in those of western European lineage who live in temperate zones.

Signs and Symptoms

Visual disturbances may be the initial presenting symptom, indicating a plaque on the optic nerve. Associated visual disturbances include diplopia, blurred vision, tunnel vision, scotoma, or amaurosis. The visual changes are usually monocular. The patient may complain of intermittent weakness, paresthesias, or numbness of the face or extremities that occurs intermittently and that may resolve for weeks to months. Patients may report episodes of falling or stumbling with gait ataxia. Hyperreflexia may be noted, particularly in the lower extremities. Other symptoms include bladder incontinence or retention. Spastic bladder may also occur. In later stages, mental status changes may be noted. Initial symptoms are typically intermittent, and the disease may go undiagnosed for months or years.

Diagnostic Studies

MS is a clinical diagnosis and a diagnosis of exclusion. A thorough neurological examination is essential. MRI of the brain and/or spine with and without gadolinium contrast reveals demyelination of the white matter of the brain, spinal cord, and optic nerves. An MRI is also helpful to rule out other causes of the symptoms such as congenital/acquired lesions or Arnold-Chiari malformation. Lumbar puncture for cerebrospinal fluid analysis may show oligoclonal band (IgG) protein greater than 55 mg/dL; however, this is not a definitive test for diagnosis.

MUSCULAR DYSTROPHIES

There are seven types of muscular dystrophy, and they are subdivided by chromosomal inheritance, age of onset, and characteristic symptoms.

Signs and Symptoms

The symptoms, which can occur in patients anywhere from a year old to late adulthood, are characterized by progressive muscle weakness and wasting. There may also be intellectual disability, skeletal deformities, and cardiac involvement.

Diagnostic Studies

Diagnosis is made by genetic testing. Creatine phosphokinase is increased in some types. An electromyogram (EMG) may be helpful to distinguish among various muscle diseases. There is no definitive treatment for muscular dystrophies. Remaining active is a critical strategy for preventing deformities and improving quality of life.

MYASTHENIA GRAVIS

Myasthenia gravis (MG) can occur at any age and may be associated with other autoimmune diseases. Limb weakness and fatigability of the affected muscles is a diagnostic sign. Symptoms are due to a variable blocking of neuromuscular transmission by autoantibodies that bind to acetylcholine receptors. Ocular, facial, masticatory, and pharyngeal muscles are most often affected. Ocular symptoms for MG are discussed in Chapter 6.

Signs and Symptoms

The eye symptoms of diplopia and ptosis are common early signs. Other symptoms include dysphagia, weakness in the extremities, and respiratory difficulties. Symptoms fluctuate during the day, and the symptoms often relapse or remit over long periods of time, but ultimately the disease is progressive. Sustained activity of the affected muscles increases the weakness, and symptoms will improve with rest. Patients may require life support if respiratory effort is significantly affected. Recent advances in treatment, however, have significantly improved the prognosis, and patients can live a longer, relatively normal life.

Diagnostic Studies

Two well-characterized autoantibodies play a role in disease pathogenesis of MG and are found in the serum of most patients with MG—anti-acetylcholine receptor (AChR) and anti-muscle-specific tyrosine kinase (MuSK) antibodies. The levels of these antibodies can be measured through a blood sample.

The Tensilon test is also useful and involves blocking acetylcholine by administering edrophonium chloride. If the patient has MG, the symptoms will temporarily worsen after the administration of edrophonium chloride (Tensilon or Enlon). Since thymomas also can be present in these patients, a CT scan of the chest should be performed.

POLYMYOSITIS AND DERMATOMYOSITIS

Polymyositis is a systemic disease of unknown etiology, although injury, infection, and autoimmune causes have been suggested. When rash is present, it is called *dermatomyositis*, and with this form, there is an increased risk of an associated malignancy, particularly ovarian cancer. It is more common in women and in those older than 60 years.

Signs and Symptoms

Bilateral proximal muscle weakness is the main symptom and occurs in all cases. Weakness of the legs precedes weakness of the arms, and weakness of the neck flexors may be seen. Symptoms may occur suddenly or be more gradual and insidious in nature. The rash typically has a butterfly pattern on the face with reddish lesions over the eyes and periorbital edema. Redness and telangiectasias of the hands and nails is highly suggestive of dermatomyositis, and Reynaud's syndrome may be associated.

Diagnostic Studies

Diagnosis is established by EMG and confirmed by a muscle biopsy of the affected proximal muscles. Biopsy is the only definitive diagnostic test and will differentiate polymyositis from dermatomyositis. Creatine phosphokinase is rarely normal in active disease and is a good indicator of disease activity. Other possible enzyme elevations include aldolase, serum glutamic oxaloacetic transaminase (SGOT), serum glutamic pyruvic transaminase (SGPT), and lactate dehydrogenase (LDH), although not specific. Testing for autoantibodies may help to differentiate polymyositis from dermatomyositis and from an underlying malignancy (Cruellas et al., 2013; Yang, Chang, & Lian, 2019).

AMYOTROPHIC LATERAL SCLEROSIS (LOU GEHRIG'S DISEASE)

Amyotrophic lateral sclerosis (ALS) actually belongs to a group of motor neuron diseases and is characterized by mixed upper and lower motor neuron deficits.

Signs and Symptoms

ALS is characterized by muscle weakness and atrophy, usually starting in the hands and then progressing randomly and asymmetrically. Other common symptoms include muscle cramps, fasciculations, spasticity, dysarthria, dysphagia, and increased DTRs. Patients may show signs of cognitive impairment. Sensory and sphincter tone generally remain intact. Over 90% of patients die within 3 to 5 years.

Diagnostic Studies

An EMG is the most helpful diagnostic test. Muscle biopsy shows histological changes owing to denervation.

GUILLAIN-BARRÉ SYNDROME

Guillain-Barré is an acute, rapidly progressive polyneuropathy that is often preceded by a virus, surgical procedure, or immunization. It is thought to have an immune etiology.

Signs and Symptoms

Symmetric weakness and paresthesias are the main symptoms. The weakness usually begins distal to proximal and in the legs then proceeding to the arms. In addition to motor symptoms, patients often complain of distal paresthesias and neuropathic pain. Over 50% develop respiratory involvement, which may require mechanical ventilation. Autonomic dysfunction can occur in severe cases and can be fatal. The maximal degree of weakness usually occurs in the first 2 to 3 weeks. Most patients will recover, but approximately 20% will have persistent disability (Douglas, Amioff, & Kerchner, 2021). Plasmapheresis and intravenous immunoglobulin can be administered to improve the course of the disease.

Diagnostic Studies

The diagnosis can be made mainly on clinical presentation. Increased protein in the cerebrospinal fluid and EMG abnormalities assist in confirmation of the diagnosis.

HYPERTHYROIDISM

Although we think of hypothyroidism as causing fatigue, hyperthyroidism can cause symptoms of muscle weakness and lead to difficulty in performing the activities of daily living. Patients have different subjective experiences of their symptoms; therefore, some may describe weakness, whereas others may describe fatigue. Graves' disease is the most common cause of hyperthyroidism, except in patients older than 55 years, in whom multinodular goiter is a more common etiology. Onset of this condition can occur at any age, but it is most common between the ages of 20 and 40 years. Often patients have a family history of Graves' disease or other autoimmune thyroid diseases, such as Hashimoto's disease. See Box 17.1 for predisposing factors for hyperthyroidism.

Signs and Symptoms

Clinical manifestations include diffuse goiter, nervousness, irritability, tremor, hyperreflexia, heat intolerance, weakness, tachycardia, palpitations, widened pulse pressure, increased sweating, weight loss, insomnia, frequent bowel movements, menstrual irregularities, exophthalmos, and infiltrative dermopathy. Patients older than 50 years often present with cardiac symptoms, such as hypertension, atrial fibrillation, or heart failure.

Diagnostic Studies

A decreased TSH and elevated free T_4 will generally make the diagnosis. Also consider an erythrocyte sedimentation rate, which can be elevated in Graves' disease; a CBC to rule out anemia or an elevated white blood cell count; and a metabolic profile, with special attention to calcium, glucose, and potassium to rule out pheochromocytoma or adrenal disease. Thyroid autoantibodies will be elevated in Graves' disease and Hashimoto's thyroiditis. Radioactive iodine (RAI) imaging should be performed to look for increased uptake and the presence of hot or cold nodules. Fine needle aspiration (FNA) is recommended. Most can

---

Box 17.1

Predisposing Factors for Hyperthyroidism

- Heredity
- Female sex assigned at birth
- Recent adverse life events causing psychological stress
- Smoking
- Pregnancy
- Parity
- Viral and bacterial infections that cause subacute thyroiditis
- Iodine supplementation or exposure to an iodine load
- Lithium, amiodarone, or antiretroviral therapy
- Type I diabetes

be managed medically or with RAI ablation. A detailed discussion of hyperthyroidism can be found in Chapter 5.

CUSHING'S DISEASE

Cushing's disease is caused by excess cortisol and corticosteroid hormones, either endogenous or exogenous. Endogenous causes of cortisol hypersecretion include pituitary adenomas; other malignancies, such as small cell lung cancer; and adrenal tumors. Exogenous causes are related to the administration of steroids for the management of other chronic diseases. A thorough medical history will alert the practitioner to chronic diseases or medications that may be causing or contributing to the cushingoid signs and symptoms.

Signs and Symptoms

Although weakness can be profound because of the muscle wasting that occurs, it is generally not the first symptom that will bring the patient to the office. For women, it may be oligomenorrhea or amenorrhea and hirsutism, and for men, impotence. Patients develop a "moon face" and "buffalo hump" with central obesity and thin extremities. Hypertension and osteoporosis develop over time. Purple striae around the thighs, breasts, and abdomen are characteristic of Cushing's; patients are prone to easy bruisability, acne, and skin infections with poor wound healing. Patients complain of excessive thirst and polyuria owing to glucose intolerance, and they are prone to renal calculi. Changes in mental health are common and range from mood swings to psychosis.

Diagnostic Studies

The most accurate way to diagnose Cushing's disease is to give intravenous dexamethasone at bedtime and then check for elevated cortisol levels 8 to 10 hours later. In patients with Cushing's disease, exogenous dexamethasone does not suppress endogenous cortisol levels.

A 24-hour urine test for cortisol and creatinine helps confirm the diagnosis. Glucose tolerance testing shows elevated glucose resulting from insulin resistance. A CBC may show leukocytosis with granulocytosis and lymphopenia. An electrolyte panel may show hypokalemia.

MALIGNANCY

Weakness caused by a malignancy may be associated with the decreased functioning of the organ involved (e.g., lung), or the weakness may be due to a secondary anemia or to weight loss. See individual chapters for specific malignancies.

■ Fever of Unknown Origin

Fever of unknown origin (FUO) is defined as a temperature of at least 101°F for at least 3 weeks without discovery of the cause (Merck Manual, 2020). In children, over 50% of fevers are due to upper respiratory or viral illness; in adults, it is prudent to be more suspicious of malignancy.

History

The history should include the timing and degree of the fever. Knowledge of recent travel or exposure to illnesses or certain animals is often very helpful. Travel outside the United States can be particularly problematic, and one should consider such diseases as malaria, typhoid, TB, mycobacterium avium complex, or HIV. Brucellosis and histoplasmosis should be considered if there is animal exposure. Weight loss might indicate a malignant process or might be due to anorexia caused by the fever. As usual, a thorough medicine history, past medical history, and family history might alert the practitioner to a possible cause. Any recent infection should be investigated first because it may not have been adequately treated. A history of frequent infections could raise the index of suspicion regarding an immunocompromised condition, such as HIV, leukemia, or lymphoma. It is important to inquire about sexual practices.

Physical Examination

The physical should include examination of the skin for lesions, redness, increased temperature, or edema, which might indicate infection or an inflammatory process. Examine the lymph nodes. If there is lymphadenopathy in a particular area, it might lead you to the point of infection. If it is generalized, consider lymphoma, leukemia, or HIV. A cardiac assessment is important, especially listening for a murmur or friction rub. Pericarditis or endocarditis has a variety of causes and may present as unexplained fever, shortness of breath, precordial pain or tenderness, and tachycardia. The lung assessment is crucial because over 50% of FUOs in children are caused by an upper respiratory illness. Observe the skin and nail beds for cyanosis. The abdomen should be palpated for tenderness or masses; smoldering cases of appendicitis, cholecystitis, pancreatitis, or hepatitis might cause a lingering fever.

INFECTION

Any infection, viral or bacterial, can cause prolonged fever. Patients usually have some other complaint that alerts you to the cause of the fever. If bacterial, it can be treated with antibiotics, which should resolve the symptoms. Viral illnesses are more problematic because supportive measures are generally all that can be provided. Be watchful for a secondary bacterial infection to develop with some prolonged viral illnesses.

Signs and Symptoms

The signs and symptoms are highly variable, depending on the source of the infection. Expected are the typical symptoms that accompany a fever, such as headache, malaise, anorexia, and possibly chills. A thorough review of systems is necessary to detect the underlying source of the fever, if it is not completely obvious by other complaints. In the pediatric and older populations, infection may present with symptoms seemingly unrelated to the source of infection (e.g., confusion as a presenting symptom for urinary tract infection in an older patient; nausea, vomiting, and diarrhea in a child with strep throat). Practitioners must be vigilant in the history and also may need to throw out a wider net for diagnostics in these populations.

Diagnostic Studies

Although the diagnostics vary with the underlying cause, ordering a CBC with differential, urinalysis, and chest x-ray is a good place to start with any complaint of FUO. Blood cultures and cultures of bodily fluids may be necessary. In babies, a lumbar puncture is recommended to rule out meningitis. Rising antibody titers for typhoid, brucellosis, and other viral infections may be helpful. Ultrasound or CT scan will identify abscesses or other infections in the abdomen, including sexually transmitted infection, diverticulitis, peritonitis, cholecystitis, possibly pancreatitis, or appendicitis. A CT scan of the chest can detect cardiac vegetation, which might suggest pericarditis or endocarditis as a cause for the fever.

MALIGNANCY

Many malignancies can cause fever, but lymphoma and leukemia should be at the top of the differential list. Acute leukemia is more common in children, and the chronic leukemias are more common in middle-aged to older adults. Hodgkin's lymphoma is more prevalent in children and young adults, although the peak for incidence is bimodal and can be seen in patients older than 60 years. Non-Hodgkin's lymphoma is more common in middle-aged to older adults. Burkitt's lymphoma is more common in HIV patients.

Signs and Symptoms

With leukemia, common symptoms include unexplained fever, easy bruising or bleeding, fatigue, bone or joint pain, and enlarged liver or spleen. With lymphoma, common symptoms include fatigue, fever, night sweats, lymphadenopathy, and weight loss.

Diagnostic Studies

A CBC is the first and easiest laboratory test to perform. The abnormalities in the CBC vary some with the type of leukemia—acute or chronic, lymphocytic or myelocytic—but in general, there is a proliferation of immature white cells (blasts), anemia, and low platelet count. In lymphoma, there is a leukocytosis, lymphocytopenia, and possibly thrombocytosis. A hypochromic, microcytic anemia is often present. A bone marrow biopsy confirms the diagnosis in both leukemia and lymphoma.

DIFFUSE CONNECTIVE TISSUE DISORDERS

The connective tissue disorders include rheumatoid arthritis, Sjögren's syndrome, Behçet's syndrome, vasculitis, systemic and discoid lupus erythematosus, polymyositis, polymyalgia rheumatica, temporal arteritis, and polyarteritis. Although fever can be present in any of the connective tissue disorders, muscle and joint pain are more common presenting symptoms. The specific signs, symptoms, and diagnostics for each of these diseases are beyond the scope of this text.

IMMUNODEFICIENCY DISORDERS

Immunodeficiency disorders are numerous and are characterized as primary or secondary, with the secondary being more common than the primary disorders. The primary disorders are classified into B-cell deficiencies (antibody), T-cell deficiencies (cellular), phagocytic disorders, and complement disorders. The secondary immunodeficiencies are classified by cause and include hereditary and metabolic diseases (e.g., chromosome abnormalities, uremia, DM, malnutrition, nephritic syndrome, myotonic dystrophy, sickle cell disease), infectious diseases (e.g., rubella; cytomegalovirus; viral exanthemas; mononucleosis; severe bacterial, viral, or fungal infections), infiltrative and hematologic diseases (e.g., histiocytosis, sarcoidosis, lymphoma, leukemia, myeloma, aplastic anemia), those caused by surgery and trauma (e.g., burns, splenectomy, anesthesia), and those caused by immunosuppressive agents (e.g., radiation, chemotherapy, corticosteroids, other immunosuppressive drugs). Specific signs, symptoms, and diagnostics are beyond the scope of this text. Some of these are discussed in other chapters.

DRUG REACTION

The most likely drugs to cause fever are the chemotherapeutic agents used to treat cancer, mainly as a result of leukopenia. The medical history should be all that is needed, along with a CBC to make this diagnosis. Allergic reactions to any drug, particularly the antibiotics, can cause fever as well as rash. The history is usually all that is necessary to identify the cause of the fever.

■ Unexplained Weight Loss

Unexplained weight loss is considered significant if it is greater than 5% of the usual body weight over a 6- to 12-month period and often indicates a serious medical or psychological illness.

History

Malignancy, diabetes, digestive diseases, thyroid disease, and depression should top the list of differential diagnoses for unexplained weight loss. A thorough history and review of systems will alert the practitioner to other complaints that could give clues to the cause, such as cough, hemoptysis, shortness of breath, nausea, vomiting, diarrhea, steatorrhea, hematemesis, melena, fatigue/weakness/lethargy, changing or new moles, persistent pain, enlarged lymph nodes, abnormal menstrual bleeding, breast discharge, and chronic headaches. A thorough medicine history is critical, especially in older patients or those with chronic diseases who are on a multitude of medicines. A psychosocial history is critical, especially in the older client who may not be eating due to the inability to shop for groceries because of financial or transportation problems, inability to prepare meals resulting from a functional limitation, poorly fitting dentures or no dentures, or loss of appetite owing to depression or medications. In the teen and young adult population, eating disorders may be the cause, and specific inquiries should be made about anorexia or bulimia. Inquire about smoking and alcohol intake because both of these can increase the risk for both weight loss and malignancies.

Physical Examination

Patients with unexplained weight loss that is due to malignancy may look cachectic, pale, and lethargic, or they may look well, depending on the amount and cause of the weight loss. Weights over the past year should be plotted out to see how much weight has been lost over what period of time. A slow weight decrease in the older patient is not uncommon and may simply be due to a lack of appetite, institutional food, or disinterest in food resulting from a decreased sense of taste or smell. A full physical examination is necessary, paying particular attention to any masses, tenderness, swelling, or lymphadenopathy. If an eating disorder is suspected, look for accompanying symptoms, such as dry, thinning hair and skin and/or teeth erosion.

MALIGNANCY

Depending on the stage of the malignancy, any are capable of causing weight loss as either a primary or a secondary symptom. However, the most common malignancies to cause weight loss are GI, lung, hematologic, and musculoskeletal.

Signs and Symptoms

The signs and symptoms will vary with the source of the malignancy, and many are asymptomatic except for the complaint of weight loss.

Diagnostic Studies

Ordering a CBC and blood chemistries is a good place to start, as are chest x-ray and hemoccult cards, depending on the age and medical history. The results of these and the history should assist the practitioner in narrowing down the search. Other diagnostics such as CT or MRI should be ordered as needed.

STRESS, ANXIETY, DEPRESSION, AND DYSTHYMIA

See Chapter 18.

EATING DISORDERS

See Chapter 18.

FUNCTIONAL AND FINANCIAL MALNUTRITION

Depending on the patient population, malnutrition may be a possibility. It is common in patients living in extreme poverty and in older patients owing to the inability to purchase, prepare, and consume a nutritious, varied diet. Eating disorders, depending on the severity, may result in malnutrition. In developing countries, malnutrition is a significant problem, but it is not common in the United States except in older persons and persons living in extreme poverty.

Signs and Symptoms

Aside from weight loss, other signs of malnutrition include dry skin and hair, pale conjunctivae, cheilosis, glossitis, bruising, lethargy, decreased vibratory sensation, decreased DTRs, bone demineralization, liver or heart enlargement, muscle wasting, lower extremity edema, and growth failure.

Diagnostic Studies

Malnutrition has a variety of consequences that can involve several body systems. A complete metabolic profile, CBC, and thyroid studies are recommended. Electrolyte imbalance is common, especially if the malnutrition is brought on by anorexia or bulimia, and it can be life-threatening. Kidney and liver functions may be affected as well. Depending on the chronicity of the problem, dual-energy x-ray absorptiometry should be considered because bone health may be at risk. In severe cases, heart failure may ensue, and an echocardiogram or more invasive cardiac testing may be needed to evaluate cardiac functioning.

DRUG REACTION

A few drugs actually cause weight loss (e.g., thyroid replacement in greater than therapeutic doses, selective serotonin reuptake inhibitors, neuroleptics, glucagon-like peptide 1 [GLP-1] agonists, sodium-glucose transporter 2 [SGLT-2 inhibitors]), but many drugs cause anorexia with weight loss as a secondary side effect. Because drug side effects vary greatly between patients, it is not possible to supply an exhaustive list of drugs that cause anorexia. A few that seem to be most problematic are digitalis, antiarrhythmics, many psychotropic medications, chemotherapeutic agents mostly as a result of nausea, stimulants such as pseudoephedrine or other drugs used to treat obesity, and drugs used to treat attention deficit/hyperactivity disorder.

A complete medication history, including over-the-counter medications, may allow the practitioner to identify the cause of the weight loss. If a drug is suspected, it should be changed if possible. For patients on multiple drugs, the suspected agents should be discontinued or substituted one at a time in order to determine the offending agent.

MALABSORPTION

Malabsorption falls into two main categories: impaired digestion and impaired absorption. Diseases and procedures that may contribute to impaired digestion include gastrectomy, bariatric surgery, chronic pancreatitis, chronic liver failure, biliary obstruction, lactose intolerance, diverticula, and Zollinger-Ellison syndrome. Diseases that fall into the impaired absorption category include intestinal infections, alcohol, celiac disease, tropical sprue, Whipple's disease, amyloidosis, ischemic or infarcted bowel, Crohn's disease, volvulus, and intussusception.

Signs and Symptoms

The signs and symptoms vary according to the underlying problem, but common symptoms include weight loss, flatulence, abdominal bloating, edema in the lower extremities resulting from protein deficiency, muscle weakness, possibly diarrhea or steatorrhea, dehydration, glossitis, and bruising. A variety of abnormal findings can be associated with malabsorption syndromes, including iron, folic acid, or B_{12} deficiency anemia; calcium deficiency; vitamins A, B, C, and D deficiencies; and niacin deficiency. A combination of weight loss, diarrhea, and anemia should raise the possibility of malabsorption.

Diagnostic Studies

There are as many diagnostics as there are causes of malabsorption. Measurement of fat in the stool is the most valuable diagnostic for diagnosing malabsorption, and a 3- to 4-day stool collection is advised. Stool specimens for ova and parasites and culture and sensitivity will help to rule out infectious causes. Absorption tests, flat plate of the abdomen, upper GI with small bowel follow-through, endoscopy, and small bowel biopsy may be necessary for definitive diagnosis.

HYPERTHYROIDISM

See p. 606 in this chapter and Chapter 5.

Pain Assessment

In the last decade, pain assessment has become the fifth vital sign, driven by studies reporting that pain was undertreated. In 2018–2019, The Joint Commission on Accreditation of Healthcare Organizations (TJC) revised pain assessment and management standards that have been incorporated into health-care facilities at all levels. The new standards call for health-care organizations to:

1. Recognize patients' rights to control pain.
2. Screen for pain.
3. Perform a complete assessment when pain is present.
4. Record the assessment in a way that facilitates regular reassessment and follow-up.
5. Set a standard for monitoring and intervention.
6. Educate providers and ensure staff competency.
7. Establish policies that support appropriate prescription or ordering of pain medicines.
8. Educate patients and families.
9. Include patient needs for symptom control in discharge planning.
10. Collect data to monitor the effectiveness and appropriateness of pain management (TJC, 2021).

While controlling pain is a worthwhile goal, encouraging providers to prescribe more pain medicine has resulted in the current opioid crisis. Dependence and addiction have skyrocketed, and the number of deaths from opioid overdose continues to rise. In 2020, overdose deaths were over 90,000, and over half involve a prescription opioid (CDC, 2020b). Patients who cannot obtain opioids legally are turning to heroin, with deadly results. Government agencies are stepping in to try and stem the rising rates of opioid abuse and addiction.

TJC continues to monitor safety standards for pain management. Opioids such as morphine, oxycodone, hydrocodone, fentanyl, and methadone can slow breathing to dangerous levels and cause other problems such as dizziness, nausea, and falls. TJC cites reasons for such adverse events, including excessive prescribing, dosing errors, improper monitoring of patients, and interactions with other drugs. Patients who have OSA, who are obese, or who are very ill may be at higher risk for harm from opioids.

Pain is a multifactorial condition and a common reason for which patients seek health care. Pain can be classified in many ways: acute, chronic, recurrent, or transient. Alternatively, it can be classified based on the quality of the pain (gnawing, burning, deep), its severity (mild, moderate, severe, excruciating), its impact (debilitating, disabling), or a related diagnosis (cardiac, neuropathic). Regardless, when pain is a presenting condition, the symptom should always be explored. When a presenting complaint of pain does not readily respond to the initial treatment, it warrants more detailed analysis.

■ Signs and Symptoms

The PQRST mnemonic (palliative/provoking, quality, radiation, severity, timing) will guide your history for the assessment of pain. In assessing pain, it is critical to identify the precipitating, palliative, and provocative factors because pain is often not constant over time. Questions on precipitating and palliative factors are also helpful in identifying how the pain limits the patient's typical activities. The quality and quantity of pain may vary, and it is essential to have the patient describe what is meant by a complaint of pain. Ask the patient to describe the pain using common words so that you can determine whether it is deep, boring, sharp, gnawing, burning, stabbing, aching, and so forth. The region where the pain is most severe and any area of radiation or secondary pain are important to identify. A body diagram may be helpful in achieving this goal, as the patient can mark where the pain is located and then rate the severity and quality of pain in various regions. Related symptoms should be explored as well.

There are many ways to measure severity of pain. The most commonly used are the numerical rating scale (NRS), with which the patient rates the pain on an 11-, 21-, or 101-point range (e.g., 0–10, 0–20, 0–100); the visual analog scale (VAS), with which the patient notes a point corresponding to the degree of pain along a 10-centimeter scale with poles of *no pain at all* to *worst possible pain*; and verbal rating scales (VRS), with which patients are asked to use verbal descriptors such as *no pain*, *mild pain*, *considerable pain*, and *most severe pain*. The timing of the pain is important because it helps to identify the situation in which onset was first recognized, including any preceding physical or emotional trauma and how the pain has progressed since first noticed. For instance, it is critical to understand whether the pain has been constant, intermittent, transient, or recurrent.

A past medical history and history of all current and recently taken medications is an important component of pain assessment. Identify the history of any neurological, cardiac, GI, musculoskeletal, respiratory, and emotional conditions. Comorbidities may affect the safety and efficacy of pain management. Ask about family history. Explore the patient's social history, including any current or recent stressors, occupational and recreational activities, and activities of daily living. Ask the patient to describe how, if at all, normal activities have been affected by the pain.

The physical examination is certainly guided by the history. In addition to basic vital signs, including BMI, the general appearance is crucial. However, it is important to remember that patients may not always exhibit behavioral indications of their pain. The physical assessment for specific types of pain (e.g., joint, chest, throat) are described in earlier chapters.

■ Diagnostic Studies

As noted earlier, common pain scales include various forms of VRS, VAS, and NRS pain ratings. There are several more detailed options, such as the Pain Faces Scale for pediatric patients and the McGill Pain Questionnaire, which include sensory and emotional aspects of pain as well as a pain diagram. Pain diaries are often helpful and should be kept for a period of at least a week. Whichever method is used should be culturally sensitive and appropriate to the patient's age and verbal/literacy abilities.

A number of diagnostic studies may be warranted for further exploration of pain and should be selected based on the history and physical findings.

REFERENCES

American Psychiatric Association. (2013). *Diagnostic and statistical manual of mental disorders* (5th ed.). American Psychiatric Association.

British Medical Journal. (2021). Covid-19: Middle aged women face greater risk of debilitating long term symptoms, *British Medical Journal, 372*. doi: https://doi.org/10.1136/bmj.n829

Centers for Disease Control and Prevention. (2020a). National diabetes statistics report: Estimates of diabetes and its burden in the United States, 2020. U.S. Department of Health and Human Services, Centers for Disease Control and Prevention. Retrieved May 17, 2021, from https://www.cdc.gov/diabetes/library/features/diabetes-stat-report.html

Centers for Disease Control and Prevention. (2020b). Increases in drug and opioid-involved overdose deaths—United States, 2015–2020. https://www.cdc.gov/nchs/nvss/vsrr/drug-overdose-data.htm

Centers for Disease Control and Prevention/Infectious Diseases Society of America. (2021). COVID-19, post-COVID conditions. https://www.cdc.gov/coronavirus/2019-ncov/long-term-effects/index.html?CDC_AA_refVal=https%3A%2F%2Fwww.cdc.gov%2Fcoronavirus%2F2019-ncov%2Flong-term-effects.html

Cruellas, M. G. P., Viana, V. S. T., Levy-Neto, M., de Souza, F. H. C., & Katsuyuki, S. (2013). Myositis-specific and myositis-associated autoantibody profiles and their clinical associations in a large series of patients with polymyositis and dermatomyositis. *Shinjo Clinics (Sao Paulo), 68*(7), 909–914.

Dirkx, T., & Woodell, T. (2021). Kidney disease. In Papadakis, M. A., McPhee, S. J. (Eds.), *CURRENT medical diagnosis & treatment* (60th ed.). Lange Medical Books/McGraw Hill.

Douglas, V., & Aminoff, M. (2021). Nervous system disorders. In S. J. McPhee, M. A. Papadakis, & M. W. Rabow (Eds.). *CURRENT medical diagnosis & treatment* (60th ed., pp. 1068–1069). Lange Medical Books/McGraw Hill.

Huang, C., Huang, L., Wang, Y., Li, X., Ren, L., Gu, X., Kang, L., Guo, L., Liu, M., Zhou, X., Luo, J., Huang, Z., Tu, S., Zhao, Y., Chen, L., Xu, D., Li, Y., Li, C., Peng, L., et al. (2021). 6-month consequences for COVID-19 in-patients discharged from the hospital: A cohort study. *The Lancet.* https://www.thelancet.com/journals/lancet/article/PIIS0140-6736(20)32656-8/fulltext

Joint Commission on Accreditation of Healthcare Organizations (TJC). (2021). Pain assessment standards. Retrieved May 17, 2021 from https://www.jointcommission.org/search/#q=pain%20assessment%20and%20management%20standards%20for%20hospitals&t=_Tab_All&sort=relevancy&f:_Sites Organizations=[The%20Joint%20Commission

Merck manual professional version, 2020. Retrieved May 16, 2021, from https://www.merckmanuals.com/professional/infectious-diseases/biology-of-infectious-disease/fever-of-unknown-origin-fuo

Yang, S-H., Chang, C., & Lian, Z-X. (2019). Polymyositis and dermatomyositis–Challenges in diagnosis and management. *Journal of Translational Autoimmunity.* https://doi.org/10.1016/j.jtauto.2019.100018

Chapter 18

Psychiatric Mental Health

Karen D. Lipford •

U nlike other clinical areas discussed in this book, the differential diagnosis of psychiatric conditions can depend less on laboratory findings and physical assessment data than on patient's complaints and reports of symptoms. As a result, the art of interviewing and the skills of active listening are critical when attempting to rule out conditions with similar symptoms (Hart, 2010). In addition, the clinician must grapple with the question of whether a presenting symptom is genuine or instead represents factitious behavior or malingering, is related to substance abuse, is a medical condition, or represents any of the overlapping symptoms within one of the categories covered in this chapter.

This chapter also looks at "medical mimics," or conditions that may easily be categorized as psychiatric in nature but that appear to have confusing medical presentations. The chapter focuses on common psychiatric disorders and common symptoms or complaints. Since many disorders have overlapping symptoms, critical indicators are presented with examples of focused questions to guide practitioners in determining the differential diagnosis. Owing to practical limitations, this is not intended to be an all-inclusive review but rather a choice of diagnostic areas most likely to be encountered by advanced practice clinicians in a primary care setting.

Diagnosis of a psychiatric illness requires attention to physical and biological indicators along with a psychiatric evaluation. Psychiatric symptoms may present in response to a medical illness, may be triggered by medications, or may be a very normative response to a stressful life event, such as in the case of grieving a loss. When a psychiatric illness is believed to be the primary problem, a comprehensive psychiatric evaluation is indicated to achieve an accurate diagnosis. For example, when a client presents with complaints of feeling tired, having difficulty sleeping, and feeling agitated and anxious, the practitioner must rule out a medical illness, determine whether the symptoms are in response to medications, and explore whether they are related to a stressful life event. When these possibilities are ruled out, a psychiatric evaluation may be indicated. Conducting a psychiatric evaluation helps prevent the frequent treatment mistake of focusing on the obvious symptoms of sleeping difficulty, anxiety, or agitation and missing an underlying depression. In such situations, a minor tranquilizer might be prescribed that could actually exacerbate depression by depleting serotonin. The basic disorder may be a depression with coexisting anxiety symptoms.

Comprehensive Psychiatric Evaluation

A comprehensive psychiatric evaluation leads to a diagnosis and a guide for treatment (Carlat, 2017). Targeted questions in the following areas aid in determining the appropriate psychiatric diagnosis. Although it is not critical to follow this guide in a lockstep manner, attention to the major areas can help prevent an inaccurate psychiatric diagnosis. This section provides a brief overview of the psychiatric evaluation. The sections that follow highlight various psychiatric problems and offer additional guides for assessment.

In 2013, the American Psychiatric Association (APA) released the fifth edition of the *Diagnostic and Statistical Manual of Mental Disorders* (*DSM-5*) at its annual meeting. It marked more than a decade of work in revising diagnostic and classification criteria of mental disorders. Historically, the manual has utilized a five-multiaxial system (formerly Axis I through Axis V), but it has been replaced by a system that essentially collapses the original first three axes into one to form a categorical system diagnosis. The system replaces Axis IV (the Global Assessment of Functioning, known as GAF) with significant psychosocial and contextual features, discontinuing Axis IV altogether. The manual states that one goal is to align with the International Classification of Diseases (ICD) system. In *DSM-5*, the phrase *general medical condition* is replaced with *another medical condition* where relevant across all disorders. This chapter will highlight the newest changes, based on *DSM-5*.

■ Problem Identification and Chief Complaint

Using the patient's own words, identify the reason for seeking care. Because many common symptoms fall within a variety of psychiatric diagnoses, the practitioner looks for specific clusters of symptoms to determine the diagnosis. So, given the chief complaint "I have been feeling tired recently; I have not been able to sleep well, and I have felt restless during the day and anxious," many more details are necessary to form an accurate diagnosis. An essential component of the psychiatric evaluation is the source of the information (patients themselves, family members, or records review) to help determine the reliability of the information (Kaplan, Sadock, & Ruiz, 2015).

■ History of Present Illness

"Can you tell me in your own words what brings you here today?" A symptom analysis similar to that done for nonpsychiatric complaints is indicated to determine the history of the specific complaint and to identify any associated problems. This analysis can be integrated into the general assessment. It should explore the timeline related to symptoms, the relationship of symptoms to life events, any recent conflicts or stressors, any drugs that are used, and how the current level of functioning differs from the client's previous level of functioning. If, at the initial presentation of a complaint, the patient indicates that the problem has existed for some time, the sequence of events leading up to the visit at this particular time may identify important triggers that have either exacerbated the problem or convinced the patient (or family member) that help was needed for the problem.

■ Pertinent Past Psychiatric History

It is important to determine whether the client has a history of any psychiatric disorders. If so, determine the extent of the illness and all prior and current treatments, medications, and outcomes or responses to the treatments. Description of past symptoms should include when they occurred, how long they lasted, and the frequency and severity of the episodes. Ask the patient whether the patient believes that prior treatments were beneficial and how well they were tolerated.

■ Pertinent Social History

The social history is an essential part of the psychiatric history. It is important to explore questions about education, family relationships, social networks, potential abuse history, and employment. This part of the history should include information on all drug and alcohol abuse because many psychiatric disorders mimic substance abuse. Psychiatric symptoms may actually stem from adverse effects of a prescribed, over the counter, or recreational drug or an herbal agent. Evaluate use of tobacco and caffeine products, as these substances can interfere in the absorption of many psychiatric medications. Often patients more readily admit to caffeine and nicotine use before use of alcohol or other substances (Kaplan, Sadock, & Ruiz, 2015). The following sections on specific complaints and problems identify medications associated with each of the complaints discussed. Obtaining a history of occupational and recreational activities and of performance of activities of daily living provides crucial information about how problems affect an individual's overall life. Finally, the social history is important in determining the disposition of a patient following assessment and diagnosis.

■ Pertinent Family History

Obtain a family history, including questions about psychiatric history as well as medical and genetic illnesses.

■ Medical History and the Review of Symptoms

Many times, psychiatric symptoms are a result of underlying medical conditions. In such cases, the focus for treatment is the medical condition. For example, the following sections identify medical conditions that can cause or exacerbate mental health symptoms, including depression, anxiety, eating disorders, and alterations in thought processes. It is important to identify all allergies or intolerances to both psychotropic and other medications. If a female patient is of childbearing age, determining the possibility of pregnancy is an essential component because of the teratogenic effects of many medications.

■ Mental Status Examination

The mental status examination comprises five major areas: (1) appearance and behavior; (2) mood and affect; (3) speech and thought processes; (4) thought content and perceptual abnormalities; and (5) sensorial, cognitive, and intellectual functioning.

Appearance and Behavior

To assess appearance and behavior, observe gait, dress, grooming, posture, gestures, and facial expressions as the history is performed. Note the patient's apparent nutritional status. Note whether the patient maintains eye contact or exhibits any unusual behaviors during the history. For example, a patient presenting with mania might exhibit psychomotor agitation, distractibility, colorful clothes or bizarre combinations of clothes, excessive makeup, and intrusiveness.

Mood and Affect

Mood is the subjective experience as self-reported. Ask clients to describe how they feel: well, happy, depressed, anxious, and so on. In contrast, affect is the practitioner's impression. Note whether your impression is that of an individual who is happy, depressed, anxious, flat, and so on.

Speech and Thought Processes

The tone, quality, quantity, and rate of speech are important indications of mental status. For instance, in mania, the speech may be pressured, loud, dramatic, and exaggerated; in depression, the speech may be soft and monotone with little or no spontaneity. In addition to noting speech patterns, consider whether the client's thought processes are clear, logical, and organized. With altered thought processes, a patient's speech may indicate irrelevant information (loose associations), frequent change of topics (flight of ideas), vagueness (circumstantiality), permanent departure from the topic of conversation (tangential thought), halted speech (thought blocking), or other signs of a formal thought disorder. If a language interpreter is used for the examination, determine if the client is fluent in their own language; this can be done by asking the interpreter.

Thought Content and Perceptual Abnormalities

During the mental status examination, it is important to determine whether the patient is experiencing abnormal content of thought, such as hallucinations or delusions. Ask whether the patient sees things that others cannot see or hears voices that others cannot hear. If so, it is important to explore what type of hallucination is experienced. Persons without a psychosis can experience a belief that their name has been called or can see shadows out of the corners of their eyes, but this is an illusion and not a hallucination. To assess for delusions, ask patients whether they have any powers or abilities that others do not have or thoughts that others would consider strange. Determine whether the patient has obsessions or compulsions or experiences feelings of hopelessness, worthlessness, or guilt.

When patients are experiencing mental health problems, it is vital to assess for past and current suicidal ideation or intent. Sixty percent of depressed clients have suicidal ideations. Patients should be asked whether they have previously performed any acts of self-harm or have any thoughts of harming or killing themselves in the future. Positive responses require more detailed assessment of current suicidal risk. Determination of violence and homicidality, past and current, to include any violent actions or intent, is a necessary component of this portion of the exam as well.

Sensorial, Cognitive, and Intellectual Functioning

Determine each patient's general level of orientation and alertness. Alertness may be affected or blunted by mental health problems such as depression. To assess the level of intelligence, ask about common knowledge issues. Often this assessment can be incorporated into the exploration of the client's history, work, and education. Judgment can be assessed in relation to how the client has handled situations in the past as well as any current challenges. Insight may be determined by evaluating the patient's understanding of current health status or living situation.

■ Assessing for Potential Medical Mimics

Whenever faced with a mental health complaint, it is vital that the differential diagnosis initially include any medical problems that could be correctable. This category includes nonpsychiatric health problems and the myriad of medications and treatments that may result in complaints similar to those of psychiatric problems. Box 18.1 provides "rules" or guidance to help spot medical conditions that may mimic mental health problems. Dr. Robert Hedeya (1996) developed the mnemonic "THINC MED," designed to help spot medical mimics. The mnemonic is useful when evaluating for underlying medical conditions that present as psychiatric symptoms, particularly anxiety disorders (Box 18.2).

Box 18.1

Rules to Follow for Spotting Medical Mimics

1. Never assume that an emotional symptom has a psychosocial cause until physical causes are fully explored.
2. Always have your patients get a complete physical if they have not had one since the onset of symptoms.
3. Look for a history that does not fit.
4. Check personal and family history thoroughly.
5. Be suspicious when the onset comes late in life (e.g., a first psychotic break after age 40) or when no stressors are present.
6. Be suspicious of a recent onset of headaches, loss of function, unusual perceptions, visual disturbances, paranormal experiences, or hallucinations.
7. Ask about all drug use, including over the counter and illicit.

Box 18.2

THINC MED

The following are major categories of medical mimics:

T Tumors
H Hormones (thyroid, adrenals, gonadal, insulin)
I Infections and immune diseases (AIDS, Lyme disease, mononucleosis, lupus, syphilis)
N Nutrition (B_{12}, B_1, B_6, manganese, iron overload)
C Central nervous system (head trauma, multiple sclerosis, seizures, Parkinson's disease, Huntington's disease)
M Miscellaneous (sleep apnea, anemia, congestive heart failure)
E Electrolyte abnormalities and toxins (K^+, NA^+, chemical exposures)
D Drugs (also include nicotine and caffeine)

Differential Diagnosis of Chief Complaints

■ Anxiety Disorders

Anxiety disorders make up the most common category of psychiatric conditions and are responsible for frequent patient use of the health-care system. Past year prevalence rates for any anxiety disorders among U.S. adults (2001–2003) noted that an estimated 19.1% of U.S. adults had any anxiety disorder in the past year, and an estimated 31.1% of U.S. adults experienced any anxiety disorder at some time in their lives. Past year prevalence rates for any anxiety disorders are higher for females at 23.4%, compared with males at 14.3% (National Institute of Mental Health, n.d.). Both functional impairment and morbidity have been linked to anxiety disorders, and recent studies suggest that chronic anxiety disorders may increase the rate of cardiovascular-related mortality. Anxiety disorders often go unrecognized and untreated in primary care (Combs & Markman, 2014). The etiology of anxiety disorders is a complex dance of genetic predisposition and environmental factors, as in many other psychiatric conditions. It is important to distinguish between *normal* anxiety, which everyone experiences, and anxiety that reaches the level of psychopathology. Anxiety is an unpleasant feeling of apprehension, often accompanied by perspiration, palpitation, stomach discomfort, restlessness, difficulty sitting still, and even tightness in the chest. Anxiety is usually differentiated from *fear* in that when one is fearful, there is an identifiable dreaded object, as opposed to anxiety, in which there is no specific focus. Whereas anxiety is a normal response to stress, pathological anxiety is distinguished by the intensity, duration, and level of impairment coping with it renders, and whether there is an environmental trigger.

More than 90% of patients with anxiety present primarily with somatic complaints in primary care and emergency department settings (Stern, Herman, & Gorrindo, 2012). Patients may initially complain of generalized and undifferentiated symptoms before they are ultimately diagnosed with a primary anxiety disorder (Combs & Markman, 2014). Patients with anxiety often present with the following symptoms: chest pain (with negative angiogram), irritable bowel, unexplained dizziness, migraine headache, and chronic fatigue. The diagnostic workup for this type of patient relies on the medical and psychiatric histories, the medication and drug histories, and the physical and neurological exams.

When assessing a patient who may be anxious, the most obvious indicators are those involving the sympathetic nervous system, such as increased heart rate, blood pressure, pallor, dry mouth, increased respiration, and sweating. These familiar signs are representations of the fight-or-flight response. Patients may also exhibit behavior connected with parasympathetic activity, such as pacing, tapping toes or fingers, and adjusting clothing (displacement activities) (Kaplan, Sadock, & Ruiz, 2015). Children and adolescents with anxiety disorders may present with headache, stomachache, or excessive worry and fears (Centers for Disease Control and Prevention [CDC], n.d.).

RED FLAG   **Medications Causing Anxiety**

- *Caffeine*
- *Respiratory medications (e.g., theophylline, albuterol)*
- *Corticosteroids*

Panic Disorder

Panic disorder is a syndrome characterized by recurrent unexpected panic attacks about which there is persistent concern. Panic attacks are discrete episodes of intense anxiety that peak within 10 minutes and are associated with autonomic arousal (cardiac, pulmonary, gastrointestinal, and neurological symptoms) and feelings of depersonalization/derealization and the fear of dying, losing control, or going crazy. After an initial attack, the apprehension of a future attack often occurs and is referred to as *anticipatory anxiety*. The anticipation is often as distressing (if not more so) to patients as the experience of an actual episode. Questions that should be included in the history in order to assess for panic disorder and panic attack are listed in Box 18.3.

Generalized Anxiety Disorder

Patients with generalized anxiety disorder are worried most of the time about many different concerns (such as work or school performance), both reasonable and unfounded. *DSM-5* requires several episodes of worry to occur on most days for at least a 6-month period of time. Patients find this worry impossible to control, and it is usually associated with somatic symptoms, such as complaints associated with sleep, muscle pain, bowel function, or mood, or problems at work or in relationships. Questions for assessing generalized anxiety disorder are listed in Box 18.4.

Box 18.3

Questions for Assessing Panic Disorder and Panic Attack

1. *"Have you had episodes when you felt nervous, frightened, anxious, or uneasy in situations when most people did not feel that way? Did the feelings peak within 10 minutes?"* **(panic disorder)**

2. *"Do you feel nervous in places where you might have a panic attack or when escape might be difficult, such as in a crowd; standing in a line; on a bridge; or in a bus, plane, or train?"* **(agoraphobia)**

Questions Related to Panic Attack

1. *"In the past, did these episodes occur unexpectedly?"*
   a. *Was your heart racing?*
   b. *Did you have difficulty breathing?*
   c. *Were your hands sweaty?*
   d. *Did you have chest pain?*
   e. *Did you fear that you were dying?*
   f. *Did you feel dizzy or think you were going to faint?*

2. *"Have you had an episode and then for a month or more feared having another episode or attack?"*

Box 18.4

Questions for Assessing Generalized Anxiety Disorder

1. *"Have you been worried about many things over the past 6 months?"*
2. *"Are these worries present most days?"*
3. *"Do you find it difficult to control your worries?"*
4. *"Do they interfere with your ability to concentrate on what you are doing?"*

Agoraphobia, Specific Phobia, and Social Anxiety Disorder (Social Phobia)

The previous diagnostic criterion, that individuals older than 18 years with agoraphobia, specific phobia, and social anxiety disorder (social phobia) recognize that their anxiety is excessive or unreasonable, is no longer used. This change is based on evidence that individuals with such disorders often overestimate the danger in phobic situations and that older individuals often misattribute phobic fears to aging. Instead, the anxiety must be out of proportion to the actual danger or threat in the situation, after taking cultural contextual factors into account. Diagnosis is based on the presence of symptoms for at least a 6-month duration, regardless of age, to minimize overdiagnosis of transient fears.

AGORAPHOBIA

Previously linked in earlier *DSM* editions to panic disorder, agoraphobia now is defined and coded as a separate diagnosis. This change recognizes that a substantial number of individuals with agoraphobia do not experience panic symptoms. Diagnostic criteria now require that symptoms or avoidance behavior must be associated with at least two settings or situations (e.g., public places, crowds, mass transportation) as a robust means for distinguishing agoraphobia from specific phobias. Also, the criteria for agoraphobia are extended to be consistent with criteria sets for other anxiety disorders (e.g., clinician judgment of the fears as being out of proportion to the actual danger in the situation, with a typical duration of 6 months or more).

SPECIFIC PHOBIA

Individuals with specific phobias develop symptoms in specific situations or exposures. Examples of specific phobias include individuals who experience extreme fear and anxiety upon encountering insects, heights, cramped quarters, or even clowns. The individual may not recognize that their fear and anxiety are excessive or unreasonable. A 6-month duration of symptoms is required for diagnosis. It is an association with symptoms to *one* situation or exposure that discriminates specific phobia from agoraphobia.

SOCIAL ANXIETY DISORDER (SOCIAL PHOBIA)

Social anxiety disorder (formerly called *social phobia*) is characterized by a marked fear of being the center of attention or behaving in a way that will result in embarrassment or humiliation (e.g., while having a conversation, meeting new individuals, being observed eating or drinking, or performing in front of others). Individuals who fear only performance situations or performing in front of an audience appear to represent a distinct subset of social anxiety disorder in terms of etiology, age at onset, physiological response, and treatment response. As with the other forms of anxiety, the individual may not recognize that the response is excessive or unreasonable, and the response to social situations should typically last for at least 6 months prior to diagnosis. In children, the fear or anxiety may be expressed with tantrums, freezing, clinging, or failing to speak in social situations.

Separation Anxiety Disorder

While separation anxiety has historically been classified in the section "Disorders Usually First Diagnosed in Infancy, Childhood, or Adolescence," it is now classified as an anxiety disorder, recognizing that the expression of anxiety symptoms is possible in adulthood as well. Previously, the diagnostic criteria included onset before age 18; however, a substantial number of adults report onset of separation anxiety after age 18, and the age requirement is no longer in place. For example, attachment figures may include the children of adults with separation anxiety disorder, and avoidance behaviors may occur in the workplace as well as at school. A duration of 6 months is required to minimize overdiagnosis of transient fears (e.g., as when a new parent returns to work and places an infant in the care of another).

Obsessive-Compulsive and Related Disorders

The chapter on obsessive-compulsive and related disorders is new in *DSM-5*, reflecting increasing evidence that these disorders are related to one another in terms of a range of diagnostic validators and the clinical utility of grouping these disorders in the same chapter. This group of disorders includes hoarding, excoriation (skin picking), trichotillomania (hair pulling), body dysmorphic syndrome, substance/medication-induced obsessive-compulsive and related disorders, and obsessive-compulsive and related disorders owing to another medical condition. Commonalities among the grouped disorders include repetitive actions and obsessive preoccupations.

Previously, the criteria for obsessive-compulsive disorders included a "with poor insight" specifier. However, it is now recognized that patients suffering from obsessive-compulsive disorder have insight ranging from "good or fair insight," in which the individual recognizes the obsessive-compulsive disorder beliefs are probably not true; to "poor insight," in which the individual thinks the obsessive-compulsive disorder beliefs are probably true; to absent insight/delusional beliefs, in which the individual is convinced the obsessive-compulsive disorder beliefs are true. This criteria change emphasizes that the presence or absence of insight/delusional beliefs warrants a diagnosis of the relevant obsessive-compulsive or related disorder, rather than a schizophrenia spectrum and other psychotic disorder.

OBSESSIVE-COMPULSIVE DISORDER

Obsessive-compulsive disorder is defined by obsessions (recurring thoughts) and compulsions (recurrent actions) over which the patient has little or no control. While the behaviors or mental acts are aimed at preventing or reducing anxiety, these defining characteristics interfere with functioning and may cause embarrassment. The most common obsession is with "contamination," which leads to excessive washing or avoidance of a particular object that is "contaminated." Another common obsession is self-doubt, associated with repeatedly checking to see that routine safety chores are done.

BODY DYSMORPHIC DISORDER

Body dysmorphic disorder involves repetitive behaviors or mental acts in response to preoccupations with perceived defects or flaws in physical appearance. Examples associated with body dysmorphic disorder include individuals who seek frequent reassurance about their appearance, perform excessive grooming, or avoid photographs. The preoccupation with appearance can affect functionality and/or quality of life. One newly identified form includes muscle dysmorphia (occurring mostly in males), which is based on a growing literature on the diagnostic validity and clinical utility of making this distinction in individuals with body dysmorphic disorder. Often these individuals will use androgenic steroids or other substances to try to make their bodies bigger and more muscular. For women and some men, repeated plastic surgery procedures, possibly starting as young as the teenage years and continuing to the point of disfigurement, are extreme examples of body dysmorphic disorder. This is often seen in professional entertainers, such as actors.

Hoarding Disorder

Hoarding disorder is newly defined as a separate diagnosis in *DSM-5*; hoarding was previously described as one of the possible symptoms of obsessive-compulsive personality disorder. However, available data do not indicate that hoarding is a variant of obsessive-compulsive disorder or another mental disorder. Instead, there is evidence for the diagnostic validity and clinical utility of a separate diagnosis of hoarding disorder, which reflects persistent difficulty with discarding or parting with possessions due to a perceived need to save the items and distress associated with discarding them. Symptoms of hoarding include impairment in functioning due to the emotional, physical, and social consequences of hoarding (Box 18.5). Hoarding disorder may have unique neurobiological correlates, is associated with significant impairment, and may respond to clinical intervention. The most notable specifier is excessive acquisition, with 80% to 90% of individuals with hoarding disorder displaying excessive acquisition (APA, 2013).

Box 18.5

Questions to Screen for Hoarding

1. *"Do you have thoughts of harming yourself?"*

2. *"Do you have ongoing difficulty discarding or parting with possessions, regardless of value others may attribute to these possessions?"*

3. *"Have you accumulated a large number of possessions that fill up and clutter active living areas of the home or workplace to the extent that their intended use is no longer possible?"* (If all living areas become decluttered, it is only because of the interventions of third parties [e.g., family members, cleaners, authorities].)

4. *"Does this problem cause any difficulty or distress with friends, at work, or in any other area of your life?"*

SUBSTANCE/MEDICATION-INDUCED OBSESSIVE-COMPULSIVE AND RELATED DISORDER AND OBSESSIVE-COMPULSIVE AND RELATED DISORDER DUE TO ANOTHER MEDICAL CONDITION

DSM-5 includes new categories for substance/medication-induced obsessive-compulsive and related disorder and for obsessive-compulsive and related disorder due to another medical condition. This change reflects the recognition that substances, medications, and medical conditions can present with symptoms similar to primary obsessive-compulsive and related disorders. For instance, behaviors consistent with obsessive-compulsive disorder could be present only while taking or during withdrawal from specific prescribed or illegal drugs. Behaviors such as hair pulling or skin picking could be associated with an undiagnosed scalp or dermatological condition. Thus, it is important to consider other medical conditions and medications or substances as potential causes of behaviors.

OTHER SPECIFIED AND UNSPECIFIED OBSESSIVE-COMPULSIVE AND RELATED DISORDERS

DSM-5 includes the diagnoses of other specified obsessive-compulsive and related disorders, which can include conditions such as body-focused repetitive behavior disorder and obsessional jealousy or unspecified obsessive-compulsive and related disorder. Body-focused repetitive behavior disorder is characterized by recurrent behaviors other than hair pulling and skin picking (e.g., nail biting, lip biting, cheek chewing) and repeated attempts to decrease or stop the behaviors. Obsessional jealousy is characterized by nondelusional preoccupation with a partner's perceived infidelity.

Medical Problems and Medications

As with all mental health symptoms, the first step in the differential diagnosis is to rule out any general medical condition (Box 18.6) or medication use as the physiological cause of the anxiety. After ruling out a medical condition, the answers to the initial questions determine the next steps.

Box 18.6

Medical Conditions Associated With Anxiety

- Hyperthyroidism
- Congestive heart failure
- Asthma
- Chronic obstructive pulmonary disease
- Malignancy
- Pheochromocytoma
- Hyperadrenalism
- Hypoglycemia
- Epilepsy
- Myocardial infarction

■ Mood Disorders

This section examines several categories of mood disorders, discussing clusters and symptoms and the process of continuing assessment. Presented are major depressive disorder, cyclothymic disorder, bipolar disorder, seasonal pattern depression, postpartum depression, and premenstrual dysphoric disorder. There are some noteworthy changes in *DSM-5* relevant to this section, including several that define new depressive disorders.

For instance, to minimize potential overdiagnosis and overtreatment of bipolar disorder in children, a new diagnosis of disruptive mood dysregulation disorder is included for any person up to age 18 years who exhibits persistent irritability and frequent episodes of extreme behavioral dyscontrol. The category of persistent depressive disorder now includes both chronic major depressive disorder and dysthymic disorder. An inability to find scientifically meaningful differences between these two conditions led to their combination, with specifiers included to identify different pathways to the diagnosis.

Suicidality always represents a critical concern with depressed patients, and *DSM-5* provides guidance on the assessment of suicidal thinking, plans, and the presence of other risk factors in order to determine the prominence of suicide prevention in treatment planning for a given individual. A new specifier to indicate the presence of *mixed symptoms* has been added across both the bipolar and the depressive disorders, allowing for the possibility of manic features in individuals with a diagnosis of unipolar depression. A substantial body of research conducted over the last two decades points to the importance of *anxiety* as relevant to prognosis and treatment decision making. The "with anxious distress" specifier gives the clinician an opportunity to rate the severity of anxious distress in all individuals with bipolar or depressive disorders and increases the likelihood that the illness exists in a bipolar spectrum; however, if the individual concerned has never met criteria for a manic or hypomanic episode, the diagnosis of major depressive disorder is retained.

Medical Problems and Medications

Several medical conditions (Box 18.7) and numerous medications (Box 18.8) can be associated with symptoms of depression. If medications are the contributing cause, switching drugs may be advised.

Major Depressive Disorder

Depression is a clinically heterogeneous disorder resulting from a combination of genetic and environmental factors. Early detection and treatment are critical, as is early intervention when signs and symptoms of recurrence are detected. There is a 5% to 11% lifetime prevalence for depression; morbidity is comparable to angina and advanced coronary artery disease. The risk of recurrence of depression is 50% after one episode, 70% after two episodes, and 90% after three episodes. Untreated and undertreated depression significantly increases the risk of suicide: 1 out of 7 people with recurrent depressive illness commit suicide;

Box 18.7

Medical Problems That Can Present With Symptoms of Depression

- Addison's disease
- AIDS
- Anemia
- Asthma
- Chronic fatigue syndrome
- Chronic infection
- Congestive heart failure
- Cushing's disease
- Diabetes
- Hyperthyroidism
- Hypothyroidism
- Infectious hepatitis
- Malignancies
- Menopause
- Multiple sclerosis
- Postpartum hormonal changes
- Premenstrual syndrome
- Rheumatoid arthritis
- Systemic lupus
- Ulcerative colitis
- Uremia

Box 18.8

Drugs That Can Cause Depression

- Antihypertensives (reserpine, propranolol, methyldopa, guanethidine monosulfate, and clonidine hydrochloride)
- Corticosteroids and hormones (cortisone acetate, estrogen, and progesterone)
- Antiparkinsonian drugs (levodopa and carbidopa, amantadine hydrochloride)
- Antianxiety drugs (diazepam, chlordiazepoxide)
- Isotretinoin
- Birth control pills

70% of suicides have depressive illness; and 70% of suicides see their primary care provider within 6 weeks of suicide. Suicide is the seventh leading cause of death in the United States (Stahl, 2013).

Depression can present in a variety of ways, and the cluster of symptoms can vary markedly from one individual to the next. For example, depression may cause severe sleep disturbance for one individual and hypersomnia in another. Some individuals with depression complain of weight gain, whereas others lose weight because they find it hard to eat. Avolition (lack of motivation to start or finish projects) is a common presenting feature in depression, but some individuals experience restlessness and agitation. Symptoms of depression include changes in mood, cognition, behavior, and motor function (Box 18.9). The accurate assessment of presenting symptoms is key to treatment. Based on diagnosis and symptoms, a combination of psychotherapy with medication is often the most effective approach.

Box 18.9

Symptoms of Depression

Mood Symptoms

- Depressed mood
- Anhedonia
- Loss of reactivity
- Loss of self-esteem
- Tears
- Loss of hope
- Loss of interest
- Social withdrawal

Psychomotor Retardation Symptoms

- Loss of energy
- Cognitive symptoms
- Subjective inability to concentrate
- Pessimism
- General rating of anxiety
- Decreased interest in activities
- Subjective inefficient thinking
- Thoughts of dying
- Free-floating anxiety
- Phobias

Behavioral Symptoms

- Psychomotor agitation
- Irritability
- Guilty ideas of reference
- Depressed mood worse in morning
- Sleep disturbances
- Early waking
- Subjectively described restlessness
- Suicidality
- Fatigue and exhaustion
- Loss of appetite or increased appetite (carbohydrate craving)
- Hypersomnia

Prevalence rates for depression are higher for individuals age 18 to 26 years, and females have 1.5- to 3-fold higher rates than males (APA, 2013). Tools such as the Hamilton Rating Scale for Depression (HAM-D) and the Patient Health Questionnaire (PHQ-9) are helpful in assessing for depression; however, they are not a replacement for skillful interviewing.

The assessment of depression includes questions designed to identify whether the person is experiencing a general loss of pleasure in life or in activities the person usually enjoys. It is important to determine whether there is any sense of being sad or a general dysphoric mood and whether any neurovegetative symptoms are evident. Manic and hypomanic symptoms should always be actively sought. As with other mental health assessments, psychiatric history and history of alcohol and/or drug use should always be elicited; they are commonly associated with depression. What appears to be major depression actually may be a result of alcohol or street drug use (APA, 2013). In addition, some prescribed medications, and several medical conditions, can be associated with depression-like phenomena (APA, 2013).

To meet the criteria for a major depressive episode, an individual must have symptoms over a 2-week period that represent a change from previous functioning, with at least one of the symptoms being a depressed mood or a loss of interest or pleasure (APA, 2013). Five of the nine criteria for major depression must be met during a 2-week period as well as either a depressed mood or diminished interest during the 2-week period:

1. Depressed mood most of the day, nearly every day, as indicated by either subjective report (e.g., feels sad or empty) or observation made by others (e.g., appears tearful). Children and adolescents may display irritability.
2. Markedly diminished interest or pleasure in all, or almost all, activities most of the day, nearly every day (as indicated by either subjective account or observation made by others).
3. Significant weight loss when not dieting, weight gain (e.g., a change of more than 5% of body weight in a month), or a decrease or increase in appetite nearly every day. In children, consider failure to make expected weight gains.
4. Insomnia or hypersomnia nearly every day.
5. Psychomotor agitation or retardation nearly every day (observable by others, not merely subjective feelings of restlessness or being slowed down).
6. Fatigue or loss of energy nearly every day.
7. Feelings of worthlessness or excessive or inappropriate guilt (which may be delusional) nearly every day (not merely self-reproach or guilt about being sick).
8. Diminished ability to think or concentrate or indecisiveness nearly every day (either by subjective account or as observed by others).
9. Recurrent thoughts of death (not just fear of dying), recurrent suicidal ideation without a specific plan, or a suicidal attempt or a specific plan for committing suicide.

If these criteria are met, additional symptom analysis is needed to explore changes in appetite, sleep, activity, energy concentration, and thoughts of self-harm. The HAM-D is a 21-item rating tool to identify the severity of depression and evaluate the patient's response to treatment. The mnemonic "SIGECAPS" is helpful for remembering criteria for depression (Box 18.10).

An individual with major depression may experience difficulty with routine personal care and present as unkempt and unclean with a slowness of movement. In contrast, an individual with the specifier of anxious distress experiences unusual restlessness and a need to move a lot (APA, 2013). Thought process and content may reflect an inability to plan and make life decisions, called "blocking

Box 18.10

SIGECAPS

S	Sleep	C	Concentration
I	Interest	A	Appetite
G	Guilt	P	Psychomotor
E	Energy	S	Suicidality

of the future." A marked slowing in thinking often occurs and is reflected in slowness in responding to questions and in long pauses. This change in cognition can be described as the stream of thought being frozen by an unexpected drop in temperature. In contrast, individuals with depression with anxious distress experience thought process as a stream of thought in a turbulent boil and have problems with concentration because of worry (APA, 2013). Restricted thought content, or "ideational caging," is the experience of having thoughts trapped within a small network of themes or ruminations.

In *DSM-IV*, there was an exclusion criterion for a major depressive episode lasting less than 2 months following the death of a loved one (i.e., the bereavement exclusion). This exclusion is omitted in *DSM-5* for several reasons. First, it is recognized that the duration for bereavement is more commonly 1 to 2 years. Second, bereavement is recognized as a severe psychosocial stressor that can precipitate a major depressive episode in a vulnerable individual, generally beginning soon after the loss. When major depressive disorder occurs in the context of bereavement, it adds an additional risk for suffering, feelings of worthlessness, suicidal ideation, poorer somatic health, worse interpersonal and work functioning, and an increased risk for persistent complex bereavement disorder. Third, bereavement-related major depression is most likely to occur in individuals with past personal and family histories of major depressive episodes. It is genetically influenced and is associated with similar personality characteristics, patterns of comorbidity, and risks of chronicity and/ or recurrence as non-bereavement-related major depressive episodes. Finally, the depressive symptoms associated with bereavement-related depression respond to the same psychosocial and medication treatments as non-bereavement-related depression. Although most people who lose a loved one experience bereavement without developing a major depressive episode, evidence does not support the separation of loss of a loved one from other stressors in terms of its likelihood of precipitating a major depressive episode or the relative likelihood that the symptoms will remit spontaneously.

The coexistence within a major depressive episode of at least three manic symptoms (insufficient to satisfy criteria for a manic episode) is now acknowledged by the specifier "with mixed features." The presence of mixed features in an episode of major depressive disorder increases the likelihood that the illness exists in a bipolar spectrum; however, if the individual concerned has never met criteria for a manic or hypomanic episode, the diagnosis of major depressive disorder is retained.

Bipolar Disorder

Assessment of depression should always be followed by an assessment of bipolar disorder. Major depressive and bipolar disorders must be distinguished from episodes of a substance-induced mood disorder or those due to a general medical condition (e.g., multiple sclerosis, stroke, hypothyroidism).

Approximately 10% to 15% of adolescents with recurrent major depressive episodes will develop bipolar I disorder. Mixed episodes are more prevalent in adolescents and young adults than in older adults. In male patients, the first episode is more likely to be manic, whereas female patients usually present first with depression. Women with bipolar I disorder have an increased risk of developing subsequent episodes during the postpartum period (APA, 2013).

Bipolar disorder is a cluster of disorders that reflect a marked flux in mood. A manic episode is a distinct period of a persistently elevated, expansive, or irritable mood lasting at least 1 week and present most of the day. This mood must coexist with at least three of the following symptoms: inflated self-esteem or grandiosity, decreased need for sleep, pressure of speech, flight of ideas, distractibility, increased involvement in goal-directed activities or psychomotor agitation, and excessive involvement in pleasurable activities with a high potential for painful consequences. Hypomanic episodes differ from manic episodes in the degree of severity. Hypomanic episodes are not usually sufficiently severe to cause marked impairment in social or occupational functioning or to require hospitalization (APA, 2013). They may, however, evolve into fully manic episodes. The mnemonic "DIG FAST" is helpful for remembering the critical criteria for mania (Box 18.11).

Bipolar I disorder is characterized by the occurrence of one or more manic episodes or mixed episodes. Mixed episodes are characterized by a period of at least 1 week in which the criteria are met both for manic episode and for a major depressive episode nearly every day. Social and occupational functioning are severely impaired as the individual experiences rapidly alternating moods (APA, 2013). To aid in the differential diagnosis for bipolar I disorder, explore whether the patient has experienced episodes of feeling "high," with noticeably increased energy and elation, requiring less sleep than normal, or experienced rapid thoughts. Ask about episodes of feeling unusually creative or productive that were noticeable to others. Also explore episodes of anger, irritability, or rage.

Completed suicides occur in 10% to 15% of individuals with bipolar I disorder. Suicidal ideations and attempts are more likely to occur in the depressive or mixed state (APA, 2013). Therefore, suicide risk should always be assessed in a psychiatric evaluation. Box 18.12 lists several questions for assessing suicide risk. If the responses identify a detailed plan for ending life, a lack of hope that things can be better in the future, or an inability to identify reasons for not dying (e.g., not wanting to leave loved ones), it is considered a psychiatric emergency, requiring immediate intervention (generally inpatient treatment).

Box 18.11

DIG FAST

D	Distractibility; leaving tasks unfinished	F	Flight of ideas
I	Insomnia; decreased need for sleep	A	Activity increased; goal directed
G	Grandiosity; increased self-worth	S	Speech pressured, hyperverbal, and rapid
		T	Thoughtless risk (sex, money)

Box 18.12

Questions for Assessing Suicide Risk

1. *"Have you been thinking that you would be better off dead or wishing that you were dead?"*
2. *"Do you have thoughts of harming yourself?"*
3. *"Have you been thinking about suicide?"*
4. *"If you have been thinking about suicide, do you have a plan? If so, describe the plan."*
5. *"Have you recently attempted suicide?"*
6. *"In the past, have you thought about or attempted suicide?"*

Bipolar II disorder is determined when the clinical course includes one or more major depressive episodes (lasting at least 2 weeks) and at least one hypomanic episode (lasting at least 4 consecutive days). The symptoms cause clinically significant distress or impairment in social, occupational, or other important areas of functioning (APA, 2013). To meet the bipolar II criteria, the individual has not experienced a manic or mixed episode. In the past, bipolar II was considered a milder form or condition than bipolar I, but that is no longer the case because individuals with bipolar II tend to spend a significant amount of time in a major depressive state. This instability of mood is generally accompanied by significant social and work problems (APA, 2013).

Cyclothymic Disorder

Cyclothymic disorder is a chronic, fluctuating mood disturbance, including hypomanic and depressive symptoms that do not meet the criteria for manic episode. In addition, the depressive symptoms lack the severity, pervasiveness, or duration to meet the criteria for depressive episode. To meet the criteria for cyclothymic disorder, symptoms must be present over a 2-year period for adults or a 1-year period for children without a lapse of symptoms longer than 2 months. Many individuals function with minor distress or impairment in social, occupational, or other areas. Individuals may present as temperamental, moody, unpredictable, inconsistent, or unreliable (APA, 2013).

Mood Disorders With Specifiers

Seasonal Pattern

Seasonal pattern depression is differentiated from the other mood disorders by the essential feature of onset and remission that is consistently related to specific times of the year. It may have features similar to those of bipolar or major depression. In most cases, episodes begin in the fall or winter and remit in the spring. A key factor is that the mood is not related to situational stressors or cyclical patterns of work or life demands. Assessment involves tracking symptoms to demonstrate clear evidence of a temporal/seasonal relationship.

Postpartum Onset

There is no simple cluster of symptoms to assess during the postpartum period. Onset may be immediate or as late as 6 months after delivery. "Baby blues" occurs in up to 70% of women postpartum. Given the social pressures to "be happy" with the birth of a new baby, women often mask their underlying depression, a phenomenon called *smiling depression*. Symptoms common in the postpartum onset include fluctuation in mood, mood lability, and preoccupation with the infant's well-being. Severity of symptoms is the key. On a continuum, thoughts can range from focused and realistic regarding the infant's well-being to obsessive or even delusional. At highest risk are women who have experienced a postpartum episode with psychotic features. Women should be screened for depression at least once during the perinatal period. The Edinburgh Postnatal Depression Scale can help identify postpartum depression (Maurer, Raymond, & Davis, 2018). See Figure 18.1 for postpartum mood conditions.

Premenstrual Dysphoric Disorder

Premenstrual dysphoric disorder (PMDD) is characterized by recurrent symptoms that occur during the luteal phase of the menstrual cycle and remit during menstruation. Even though many women express mood changes and other symptoms during the premenstrual phase, 5% to 9% fully meet the criteria for PMDD. Differential diagnosis includes dysmenorrhea, bipolar disorder, thyroid dysfunction, use of hormonal treatments, premenstrual syndrome, exacerbation of unipolar depression, anxiety disorder, and cyclothymic disorder. Careful tracking of symptoms for at least 2 symptomatic cycles is required to determine a diagnosis of PMDD (Box 18.13).

■ Substance-Related Disorders

While substance abuse and substance dependence have historically been separate diagnoses, they are now combined in *DSM-5* as *substance use disorders*, with a separate substance use disorder for each substance of abuse. Each substance use disorder is then divided into mild, moderate, and severe subtypes. Even mild substance use disorder requires at least two symptoms; owing to the effect of certain substances on mood, cognition, perception, and behavior, patients may present with a confusing array of symptoms. Comorbidity with other psychiatric conditions is high in this population. Almost 25% of individuals with a severe mental illness also have a substance use disorder (National Institutes of Health, 2020). The recent diagnostic revisions are intended to strengthen the reliability of substance use diagnoses by increasing the number of required symptoms and clarifying the definition of "dependence," which is often misinterpreted as implying addiction and has at its core compulsive drug-seeking behaviors. In contrast, features of physical dependence, such as tolerance and withdrawal, can be normal responses to prescribed medications that affect the central nervous system and need to be differentiated from addiction. Moreover, although marijuana

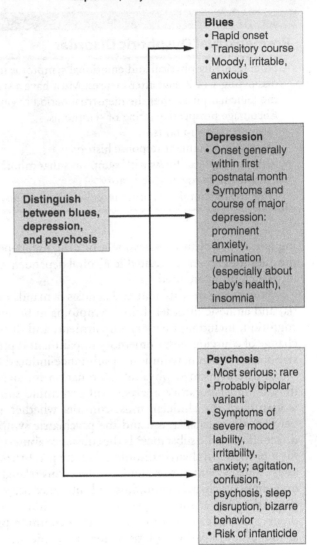

Figure 18.1 Postpartum mood disorders.

abuse can be functionally impairing, physical dependence is not part of the clinical picture. These mental and behavioral aspects are more specific to substance use disorders than the physical domains of tolerance and withdrawal, which are not unique to addiction (Kaplan, Sadock, & Ruiz, 2015).

Similarly, the terms *use* and *abuse* are often confused. Sanctioned uses of drugs (e.g., caffeine) have been defined by a culture, vary among cultures, and can change over time. Abuse from a cultural perspective is the self-administration of any drug in a culturally disapproved manner that causes adverse consequences. From a physiological standpoint, *use* and *abuse* take on different meanings, with a focus on the chemical neurotransmission and the degree of clinically significant

Box 18.13

Premenstrual Dysphoric Disorder

- Note recurring physical and emotional symptoms in late luteal phase, dissipating 1 or 2 days after menses. Must have a symptom-free period during the follicular phase after the menstrual period begins.
- Encourage prospective rating of symptoms.
- Document precipitants.
- Document treatment response history.
- Rule out medical illness with symptoms that mimic premenstrual syndrome.
- Obtain family psychiatric history.
- Note use of stimulants, other mood-altering agents, water-retaining drugs.

impairment or distress. Assessment of drug use, dependence, and abuse follows the questions presented related to alcohol dependence and abuse, after determining which drugs are used.

Prioritizing the differential diagnosis demands ruling out delirium, dementia, and amnesic disorder. Initial symptoms to be aware of include a change in cognition, including memory impairment, and disturbed consciousness. If no change of consciousness or memory impairment is present, then look for specific symptoms, which may indicate a substance-induced disorder.

A careful history, physical examination for signs of intoxication or withdrawal, and laboratory analysis will determine substance use. If a substance is identified, the clinician must consider whether a causal relationship exists between the substance use and the psychiatric symptom. Are the symptoms a direct effect of the substance? Is the substance abuse a means of "self-medicating" for a primary psychiatric disorder? Are the psychiatric symptoms and substance abuse independent of one another? Questions related to the timing of the development of psychiatric symptoms and substance use will help determine whether the patient has a primary psychiatric condition or a true substance abuse disorder. Substance abuse can mimic many common psychiatric symptoms, such as depression, apathy, agitation, anxiety, panic attacks, thought disturbances, paranoia, and psychosis. Thus, during the assessment of *any* psychiatric illness, the use and possible abuse of substances must be evaluated.

The growing opioid epidemic is a current public health crisis. The number of deaths related to drug overdoses has quadrupled between 1999 and 2019, increasing nearly 5% from 2018 to 2019. In 2019, 70% of the overdose deaths involved an opioid. Assessment of risk factors for opioid-related harm is an essential skill for clinicians who treat patients on opioids (CDC, 2021).

The National Institute on Drug Abuse Web site (www.drugabuse.gov) provides information regarding screening tools specific to the primary care setting. It provides resources for both providers and patients with regard to alcohol and drug assessment and patient education materials.

■ Eating Disorders

Eating disorders encompass much more than a list of symptoms. The lifetime prevalence rates for anorexia are 0.3% to 3% for female patients and 0.24% to 0.3% for male patients. The lifetime prevalence rates for bulimia are 0.88% to 4.6% for female patients and 0.1% to 1.5% for male patients (Mayhew et al., 2018). With *DSM-5*, binge eating disorder now has its own category as an eating disorder. Lifetime prevalence of binge eating disorder is around 2.6% in the United States (Kornstein, 2017).

Although both men and women are affected by cultural norms of physical attractiveness, the impact on self-esteem is greater for women. Anorexia and bulimia have different profiles, even though many symptoms can overlap. In fact, clients who have been initially diagnosed with one eating disorder can evolve over time into another eating disorder. Approximately 25% to 30% of people receiving treatment for bulimia had been previously diagnosed with anorexia (Mayhew et al., 2018). The dominant feature of anorexia is the drive to lose weight. Common patterns include restricting food intake and exercising excessively. The dominant features of bulimia are binge eating, inappropriate measures to prevent weight gain, and a self-evaluation predominantly influenced by body shape and weight (APA, 2013). The aspects that differentiate eating disorders from the "normal" cultural obsessions with weight and thinness are the amount of time and energy involved in the thinking and behaviors associated with an eating disorder and the degree to which they interfere with social functioning.

Many adolescents and young adults do not meet the full criteria for anorexia or bulimia but exhibit many of the characteristics. As explained in Schwitzer et al. (2001, p. 158), eating disorders are driven by "(1) perfectionism regarding body image, romantic and other personal relationships, and grades; (2) a fragile sense of self, feelings of inadequacy, and a need to be bolstered by others; (3) self-doubt expressed as sexual intimacy questions and ambivalence about whether one is thin enough to attract a romantic partner and whether one should want to please a partner at all; and (4) a sense of powerlessness in intimate relationships and the world generally." There exists a "high incidence of diagnostically subthreshold problems centering on dissatisfaction with body image."

Anorexia Nervosa

Individuals with this disorder are required to be at a significantly low body weight for their developmental stage, have an overtly expressed fear of weight gain, and also have persistent behavior that interferes with weight gain.

Individuals with anorexia are below 85% of the normal weight for their height, not attributable to a medical condition. Below-normal weight can also be described as a body mass index equal to or below 17.5 kg/m^2 (APA, 2013). Individuals with anorexia do not believe they need to gain weight and have an intense fear of becoming fat even though they are underweight. This fear is not

Box 18.14

Questions to Screen for Anorexia

1. *"Do you think your current weight is normal or excessive?"*

2. *"Do you think that any part of your body is still too fat?"*

3. *"Do you have concern or fear about gaining weight even though you are underweight?"*

relieved if additional weight is lost. More often, weight loss is accomplished through a reduction in total food intake, particularly high-calorie foods, leading to a diet limited to very few foods.

While the restricting pattern is more common in anorexia, binge–purge behavior may also exist. Although purging may follow a binge episode, purging may also be used even after the consumption of small amounts of food. A significant physical finding in anorexia is an irregular menstrual cycle or amenorrhea. The core diagnostic criteria for amenorrhea were eliminated with *DSM-5*. Questions used to screen for anorexia are listed in Box 18.14.

Bulimia Nervosa

Individuals with bulimia are characterized by cycles of binge eating followed by purging; the severity of the disorder is determined by the frequency of the binge–purge cycles. In severe cases, the bulimia becomes the center of the person's life, and all other aspects of life revolve around the binge–purge cycles. With publication of *DSM-5*, the frequency criteria for binge eating and inappropriate compensatory behavior associated with bulimia nervosa decreased from twice weekly to once weekly within a 3-month period. Individuals with bulimia are usually within the normal range for weight. The essential features of bulimia nervosa are binge eating and the use of inappropriate compensatory methods to prevent weight gain, such as vomiting or purging. Binge eating is the consumption of a large amount of food in a "discrete period of time" (APA, 2013). High-calorie foods are often preferred, and binging is associated with the abnormally large amounts of food consumed rather than with a craving for a specific type of food, such as carbohydrate. A feature of bulimia is an inability to control binges. Individuals with bulimia have a high degree of dissatisfaction with appearance and often have low self-esteem.

Physical findings may be a noticeable loss of dental enamel on the lingual surfaces of the front teeth as a result of recurrent vomiting. Teeth may become chipped, and there may also be an increase in dental cavities. The parotid glands may also be enlarged. Calluses or scars may be noted on the dorsal surface of the hand from inducing vomiting. If the dominant hand is used, calluses or scars may be evident on only that hand. There may be electrolyte imbalances—frequently hypokalemia, hyponatremia, and hypochloremia. Assessment for bulimia nervosa includes the questions listed in Box 18.15.

Box 18.15

Questions to Screen for Bulimia

1. *"In the past 3 months, were there times when you ate very large amounts of food, more than most people would eat, within a short period of time (2 hours)?"*

2. *"Has this occurred at least once a week over the last 3 months?"*

3. *"Did you feel as if you could not stop eating or control what or how much you were eating?"*

4. *"Have you used any of the following methods to prevent weight gain?"*
   a. *Purging: self-induced vomiting, laxatives, diuretics, enemas, and other medications*
   b. *Nonpurging: fasting or excessive exercise*

Binge Eating Disorder

Binge eating is often done alone, is not associated with hunger, and is done to the point of feeling uncomfortable. The minimum average frequency of binge eating required for diagnosis is once weekly over the past 3 months (compared to at least twice weekly for 6 months in *DSM-IV*). Patients present as overweight with marked distress associated with the binge episodes. The degree of severity is based on the number of binge eating episodes per week. For example, mild would be 1 to 3 binge eating episodes per week, and extreme would be 14 or more binge eating episodes per week.

■ Thought Disorders

Thought disorders are evaluated as they relate to (1) content of thought, (2) form of thought, and (3) perception. In psychiatry, thought disorders are commonly associated with schizophrenia and psychosis. However, the severity and the range of symptoms can vary significantly and often do not result from a primary psychiatric illness. Medical conditions, medications, and medical mimics often present with a clinical picture of a thought disorder.

Assessment of the *content of thought* relates to the client's ability to form an accurate assessment of reality. Major difficulties in this area may include delusions, which involve false beliefs held to be true despite proof that they are false or irrational. Examples of delusional thinking include delusions of persecution or of grandeur, somatic delusions, paranoia, and magical thinking.

The second category, *form of thought*, is assessed by listening to how the client presents ideas. Does the client present with looseness of associations? In such situations, the client is unaware that the topics are unconnected. When this is extreme, the practitioner may be unable to understand what the client is talking about. Other difficulties with form of thought include circumstantiality and tangentiality. Circumstantiality is the delay in presenting a point because of numerous unnecessary and tedious details. Tangentiality is the inability to get to the point owing to the introduction of unrelated topics. The degree of circumstantiality and tangentiality can vary significantly. For example, an anxious patient might shift from topic to topic with some awareness of doing so. This would not be considered a thought disorder problem. Serious thought disorder might include neologisms (invented words), word salad (a group of words put together randomly), and clang associations (choice of words based on rhyming).

The third category, *perception*, refers to hallucinations and illusions. Hallucinations are false sensory perceptions that are not associated with external stimuli and may involve any of the five senses. Illusions are misperceptions or misinterpretations of real external stimuli (when an actual object appears to be something else, such as a stick mistaken for a snake).

Psychotic Disorders

In schizophrenia, psychotic features are evident with two or more of the following characteristics: delusions, hallucinations (must be experienced in the context of a clear sensorium), disorganized speech, grossly disorganized or catatonic behavior, and negative symptoms. The last of these characteristics, negative symptoms, refers to affective flattening, poverty of speech, avolition, anhedonia, and social isolation. Differential diagnoses include schizophreniform disorder, characterized by schizophrenic symptoms of 1 to 6 months; schizoaffective disorder, characterized by a prominent mood component coexisting with the schizophrenic symptoms; delusional disorder, characterized by at least 1 month of no bizarre delusions without an active phase of symptoms of schizophrenia; brief psychotic disorder, characterized by symptoms that last more than 1 day but remit by 1 month; and substance-induced psychotic disorder, characterized by symptoms directly related to an abused substance, toxin, or medication. Although it is difficult to absolutely differentiate psychosis associated with schizophrenia or bipolar disorder from psychosis originating from a general medical process, there are some common organic causes that should be explored (Box 18.16).

The assessment of psychotic disorders can be guided by the diagnostic questions listed in Box 18.17. If the patient answers yes to any of the questions, further probing can be accomplished by asking the patient to give an example to determine the distortion of perception and thought and whether they can be considered "bizarre." In addition, check for evidence of thoughts that are based in reality. For example, if you ask, "Have you ever believed people are out to get you or have been spying on you?" and in reality the person was actually being stalked, it would not be a case of delusional thinking. Delusions are considered bizarre when they are absurd, implausible, and not understandable and clearly do not relate to ordinary life experiences (Kaplan, Sadock, & Ruiz, 2015).

The nature of hallucinations varies. Understanding the differences may help in determining whether the psychosis has medical origins, is in response to substance abuse, or is psychiatric in nature. A true visual hallucination is a perceptual image that arises from an open space and is not being triggered by an environmental stimulus. Illusions are images that *are* triggered by an actual object or stimulus. A visual hallucination in patients whose psychosis is related to delirium

Box 18.16

Common Causes of Delirium and Organic Psychosis

Metabolic

Electrolyte abnormalities (e.g., altered sodium, calcium, bicarbonate)
Advanced hepatic or renal disease
Nutritional disorders (e.g., deficits in thiamine, niacin)
Endocrine disorders (e.g., glucose abnormalities, disorders of the thyroid, adrenals, parathyroid)

Infections

Systemic (e.g., pneumonia, septicemia, malaria, and syphilis)
Intercranial (e.g., meningitis, encephalitis)

Neurological Disorders

Neurovascular (e.g., hypertensive crisis, stroke, subarachnoid hemorrhage)
Seizures
Trauma
Space-occupying lesions

Substances

Withdrawal (e.g., alcohol, stimulants, sedatives)
Intoxication (e.g., alcohol, stimulants, sedatives)
Adverse effects (e.g., digoxin, anticholinergics, levodopa, corticosteroids, barbiturates, antipsychotics, antidepressants)

Postoperative Sequelae

Greenberg, Aminoff, & Simon. (2013); Ropper, Samuels, & Klein. (2014).

differs from the classic psychosis in the following ways: (1) more often occurs at night, (2) is frequently perceived as moving, (3) is briefer in duration, and (4) has no personal significance to the patient. A patient with delirium may see a snake, whereas a patient with schizophrenia may hallucinate about a deceased relative. Asking the client to state the time of day or night when the hallucination is seen helps in the differentiation. In medical conditions, hallucinations are often seen at night and when the patient closes the eyes. In schizophrenia, visual hallucinations are usually present with auditory hallucinations, occur in an otherwise normal-appearing environment, and appear somewhat suddenly.

Substance abuse can produce psychotic episodes. Among the common agents are "speed," lysergic acid diethylamide (LSD), hallucinogens, marijuana, cocaine, crack, and phencyclidine (PCP). In a drug-induced psychosis, the environment appears distorted with numerous illusions and hallucinations. From a behavioral perspective, psychotic symptoms tend to be very bizarre and can be violent. On physical examination, nystagmus and hypertension may be present.

Box 18.17

Diagnostic Questions for Psychotic Disorders

1. *"Have you ever believed people are out to get you or have been spying on you?"*
   If yes: *"Do you currently believe this?"* **Example:**

2. *"Have you ever thought that someone could read your mind or that you could read someone's mind?"*
   If yes: *"Do you currently believe this?"* **Example:**

3. *"Have you ever believed that a force outside of you had control over your thoughts or actions?"*
   If yes: *"Do you currently believe this?"* **Example:**

4. *"Have you ever believed you were being sent messages through the TV, radio, newspaper, or computer?"*
   If yes: *"Do you currently believe this?"* **Example:**

5. *"Have you ever heard voices that others around you could not hear?"*
   If yes: *"Do you currently hear them?"* **Example:**

Unlike schizophrenia, drug-induced psychosis usually presents with rapid-onset psychotic symptoms.

In addition to street drugs or commonly abused drugs, anticholinergic agents can precipitate delirium, especially in older patients. Anticholinergic medications can cause a patient to present with hyperthermia, blurred vision, dry skin, facial flushing, and delirium. The mnemonic "hot as a pepper, blind as a bat, dry as a bone, red as a beet, and mad as a hatter" can be used to describe this toxic state (Broderick, Metheny, & Crosby, 2020). It is important to note that anticholinergic syndrome may be incomplete or hidden by other medications, such as opiates, and may not present as a classic anticholinergic syndrome.

■ Trauma- and Stressor-Related Disorders

Acute Stress Disorder

In *DSM-5*, the stressor criterion is changed and requires being explicit as to whether qualifying traumatic events were experienced directly, witnessed, or experienced indirectly. Also, the criterion regarding the subjective reaction to the traumatic event (e.g., "the person's response involved intense fear, helplessness, or horror") has been eliminated. Based on evidence that acute posttraumatic reactions are very heterogeneous, individuals now may meet diagnostic criteria in *DSM-5* for acute stress disorder if they exhibit any 9 of 14 listed symptoms in these categories: intrusion, negative mood, dissociation, avoidance, and arousal.

Adjustment Disorder

In *DSM-5*, adjustment disorders are reconceptualized as a heterogeneous array of stress-response syndromes that occur after exposure to a distressing (traumatic or nontraumatic) event, rather than as a residual category for individuals who exhibit clinically significant distress without meeting criteria for a more discrete disorder (as in *DSM-IV*). *DSM-IV* subtypes marked by depressed mood, anxious symptoms, or disturbances in conduct have been unchanged.

Posttraumatic Stress Disorder

DSM-5 criteria for posttraumatic stress disorder differ significantly from those in *DSM-IV*. The stressor criterion is more explicit with regard to how an individual experienced "traumatic" events, and the subjective reaction criterion has been eliminated. Whereas there were previously three major symptom clusters (re-experiencing, avoidance/numbing, and arousal), there are now four in *DSM-5*, with the avoidance/numbing cluster divided into two distinct clusters: avoidance and persistent negative alterations in cognitions and mood. This latter category, which retains most of the *DSM-IV* numbing symptoms, also includes new or reconceptualized symptoms, such as persistent negative emotional states. The final cluster—alterations in arousal and reactivity—retains most of the *DSM-IV* arousal symptoms. It also includes irritable or aggressive behavior and reckless or self-destructive behavior. Posttraumatic stress disorder is now developmentally sensitive in that diagnostic thresholds have been lowered for children and adolescents. Furthermore, separate criteria have been added for children age 6 years or younger with this disorder.

Reactive Attachment Disorder

The *DSM-IV* childhood diagnosis reactive attachment disorder had two subtypes: emotionally withdrawn/inhibited and indiscriminately social/disinhibited. In *DSM-5*, these subtypes are defined as *distinct disorders*: reactive attachment disorder and disinhibited social engagement disorder. Both of these disorders are the result of social neglect or other situations that limit a young child's opportunity to form selective attachments. Although sharing this etiological pathway, the two disorders differ in important ways. Because of dampened positive affect, reactive attachment disorder more closely resembles internalizing disorders; it is essentially equivalent to a lack of or incompletely formed preferred attachments to caregiving adults. In contrast, disinhibited social engagement disorder more closely resembles attention-deficit/hyperactivity disorder (ADHD); it may occur in children who do not necessarily lack attachments and may have established or even secure attachments. The two disorders differ in other important ways, including correlates, course, and response to intervention; for these reasons, they are considered separate disorders.

■ Medically Unexplained Symptoms

According to the APA, *DSM-IV* criteria "overemphasized" the importance of an absence of a medical explanation for the somatic symptoms. Unexplained symptoms are present to various degrees, particularly in conversion disorder, but somatic symptom disorders can also accompany diagnosed medical disorders. The reliability of medically unexplained symptoms is limited, and grounding a diagnosis on the absence of an explanation is problematic and reinforces mind–body dualism. The *DSM-5* classification defines disorders on the basis of positive symptoms (i.e., distressing somatic symptoms plus abnormal thoughts, feelings, and behaviors in response to these symptoms). Medically unexplained symptoms do remain a key feature in conversion disorder and pseudocyesis because it is possible to demonstrate definitively in such disorders that the symptoms are not consistent with medical pathophysiology.

Hypochondriasis and Illness Anxiety Disorder

Hypochondriasis has been eliminated as a disorder, in part because the name was perceived as pejorative and not conducive to an effective therapeutic relationship. Most individuals who would previously have been diagnosed with hypochondriasis have significant somatic symptoms in addition to their high health anxiety and would now receive a *DSM-5* diagnosis of somatic symptom disorder. In *DSM-5*, individuals with high health anxiety without somatic symptoms would receive a diagnosis of illness anxiety disorder (unless their health anxiety was better explained by a primary anxiety disorder, such as generalized anxiety disorder).

Pain Disorder

DSM-5 takes a different approach to the important clinical realm of individuals with pain in that this diagnosis assumes that some pains are associated solely with psychological factors, some with medical diseases or injuries, and some with both. Most individuals with chronic pain attribute their pain to a combination of factors, including somatic, psychological, and environmental influences. In *DSM-5*, some individuals with chronic pain would be appropriately diagnosed as having somatic symptom disorder, with predominant pain. For others, psychological factors affecting other medical conditions or an adjustment disorder would be more appropriate.

■ Psychological Factors Affecting Other Medical Conditions and Factitious Disorder

Psychological factors affecting other medical conditions is a new mental disorder in *DSM-5*. This disorder and factitious disorder are placed among the somatic symptom and related disorders because somatic symptoms are predominant in both disorders and both are most often encountered in medical settings.

Issues Related to Older Adults

The presence of coexisting medical conditions makes accurate psychiatric diagnosis and treatment a complex matter. History taking and the mental status examination of older adults is similar to those for younger patients, but cognitive impairments make verification from a family member an important difference.

Psychiatric history includes identification (e.g., name, sex, marital status), chief complaint, and history of present illness; history of previous illnesses; personal and family history; and current medication review. Past history can provide invaluable information about personality organization, coping styles, and defense mechanisms during times of stress. Family history includes adaptation to older age and the presence of Alzheimer's disease if known.

Mental disorders of old age include depressive disorders, cognitive disorders, phobias, and substance abuse, particularly alcohol. Psychosocial risk factors that predispose older adults to mental illness include social isolation and loss of friends, social roles, autonomy, and health. In 2014, the suicide rates per 100,000 men aged 65 to 74 and 75 and older were 26.6 and 38.9, respectively; the suicide rates per 100,000 women aged 65 to 74 and 75 and older were 5.9 and 4.0, respectively (CDC, 2016).

Several studies have shown that many older adults who commit suicide visit their primary care physician close to the act. In the year prior to committing suicide, 64% of older adults saw a primary care provider and 62% saw a non–mental health specialist. Recent statistics confirm that while only 22.7% of older adults scheduled a visit for mental health reasons during the 4 weeks prior to committing suicide, 67% of older adults were seen by at least one health-care provider during the 4-week period. Many (39.9%) saw their primary care provider for non–mental health reasons during the 4-week period preceding suicide (Ahmedani, Simon, & Stewart et al., 2014).

Depression coexists with other medical conditions (e.g., cancer, diabetes, stroke, cardiovascular disease). Clinicians and patients may often feel that depression is a natural consequence of these problems. This allows depression to be both underdiagnosed and undertreated. Depression is not a natural consequence of aging. This false belief may help explain the high rates of successful suicide in older persons. Other common conditions related to this age group are vertigo, syncope, hearing loss, elder abuse, spousal bereavement, and sleep disorders. The very real possibility for psychiatric symptoms related to either a response to medications or a medical condition is an important concept with older patients.

REFERENCES

Ahmedani, B. K., Simon, G. E., Stewart, C., Beck, A., Waitzfelder, B. E., Rossom, R., Lynch, F., Owen-Smith, A., Hunkeler, E. M., Whiteside, U., Operskalski, B., Coffey, M. J., & Solberg, L. I. (2014). Health care contacts in the year before suicide death. *Journal of General Internal Medicine, 29*(6), 870–877. http://doi.org/10.1007/s11606-014-2767-3

American Psychiatric Association. (2013). *Diagnostic and statistical manual of mental disorders (DSM-5)* (5th ed.). American Psychiatric Association.

Broderick, E. D., Metheny, H., & Crosby, B. (2020). Anticholinergic toxicity. *National Institute of Health StatPearls.* Accessed May 23, 2021, from https://www.ncbi.nlm.nih.gov/books/NBK534798/

Carlat, D. (2017). *The psychiatric interview* (4th ed.). Wolters Kluwer.

Centers for Disease Control and Prevention. (n.d.). Children's mental health: Anxiety & depression. www.cdc.gov/childrensmentalhealth/depression.html

Centers for Disease Control and Prevention. (2016). Increase in suicide in the United States: 1999–2014. Retrieved from https://stacks.cdc.gov/view/cdc/39008.

Centers for Disease Control and Prevention. (2017). CDC guideline for prescribing opioids for chronic pain. Retrieved from https://www.cdc.gov/drugoverdose/prescribing/guideline.html.

Combs, H., & Markman, J. (2014). Anxiety disorders in primary care. *Medical Clinics of North America, 98*(5), 1007–1023.

Greenberg, D., Aminoff, M., & Simon, R. (2015). *Clinical neurology* (9th ed.). McGraw-Hill.

Hart, V. (2010). *Patient-provider communications: Caring to listen.* Jones & Bartlett Publishers.

Hedeya, R. J. (1996). *Understanding biological psychiatry.* W.W. Norton.

Kaplan, B. J., Sadock, V. A., & Ruiz, P. (2015). *Kaplan & Sadock's synopsis of psychiatry* (11th ed). Wolters Kluwer.

Kornstein, S. G. (2017). Epidemiology and recognition of binge-eating disorder in psychiatry and primary care. *Journal of Clinical Psychiatry, 78*(1), 3–8. doi: 10.4088/JCP.sh16003su1c.01

Maurer, D. M., Raymond, T. J., & Davis, B. N. (2018). Depression: Screening and diagnosis. *American Family Physician, 98*(8), 508–515.

Mayhew, A. J., Pigeyre, M., Couturier, J., & Meyre, D. (2018). An evolutionary genetic perspective of eating disorders. *Neuroendocrinology, 106*, 292–306. https://doi.org/10.1159/000484525

National Institutes of Health. (2021). Substance use and co-occurring mental disorders. Retrieved May 6, 2022, from nimh.nih.gov/health/topics/substance-use-and-mental-health/

National Institute of Mental Health. (n.d.). *Any anxiety disorders.* Bethesda, MD: National Institute of Mental Health. Retrieved from nimh.nih.gov/health/statistics/any-anxiety-disorder.shtml

Ropper, A. H., Samuels, M. A., & Klein, J. P. (2014). *Adams and Victor's principles of neurology* (10th ed.). McGraw-Hill.

Schwitzer, A. M., Rodriguez, L. E., Thomas, C., & Salimi, L. (2001). The eating disorders NOS diagnostic profile among college women. *Journal of American College Health, 49*(4), 157–166.

Stahl, S. M. (2013). *Stahl's essential psychopharmacology: Neuroscientific basis and practical applications* (4th ed.). Cambridge University Press.

Stern, T. A., Herman, J. B., & Gorrindo, T. (2012). *Massachusetts General Hospital psychiatry: Update and board preparation* (3rd ed.). McGraw-Hill.

Assessment and Differential Diagnosis in Special Patient Populations

Chapter 19

Pediatric Patients

Sara F. Barber •

Communicating With Infants and Children During the Pediatric Assessment

When assessing infants and children, it is crucial to remember that they are not merely "little adults." Obviously, infants and children have varying communication abilities and interaction skills. Pediatric assessments are more successful when providers take the time to communicate with children in an age-appropriate manner.

■ Infants

Infants are in the midst of the developmental stage of trust and mistrust, so they should be approached slowly. Be prepared for stranger anxiety in an infant of 6 to 7 months and for separation anxiety in an infant just slightly older. Owing to these normal fears, it is best to conduct most, or all, of your examination with the infant on the parent's lap. During the assessment, integrate distraction techniques, such as singing or making funny faces, or allow the child to hold on to a familiar security item if present. Rather than a head-to-toe approach, plan your examination in order from noninvasive to invasive (e.g., auscultate the heart and lung sounds first, and examine the ears and throat last). Remember to talk in a soothing voice and to avoid sudden movements.

■ Toddlers

Toddlers are at the height of negativism and are developmentally struggling for independence. They still have fears of parental separation, and they also fear any intrusion to their bodies. Their attention spans are short, and they can be strong-willed and uncooperative, especially when tired or ill. Allow toddlers to touch or hold some of your equipment before you begin the physical examination. Demonstrate what you are going to do on a doll or stuffed animal or parent before doing it on the child. Use distraction as much as possible and give the child choices when they exist, such as, "Which ear should I look in first?" Be direct but friendly—tell the child what you are going to do instead of asking permission. At this age, continue to conduct as much of the examination as you can with the child on a parent's lap, working from noninvasive to invasive procedures.

■ Preschoolers

Preschoolers are magical thinkers and may have fears of pain and body mutilation. They believe that everything is "alive" and may fear unknown equipment or procedures. Involve the child in the examination by describing what you are doing and letting the child practice on a doll or stuffed animal first. Move slowly and systematically and explain in simple terms what you are doing. Choose your words carefully because preschoolers are very literal. Allow choices when possible and praise the child frequently for helping and cooperating. A head-to-toe sequence may be possible at this age.

■ School-Age Children

School-age children generally want to be brave and cooperate, although they still fear pain and the loss of control. They often ask lots of questions and are curious about using your equipment. Allow them to examine the equipment and provide concrete answers to their questions whenever possible because children at this age become very logical. Teach them the proper names for equipment and body parts. Modesty may begin to appear in this age group, so be sensitive to this. A head-to-toe sequence is possible for this age.

■ Adolescents

Adolescents are at the height of trying to fit in and be "normal." They worry about how they stack up alongside their peers and may have concerns about their physical appearance, including height, weight, or the presence of acne. They are striving to be independent and fear the loss of control and possibly even death. Privacy is very important at this age, so offer to examine the child without the parent unless the child prefers it otherwise. Remember to keep body parts covered when you are not examining them. Explain each step of your examination and give the child a chance to ask questions or make choices as you progress. Be very nonjudgmental and talk professionally but casually with them. Teach adolescents about their bodies and stress the normalcy of their features and appearance. Reassure them that others their age feel the same way and try to initiate discussion of sensitive subjects by utilizing this fact (e.g., "Lots of kids your age are faced with tough decisions, like whether to try drugs and alcohol. Have you been faced with any situations like that?"). Teach self-breast and testicular examinations. Give concrete information on sexually transmitted infections, safe sex, and HIV. Give adolescents an opportunity to ask questions.

Pediatric History and Physical Examination

Much of the content of earlier chapters regarding the assessment of specific systems is relevant to the pediatric assessment. However, the assessment of infants and children should be based on knowledge of the anticipated problems of childhood, developmental stages, and potential risks. The following section summarizes specific questions or examinations that should be considered during pediatric assessment, along with the potential findings that should be considered as red flags, warranting further assessment or consultation.

■ Head

When assessing pediatric patients, remember to ask about head trauma, head growth, and the history of headaches. The head circumference should be measured at all well-child visits up to age 2 years to assess for macro- or microcephaly and to ensure that sutures are not fusing prematurely (craniosynostosis). Assess the head symmetry and look for plagiocephaly. For the fontanel to be accurately assessed, the child should be sitting upright and not crying. Some variants that might be noted in newborns include the following:

- *Caput succedaneum*—Seen at birth, usually following a traumatic vaginal delivery or vacuum-assisted delivery; edema of the soft tissue of the scalp that usually crosses the suture lines; no specific treatment; should resolve in a few days.
- *Cephalohematoma*—Often appears several hours after birth and may increase for the first 24 hours; subperiosteal collection of blood that does not cross the suture lines; may take weeks to months to resolve; watch for hyperbilirubinemia.

Common Diagnoses for the Head

- Headache
- Head trauma
- Plagiocephaly

RED FLAG ◀ **Red Flags for the Head Examination**

- *No growth in head circumference between well-child visits.*
- *Enlarged head size or excessive growth between well-child visits.*

Common Diagnoses for the Eye

- Conjunctivitis
- Allergies
- Corneal abrasion
- Lacrimal duct stenosis
- Strabismus

RED FLAG ◀   **Red Flags for the Eye Examination**

- *Presence of white instead of red reflex may indicate retinoblastoma; an absent red reflex or opacity of the lens may indicate cataracts*

- *Dilated and fixed pupils, which indicate severe brain damage*

- *Strabismus, which requires referral to ophthalmology for further evaluation*

■ Eyes

Ask about vision problems or history of eye drainage. The vision portion of the "Growth and Development" section of this chapter (see pp. 682–684 provides details on specific vision assessments and screening for children of various ages. Some variations that may be noted in newborns include the presence of "stork bites" (telangiectatic nevi) on the eyelids, nasolabial area, or nape of the neck; they appear as a purplish red color and generally diminish or disappear by age 12 months. Strabismus is considered normal until about 4 to 6 months.

Eye Examination Tips for Infants and Younger Children

Infants and younger children may be better examined while they are being held by their parents or caregivers. The examination may be facilitated by using a colorful toy or sticker. Bright lights lack spatial orientation and should not be used. Ocular misalignment, or intermittent strabismic gaze, may be normal during a child's first few months, but if the deviations persist after 4 months, the child should be referred to an ophthalmologist for further evaluation and treatment.

In infants and toddlers younger than 2 to 3 years, visual behavior is assessed. Parents are often aware of a child's vision problem before it is readily apparent. Parents should therefore be asked if they have any concerns regarding their child's vision, if the child's eyes seem to cross or wander, if the child often squints or holds objects close, or if the eyelids droop. Infants' vision acuity may be assessed by inquiring about or observing their ability to focus on an object or their parent's face. Most infants should develop the ability to follow an object by age 3 months. Visual acuity should be performed in an environment with minimal distractions. Visual acuity in children 3 to 4 years or older can be assessed using LEA Symbols, which are four simple and familiar objects (a circle, square, house, and apple), or the HOTV test, which uses only the letters H, O, T, and V, or the tumbling E. Standardized eye charts (Snellen or Sloan) use letters and can be used once the child has mastered the alphabet. If the child is unable to cooperate with a visual acuity screening, a repeat screening can be done within 1 to 6 months. If the child is unable to be tested after two attempts, or if an abnormality is suspected, an ophthalmologist or optometrist referral should be completed. Visual acuity measurement should be done at regular well-child visits beginning at age 3 to 5 years or if the child exhibits a school performance decline or reading difficulty or complains of headaches, eye strain, or blurred or double vision (AAP, 2012).

While the visual acuity may vary with the child's age, the "rule of 8s" is helpful to determine if a referral is warranted (Table 19.1).

Ocular alignment and strabismus may be assessed with the cover-uncover test. This is done by having the child look at a near object. One eye is then covered for 5 seconds. The cover is then removed, and the alignment of the covered eye is observed. The opposite eye is tested in the same fashion. The test is repeated for both eyes while they are fixating on a far object. A normal test occurs when neither eye moves out of alignment or "drifts." Box 19.1 indicates reasons for referral. If a problem is suspected, it is imperative that eye referrals be made in a timely manner to avoid long-term morbidities.

Table 19.1

Rule of 8s (Shen & Bhatt [2017])

Age (years)	Rule of 8s	Normal Visual Acuity	Referral Level
2	$2+6=8$	20/60	20/70
3	$3+5=8$	20/50	20/60
4	$4+4=8$	20/40	20/50
5	$5+3=8$	20/30	20/40
6	$6+2=8$	20/20	20/30

The child's age plus the tens digit of the denominator of the visual acuity should be ≤8. If the child's age plus the tens digit of the denominator of the visual acuity is nine or more, a referral is warranted.

Box 19.1

Indications for Childhood Ophthalmologist/Optometrist Referral

- Abnormal red reflex (white reflex should have immediate referral)
- Prematurity (if not already cleared by ophthalmologist)
- Family history of childhood eye condition (i.e., cataract, glaucoma, retinoblastoma, retinal dysplasia)
- Pupillary or corneal asymmetry
- Visual acuity difference of two or more lines between eyes
- Nystagmus (may be horizontal, vertical, rotary, or combination; latent nystagmus occurs only when one eye is covered)
- Inability to fix and follow by 3 months of age
- Abnormal ocular alignment in children older than 4 months
- Ptosis or eyelid lesions (i.e., hemangiomas)
- Presence of handicap

Common Diagnoses for the Ear

- Acute otitis media
- Middle ear effusions
- Otitis externa
- Wax impaction
- Foreign body

RED FLAG ◄ **Red Flags for the Ear Examination**

- *Pain over the mastoid process, which may indicate mastoiditis*
- *Foreign bodies, which should be considered if the child complains of strange sounds or sensations in one ear or if there is an obvious blockage or odd color noted on otoscopic examination*
- *Hearing deficit*

■ Ears

Ask about hearing ability or difficulties, ear pain, and ear drainage. The general appearance and placement of the ears is important in pediatric assessment. Ears that are set low may indicate genitourinary or chromosomal abnormalities or a multisystem syndrome such as Turner syndrome. Assess for preauricular sinuses.

The otoscopic examination is described in detail in Chapter 7. This examination should be saved for last in infants and young children because of the distress it often causes. To examine the inner ear in an infant or young child, pull the pinna down and out. For examination in an older child, pull up and back as you would with an adult. As with adults, the tympanic membrane (TM) should be mobile and intact and should appear thin, smooth, and pearly gray with bright light reflexes. The mobility of the TM should be assessed by pneumatic otoscopy if a diagnosis of acute otitis media is expected. Although crying will cause erythema of the TMs, the light reflexes and mobility should remain intact. Diagnosis of acute otitis media should not be based solely on a reddened TM. Also observe for bubbles or an obvious fluid level line behind the TM, which indicates middle ear effusion.

A young child who frequently asks for things to be repeated, seems markedly inattentive, and responds inappropriately to questions should be investigated for hearing deficit. Middle ear effusions and acute otitis media may cause hearing deficits. The "Hearing" portion of the growth and development section of this chapter provides details on hearing screening (see pp. 682–683).

■ Nose and Sinuses

Ask about nasal drainage, nosebleeds, and breathing interference. Note the characteristics of any drainage. Clear, watery drainage may indicate allergies, especially when coupled with pale, boggy mucosa. Persistent, copious, or

Common Diagnoses for the Nose and Sinuses

- Upper respiratory
  infection
- Allergic rhinitis
- Foreign body
- Sinusitis

Red Flags for the Nose and Sinus Examination

- *Reports of apnea should be investigated fully and may require hospitalization for monitoring.*

- *Foreign bodies should be removed as soon as possible, and referral to a specialist should be considered if removal in the office is impossible.*

Common Diagnoses for the Mouth and Throat

- Stomatitis
- Oral candidiasis
- Viral pharyngitis/
  tonsillitis
- Strep pharyngitis
- Dental caries

Red Flags for the Mouth and Throat Examination

- *An absent suck in a newborn, an obvious communication between the nose and mouth, or a bifid uvula should be investigated for cleft palate.*

- *A unilateral enlarged tonsil should be further evaluated to rule out abscess or lymphoma.*

---

purulent drainage may indicate sinusitis. Unilateral, purulent drainage is seen with foreign bodies. Bloody discharge indicates irritation that may be caused by a foreign body, infection, or excessive nose picking.

Newborns frequently have nasal congestion without other symptoms of illness ("newborn congestion"); this should resolve after 2 to 3 months. Newborns are obligate nose breathers.

■ Mouth and Throat

Ask children or parents about throat pain, difficulty swallowing, tooth eruption, dental trauma, and brushing habits. Table 19.13 in the "Growth and Development" section identifies the typical age of tooth eruption (see p. 689).

Common Diagnoses for the Lung

- Asthma
- Upper respiratory infection
- Croup
- Pneumonia
- Bronchitis
- Bronchiolitis

- Gastroesophageal reflux disease (may be a cause of cough although not an obvious lung problem)
- Allergies
- Sinusitis

RED FLAG ◀ **Red Flags for the Lung Examination**

- *Any abnormal breath sounds should be evaluated further with pulse oximeter monitoring and possibly a chest x-ray.*

- *Cough in the middle of the night or with exertion may indicate asthma, even in a child who does not wheeze.*

- *Retractions, grunting, and/or nasal flaring should be taken seriously. Any work of breathing should be evaluated emergently.*

■ Lungs

Ask about breathing patterns, blue spells or apnea, and cough. Children under age 7 are diaphragmatic (abdominal) breathers—this is particularly pronounced in infancy; after age 7, children become more thoracic breathers. Observe the general work of breathing, noting any use of accessory muscles, nasal flaring, and retractions. Breath sounds are heard best by having the child breathe through the mouth. Asking the child to pretend may help with breath sound auscultation; for example, to hear inspiratory sounds, have the child pretend to hold the breath as if preparing to go under water. Alternatively, have the child pretend to blow bubbles or "birthday candles" as you listen to both inspiratory and expiratory sounds.

A common complaint from parents of infants and toddlers is that their child's chest sounds "rattly." These vibrations that can be felt (and sometimes heard) over the chest are rhonchi produced by excess mucus caught in a younger child's throat. Although it sounds odd, it is not dangerous and will typically clear the next time the child coughs. Use this parental concern to educate parents about what types of respiratory symptoms could be worrisome (e.g., retractions, wheezing, apnea).

■ Heart

Ask about a history of heart murmur, cyanosis, activity intolerance, or syncope. Measure vital signs, with blood pressure measurement beginning at age 3 years. Always assess pulse for rate and rhythm; an apical pulse should be determined in infants.

A common variation of heart rhythm is sinus arrhythmia, in which the heart rate increases with inspiration and decreases with expiration. This fluctuation in rhythm will cease if the child is instructed to hold the breath. Assess carefully for murmurs. Up to one-half of all children have an innocent (functional) murmur. Box 19.2 includes characteristics common to innocent murmurs in general. Table 19.2 identifies characteristics of select innocent murmurs.

Box 19.2

Characteristics Common to Innocent Murmurs

- Soft, grade III or lower
- Systolic timing
- Short duration
- Low-pitched, vibratory, and musical
- Rarely transmitted
- Loudest in left lower sternal border or at second/third intercostal space
- Loudest when lying down, during expiration, and after exercise
- Sound diminishes with position change from recumbent to sitting
- Intensity and presence may vary over time
- Child has normal growth and development, blood pressure, respiratory rate, and pulses
- No associated thrill or cyanosis

Table 19.2

Types of Innocent Murmurs

Type of Murmur	Characteristics
Still's murmur	Most common; heard most frequently from 3 to 7 years of age; described as vibratory or musical; heard best between lower left sternal border and apex with child supine; probably caused by turbulence in left ventricular outflow tract
Basal systolic ejection murmur	High-pitched, blowing sounds heard best at the pulmonic area with child supine
Physiological peripheral pulmonic stenosis (pulmonary outflow murmur)	Short, systolic; heard best in the axillae and back; usually disappears during infancy
Venous hum	Humming, continuous murmur; heard best in the supraclavicular areas with the child sitting; can be diminished by having the child lie down, turning the head or occluding the jugular vessels

---

Common Diagnosis for the Heart

- Innocent murmur

RED FLAG ◀ **Red Flags for the Heart Examination**

- *Pathological murmur*
- *Unequal or absent pulses*
- *Cyanosis*

Common Diagnoses for the Breasts

- Normal breast bud
- Gynecomastia

RED FLAG ◀ **Red Flags for the Breast Examination**

- *Firm, unmovable masses*
- *Galactorrhea, which may indicate hypothyroidism or pituitary tumor*

In newborns, innocent murmurs are common and are usually systolic, grade I or II, and not associated with other symptoms. The transition period from fetal to maternal conditions may take 48 hours. Patent ductus arteriosus is a fetal vascular connection that directs blood from the pulmonary artery to the aorta. It typically closes by day 4 following birth. However, if it remains patent, the direction of blood flow is reversed through the ductus owing to the higher pressure in the aorta. Clinical findings in a newborn with a still-patent ductus arteriosus include diaphoresis (especially during feedings) and poor feedings with easy tiring that may result in failure to thrive. Immediately postnatally, the associated murmur is soft and systolic, heard along the left lower sternal border. Soon thereafter, the sound is described as a harsh, rumbling, continuous murmur heard in the left infraclavicular and pulmonic areas. When patent ductus arteriosus is suspected, evaluation by a pediatric cardiologist is essential.

■ Breasts

Ask about tenderness, nipple discharge, and masses. Asymmetric breast development is normal in an adolescent girl. Gynecomastia may be normal in boys during puberty. It usually occurs during Tanner stages II and III and may last up to 2 years. Gynecomastia typically presents as a small, tender, oval mass directly under the areola that may measure up to 2 to 3 cm. If imaging of adolescent breast tissue is desired, an ultrasound should be chosen over mammogram because of the dense nature of adolescent breast tissue.

Common Diagnoses for the Abdomen

- Abdominal pain, unknown etiology (possibly related to stress or anxiety)
- Gastroenteritis
- Pyloric stenosis

- Constipation
- Lactose intolerance
- Gas
- Gastroesophageal reflux disease

RED FLAG ◄ **Red Flags for the Abdominal Examination**

- *Failure to pass first meconium stool in first 24 hours of life*

- *Projectile vomiting*

- *Blood in stool or emesis*

- *Chronic diarrhea or constipation*

- *Severe abdominal pain or guarding*

- *Abdominal mass*

■ Abdomen

Ask about diarrhea, constipation, bowel habits, reflux or spitting up, and stomach aches. A "potbellied" look is common in early childhood owing to poorly developed muscles. Bowel sounds should be assessed. The liver edge may be palpable 1 to 2 cm below the right costal margin with deep inspiration, and the spleen tip may be palpable 1 to 2 cm below the left costal margin with deep inspiration. Constipation may cause a palpable fecal mass in the lower left quadrant, and a rectal examination may be indicated if constipation is suspected. To aid in the abdominal assessment of a ticklish child, have the child lie with knees bent or use the child's smaller hand under your own to palpate the belly. It is also helpful to engage the child in conversation to provide distraction from what you are doing.

■ Genitourinary System

Ask about voiding patterns (number of wet diapers in infants, frequency of urination in older children), pain, discharge, and menstrual cycle if applicable. A clean-catch urine sample should be obtained for urinalysis at all well-child checkups beginning at age 3 years, with further testing warranted with abnormal findings.

Female Genitalia

Enlarged labia or mild vaginal bleeding in a female newborn is considered a normal response to maternal hormones. Observe for labial adhesions, which occur mostly in girls 3 months to 6 years of age. No treatment is needed as long as urine and vaginal secretions are not obstructed. Observe the presence and distribution of pubic hair.

Male Genitalia

Observe the location of the urethral meatus. Hypospadias is a congenital defect that causes the meatus to be on the ventral surface of the penis, and epispadias results in dorsal placement of the meatus. Palpate the scrotum for the presence of testes; *cryptorchidism* is the term for an undescended testicle. If the testes are not immediately palpable in the scrotum but can be "milked" down into the scrotum, consider them descended. If one or both testes are undescended at age 1 year, referral to a specialist is indicated. Male newborns frequently have an enlarged scrotum as a normal finding.

At any age, if a male child complains of pain in the scrotal area, it should be thoroughly evaluated. Testicular torsion occurs mostly in adolescents but can occur at any age. It will present with severe pain in the scrotal area. Even pain that occurs and resolves on its own should be evaluated for torsion since a testicle

---

Common Diagnoses for the Genitourinary System

- Urinary tract infection
- Enuresis (most common is primary nocturnal enuresis—a child who has never stayed dry through the night)
- Labial adhesion
- Yeast dermatitis
- Diaper dermatitis
- Vaginitis
- Balanitis
- Retractile testes

| RED FLAG | Red Flags for the Genitourinary Examination |

- *Ambiguous genitalia*
- *Premature puberty*
- *Hypospadias or epispadias*
- *Scrotal pain*

can twist and untwist on its own. Prompt surgical intervention is often needed to prevent recurrence, which could result in testicular ischemia.

■ Musculoskeletal System

Ask about pain or limited movement, joint pain, and history of fractures. Although a comprehensive musculoskeletal assessment should be performed, an emphasis should be placed on specific joints.

Hips

Assessment for developmental dysplasia of the hip is extremely important in all infants and children under 2 years. Risk factors for hip dysplasia include female sex, breech position in utero, first-born child, and family history. It is more prevalent in white, Inuit, and Navajo people. A variety of specialized maneuvers are useful in assessment for hip dislocation. Table 19.3 differentiates between the Barlow's, Ortolani's, and Galeazzi's maneuvers.

When assessing for hip dislocation or dysplasia, it is essential to differentiate between normal "clicks" and the worrisome "clunk." Normal clicks may be felt when doing some hip manipulation as a result of laxity and movement of ligaments. A definitive clunk is felt when a bone (the femur) actually comes out of its socket. Even though doing these maneuvers is extremely important, it is also important to remember that as the infant ages, limited abduction becomes an increasingly definitive sign of hip dysplasia. Limited abduction (less than 60%) is also the key sign to look for in bilateral dislocation. If hip dysplasia is suspected, further evaluation is warranted. In an infant older than 6 weeks but

Common Diagnoses for the Musculoskeletal System

- Trauma or injury
- Local sprain or strain
- Torticollis
- Tibial torsion
- Osgood-Schlatter disease
- Growing pains

RED FLAG ◀ Red Flags for the Musculoskeletal Examination

- *Refusal to bear weight or walk*
- *Refusal to use or bend an arm*
- *Heat, redness, or swelling of one or more joints*
- *Hip clunks*
- *Toe walking—can be a normal phase and also can be associated with cerebral palsy, tight heel cords, autism, or muscular dystrophy*

Table 19.3

Special Maneuvers

Barlow's Maneuver

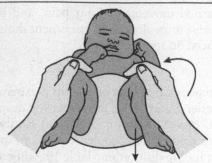

Dislocates a dislocatable hip posteriorly. With the infant supine, flex the hip, adduct the thigh, and feel for a palpable dislocation. As the thigh is adducted, the femoral head drops (or can be gently pushed) out of the acetabulum. Do the maneuver gently on an infant who is not crying.

Ortolani's Maneuver

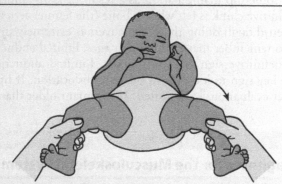

Reduces a posteriorly dislocated hip. With the infant supine, place fingers posteriorly over the greater trochanter, flex the hip 90 degrees, and abduct the thigh while pushing up with the fingers. Feel for a clunk and palpable jerk as the femur is relocated. Do the maneuver gently on an infant who is not crying.

Galeazzi's Maneuver

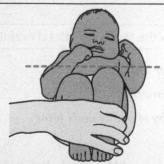

Assesses knee height for equality. With the infant supine, flex the hips and knees and place the soles of the child's feet on the table near the buttocks. Observe the knees for equal height. The sign is considered positive if the knee heights are unequal. A dislocatable hip will fall out of socket in this position and will cause the knee on the affected side to appear lower.

younger than 6 months, ultrasound is the usual choice. After 6 months, the preferred method of evaluation is anteroposterior and frog lateral x-rays (Yang et al., 2019). (In some institutions, x-rays may be used for evaluation in infants as young as 4 months.)

Gait

Observe a child's gait during the well-child examination. Toddlers commonly walk with a wide-based gait and a bowlegged (genu varum) appearance. A knock-kneed (genu valgum) appearance is common in preschoolers.

Back

Assessment for scoliosis (a lateral curvature of the spine) should be performed at each well-child visit starting at age 10 years. With the child standing straight with arms at the sides, observe for equal shoulder height. While the child bends forward, assess for curvature of the spine as well as rib humps. If abnormal findings are present, radiographs should be obtained for confirmation and to guide possible referral. Both the age of the child and the degree of the curve will guide treatment, if any. Scoliosis is more worrisome in a child who is prepubertal because there is more growth to occur and therefore more time for a curve to worsen.

Joints

Assess joints by palpating for pain, heat, or deformity. Active range of motion gives information about how muscles and bones are working together for functional movement. Assess active range of motion by engaging a child in games in the examination room. For example, have the child perform jumping jacks, clap, pretend to be a certain animal, and walk heel to toe on a line on the floor. Passive range of motion gives information about joint mobility and stability and the limits of tendons and muscles. Excessive range of motion may indicate an unstable joint. Assess passive range of motion by flexing and extending the joints through various movements with the child relaxed or lying supine.

Elbow

A child's elbow is commonly and easily dislocated (nursemaid's elbow or toddler's elbow). Dislocation is indicated by refusal to use an arm, especially when accompanied by crying and an appropriate history.

Knees

Knee pain is a common complaint in older children and adolescents, especially in athletes. Some knee pain is normal due to rapid growth of the long bones and the efforts of the supporting tendons/ligaments to match bone growth. Osgood-Schlatter disease should be suspected if a child complains of pain and mild swelling directly over the tibial tubercle. This may be unilateral or bilateral. Management includes activity only as tolerated, ice after activity, and NSAIDs. If there is fluctuance around the knee or severe swelling and decreased range of motion, then a referral to an orthopedist may be necessary, especially if symptoms persist after trying ice/rest/immobilization.

■ Integumentary System

Ask about birthmarks, lesions, and skin conditions. Common birthmarks are listed here:

- *Stork bites* commonly appear on eyelids, nasolabial area, or nape of neck and usually disappear by 12 months.
- *Nevus flammeus* (port-wine stain) is pinkish red in color and grows as the child grows.
- *Strawberry nevus* (raised hemangioma) may not be present at birth; it usually starts out as a grayish white area and later becomes red and raised; most resolve spontaneously by age 10 years.
- *Mongolian spots* are usually seen in newborns of African American, Latin, or Asian descent; they are generally found in the sacral or gluteal region.

Assess all skin for color, texture, and turgor; check for any rashes, lesions, pruritus, or bruising. Observe for skin conditions that may indicate underlying pathology, such as depigmented nevi, café au lait spots, and hemangiomas on the scalp.

The incidence of community-acquired methicillin-resistant staphylococcus aureus (MRSA) is prevalent and is now managed quite frequently in the primary care setting. In children, a common presentation is a small bump that may resemble a bug bite and then quickly enlarges and turns into a pustule. In infants, this is commonly seen in the diaper area, but it can occur anywhere. A culture and sensitivity should be obtained on any questionable lesions or abscesses to confirm diagnosis.

■ Neurological System

Ask about episodes of seizure or loss of consciousness, tremors, or tics. A large part of the assessment of the neurological system in a child can be accomplished by observation during the visit. Watch for symmetry and quality of movement;

Common Diagnoses for the Skin

- Viral exanthem
- Atopic dermatitis (eczema)
- Contact dermatitis
- Tinea

- Impetigo
- Cellulitis
- MRSA

RED FLAG ◀ **Red Flags for the Skin Examination**

- *Any mole or lesion that is changing, has irregular borders, or is growing should be examined by a dermatologist.*

observe gait, posture, coordination, balance, strength, and tone. Children are generally very active, and by watching the way they climb on the examination table, hop around the room, and manipulate objects and toys, you can gain a lot of information. In a newborn or small infant, observe for symmetry of movements, muscle tone, and pitch of the cry. Test deep tendon reflexes. Assess newborn reflexes—absence or persistence past expected age of disappearance may indicate severe central nervous system dysfunction and should be investigated fully. Table 19.4 details newborn reflexes.

The pediatric assessment should integrate cranial nerve evaluation. Table 19.5 describes the pediatric assessment of cranial nerves.

During the neurological examination, assess for developmental milestones. Although children develop at their own speed, any regression in developmental milestones is a major concern. The Denver II Developmental Screening Test is a useful tool when evaluating developmental milestones. See information on developmental milestones elsewhere in this chapter.

Practitioners caring for children should be aware of the following three neurological disorders and conditions and the signs and symptoms that children may exhibit that indicate the need for further evaluation.

Autism

Autism is a bioneurological developmental disorder and generally presents before the age of 3 years. It is characterized by marked impairment in skills related to social interaction, language development and communication, and imagination

---

Common Diagnoses for the Neurological System

- Cognitive delay
- Developmental delay
- Attention deficit/hyperactivity disorder and autism
- Neuromuscular diseases/ dystrophies
- Seizure/epilepsy
- Concussion

RED FLAG ◄ **Red Flags for the Neurological Examination**

- *Absence, or persistence past the expected age, of newborn reflexes*

- *Spasticity or poor muscle tone*

- *Unresponsiveness or depressed level of consciousness*

- *Any loss or regression of developmental milestones*

- *Abnormal cranial nerve responses*

Table 19.4

Newborn Reflexes

	Age Appears	Age Disappears	How to Test	Response	Meaning
Rooting	Birth	3–4 mo	With head midline, stroke perioral area.	Infant should open mouth and turn head toward stimulated side.	Absence indicates central nervous system disease or depression; sleepy infant may not respond.
Sucking	Birth	3–4 mo	Place nipple or finger 3–4 cm into mouth; may stroke roof of mouth.	Infant should have strong suck.	Absence indicates central nervous system depression; sleepy baby may not respond.
Palmar Grasp	Birth	3–6 mo	Place finger in infant's palm and press gently.	Infant should flex all fingers around examiner's finger.	Grasp should be strong and symmetrical.
Stepping	Birth	6–8 wk	Hold infant in a standing position with feet against firm surface.	Infant should "step" along, raising one foot at a time.	Absence indicates paralysis or a depressed infant.
Moro	Birth	4–5 mo	Make a loud noise or allow infant's head to drop down slightly.	Infant's arms should spread, fingers should extend and then flex, and arms should come together; may elicit a cry.	Asymmetry may indicate paralysis or a fractured clavicle; absence indicates a brainstem problem.

and play. Abnormal social skill development is the classic indicator of autism or autism spectrum disorders (ASDs). These children lack social reciprocity and are not fluent in nonverbal communication. These social skill deficits may include abnormal eye contact, failure to respond to name, failure to use gestures or pointing, and lack of interest in other children. Language development is typically delayed in autistic children. Such children also frequently exhibit an inability to adjust to new surroundings and show an absence of imaginary play. They commonly engage in unusual or repetitive behaviors and often do not "play" with toys but instead spend hours arranging them or organizing them in a certain way. Their interests and activities are generally restricted and repetitive.

The American Psychiatric Association released the fifth edition of the *Diagnostic and Statistical Manual of Mental Disorders* (*DSM-5*) in May 2013 with some revisions to the diagnostic criteria for autism. Several disorders that were defined separately in the previous manual have been grouped together under ASD. While a nurse practitioner is generally not expected to be the sole healthcare provider rendering a diagnosis of autism, it is important to be aware of

Table 19.5

Pediatric Assessment of the Cranial Nerves

I, Olfactory	Occlude one nostril and offer odors for identification (not frequently tested in the office unless specific concern).
II, Optic	Test visual acuity and visual fields and examine fundi; test blink reflex in an infant.
III, Oculomotor	Test extraocular movements by having child follow a light or a toy in all visual fields and observe infants for tracking abilities; observe for asymmetry of eyelids; pupils should both constrict when light is shined in one eye.
IV, Trochlear	Tested in the same way and at the same time as CN III.
V, Trigeminal	For sensory, apply light touch and pressure to points across forehead, cheeks, and jaw; for motor, have child bite hard on tongue blade or observe an infant chewing on a teething toy.
VI, Abducens	Tested in the same way and at the same time as CN III and CN IV.
VII, Facial	For sensory, observe for eyes tearing; can offer samples for taste. For motor, have child imitate you smiling big, grimacing, puffing out cheeks, and raising eyebrows; observe for facial grimaces in an infant.
VIII, Acoustic	Observe balance, do auditory testing as needed, question parents regarding hearing.
IX, Glossopharyngeal	Elicit gag reflex or have child say "ah"; observe swallowing.
X, Vagus	Tested along with CN IX.
XI, Accessory	Have child shrug shoulders against pressure, turn head against resistance, stick tongue out.
XII, Hypoglossal	Have child move tongue back and forth or push against a tongue blade; may observe this behavior only during examination of oropharynx in an infant.

CN = cranial nerve

the diagnostic criteria and presentation that should prompt further evaluation or referral. The American Academy of Pediatrics (2012) recommends that all children be screened for ASDs at 18 and 24 months of age.

Ask parents if their infant studies their faces by 2 months, smiles at them by 6 months, and babbles by 1 year. Ask if their 1-year-old points to things to indicate wants or just for a parent to notice the object. Does their 18-month-old imitate play with objects like a hairbrush or a phone? Does their 2-year-old put two words together meaningfully on their own? If a child exhibits any of the following red flags, the child should be referred for further evaluation.

The Modified Checklist for Autism in Toddlers, Revised (MCHAT-R) is a 20-question screening instrument intended for use with children between 16 and 30 months of age. It is a good starting place when deciding if further evaluation is needed. Parents can access it free online or fill it out in the office in a short period of time. It is a useful tool to guide the discussion of child development and can help uncover some parental concerns and/or direct parents to tune in more to certain milestones and skills. The Autism Speaks (2013) website gives parents access to the screening tool. The M-CHAT Autism Screening Web site has helpful information for providers.

RED FLAG ◄   **Red Flags for Autism**

- *No big smiles or expressions of happiness by 6 months*
- *Limited or no eye contact by 6 months*
- *No back-and-forth sounds, gestures, or facial expressions by 9 months*
- *No babbling by 12 months*
- *Little or no response to name by 12 months*
- *No pointing, waving, or reaching by 12 months*
- *No words by 16 months*
- *No two-word phrases by 24 months (without imitating)*
- *Any language regression or unusual use of language*

An online resource that may be helpful to parents and practitioners is Autism Navigator. This Web site provides written information as well as video footage of children with ASD that illustrates some of the traits and characteristics commonly found in children with this disorder.

Attention Deficit/Hyperactivity Disorder

Attention deficit/hyperactivity disorder (ADHD) is a neurobehavioral disorder that affects an estimated 5% to 10% of the school-age population. Its main symptoms are inattention with increased distractibility, poor impulse control, and motor restlessness and hyperactivity. There are three subtypes of ADHD: The predominantly inattentive type of ADHD is more common in females, and the predominantly hyperactive-impulsive type and combined type are more frequently diagnosed in males. When assessing a child for ADHD, it is important to ascertain the degree of symptoms, when they were first noticed, and in what settings they are present. It is also important to remember that many children with ADHD have comorbid psychiatric diagnoses.

According to the *DSM-5*, a child with ADHD must exhibit behavior that is developmentally inappropriate and clearly interferes with the quality of social, school, or work functions. The behavior must also meet the following criteria:

- Has been present before the age of 12 years
- Has been present for at least 6 months
- Is present in at least two settings
- Is not related to another disorder

A diagnosis of ADHD should not be made quickly or without a complete evaluation. A thorough history should include any injury to the central nervous system, any medications the child takes, any family history of similar symptoms, and any social or family situations that might contribute to the inappropriate behaviors. Because of the importance of symptoms being present in more than one setting, it is a good idea to use a behavior rating scale that compares answers from both a parent and another caregiver like a teacher. The Connor Rating Scale is an example of this type of checklist. The older the child, the more helpful it may be to involve a psychologist or psychiatrist specifically trained in the diagnosis of this disorder. This is mostly because there may be a variety of comorbid conditions occurring and presenting with similar symptoms. Other diagnoses to consider when evaluating a child with ADHD-like symptoms include anxiety disorders, depression, sleep disorders, and learning disabilities.

Concussion

According to researchers in the field of concussion management, 1 in 10 adolescents who play high school contact sports will suffer from a concussion annually. The field of concussion research is constantly evolving, which makes it essential that providers stay up-to-date on the most current recommendations. At the time of this publication, the most recent information and recommendations come from a consensus statement put out by the international Concussion in Sport Group (2017).

Signs and Symptoms

A good starting point for anyone who may care for children with concussions is to be fully aware of what defines this type of injury. A sport-related concussion may have the following characteristics:

- Injury caused by direct blow to the head, face, neck, or elsewhere on the body with an impulsive force transmitted to the head.
- Rapid onset of signs and symptoms of neurological impairment post injury. Symptoms may evolve over few hours, are typically short-lived, and resolve spontaneously.
- Acute signs and symptoms are typically due to functional impairment rather than structural impairment and are usually not seen on standard structural imaging studies.
- Injury may or may not involve loss of consciousness.
- Resolution of clinical and cognitive features typically follows a sequential course, although some may have prolonged problems.

Concussion symptoms can be divided into four main categories: physical, cognitive, sleep-related, and emotional. Box 19.3 lists various symptoms that fall into each category and should guide your interview with patients suspected of experiencing a concussion. In addition to a thorough history and detailed neurological examination, the provider should also assess whether the patient has gotten better or worse since the event and determine whether any imaging is necessary to exclude a more severe injury.

A full evaluation and history remain essential even if the child was evaluated in the emergency department or on the "sidelines" before presenting for follow-up. The most important thing when caring for a patient with a concussion

Box 19.3

Types and Symptomatology of Concussion

Physical:

- Headache
- Visual problems
- Light sensitivity
- Noise sensitivity

- Nausea/vomiting
- Dizziness/balance issues
- Fatigue

Cognitive:

- Attention problems
- Memory dysfunction
- Cognitive fogginess

- Cognitive slowing/difficulty thinking
- Dazed

Sleep-related:

- Difficulty sleeping
- Sleeping less than normal

- Sleeping more than normal
- Sleepiness/drowsiness

Emotional:

- Increased emotionality
- Sadness
- Irritability
- Nervousness

- Impulsive behavior
- Change in personality
- Outbursts of anger
- Poor coping skills

is to prevent another head injury. Anticipatory guidance recommendations by the Concussion in Sport Group (2017) include the following:

- A period of 24 to 48 hours of initial physical and cognitive rest is recommended followed by gradual and progressive return to activity, as tolerated, with frequent assessment to evaluate for any exacerbation of symptoms.
- Avoiding vigorous activity during recovery is suggested. No activity should bring on or worsen symptoms, so the exact level of reengagement differs for each patient.
- Restrictions on electronics or reading may be necessary, as well as special accommodations when students transition back to school.

The Web sites for the Centers for Disease Control and Prevention and Rocky Mountain Orthopedics are good resources for return to play and return to school schedules:

Parents and patients should be informed that every concussion is different and that each person recovers on his or her own schedule. On average, an adolescent will take 2 to 3 weeks to recover from a concussion. The severity of initial symptoms in the first day, or days, of a concussion is a strong predictor of recovery time. The more severe the symptoms, the longer recovery should be expected to take (Concussion in Sport Group, 2017).

Recovery also may be predicted by early exercise tolerance. Research has shown that adolescents who return to (and tolerate) some level of physical activity by 7 days post concussion are less likely to have symptoms at 28 days (Guthrie, 2018). There is some data suggesting that teens with a history of mental health problems or migraines may be at greater risk for symptoms lingering for more than a month. If symptoms are lingering longer than this time frame, or seem to be worsening instead of gradually improving, a referral to a specialist is recommended (Concussion in Sport Group, 2017).

■ Mental Health

Anxiety/Depression

In addition to a full physical examination, a complete assessment of a child or teen should include questions regarding mental health. Both anxiety and depression are on the rise in teenagers, and it is necessary for clinicians to be vigilant for the signs of one or both of these conditions. Recent studies show that almost 1 in 5 teenagers will suffer from clinical depression; 25% of teens between the ages of 13 and 18 years will suffer from anxiety—with females slightly more affected than males (Merikangus et al., 2010).

Include in your assessment questions regarding a teen's schedule, activities, grades, and hobbies. Try to get a sense of how involved and connected the teen feels. Ask about friends and social media usage. Involve parents in this discussion and be alert to any suggestion that the teen has become more withdrawn or is losing motivation or interest in previously enjoyed activities. There are surveys and questionnaires that can be used to ask more specific questions about depression and/or anxiety if necessary. Two widely known surveys are the PHQ-9 for depression (Kroenke, Spitzer, & Williams, 2001) and the GAD-7 for anxiety (Spitzer et al., 2006). New surveys are frequently introduced or updated; it is recommended to research the most current options. While these surveys can be helpful, a thorough history is still essential.

Signs and Symptoms

Assessing for anxiety is also important in this age group. With adolescence comes an increase in school performance pressure, family responsibilities, and social pressure. Like adults, teenagers suffering from anxiety can become almost paralyzed in certain situations. They may describe physical symptoms such as

- increased heart rate
- nausea
- diarrhea
- sweaty palms
- dizziness
- inability to focus

- restlessness
- insomnia
- appetite changes
- tingling or numbness in hands/feet

Often an adolescent will present with complaints of physical symptoms such as those listed above, but through the course of the history and examination it is discovered that the root of these symptoms is really anxiety. As with depression, it then becomes essential to assess how disruptive these symptoms are to the teenager's life. Anxiety or depression in teens should not be dismissed or minimized. Therapy/counseling should be recommended. Medication should be considered.

If a diagnosis of depression is suspected, then determining the severity of symptoms is critical, as suicide rates have tripled in the United States in this age group over the last several decades. Be direct when questioning teenagers about suicidal ideation. Ask if the teenage patient has thoughts of self-harming or of harming others, as well as if the patient has a plan. If the answer to these questions is yes, then immediate medical and psychiatric attention is needed. If the teen admits to occasional depressive thoughts but seems stable in the office, then the discussion should continue to include how to best keep the patient safe.

- Encourage a safe environment and inquire about the presence of firearms and medications.
- Discuss coping mechanisms that the teenager can use if these thoughts occur.
- Identify friends or family members that the teenager can call on if these thoughts persist or worsen.
- Reiterate the seriousness and permanence of suicide and identify/remind the teen of how to get help if needed emergently.

At this point a recommendation for therapy and/or medication should be considered. While ideally a mental health professional would be able to assess and evaluate these teens and aid in the plan of care, in reality primary care and pediatric providers are practicing more and more mental health care all the time. Stay up-to-date on mental health providers in your area that serve adolescents. Therapy/counseling is essential to helping these teens. Medication may also be warranted, but the coping skills that can be taught in therapy are the tools that will help into the future.

The number of children and adolescents suffering from mental health issues, such as anxiety and depression, increased during the COVID-19 pandemic. School closures and social distancing led to loneliness and isolation from peers—both known factors that negatively affect the mental health of young people. The additional burden of parents suffering from their own mental health issues related to job insecurity and financial strain only compounded these issues for children and adolescents. Some data indicate that 25% to 30% of students described their emotional health as worse during the pandemic, and parents concurred that their children were exhibiting more psychological stress and signs of depression and anxiety. Parental responses to surveys indicate the same (Henry J. Kaiser Family Foundation, 2021).

Additionally, access to mental health care declined for many young people during the pandemic. While telehealth increased in some areas, many children who may have been receiving care through their schools were no longer able to receive it due to school closures. This issue of access may have disproportionately affected children of color and children in rural areas (Henry J. Kaiser Family Foundation, 2021). What we learned during this period has application to the persistent upheaval during ongoing or resurgent COVID-19 and to other crises that may occur in the future.

■ Social Media

Today's teens are connected to each other and to the Internet more than any previous generation. Texting and social media applications (apps) are used more for communication than e-mail in this age group. Asking adolescent patients about their social media usage should become a part of the full assessment. Again, involve parents in this discussion, as they may not be aware of some of the apps their children are using.

Because digital usage is starting younger and younger, providers should start asking these questions even with elementary school-age children. Ask about what types of devices they use and what games they play that may encourage them to create an online profile. It is never too early to teach about not providing personal information to others online!

Anticipatory guidance includes

- Encourage parents to be aware of what apps their kids are using by having an account themselves, talking with other parents, and asking their kids directly to show them on their own devices.
- Encourage families to keep computers in a "public" part of the home so that parents can observe what their children are doing online and how much time they are spending. "Parking" phones in the kitchen or other public place at night should also be encouraged.
- Remind children that anything texted or sent online to others can be shared, so good judgment is essential.
- Have a frank discussion regarding sexting. Not only can this lead to emotional pain for the people involved, it is illegal in many places. Tell young children that they should never receive pictures or messages from people they don't know. Encourage older children never to initiate or pass along pictures of this nature and remind older teens of the emotional and legal ramifications of sexting.

Growth and Development

The growth and development of a child is one of the most important things to consider when assessing and caring for pediatric patients. Parents are very interested in how their child is growing, both physically and developmentally, and assessments of these areas by trained professionals can help indicate possible problems and the need for referral or more intensive evaluation.

■ Physical Growth

The measurement of a child's weight and height is done at every well-child visit. If the child is not routinely seen for well-child visits, this must be incorporated into visits for specific complaints/illness. The head circumference is measured at every well-child visit from birth to age 2 years. Each of these measurements is plotted on a growth chart. Other charts have been developed to measure a child's body mass index (BMI) and plot a child's weight versus height. These charts allow for a visual representation that enables practitioners to watch how a child develops in each area over time. Although parents often become interested in what percentile their child "ranks in," providers should stress the importance of watching the growth curves to compare the child against the child's own progress, not against others. For example, it is much more worrisome for a child's weight or head size to drop from the 75th to the 25th percentile than it is for a child to continuously grow along the 25th percentile curve. A child whose growth is at the extremes of the growth curves but whose growth rate is normal and consistent is likely to be very healthy.

Trends

The following trends are generalizations that can be used as rules of thumb in assessing pediatric growth and development in the United States. An average American newborn weighs around 7 pounds and is 20 to 21 inches long. The average head circumference of an American newborn is 13 to 14 inches, with a chest circumference of 2 cm less than that of the head. The head circumference generally increases by a half inch per month during the first 6 months of life and a quarter inch per month during the second 6 months.

Weight

Up to an initial 10% loss of weight can be expected in the first 3 to 4 days of life. This is typically regained by age 2 weeks. For the first 1 to 2 months of life, an infant is expected to gain 0.5 to 1 ounce per day. A child's weight typically doubles around 4 to 6 months, triples at a year, and quadruples around age 2 years. Typically, in the first 6 months of life, a baby gains 5 to 8 ounces a week. Between 6 and 12 months, this decreases to 3 to 5 ounces a week. During the second year of life, a child gains 8 to 9 ounces a month. Toddlers and preschoolers gain 4.5 to 6.5 pounds a year. A school-age child gains 5 to 6 pounds a year. During the pubertal growth spurt, an average American girl gains 38 pounds, and an average American boy gains 42 pounds.

Length/Height

The length of a child typically increases by 50% at age 12 months, doubles around age 4 years, and triples by age 13 years. The average gain in length in infancy is 1 inch per month during the first 6 months and then 0.5 inch per month during the second 6 months. Toddlers, preschoolers, and school-age children grow 2 to 3 inches per year. During the pubertal growth spurt, American girls grow an average of 8 to 9 inches and reach 95% of their mature height by the onset of menarche or the skeletal age of 13. Boys grow an average of 9.5 to 11 inches and reach 95% of their mature height by the skeletal age of 15.

■ Development by Age

The tables in this subsection illustrate age-by-age behaviors and skills that babies and children should develop. Because every child is different, it is impossible to say that these behaviors will occur in all children at the given age. Milestones occur along a wide spectrum, and patterns considered "normal" have wide parameters. The "whole picture" of the child must be taken into consideration when comparing a child with a given standard. However, knowledge of the developmental milestones is essential when assessing infants and children. Behavioral observations and parents' questions can be used to determine the child's developmental progress.

Newborns/Infants

The term *newborn* is typically applied to babies from birth until 1 month of age. The period from 1 month to 12 months is infancy. The first 12 months of life represent the period of the most rapid change and maturation—both physically and emotionally. See Table 19.6 for infant developmental milestones.

Infant Developmental Red Flags

Because of the importance of early intervention in preventing or minimizing long-term consequences of sensory deficits, Table 19.7 is included to provide developmental red flags in infants. As always, there is some parameter for "normal," and the gestational age of the child at birth must be taken into account. However, in terms of early intervention and evaluation, it is much better to err on the side of caution and refer for further evaluation if any suspicions arise regarding the development of a child.

Toddlers

The period of toddlerhood lasts from the first birthday until age 3 years. During this stage, the child's rate of physical growth slows down, but the process of moving toward independence continues rapidly as toddlers acquire many new motor, cognitive, and psychosocial skills. Behavioral challenges frequently arise during this period owing to both the toddler's attempts to test limits and their own frustration at trying to communicate. See Table 19.8 for toddler developmental milestones.

Preschoolers

The period from age 3 to 5 years is known as the preschool stage of development. Children in this stage are usually very active, energetic, imaginative, inquisitive,

Table 19.6

Newborn/Infant Development Milestones

Time Period	Sensory	Emotional/ Behavioral	Motor	Language
Newborn–1 mo	Sees best at 8–10 inches; cannot focus clearly; startles to loud noises	Cries a lot but responds positively to soft voice and being held	Jerky movements; grasps whatever is placed in hand; turns head	Has varying cries for different needs; may start making gurgling sounds
1–2 mo	May follow some objects with eyes (at least to midline); turns toward some sounds	May smile socially to caregiver; may quiet down in response to human face	Movements become more controlled; lifts chin for a few seconds while on tummy	Makes variety of cooing and gurgling sounds when content
2–4 mo	Focuses better but no more than 12 inches; follows objects 180 degrees by turning head side to side; prefers bright objects	Crying decreases; displays more emotions	Movements are smoother; discovers hands; may lift chest slightly while prone; may bat at dangling objects	Smiles, gurgles, and coos—especially interactively
4–6 mo	Focuses clearly; fascinated by mirror image; turns purposefully in response to voice	Very active and playful; basks in attention; acknowledges breast or bottle excitedly	Rolls from side to side; holds up chest when prone; supports head well when held in sitting position; no head lag at 6 mo	Laughs and giggles; imitates speech sounds
6–9 mo	Begins to recognize sound of own name; puts everything in mouth	May show sharp mood changes; strong attachment to mother; stranger anxiety	Rakes objects; transfers objects from hand to hand; begins to sit alone; crawling motions	Babbles and squeals; repeats sounds over and over; frequently uses syllables such as *ba, da, ka*
9–12 mo	Scrutinizes toys and objects; still puts everything in mouth	May cry when parent leaves; may resist diapering or other things they do not want to do; plays peek-a-boo	Refined pincer grasp; goes from sitting to lying; crawls well; may pull self to stand; cruises; may begin to walk	Imitates inflection of conversation; imitates speech sounds; says "mama" and "dada"; may say 2–3 other words; points to objects to indicate wants

and social. They also become increasingly independent with tasks such as self-care. They acquire more language skills and, as a result, can respond more verbally, which often decreases previous behavioral challenges. See Table 19.9 for preschooler developmental milestones.

School-Age Children

The school-age period of development begins with entry into school (around age 5 years) and lasts until adolescence. This is a period of extensive development.

Table 19.7

Infant Developmental Red Flags

Age	Social/ Emotional	Cognitive/ Visual	Language/ Hearing	Fine Motor	Gross Motor
1 mo	Excessive irritability	Doll's eyes; questionable or no red light reflex; poor alert state	No startle to sound; no quieting to voice	Absent or asymmetrical palmar grasp	Asymmetric movements; increased or decreased tone; asymmetric primitive reflexes
4 mo	Lack of social smile; depressed/ withdrawn affect	No tracking; no ability to fixate on face or object	No turning to voice or sound; no cooing or squeals	No hand-to-mouth activity	Same as above; no attempt to raise head when prone
6 mo	No smiling or response to play	No looking at caregiver; no reaching for objects; no tracking	No babbling; no response to rattles, sounds, or loud noises	No grasping of objects; no holding hands together	No attempt to sit with support; head lag when pulled to a sit; persistence of primitive reflexes
9 mo	No eye contact or interactive play	No reaching for toys; no visual or oral investigation of toys	No response to name or voice; no single or double consonant sounds	No self-feeding; no solids; no picking up of toys with one hand	No sitting (including tripod sit); unequal movements or excessive one-handedness
12 mo	No response to games, books, or interactive play	No visual involvement in environment	No speech imitation	No attempt to self-feed or hold cup; no transfer of objects	No pulling self to stand; no exploring of environment

Table 19.8

Toddler Development Milestones

Age	Cognitive	Emotional/ Behavioral	Motor	Language
18 mo	Learns cause and effect; looks for hidden objects; recognizes pictures of familiar people and objects; points to a few body parts	Likes to feed self; likes water play; prefers adults to other children	Likes to throw, roll, push, and pull toys; walks unassisted with wide stance; stoops and recovers; imitates scribbling; makes tower of 3–4 cubes	Adds gestures to speech; likes to imitate activities and speech; uses 10–20 words; may start combining two words; understands "no"
2 yr	Cannot be reasoned with; can picture objects and events mentally; concrete thinking; identifies body parts; matches some colors	"Do-it-myself" stage; may resist bedtime; gets frustrated easily; may respond with "no" constantly; learns to hold up fingers to show age; tries to get adult attention	Runs and climbs; goes up and down stairs alone; scribbling turns into more controlled movements; turns pages one at a time; builds tower of 8 cubes	Uses simple sentences; seems to understand most of what is said; uses more pronouns; learns songs/rhymes

Table 19.9

Preschooler Development Milestones

Age	Cognitive	Emotional/ Behavioral	Motor	Language
3 yr	Develops more stable sense of self; egocentric thinking; knows names of time components but does not understand sequencing; may identify some colors, letters, numbers	Learns to share and take turns; tests limits; seeks approval from adults; likes hearing stories over and over; likes imaginative and imitative play; increased curiosity about bodies	Tiptoes; rides a tricycle; kicks a ball; stands briefly on one foot; undresses self; copies a circle; can brush teeth (although not well)	Speaks about 1,000 words; tells simple stories; asks lots of questions; responds to three-part commands; may have a stuttering phase; can consistently produce *m, n, p, f, h, b,* and *w* sounds
4 yr	Uses words to solve problems; begins to understand some concepts of time; knows difference between right and wrong; begins to discern real life from make-believe; identifies shapes and colors	Has penchant for silliness; shows new fears, which shows awareness of new dangers; likes to help; imitates adults; shares grudgingly; enjoys group activities and fantasy play	Runs, skips, climbs, hops with better skill; uses scissors; dresses self; holds a pencil correctly; draws recognizable shapes; draws a person with three parts; catches a large ball	Tells stories; uses four- to five-word sentences; uses prepositions; asks "how" questions; starts using past and future tenses correctly; adds approximately 50 words a month to vocabulary

Children become more influenced by peers and groups outside the home, and they are expected to follow certain rules and adhere to some degree of structure in the school setting. Children often remain very imaginative as they learn new things. This is the period when a child develops a sense of self and self-worth, so accomplishment and confidence become important tasks. Refer to Table 19.10 for school-age developmental milestones.

Adolescents

The period of adolescence is the transition from childhood to adulthood. Typically beginning at age 12 or 13 years, adolescence is a time of change and new responsibilities. With the initiation of puberty, children experience a wide array of physical, emotional, and social changes. The peer group is of utmost importance to an adolescent, and many challenges and temptations arise during this time period. During middle and late adolescence, focus on the future becomes significant, and teens gain a sense of morality as they prepare to enter the adult world. Table 19.11 lists adolescent developmental milestones.

■ Hearing/Speech

Assessment of an infant's hearing is somewhat subjective (unless specific audiological testing is done), but it is essential to be aware of the signs of a hearing deficit. Hearing is critical to language development, and the failure to recognize

Table 19.10

School-Age Development Milestones

Age	Cognitive	Emotional/ Behavioral	Motor	Language
5 yr	Understands time concepts; recognizes letters and some words; can learn address and phone number; begins to understand opposites; has overall image of self	Likes to please adults; enjoys family activities; embarrasses easily; submits to more rules and shows guilt over misbehavior; can participate in informal games	Displays handedness; can bathe independently; builds elaborate structures; walks downstairs alternating feet; may print name; cuts out simple shapes; copies a square	Speaks in good sentences; uses conjunctions to string thoughts together; has a vocabulary of over 2,000 words and continues to add more; masters most consonant combinations
6 yr	Loses magical thinking; starts to understand concepts of measurement (weight, length, mass); can group things into subgroups based on a common attribute; knows right from left; knows days of the week	Develops better impulse control; may enjoy and succeed at sports and arts & crafts programs; is sensitive to criticism; may resist baths; prefers socializing with same sex	Loves active play; still somewhat uncoordinated; may be reckless; can tie shoes; copies a triangle; very active	Well-developed vocabulary with increasingly improved semantics; speaks with good intelligibility; may still distort some sounds/ blends (*thr, sk, st, shr, s, z, sh, ch, j*)
7 yr	Begins to use simple logic; can tell time; can group objects in ascending order; understands basic addition and subtraction principles	Less egocentric; more cooperative; usually has a best friend of same sex; seeks approval from peers; tends to be critical; tattles on others for not following rules	Has refined hand–eye coordination; rides a bike; swims; printing gets smaller; activity level decreases slightly	Produces all language sounds; uses adultlike grammar; rapid language development
8 yr	Memory span increases; understands causal relationships; can be idealistic	Adheres to simple rules; often idolizes someone; begins to show sense of loyalty; likes secrets and clubs; enjoys projects and collections	Gains better control over small muscles; writes in cursive and draws better; movements are more graceful	Articulation nears adult level; better use of pronouns; understands complex directions; better storytelling skills; likes to tell jokes and enjoys bathroom humor
9–10 yr	Understands explanations; can use reference books and resources; classifies objects	Succumbs more easily to peer pressure; does not want to be different; tends to be self-critical; develops internal standards of right and wrong	Eagerly learns new skills; enjoys team competition; well coordinated with increasing dexterity and eye–hand coordination	Uses language to convey thoughts and looks at another's point of view
11–12 yr	Begins abstract thinking; increasing spans of attention and concentration	Peer acceptance is very important; critical of parents; acutely aware of opposite sex; vacillates between dependent child and independent preteen	Refines gross and fine motor skills; can do crafts and use tools well	Reading vocabulary of 50,000 words; oral vocabulary of 7,200 words; speech is grammatically correct

Table 19.11

Adolescent Development Milestones

Age	Cognitive	Emotional/ Behavioral	Motor	Language
12–15 yr	Increase in abstract thinking and decrease in concrete thinking; increased ability to relate actions to consequences	Very focused on social life, peer acceptance, physical appearance; grades may suffer; interest in sexuality increases; wide mood swings; values privacy	May enjoy and excel at a specific sport or activity; enjoys video/computer games	Increasing ability for self-expression; may enjoy keeping a journal or diary
15–18 yr	Beginning interest in social problems; may become idealistic and altruistic; inductive and deductive reasoning; may be very introspective; increased creative ability	Risk taking is common; rejection or questioning of parental authority; may experiment with sex, alcohol, or drugs; confusion over self-image may persist	Periods of high energy alternate with periods of lethargy; may enjoy and excel at a specific sport or activity	Language skills at or near adult level

and address a hearing deficit in infancy can be detrimental to a child's development. Basic hearing screenings should be done at each well-child visit. Parents should be specifically questioned regarding behaviors that indicate normal hearing. Any concerns regarding hearing should be thoroughly addressed. Part of assessing hearing is to check for any factors that may increase the risk of a hearing deficit. See Box 19.4 regarding the risk factors for hearing deficit.

The development of language skills may provide evidence of intact hearing, and parents can be asked to identify the infant's level of interaction and language development. As long as the child is progressing (and not regressing) in language skills and there are no physical abnormalities, monitoring and intermittent assessment is acceptable during this stage. However, formal audiometry should be considered if parents express concerns about the child's hearing abilities or if there are no recognizable, meaningful sounds or words at age 18 months. See Box 19.5 for reasons for referral.

■ Vision

Vision is the least-developed sense in a newborn, but the amazing pace at which visual acuity develops is obvious when watching the overall development of an infant's actions. At 1 month, an infant will stare at large objects. By 2 months, more detail is noticed and babies begin to enjoy gazing at a caregiver's face. As the baby reaches 3 to 4 months of age, the eyes begin to converge, and the infant starts to bring things to the mouth and develop eye–hand coordination.

Box 19.4

Risk Factors for Hearing Deficit

- An affected family member
- Newborn bilirubin greater than 20 mg/dL
- Congenital cytomegalovirus, herpes, or rubella
- Defects in ear-nose-throat structures
- Birth weight less than 1,500 g
- Bacterial meningitis
- Use of ototoxic medications
- Intracranial hemorrhage
- Use of mechanical ventilation for more than 48 hours
- Head trauma or temporal bone fracture
- Infections such as mumps/measles associated with sensorineural hearing loss
- Recurrent acute otitis media or middle ear infection

Box 19.5

Reasons for Audiology Referral

- Hearing threshold levels greater than 20 dB at 500, 1,000, 2,000, or 4,000 Hz
- Presence of middle ear fluid documented for longer than 3 months
- Hearing or language skills seem to regress at any point

At this age, an infant should be able to track an object 180 degrees. Around 6 to 7 months of age, a baby can recognize different faces.

Like hearing, it is essential to assess visual acuity at all well-child checkups. Again, parents are the best evaluators, so they should be questioned about a baby's or child's behaviors, including tracking ability, presence of eye crossing or wandering, response to new and familiar faces, distance a child sits from a book or television, and ability to notice details far away. Risk factors for decreased visual acuity should also be assessed (Box 19.6).

Assessment of the red reflex should be a part of each well-child visit. Other things that should be assessed in a young infant include the pupillary response to light, the blink reflex, and the ability to fix and follow. An older infant or toddler should also be assessed using the corneal light reflex test and the cover/uncover test. Starting at preschool age, children should be assessed using visual acuity charts (Allen, illiterate E, or Sjögren hand). The school-age child and adolescent should be assessed using these measures as well as the Snellen chart for far vision. The Ishihara test should be used for color perception. See Box 19.7 for reasons for referral.

Box 19.6

Risk Factors for Decreased Visual Acuity

- Prenatal infections
- Congenital cyanotic heart disease
- Structural malformation
- Family history of vision problems
- Excessive oxygenation in neonatal period
- Hearing problems

Box 19.7

Reasons for Ophthalmology Referral

- Prematurity
- Searching nystagmus
- Strabismus (intermittent strabismus is normal until age 4 to 6 months)
- Absence of blinking to a threat
- Lack of vertical and horizontal following by age 2 months
- Inability to fix and follow by age 3 months
- Abnormal or asymmetric red reflex
- Asymmetric corneal light reflex
- Abnormal cover/uncover test
- Visual acuity 20/50 or worse at age 3 years
- Visual acuity of 20/30 or worse at age 5 years
- Difference in score of two lines or more between eyes on visual acuity chart
- Structural abnormality

■ Nutrition

Assessing an infant's or child's nutrition and diet is an important part of an over-all well-child evaluation and requires knowledge of anticipated intake and weight change. For infants, parents should be questioned regarding the frequency of feedings, the type and amount of formula if bottle-fed, and the baby's tolerance of feedings. Once solids are initiated (around age 4 to 6 months), parents should be asked about what types of foods the baby is taking, how much and at what times of the day, and how much fluid the infant is drinking now that solids have been started. As the child progresses to more table foods, part of the assessment is determining whether the child is getting a good variety of foods, is transitioning well to table foods, and is maintaining adequate fluid intake. Encourage establishing a good habit of drinking water once the child is drinking from a cup or sippy cup, and discourage juice intake until at least age 1 year (and then only one 4-ounce serving per day). Table 19.12 includes information to guide the nutrition questions posed at various ages.

Table 19.12

Age-Appropriate Nutritional Guidelines

Age	Intake	Anticipated Weight Change
Newborn	Requires 110–120 kcal/kg^{-1}/day^{-1} Eats every 1.5–3 hr 20–24 oz/day	Gains 0.5–1 oz/day
2 mo	Requires 120–130 kcal/kg^{-1}/day^{-1} Eats 6–9 times/day 20–24 oz/day	Gains 0.5–1 oz/day
4 mo	Requires 120–130 kcal/kg^{-1}/day^{-1} Eats 24–32 oz/day	Gains 5–8 oz/week
6 mo	Requires approx. 100 kcal/kg^{-1}/day^{-1} Eats 24–32 oz/day Solids include iron-fortified single-grain cereal mixed with water, formula, or breast milk Only one new food introduced every 3–7 days No additives, such as honey, sugar, or seasonings	Gains 3–5 oz/week Weight usually doubles by 5–6 months
8–9 mo	Requires approx. 100 kcal/kg^{-1}/day^{-1} Drinks 24–32 oz/day, often with sippy cup; introduce water in a sippy cup Menu slowly expanded to include tender meats and finger foods	Gains 3–5 oz/week
10–12 mo	Drinks 20–32 oz/day Menu expanded to more table and finger foods Meal pattern resembles family's (three meals/day plus snacks) Whole milk at 12 months No juice until 12 months, and then only one 4-ounce serving a day (ideally diluted with water)	Gains 3–5 oz/week Weight usually triples by 12 months

In addition to identifying the daily intake of meals and snacks, include questions to identify nutritional supplements and vitamins. Of particular interest is the intake of vitamin D and fluoride. Breastfed infants who do not receive vitamin D supplementation or adequate exposure to sunlight are at risk for developing rickets. All breastfed infants should receive a supplement of 200 IU per day of vitamin D unless they are consuming at least 500 mL a day of vitamin D–fortified formula. This practice should begin within the first 2 months of life.

Because new evidence indicates early introduction of peanut-containing foods may help prevent the development of peanut allergy, ask parents about whether and/or how peanut-containing foods have been introduced and how they have been tolerated. Assess whether an assessment of allergy risk was first conducted. The recommendation, which comes from the National Institute of Allergy and Infectious Diseases (Togias et al., 2017), advises that infants at higher risk (e.g., those infants with eczema or an egg allergy) have peanut-containing foods introduced at age 4 to 6 months. Infants deemed at mild or moderate risk should have these types of foods introduced around age 6 months. Infants with no known risk should have foods containing peanuts introduced as a normal progression of their diet as parents see fit. Ask parents to check with their child's primary care provider before initiating these foods, in case allergy testing or a food challenge is indicated.

Toddlers and Preschoolers

As a child reaches the toddler stage, the appetite naturally starts to decrease as growth starts to slow down. Toddlers are frequently easily distracted and are picky about what they eat, so mealtimes can be a challenge. Parents should be encouraged to look at their child's diet on a week-by-week rather than day-by-day basis because toddlers frequently have days when they eat very little or eat only two or three things and then may make up for it the next day. When assessing toddlers, ask about the child's typical diet, including overall intake and any self-imposed limitations. Preschoolers frequently go on food jags, insisting on eating the same food over and over. As long as the food is not a high-sugar or empty-calorie item, parents should allow the food choice and remember that the phase usually does not last too long.

School-Age Children

Energy needs for school-age children depend somewhat on the individual's body size, growth pattern, and activity level. Children age 6 to 7 years require approximately 90 kcal/kg^{-1}/day^{-1}; 7 to 10 years approximately 70 kcal/kg^{-1}/day^{-1}; and 10 to 12 years 40 to 55 kcal/kg^{-1}/day^{-1}, depending on their size and activity. The school-age period is a time of busy schedules, and children at this age tend to skip meals and to snack more often. Also, because children spend a good part of the day away from home, parents become somewhat out of touch with what their child is eating throughout the day. Because of these habits, problems with obesity can begin at this stage. Parents should make an effort to have easy, healthy snacks available. Healthy meals and family mealtime routines should be reinforced during this period to help prevent obesity.

Adolescents

As for school-age children, energy requirements for adolescents vary somewhat, depending on body size and activity level. However, owing to the rapid growth and development during this stage, it is essential that all adolescents consume an adequate amount of calories, protein, vitamins, and minerals. Boys typically require more kilocalories per day than girls because of their larger body mass and prolonged period of growth. Teens involved in athletics also have an increased need for calories. Twelve- to 14-year-old boys need approximately 60 kcal/kg^{-1}/day^{-1}, whereas girls at this age need 45 to 50 kcal/kg^{-1}/day^{-1}. At age 15 years, daily caloric intake decreases to 40 to 45 kcal/kg^{-1}/day^{-1} for boys and 35 to 40 kcal/kg^{-1}/day^{-1} for girls. Daily calcium intake during adolescence should be a minimum of 1,300 mg per day.

Because of the teenage lifestyle, healthy eating habits are sometimes difficult to maintain in adolescents. The nutritional history should be considered in the context of overall lifestyle and activity. Because issues of body image and peer influence are at their peak during this age, it is essential to watch for signs of eating disorders and to caution parents on how to carefully discuss the importance of diet with their teen.

■ Obesity

The topic of obesity cannot be ignored when caring for children and adolescents, and it is the responsibility of the provider to address obesity, despite the sensitive nature of the topic. The percentage of U.S. children with obesity has tripled over the last 40 to 50 years, and roughly 19% of children between the ages of 2 and 19 years are considered obese today (Fryar et al., 2020). (Obesity is defined as an age- and sex-specific BMI in the 95th percentile or greater.) The overall rate of childhood obesity has leveled off over the past decade, although it is still on the rise in certain pediatric patient populations, specifically African American girls and Hispanic boys.

Children and adolescents affected by weight problems may face an array of physical, mental, and emotional problems. Physical ailments such as asthma, obstructive sleep apnea, orthopedic problems, high blood pressure, abnormal lipid levels, and insulin resistance are associated with obesity in these age groups. In addition, these children may suffer from teasing and bullying from their peers that may lead to anxiety, depression, and other emotional issues. While approaching the topic of obesity with parents can seem tricky, it is important and can be done respectfully by using data and facts.

Incorporating the child's growth charts into the conversation can be helpful and is a visual representation of a child's growth that can be easily explained to parents. A child's own growth chart can be compared to itself over time. The curves that represent overweight (85%) and obese (95%) are clearly marked. The BMI chart is also a helpful tool for measuring children's weight and growth by sex, as it takes into account that they are still growing and at various rates. This chart is the preferred tool for screening for obesity in the pediatric population.

Inquiring about nutrition and daily intake of certain food groups is a good way to assess risk factors for obesity and habits that may lead to weight gain. Asking young children what their favorite foods are can be a fun place to start. Or ask teenagers if they eat breakfast and, if so, what do they eat? Ask if they like fruits and/or vegetables, but follow up by asking if they eat them very often. Just liking them is not enough if they are never actually eating them. Also ask about frequency of fast-food meals and how often families eat at home together. Definitely ask about what the child drinks; liquids can be a hidden source of high amounts of calories. Just getting a child to limit juice, give up soda, drink lower-fat milk, and increase water can make a huge difference in daily calorie intake.

Below is a list of eating-related behaviors that have been shown to be associated with childhood obesity. Being aware of some of these can help guide your assessment and questions for parents and families.

- Skipping breakfast
- Eating meals away from home (especially fast food)
- Eating quickly

- Ingesting larger portions
- Eating in the absence of hunger
- Drinking sugar-sweetened beverages

Asking parents about family health history is another helpful way to assess for obesity risk. A child with obese parents is more likely to become obese. If many older family members are struggling with diabetes, heart disease, or hypertension, you can use these examples of illnesses that we would like to limit in the next generation. Reinforce with parents that overweight and obese children may grow into overweight and obese adults—with the heart problems and metabolic diseases that may come along with that. Studies show that nearly 80% of adolescents with obesity will also be obese as adults. Starting healthy habits with children is the best way to create healthy adults.

Include an assessment of physical activity in your discussion of healthy weight with parents and patients. Increased sedentary behavior is linked to obesity. In this age group, that means asking specifically about screen time and time allowed for electronics of any kind. Question children about what kinds of games or sports they enjoy, and teach them about the importance of being active every day. Children who live farther away from parks or in perceived "dangerous" neighborhoods have been shown to have an increased risk of being overweight or obese, so helping those families come up with creative ways to get kids active is essential.

Overall, providers caring for children are in an ideal position to assess and counsel families about childhood obesity. By following children closely and measuring height, weight, and BMI at least annually, providers can pick up on changing trends (like a rapid increase in BMI) and intervene early, as necessary. Obesity in children is a complex issue and, as a result, a comprehensive assessment is necessary to catch risk factors early and reverse unhealthy habits before they become permanent behaviors.

■ Anticipatory Guidance and Safety

Well-child checkups are not solely conducted to examine the patient physically but also to offer advice and insight into upcoming stages and safety issues. A focus of the assessment should include identifying a child's potential risks in order to appropriately counsel parents.

Create an open dialogue with parents that addresses safety topics by asking about daily practices and home environment. Table 19.13 is an age-by-age list of anticipatory guidance and safety topics, which should be covered at each well-child checkup, regarding feeding, sleeping, elimination, safety, and illness. Other issues may arise, and discussion during the visits should be based on parental concerns and questions.

■ Teething and Tooth Eruption

Assess the child's history of teething and tooth eruption. The primary teeth begin to erupt around age 6 months. Table 19.14 identifies the typical age of tooth eruption. The eruption pattern may vary from the expected norm.

Table 19.13

Anticipatory Guidance

Age	Feeding	Sleeping	Elimination	Safety	Illness
Newborn–1 mo	Feed on demand; ask about duration of feeds (or amount per feeding if on formula); always hold bottle—don't prop	Place on back to sleep; firm mattress; avoid pillows and blankets; ask about where baby is sleeping and in what position	Breastfed stool is yellow and pasty; normal bowel frequency varies from after each feeding to every other day; ask about stool frequency and consistency	Do not leave infant alone on high surfaces; set water heater thermostat to 120 degrees; always use a proper rear-facing car seat; smoke detectors; sun protection	Call office for rectal temp higher than 100.4°F; persistent vomiting or diarrhea; refusal to feed, prolonged irritability, bulging fontanel, or yellow tinge to skin or eyes
1–2 mo	Feed on demand; may stretch out time between feeds	Same as above; some routine may slowly develop; may sleep 16–18 hr/day	Babies frequently grunt and strain while stooling; as long as stool is soft, then baby is not constipated	Same as above; learn infant/child CPR	Same as above
2–4 mo	Same as above; more routine develops; may slowly increase amount of formula; no solids needed yet; avoid adding cereal to bottle	Same as above	Same as above	Same as above	Same as above
4–6 mo	Night feedings should decrease or stop; may start solids close to 6 mo	Should sleep longer stretches at night; routine nap schedule develops; if infant rolls to stomach to sleep, it is okay	Same as above	Watch for choking hazards; watch for burns from infant grabbing at hot food or liquids	Call for rectal temp over 101°F; decreased urination (no wet diaper in 8 hr); prolonged inconsolability; wheezing; cold symptoms (without fever) for over 5–7 days
6–9 mo	Start solids—infant rice cereal or any store bought or homemade single food; add foods slowly and one at a time (stick with one new food for 3–4 days); night feedings should stop	Establish consistent nighttime rituals, including reading	Stools will change in consistency with addition of solids; rice cereal can be constipating; give diluted juice if constipation is a problem	Make sure house is completely baby-proofed. Lock up poisons; cover outlets; pool safety if applicable; choking hazards with new foods; sunscreen	Same as above

(cont. on page 690)

Table 19.13

Anticipatory Guidance—cont'd

Age	Feeding	Sleeping	Elimination	Safety	Illness
9–12 mo	Increase table/finger foods; offer cup with water (no juice until 12 months); establish mealtime routines	Stick with nighttime rituals; security item may help with bedtime	Same as above	Same as above	
Stage	**Feeding**	**Sleeping**	**Elimination**	**Safety**	
Toddler	Appetite slows; child becomes pickier; offer new foods; avoid battles	Transition to regular bed; consistent nighttime ritual; nightmares may occur; usually one nap during the day	Interest in potty training emerges; most children demonstrate readiness between 24 and 30 mo	Always use proper car seat; teach street safety; have a fire escape plan; lock guns away; lock poisons and medications; use sunscreen and bug repellent; caution about burns and falls	
Preschooler	Encourage balanced diet; child should use utensils correctly; pickiness may continue	Naps may decrease or stop; bedtime may be moved up when napping ceases; nightmares and terrors may occur	By age 3, 90% of children are bowel trained, 85% are dry during the day, and 60%—70% are dry at night; no interventions if still wetting at night	Same as above; water safety; begin stranger awareness and safety; continue using car or booster seat	
School age	Encourage balanced diet, limiting junk foods; eat as a family; involve child in food preparation	Continue consistent nighttime ritual; average 8-year-old sleeps 9–12 hours a night	Consider interventions (pharmacological or behavioral) if nocturnal enuresis occurs	Same as above; bike safety; fire safety; child should remain in a booster car seat until age 8 or 80 pounds	
Adolescent	Encourage balanced diet and healthy food choices; limit junk and fast food	Erratic sleep patterns; napping may increase; need average of 8–9 hours of sleep per night		Seat belts; car safety; safe sex; discourage drug and alcohol usage; reinforce sunscreen usage; keep firearms locked	

Table 19.14

Patterns of Tooth Eruption

Primary Teeth	Maxillary	Mandibular
Central incisors	6–8 mo	5–7 mo
Lateral incisors	8–11 mo	7–10 mo
Cuspids/canines	16–20 mo	16–20 mo
First molars	10–16 mo	10–16 mo
Second molars	20–30 mo	20–30 mo
Permanent Teeth	Maxillary	Mandibular
Central incisors	7–8 yr	6–7 yr
Lateral incisors	8–9 yr	7–8 yr
Cuspids/canines	11–12 yr	9–11 yr
First premolars	10–11 yr	10–12 yr
Second premolars	10–12 yr	11–13 yr
First molars	6–7 yr	6–7 yr
Second molars	12–13 yr	12–13 yr
Third molars	17–22 yr	17–22 yr

Table 19.15

Fluoride Concentration in Community Drinking Water

Age	Less Than 0.3 ppm	0.3–0.6 ppm	More Than 0.6 ppm
Birth–6 mo	None	None	None
6 mo–3 yr	0.25 mg/day	None	None
3–6 yr	0.50 mg/day	0.25 mg/day	None
6–16 yr	1 mg/day	0.5 mg/day	None

ppm = parts per million.
From Centers for Disease Control and Prevention (2001).

During the assessment of teething and tooth eruption, determine the level of fluoride present in the child's drinking water. It is helpful for providers to know the amount of fluoride in a community's drinking water because any recommendations for supplementation are based on those amounts. Children who do not live in a fluoridated water area but who attend school or day care in such an area (and drink water while at school) may not need additional supplementation. The guidelines in Table 19.15 should be incorporated into the care of pediatric patients.

REFERENCES

American Academy of Pediatrics. (2012). Instrument-based pediatric vision screening policy statement. *Pediatrics, 130*(5), 983–986.

American Psychiatric Association. (2013). *Diagnostic and statistical manual of mental disorders* (5th ed.). American Psychiatric Publishing.

Concussion in Sport Group. (2017). Consensus statement on concussion in sport—the 5th international conference on concussion in sport, Berlin, October 2016. *British Medical Journal, 51*(11). http://dx.doi:org/10.1136/bjsports-2017-097699

Fryan, C. D., Carroll, M. D., & Afful, J. (2020). Prevalence of overweight, obesity, and severe obesity among children and adolescents aged 2–19 years: United States, 1963–1965 through 2017–2018. NCHS Health E-Stats. https://www.cdc.gov/nchs/data/hestat/obesity-adult-17-18/obesity-adult.htm

Guthrie, R. (2018). Physical activity following acute concussion and persistent postconcussive symptoms in children and adolescents. *The Physician and Sports Medicine, 46*(4), 416–419. http://doi.org/10.1080/00913847.2018.1516479

Henry J. Kaiser Family Foundation. (2021). Mental health and substance use considerations among children during the COVID-19 pandemic, KFF COVID-19 Vaccine Monitor. https://urldefense.com/v3/__https://www.kff.org/coronavirus-covid-19/issue-brief/mental-health-and-substance-use-considerations-among-children-during-the-covid-19-pandemic/__;!!PhOWcWs!jDGqR8OXOX4O7WfjPIs_-LzKYxDyg6Xy5ny6gePub671eg4vgtZ-JELI7403rZw$

Kroenke, K., Spitzer, R., & Williams, J. (2001). The PHQ-9: Validity of a brief depression severity measure. *Journal of General Internal Medicine, 16*, 606–613. doi:10.1046/j.1525-1497.2001.016009606.x

Merikangas, K., He, J., Burstein, M., Benjet, C., Georgiades, K., & Swenden, J. (2010). Lifetime prevalence of mental disorders in U.S. adolescents: Results from the National Comorbidity Survey Replication – Adolescent Supplement (NCS-A). *Child and Adolescent Psychology. 49*(10); 980–989. https://doi.org/10.1016/j.jaac.2010.05.017

Shen, K., & Bhatt, A. (2017). Clinical pearl: The "rule of 8." *Journal of Pediatric Ophthalmology & Strabismus.* https://doi.org/10.3928/01913913-20170907-08

Spitzer, R. L., Kroenke, K., Janet, B. W., Williams, J. B. W., & Lowe, B. (2006). A brief measure for assessing generalized anxiety disorder: The GAD-7. *Archives of Internal Medicine, 166*, 1092–1097. https://doi:10.1001/archinte.166.10.1092

Togias, A., Cooper, S. F., Acebal, M. L., Assa'ad, A., Baker, Jr., J. R., Beck, L. A., Block, J., Byrd-Bredbenner, C., Chan, E. S., Eichenfield, L. F., Fleischer, D. M., Fuchs, III, G. J., Furuta, G. T., Greenhawt, M. J., Gupta, R. S., Habich, M., Jones, S. M., Keaton, K., Muraro, A., . . . Boyce. J. A. (2017). Addendum guidelines for the prevention of peanut allergy in the United States: Report of the National Institute of Allergy and Infectious Diseases-sponsored expert panel. *Journal of Allergy and Clinical Immunology. 139*(1), 29–44. https://doi: 10.1016/j.jaci.2016.10.010

Yang, S., Zusman, N., Lieberman, E., & Goldstein, R. (2019). Developmental dysplasia of the hip. *Pediatrics, 143*(1). https://doi.org/10.1542/peds.2018-1147

Chapter 20

Pregnant Patients

Kelley Stallworth Borella ·
Janatha S. Grant ·
Brandy Tanner ·

P regnancy is considered a wellness condition and not a disease entity. The focus of care during a low-risk pregnancy is therefore on health promotion and maintenance while achieving a healthy outcome for both the pregnant patient and the child. Advanced practice nurses—specifically, nurse practitioners—have a strong tradition of delivering wellness care throughout the life span in a cost-effective manner and with a high level of patient satisfaction. Caring for pregnant patients is therefore congruent with the advanced practice nursing model.

Pregnancy care from nurse practitioners should ideally begin with preconception care and continue throughout pregnancy. Childbirth is typically the role of a physician or certified nurse midwife with the nurse practitioner resuming care during the postpartum period.

The status of the patient's health directly affects the pregnancy outcome. Basic prenatal care is a "coordinated approach to medical care, continuous risk assessment and psychological support that optimally begins before pregnancy and extends throughout the postpartum and the interpregnancy period" (AAP & ACOG, 2017, p. 149). Preconception care should be used to maximize the patient's physical and psychosocial health and to allow the patient to make informed decisions regarding any potential health or lifestyle adjustments that may affect future pregnancies.

History

After pregnancy is confirmed, a complete medical, psychosocial (including the current living situation and social support and abuse information), family (including genetic), and reproductive history is obtained. This includes a menstrual, contraceptive, gynecological, sexual, surgical, nutritional (including prepregnancy weight), and medication (including over-the-counter, herbal, and recreational drug use) history, as well as alcohol and tobacco use. An estimated date of delivery (EDD) is projected at this time by using the last menstrual

Table 20.1

Pregnancy Nomenclature

Letter	Meaning	Definition
G	Gravidity	Total number of pregnancies, regardless of duration or outcome
P	Parity	Number of pregnancies after 20 weeks of gestation
T	Term	Number of pregnancies considered to be 37–40 weeks of gestation
P	Premature/preterm deliveries	Number of pregnancies between 20 and 37 weeks of gestation
A	Abortions	Number of induced or spontaneous terminations of pregnancy before 20 weeks of gestation
L	Live births	Number of living children who are alive at the time of data collection

period. This estimation can be made with either a pregnancy wheel or a calculator or by applying Naegele's rule of adding 7 days to the first day of the last menstrual period and then subtracting 3 months (Cunningham et al., 2018). This method of estimating the EDD depends on the patient having regular menstrual cycles of 28, plus or minus 7 days. If available, an ultrasound in the first trimester is the most accurate tool for dating criteria and should be used to establish or confirm the EDD. An EDD determined without ultrasound is considered suboptimal (AAP & ACOG, 2017).

The reproductive history includes the contraceptive, sexual, and obstetric history. The contraceptive history elicits the last time contraceptives have been used, what types of contraceptives were used, and the dates of any unprotected intercourse. The sexual history helps identify risks for sexually transmitted infections or ectopic pregnancies. The obstetric history consists of the number of pregnancies and their outcomes using the gravida–para–TPAL nomenclature (Table 20.1). This portion of the history also includes the year of each pregnancy, infant birth weight, gestational age at birth, type of delivery (vaginal or caesarean), length of labor, anesthesia received, and any maternal or fetal complications during the pregnancy.

Physical Examination

The initial physical examination is a systematic, complete, head-to-toe examination that is usually performed at the time of the first visit to provide baseline information. The clinical pelvimetry assessment is done at this time to ensure pelvic adequacy for vaginal delivery. Vital signs, especially blood pressure and weight, are included with each assessment. Subsequent visits are abbreviated in that they focus on the developmental stage of the pregnancy and the overall health of the pregnant patient and fetus. Components of these targeted examinations (depending on the week of gestation) include fundal height, presentation, fetal heart rate (FHR), fetal movement, the presence or absence of preterm labor signs and symptoms, cervical examination (including dilatation and effacement), urine dipstick, and timing of the next appointment.

Monitoring FHR is a vital component of fetal surveillance, providing important information on placental function, fetal hypoxia, and whether the intrauterine environment can support and sustain the fetus. The FHR can usually be auscultated by 10 weeks with an electronic Doppler and by 20 weeks with a fetoscope (Cunningham et al., 2018). A normal FHR is 110 to 160 beats per minute. A sustained FHR of below 100 beats per minute is indicative of fetal jeopardy. If there is a question of whether the FHR is being adequately evaluated, the maternal pulse should simultaneously be assessed to ensure that the FHR and not the maternal heart rate is actually being auscultated.

Leopold's maneuvers should be integrated into the prenatal assessment after 28 weeks of gestation in order to locate the most appropriate area for FHR auscultation (Fig. 20.1). The location where the fetal heart tones (FHTs) are best heard or the point of maximal intensity should be documented. This procedure can reinforce the accuracy of the fetal position as assessed by the examiner through palpation. FHTs are best auscultated through the fetal back in vertex and breech presentations and toward the patient's flank when the fetus is in a transverse lie. In vertex presentations, FHTs are usually best heard below the patient's umbilicus, in the lower abdomen, whereas for breech presentations, they are best heard at or slightly above the umbilicus, in the patient's upper abdomen.

Fundal height provides an estimation of gestational age in relationship to uterine size. Before 20 weeks, the anatomic location of the fundus provides an estimation of gestational age. The uterus is usually palpable above the symphysis at 12 weeks of gestation, midway between the symphysis pubis and umbilicus at 16 weeks, and at the umbilicus at 20 weeks. Fundal height measurement and changes correlate closely with the number of weeks of pregnancy

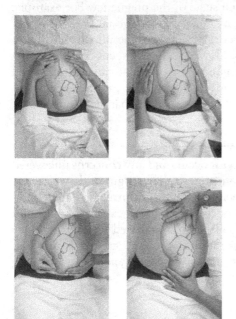

Figure 20.1 Leopold's maneuver.

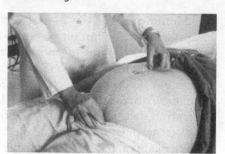

Figure 20.2 Measuring fundal heights: Fundal height in centimeters should correlate closely with number of weeks' gestation. From Dillon (2007), p. 838.

from 20 to 34 weeks of gestation (i.e., a fundal height of 32 cm correlates with 32 weeks of pregnancy) and provide an estimation of gestational age in relationship to uterine size (Cunningham et al., 2018). Fundal height is measured by placing the end of a tape measure at the symphysis pubis and extending it to the fundus (Fig. 20.2). Small uterine size for dates may be indicative of inaccurate pregnancy dating, intrauterine growth restriction, or oligohydramnios (low amount of amniotic fluid). Large uterine size for dates may be associated with inaccurate dates, macrosomia, polyhydramnios (excessive amount of amniotic fluid) or multiple gestations (more than one fetus).

Laboratory Studies

Laboratory studies during the initial visit are quite extensive. These screening tests are dependent on the disease prevalence within the screened population (Table 20.2). Laboratory testing throughout the pregnancy is dependent on presenting complaints and the developmental stage of the pregnancy. For example, a glucose screen should be done between 24 to 28 weeks of gestation, whereas an anemia screen (hemoglobin and hematocrit) should be done initially and again at 24 to 28 weeks and at 32 to 36 weeks. However, if the patient complains of a vaginal discharge later in the pregnancy, a gonorrhea and chlamydia culture could be done even if the initial screen was negative. A culture for group beta streptococcus should be obtained at 36 0/7 to 37 6/7 weeks in preparation for delivery.

Prenatal Education

Prenatal education depends on when the visit occurs and any concerns uncovered during the visit, but it usually focuses on preterm labor signs and symptoms, danger signs of pregnancy, fetal movement awareness, information about prenatal classes, nutrition, exercise, weight goals, teratogens, sexuality, and infant feeding choices. Education on weight goals should be based on prepregnancy weight, allowing for slower gain during the first trimester compared to later. Table 20.3 depicts recommended weight gain for pregnancy, adjusted according to the patient's body mass index.

Table 20.2

Recommended Pregnancy Screening Tests

Initial Routine Tests for All Pregnant Patients	Additional Tests Depending on the Patient's History	Tests for Subsequent Pregnancy Visits
• CBC • Blood type, Rh, and antibody screen • Urine culture • Aneuploidy screen (PAPP-A and hCG) with nuchal translucency ultrasound • Rubella titer • Serology for syphilis • Hepatitis B surface antigen • Pap smear if indicated per ASCCP guidelines • Chlamydia/gonorrhea screening	• Sickle cell screen (Sickledex) or hemoglobin electrophoresis for African Americans • Tuberculosis screen • HIV screen • Hepatitis C antibody • Urine toxicology screen • Diabetes screening • Herpes culture • Serum iron studies • Thyroid studies • Toxoplasmosis titer • Potassium hydroxide (KOH)/wet prep	• CBC or hemoglobin at 24–28 wk and 32–36 wk • Diabetes screening: 24–28 wk • Urine dipstick every visit • Quad screen (MSAFP, hCG, estriol, and inhibin A) in second trimester to complete integrated aneuploidy screen • Antibody screen for Rh-negative patients: 28 wk • Retest chlamydia/gonorrhea if positive earlier: 34–36 wk based on patient population and risk factors • Group beta strep culture (vaginal/anorectal): 35–37 wk • Repeat syphilis and HIV testing in third trimester based on patient population and risk factors

CBC = complete blood count; PAPP-A = pregnancy-associated plasma protein-A; hCG, human chorionic gonadotropin; MSAFP = maternal serum alpha-fetoprotein; ASCCP = American Society for Colposcopy and Cervical Pathology

Table 20.3

New Recommendations for Total and Rate of Weight Gain During Pregnancy by Prepregnancy Body Mass Index

	Total Weight Gain		Rates of Weight Gain* Second and Third Trimester	
Body Mass Index	Range in kg	Range in lbs	Mean (range) in kg/week	Mean (range) in lbs/week
Underweight (<18.5 kg/m²)	12.5–18	28–40	0.51 (0.44–0.58)	1 (1–3)
Normal weight (18.5–24.9 kg/m²)	11.4–15.9	25–35	0.42 (0.35–0.50)	1 (0.8–1)
Overweight (25.0–29.9 kg/m²)	6.8–11.4	15–25	0.28 (0.23–0.33)	0.6 (0.5–0.7)
Obese (>30 kg/m²)	6.8	11–20	0.22 (0.17–0.27)	0.5 (0.4–0.6)

Institute of Medicine and National Research Council Committee to Reexamine IOM Pregnancy Weight Guidelines (2009). Weight gain during pregnancy: Reexamining the guidelines. Washington DC: National Academies Press, with permission.

*Calculations assume a 0.5–2.0 kg (1.1–1.4 lb) weight gain in the first trimester.

If prenatal vitamins are not already being taken during the preconception period, during the initial visit educate the patient to start taking them. Instruct the patient regarding other medications as indicated by the history or physical examination (e.g., iron or calcium supplementation).

Educate the patient regarding the follow-up plan. For routine pregnancies, prenatal visits are usually scheduled every 4 weeks until 28 weeks of gestation. At that time, visits are scheduled every 2 weeks from 28 to 36 weeks and then weekly until childbirth occurs (Cunningham et al., 2018).

Common Chief Complaints of Pregnancy

■ Gastrointestinal Complaints

Gastrointestinal (GI) complaints are common in pregnancy. These ailments include mild to severe nausea, vomiting, and dyspepsia, which are associated with increased levels of human chorionic gonadotropin (hCG), or the effects of increased progesterone on smooth muscles in the GI tract. Evidence supporting GI ailments caused by the uterine displacement of abdominal organs is limited. Other GI conditions such as cholestasis and cholelithiasis and constipation are also associated with pregnancy, with the risk of gallstones increasing with number of pregnancies. It is important to differentiate normal changes associated with pregnancy from more serious disease states, and the practitioner must know which diagnostic tests will not be harmful to either the patient or the fetus.

When assessing abdominal complaints, issues regarding imaging during pregnancy arise. There is no "safe" threshold for radiation during pregnancy. Decisions must be made balancing the potential benefit related to specific imaging with the potential risks. The American College of Radiology (ACR) does provide reference of the suspected in utero effects of radiation by weeks of pregnancy, suggesting that <5 rad are likely to have no effects, regardless of gestational age. Abdominal imaging is associated with exposure to the fetus and should be carefully considered (ACR, 2018). Furthermore, it is important to consider not only an individual exposure but also cumulative exposure if multiple procedures are required, particularly between 8 and 15 weeks of gestation (Cunningham et al., 2018).

Upper endoscopy is a safe diagnostic procedure during pregnancy and does not carry an increased risk of preterm labor or other complications as compared to other diagnostic modalities such as diagnostic radiology studies (Sadro & Dubinsky, 2013). However, as a general rule, any procedures during pregnancy are usually postponed until after delivery or at least until after the first trimester unless the risk of the disease outweighs the risk of the procedure and definitive evaluation is needed.

If radiology studies are warranted, ultrasound is safe and effective in diagnosing intra-abdominal conditions during pregnancy. Current knowledge indicates that magnetic resonance imaging (MRI) is safe during pregnancy, but computed tomography (CT) imaging exposes the fetus to doses of ionizing radiation and should only be done in cases of extreme nonobstetrical emergencies (Sadro & Dubinsky, 2013).

NAUSEA AND VOMITING

Onset of pregnancy-related nausea and vomiting is usually between the 4th and 6th weeks, peaking between the 8th and 12th weeks. Resolution is common by week 20 (Gomes et al., 2018).

Causes of nausea and vomiting associated with pregnancy are unknown, although elevations of hCG and progesterone are believed to play a role. Psychological factors may be involved, including anxiety and depression (Gomes et al., 2018).

Hyperemesis gravidarum is characterized by persistent or severe nausea and vomiting to the point of affecting the patient's nutritional status. It is not controlled by dietary changes or antiemetics and can lead to problems such as weight loss, electrolyte disruptions, vitamin deficiencies, and dehydration. This is a diagnosis of exclusion (Cunningham et al., 2018). Treatment may require hospitalization. The onset of hyperemesis gravidarum is later than typical pregnancy nausea and vomiting, but it usually occurs by week 22. The cause is unknown, although suggested etiologies relate to effects of pregnancy-related hormonal changes (Gomes et al. [2018]).

Subjective

Initial questions regarding pregnancy-induced nausea and vomiting should include whether these symptoms occur more frequently during certain times of the day. Any pain should be assessed as to whether it has a gradual or rapid onset and whether eating either alleviates or exacerbates the condition. For example, nausea with pain that occurs with eating may indicate esophagitis, whereas symptoms that occur several hours postprandially suggest a duodenal ulcer. Hydration status can be assessed by asking about dark-colored urine and excessive thirst. Psychosocial distress also should be evaluated. Worrisome features in the history include fever, abdominal pain, abdominal cramping, diarrhea, jaundice, vaginal bleeding, headaches, neurological signs, projectile vomiting, hematemesis, and melena.

Objective

Vital signs should be within normal limits and not be indicative of dehydration. There should not be any weight loss. The thyroid should be of normal size and shape. Uterine size should be appropriate for dates, and the presence of FHTs (after 12 weeks) is a reassuring sign. A complete blood count (CBC), complete metabolic panel containing liver enzymes and a calcium level, and a hemoccult of the stool may eliminate other causes for the nausea and vomiting. Urine ketones and specific gravity should not indicate dehydration, and urine dipstick or urinalysis should be negative for infection or hematuria (to rule out renal calculus). Stool antigen for *Helicobacter pylori* can be attained to evaluate for current infection, since a serum titer will not differentiate between past and current infections.

Differential Diagnoses

Differential diagnoses include hyperemesis gravidarum, multiple gestation, hydatidiform gestation, molar pregnancy, intestinal obstruction, gastroenteritis, cholecystitis, pancreatitis, hepatitis, diabetes, thyroid dysfunction, migraine, food poisoning, emotional problems, eating disorders, and normal pregnancy.

HEARTBURN

Heartburn is associated with a number of pregnancy-related factors. Progesterone is associated with decreased gastric emptying. Furthermore, fetal growth may alter the relationships between organs, compressing the stomach, while the lower esophageal sphincter relaxes (Gomes et al., 2018; Cunningham et al., 2018). Unlike nausea and vomiting, heartburn may not resolve until after delivery.

Subjective

Heartburn and epigastric/upper abdominal pain are often associated with heavy, high-fat, fried, spicy, or gas-producing meals and with positional changes, such as bending over. Ask about diet and any other triggers. Another common symptom includes a sense of abdominal bloating or distention. Any psychosocial stressors or depression should be explored. Differentiate between dyspepsia or heartburn and dysphagia. Ask about associated symptoms such as chest pain, dyspnea, exercise intolerance, palpitations, diaphoresis, fatty stools, foul-smelling stools, melena, nausea, vomiting, diarrhea or constipation, or fever and chills.

Objective

Diagnosis for heartburn is usually based on history and physical examination. A CBC, complete metabolic panel and a hemoccult for blood in the stool may eliminate other causes for the dyspepsia. The presence of *H. pylori* can be addressed.

Differential Diagnoses

Differential diagnoses include pregnancy-related heartburn, cholecystitis, pancreatitis, cardiac etiology, ulcer, and hiatal hernia.

ABDOMINAL PAIN

Uterine pressure increases as a result of the growing fetus and placenta and the increase in amniotic fluid volume. At 12 weeks, the fundus rises above the symphysis. When the pregnant patient is in an upright position, the broad and round ligaments anchor the uterus to the anterior abdominal wall in order to provide uterine stability (Davidson et al., 2016). The weight of the uterus may cause tension on these ligaments, creating inflammation and discomfort. This pain is often exacerbated with movement and is more often present on the right side. This ligament pain usually resolves when the patient assumes a supine position as the uterus descends backward.

Subjective

Determine whether the abdominal pain is acute, chronic, or recurrent; whether it has a gradual or rapid onset; and whether the pain has ever occurred before.

The severity of the pain (on a scale of 1 to 10) and the progression or resolution of the pain should be noted. Determine the quality of the pain (e.g., sharp or dull) and any precipitating factors such as eating or movement. Identify the location of pain (e.g., periumbilical, right lower quadrant, suprapubic). If there is a sense of tightening or pressure in the uterus, ask whether the pressure resolves with position change or with bladder emptying. Ask about the timing and consistency of the last bowel movement. Identify any associated symptoms such as regular contractions that do not improve with position change or bladder emptying, nausea, vomiting, diarrhea, melena, hematochezia, hematemesis, fever, anorexia, urinary tract infection (UTI) symptoms, a tender lump in the groin that worsens with prolonged standing, vaginal bleeding or bloody show, or vaginal fluid leaking.

Objective
Vital signs and physical examination should be appropriate for the gestational age of the pregnancy. There should be no reproducible tenderness with palpation to the chest wall or pain with deep breathing. There should be no regular contractions felt; no cervical dilatation or effacement; no fluid leakage, possibly indicating rupture of membranes, or bleeding from the os; and no adnexal, abdominal, or pelvic masses or tenderness. Bowel sounds should be normal. A rectal examination may be done to check for impaction. Fetal activity should be present. Fetal heart sounds should be heard by Doppler if gestation is over 10 to 12 weeks. Ultrasonography should show a normal fetal heart motion and no worrisome signs, such as decreased fetal movement, abnormal placenta placement, or abnormal amniotic fluid levels. If the pregnancy is between weeks 4 and 8, the hCG levels should correspond with the gestational age of the fetus and should double every 2 to 3 days (Cunningham et al., 2018).

Differential Diagnoses
Differential diagnoses include normal fetal activity, ligament pain, Braxton Hicks contractions, preterm or true labor, ectopic pregnancy, abruptio placentae, placenta previa, threatened abortion, complete abortion, missed (incomplete) abortion, premature rupture of membranes, pre-eclampsia, vaginitis, pelvic inflammatory disease, ovarian cyst rupture, constipation, intestinal obstruction, ulcer, diverticulitis, appendicitis, kidney stone, inguinal hernia, gastroenteritis, UTI, and costochondritis.

▪ Musculoskeletal Complaints

Common musculoskeletal complaints include back pain, leg pain and cramps, and pain or tingling of the hands.

BACK PAIN

Low back pain occurs in up to 70% of pregnancies. Back pain usually results from the exaggeration of the lumbar spine curvature that balances the patient's center of gravity over the lower extremities in response to the growing uterus. The release of the hormone relaxin causes ligaments in the pubic symphysis and sacroiliac joints to soften in preparation for vaginal delivery. An increased breast size may also result in upper back pain. Patients who are obese or have a history of back pain are more likely to experience it during pregnancy. A thorough musculoskeletal examination should be performed prior to labeling severe back pain as pregnancy related (Cunningham et al., 2018).

Subjective

The PQRST process for exploring a complaint (see Chapter 1) should be used to identify critical information such as the location, quality, rating, and radiation of the pain, as well as associated symptoms and any triggers. Identify any history of back injuries, problems, or surgeries. Ask about associated symptoms including those consistent with a UTI or vaginal infection. Determine whether the patient has experienced bowel changes; uterine contractions; pain, numbness, or tingling that radiates either into the abdomen or down into the legs; and any neurological deficits.

Objective

Note the patient's weight and body mass index. Observe posture for lordosis and gait. Assess presence of paraspinal or costal vertebral angle tenderness to palpation, and response to straight leg raises. Reflexes and a neurological examination should be assessed. A rectal examination may be done to assess for rectal tone and impaction. Urinary tract symptoms, vaginal discharge, or uterine contractions, as well as weakness and/or severe pain, necessitate appropriate evaluation.

Differential Diagnoses

Differential diagnoses include backache related to pregnancy, muscle sprain or strain, sciatica, arthritis, herniated disk, uterine contractions, vaginal infection, UTI, kidney stone, pancreatitis, gallstones, and ulcer.

LEG MUSCLE CRAMPS AND PAIN

Pregnancy-associated cramping typically occurs at night or in early morning. However, sudden development of pain with edema of the leg or thigh may indicate thrombosis. Pregnant patients are 4 to 5 times more likely to experience a thromboembolism than nonpregnant patients. In the United States, thromboembolisms account for approximately 9% of deaths among pregnant patients (ACOG, 2018a). Causes other than thrombosis include electrolyte disturbances and injury.

Subjective

Investigate the symptom of muscle cramps or pain, determining location, timing, quality, and precipitating factors. Ask about recent excessive exercise or walking. Fluid and calcium intake should be checked through a diet recall. Ask about history of previous deep vein thrombosis (DVT) and a personal or family history of thrombophilic disorders (Table 20.4). Prior thrombosis is an important risk factor for pregnancy-related events. Also identify any recent trauma or surgery, lower back pain or arthritis, or neurological complaints.

Table 20.4

Thrombophilic States in Pregnancy

Inherited Thrombophilias	Acquired Thrombophilias
Factor V Leiden	Pregnancy/postpartum
Prothrombin A20210	Immobilization
AT III	Trauma
Protein C	Postoperative state
Protein S	High estrogen levels
Homocysteine	Malignancy
	Nephrotic syndrome
	Heparin-induced thrombocytopenia
	Myeloproliferative disorders
	Paroxysmal nocturnal hematuria
	Congestive heart failure and atrial fibrillation
	Antiphospholipid antibody syndrome

AT = antithrombin.

Objective

The physical examination should include Homan's sign, skin color, edema, and pulses. A clinical assessment of the probability of having a DVT can be determined by calculating a modified Wells' criteria score (Table 20.5). Worrisome findings include unilateral calf swelling or tenderness, diminished pulses in the lower extremities, redness, abnormal warmth or coldness, numbness, or pale-appearing calf or leg. Orthostatic blood pressures and pulses should be taken if indicated. Electrolytes and serum calcium levels may need to be checked. If DVT is suspected, a compression ultrasound is recommended (AAP & ACOG, 2017).

Differential Diagnoses

Differential diagnoses include muscle cramps, electrolyte imbalances, thromboembolic disease, varicosities, dehydration, arthritis, sciatica, and nerve root compression.

NUMBNESS OR TINGLING IN HANDS

Several conditions may be associated with numbness, tingling, and/or pain in the hands, including cervical radiculopathy and de Quervain's tendonitis. However, carpal tunnel syndrome is the most common pregnancy-related mononeuropathy, occurring in 7% to 43% of pregnancies. Among pregnant patients with carpal tunnel syndrome, up to 80% describe bilateral symptoms (Cunningham et al., 2018).

Table 20.5

Modified Wells' Score

1. Active cancer or cancer treated within last 6 months (+1 point)
2. Bedridden recently >3 days or major surgery within the past 4 weeks (+1 point)
3. Calf swelling >3 cm compared to other leg, measured 10 cm below the tibial tuberosity (+1 point)
4. Collateral nonvaricose superficial veins present (+1 point)
5. Swelling of entire leg (+1 point)
6. Localized tenderness in the deep vein system (+1 point)
7. Pitting edema greater in the symptomatic leg (+1 point)
8. Paralysis, paresis, or recent orthopedic casting/immobilization of the lower extremity (+1 point)
9. Previously documented history of DVT (+1 point)
10. Alternative diagnosis more likely than DVT (−2 points)

Note: Possible score: −2 to 9; score denotes risk for DVT
- 0 or less—low probability (3%–5%)
- 1–2—moderate probability (17%)
- 3–9—high probability (17%–75%)

DVT = deep vein thrombosis.

Subjective

Ask about quality, location, and timing of symptoms such as dull aching pain, tingling, or numbness. Determine whether the symptoms are limited to the wrist and hand or extend up the arm. Ask about any weakness in the hand. Edema in the hands or upper extremities may be noted. A history of repetitive activity of the upper extremity may be reported. Sitting, standing, and sleep posture (especially if the patient sleeps with the arm extended against the head) should be investigated.

Objective

Tinel's sign and Phalen's test should be performed. Upper extremity, grip, and finger strength should be assessed along with the ability to oppose the thumb to the fingers. An evaluation for thenar atrophy and dry skin on the thumb and index and middle fingers (median nerve distribution) should be completed. The size and shape of joints, skin color, pulses, and capillary refill should be noted.

Differential Diagnoses

Differential diagnoses include carpal tunnel syndrome, musculoskeletal pain, arthritis, infection, cervical neck injury or disease, nerve damage in the hand, cardiac problems, thoracic outlet syndrome, and hyperventilation.

■ Respiratory Complaints

Pregnant patients are at risk for many of the same respiratory conditions that others experience. However, pregnancy is associated with significant alterations of the respiratory structures. As the uterus enlarges, it presses against the abdominal organs and diaphragm, and this prevents the lungs from fully expanding and results in a decreased residual volume and functional residual capacity. Nasal congestion or stuffiness may result from increased estrogen and progesterone levels, which increase perivascular edema and enlargement of the nasal turbinates (Davidson et al., 2016). These changes may also lead to episodes of epistaxis.

DYSPNEA (SHORTNESS OF BREATH)

Pregnancy is associated with a rise in the diaphragm, widening of the subcostal angle, and lengthening of thoracic cage and circumference; at the same time, pregnancy has increased oxygen requirements. Conditions such as asthma, pneumonia, or other respiratory conditions, added to the pregnancy-induced pulmonary changes, can result in poor tolerance of lung conditions (Cunningham et al., 2018). Pregnant patients are at risk of many respiratory conditions not specifically associated with pregnancy, including asthma, bronchitis, and pneumonia. As noted earlier, pregnancy is associated with heightened risk of thromboembolism and associated pulmonary emboli. Severe dyspnea and significant oxygen deprivation require an immediate assessment and referral.

Subjective

Explore any complaint of labored or heavy breathing by asking about the onset (either acute or chronic), association with activity, progression, and any prior episodes. Depending on the description, ask whether associated symptoms such as dizziness or light-headedness were experienced. Explore potential triggers such as eating, drinking, or potential allergen exposure, such as an insect bite. Identify related fever, cough, trauma, hemoptysis, night sweats, wheezing, chest pain, or GI symptoms. The patient's smoking history should be obtained. Past medical and family history should include assessment for DVT, recent immobilization or prolonged sitting, and thrombophilias such as factor V Leiden, protein C or S deficiency, and antiphospholipid syndrome.

Objective

Vital signs, pulse oximetry, and physical examination, especially of the upper and lower respiratory tracts and cardiac system, should be within normal limits for gestational age. There may be dependent edema that accumulates during the day related to the patient's weight, profession (prolonged standing or sitting), and activity level. Edema that does not subside overnight or with leg elevation is cause for concern. As indicated, further diagnostic studies may be warranted. A CBC should not indicate anemia. If pneumonia is suspected, the CURB-65 Severity Score for Community-Acquired Pneumonia can be calculated to help determine whether inpatient or outpatient treatment is warranted if pneumonia is present (Table 20.6), although it has not been studied in the pregnant population. If asthma is suspected, pulmonary functions are warranted. When a pulmonary embolism cannot be ruled out, the patient should be emergently transferred to an acute-care setting for further evaluation and treatment.

Radiologic images are not indicated unless absolutely necessary. According to the ACR (2013), a dose of more than 5 rads is unlikely to have health effects. The potential for risk associated with higher doses varies with fetal age.

Table 20.6

CURB-65/CRB-65 Score

- **C**onfusion
- **U**rea (BUN) >20 mg/dL (>7 mmol/L)
- **R**espiratory rate >30 breaths/min
- **B**lood pressure: systolic <90 mm Hg or diastolic <60 mm Hg
- Age >**65**

Note: CRB-65 score does not require testing for blood urea nitrogen (BUN).

A risk-versus-benefit assessment should be documented in the provider's note, along with documentation that the abdomen had lead shielding and that the lowest exposure technique possible was used.

Differential Diagnoses

Differential diagnoses include pregnancy-related dyspnea, upper respiratory infection, nasal congestion, asthma, bronchitis, pneumonia, pulmonary embolus, cardiac disease such as congestive heart failure (CHF), anemia, anxiety, hyperventilation, aspiration, and anaphylaxis.

NASAL CONGESTION

Subjective

The patient may report nasal stuffiness, rhinorrhea, sneezing, postnasal drip, or cough. The history may be positive for epistaxis. Worrisome symptoms include frontal headaches or sensation of fullness or pressure, teeth pain, or fever. Nasal spray and intranasal drug use should be investigated. Past medical history should include inquiries regarding allergic rhinitis, seasonal allergies, sinusitis, nasal or facial trauma, and hypertension (HTN).

Objective

Vital signs, particularly temperature and blood pressure, should be normal. Nasal turbinates may be pale to red and edematous and may either be dry or have discharge. Clotted blood may be noted if epistaxis has occurred. Sinuses should be percussed and palpated. There should be no pain with forward head motion. No polyps should be noted, and the septum should be intact and not deviated.

Differential Diagnoses

Differential diagnoses include nasal congestion related to pregnancy, epistaxis, upper respiratory infection, sinusitis, allergic rhinitis, nasal polyps, cocaine or chronic nasal spray use, HTN, and facial trauma.

FATIGUE

Fatigue usually occurs during the first and third trimesters of pregnancy. First-trimester fatigue is often associated with physical and psychosocial pregnancy changes. While nausea and vomiting can lead to fatigue early in the pregnancy, later factors such as urinary frequency and dyspnea may affect sleep. Fatigue may also be indicative of a more serious physical, emotional, or dietary problem.

Subjective

Ask about degree of fatigue and potential effects on activities of daily living. Obtain history of sleep, including naps. Ask the patient about any suspected contributing factors. In the review of systems, ask about depression, anxiety, anorexia, exercise intolerance compared to prepregnancy state, chest pain or discomfort, and dyspnea. If anemia is suspected, ask about pica or other clues that may indicate an underlying cause.

Objective

Obtain vital signs and physical examination, with attention to the thyroid and cardiac and pulmonary systems. Weight gain during the pregnancy should be noted. A CBC and thyroid function tests (thyroid-stimulating hormone [TSH] and free T_4) are reasonable choices for screening. Other laboratory tests should be conducted as indicated by history or physical examination findings.

Differential Diagnoses

Differential diagnoses include fatigue due to pregnancy, anemia, thyroid disorder, or other pathologic states.

■ Genitourinary Complaints

Urinary frequency is often at the top of the list of common pregnancy complaints. Renal enlargement occurs shortly after conception. Glomerular filtration rate increases 20% by week 12. Increases in circulating fluid volume and the glomerular filtration rate may contribute to urinary frequency (Cunningham et al., 2018). Uterine displacement of the bladder by the end of the second trimester can result in urinary frequency and incontinence. Urinary infections and risk of trauma are greater owing to increased bladder tone relaxation, enlarged bladder capacity, increased bladder pressure, and increased edema of the bladder mucosa.

URINARY FREQUENCY

Subjective

Ask about general increased urination, nocturia, and episodes of incontinence. Determine whether associated symptoms are present, including fever, back or flank pain, suprapubic pain, dysuria, urgency, hematuria, dark or cloudy urine, polyuria, polyphagia, or polydipsia.

Objective

Vital signs and examination may be normal. An abdominal examination should assess for uterine contractions or irritability, as well as costal vertebral angle and/or suprapubic tenderness. CBC and glucose levels should be within normal limits. Urine dipstick, urinalysis, and/or culture and sensitivity tests should be normal.

Differential Diagnoses

Differential diagnoses include pregnancy-related urinary frequency, UTI, pyelonephritis, kidney stone, and diabetes.

URINARY INCONTINENCE

Pregnancy-related incontinence is usually caused by a combination of increased intra-abdominal pressure associated with certain activities (e.g., sneezing, bending, lifting), and the pressure of the uterus against the bladder. Multigravidas may experience incontinence more often because of poor perineal muscle tone.

Subjective

The main complaint is usually consistent with stress incontinence, that is, an involuntary loss of urine possibly associated with exertion, coughing, sneezing, or laughing. Rule out associated symptom of UTI such as burning with urination, abdominal tenderness, etc. Ask about fluid that does not smell like urine, increases with lying down, or gushes with initial standing. These patterns of fluid release may indicate rupture of membranes.

Objective

Obtain vital signs and complete abdominal examination, ruling out any uterine contractions or irritability. Conduct vaginal examination for signs of amniotic fluid pooling. Conduct dipstick urine test. Nitrazine and fern tests can differentiate between vaginal discharge and amniotic fluid. A sterile cotton-tipped applicator is used to place vaginal discharge either on nitrazine paper or on a clean microscope slide. If the nitrazine paper changes color and indicates a pH of 7, the discharge may be amniotic fluid. With a fern test, the discharge is allowed to dry on the slide and examined under a microscope. Amniotic fluid forms a fernlike pattern.

Differential Diagnoses

Differential diagnoses include stress urinary incontinence, UTI, rupture of membranes, leukorrhea, and vaginitis.

■ Circulatory Complaints

An increase in cardiac output occurs early during pregnancy and increases by about 40% by delivery. On average, the resting heart rate increases 10 beats per minute. The plasma volume expands as early as 10 weeks of gestation. Even in normal pregnancy, the cardiovascular changes may result in functional murmurs, edema, activity intolerance, and a degree of dyspnea. These changes may make it more difficult to detect and diagnose functional heart disease (Cunningham et al., 2018).

DIZZINESS OR SYNCOPE

Subjective

For complaints of dizziness or faintness, determine whether episodes occur when the patient is standing, performing physical activity, lying on the back, or changing positions. Ask about caloric and fluid intake and all medications taken, as well as substance abuse. To differentiate between dizziness and syncope, ask whether the patient experiences disorientation to spatial relation (i.e., feels like the patient is spinning or the room is spinning) versus about to "pass out." Ask about precipitating and associated factors, such as micturition, defecation, hyperventilation, coughing, dyspnea, chest pain, palpitations, or exposure to a stressful event.

Objective

Vital signs with postural (orthostatic) blood pressures should be obtained with a physical examination (cardiovascular, ear-nose-throat, neurological, extremities). A CBC should be considered to rule out anemia. Blood glucose, urine-specific gravity, and electrolytes should be obtained.

Differential Diagnoses

Differential diagnoses include compression of the vena cava, orthostatic hypotension, dehydration, anemia, hypoglycemia, hyperventilation, psychosocial stress, inner ear or sinus disease, substance abuse, neurological disorders, cardiopulmonary disorders, and positional dizziness.

EDEMA

Subjective

Ask whether swelling worsens as the day progresses, worsens with prolonged sitting or standing, and/or improves with rest and elevation. Question about the use of any type of constrictive clothing (pantyhose, girdles, or tight belts), nutrition (sodium and sugar intake), and medication use. During review of systems, ask about any numbness, decreased strength, sensation loss, mental status changes, headaches, flashing lights, upper abdominal pain, nausea or vomiting, dyspnea, decreased fetal movement, or decreased urine output.

Objective

Vital signs, especially blood pressure, should be normal for gestational age. According to the American College of Obstetricians and Gynecologists (ACOG), a normal blood pressure during pregnancy is less than 120/80 mm Hg (ACOG, 2019). The weight gain should be noted and an increase of more than 2 pounds per week investigated. Cardiac and pulmonary status should be evaluated, along with deep tendon reflexes. The location, amount, and extent of the edema should be documented. Determine whether edema decreases with leg elevation. Note the presence of hard or painful veins or legs and temperature changes to the extremities. A urine dipstick test should be obtained to test for protein.

Differential Diagnoses

Differential diagnoses include uncomplicated pregnancy-related lower extremity edema; pre-eclampsia; hemolysis, elevated liver enzymes, low platelets (HELLP) syndrome; superficial varicosities; phlebitis, renal, or liver disease; local trauma or infection in an extremity; and CHF.

Pregnancy Complications

■ Anemia

Anemia is not a disease unto itself but rather is a sign of an underlying disorder, which is common among pregnant patients. A hemoglobin less than 11 g/dL in either the first or the third trimester or less than 10.5 g/dL in the second trimester is considered anemia (Cunningham et al., 2018). Patients with hemoglobin values below these levels should have the etiology evaluated since anemia during pregnancy is associated with high-output CHF, premature delivery, low birth weight, and fetal demise.

The anemias diagnosed during pregnancy are usually associated with either iron deficiency, folic acid deficiency, or acute blood loss (Cunningham et al., 2018). The demand for both iron and folic acid increase significantly during pregnancy, usually requiring supplementation.

Subjective

Identify any complaint of fatigue and dyspnea on exertion. Folic acid deficiency is associated with anorexia, so dietary intake is important for this fact, as well as determining the dietary sources of both iron and folic acid.

Objective

Obtain vital signs, noting heart rate. Examine for skin pallor, tachycardia, grade II/VI systolic heart murmur, and/or increased respiratory rate. The CBC will confirm anemia, as well as indicate potential causes and guide selection of additional diagnostic studies, such as iron panel, folate level, sickle cell screen or hemoglobin electrophoresis, and liver function tests.

Differential Diagnoses

The differential diagnosis includes iron deficiency, folate deficiency, vitamin B_{12} deficiency, sickle cell trait/anemia, and thalassemia.

■ Gestational Diabetes Mellitus

Gestational diabetes mellitus (GDM) involves glucose intolerance that develops or is first discovered during pregnancy and hence may include patients who have undiagnosed pregestational diabetes. GDM complications include large for gestational age, preterm birth, still birth, C-section, HTN and preeclampsia, macrosomia, shoulder dystocia, or other birth trauma. Over half of patients with GDM will develop diabetes later in life (Cunningham et al., 2018). Development of overt diabetes is most likely among patients who are autoantibody positive, require insulin treatment during pregnancy, have a body mass index greater than 30 kg/m², or have more than two prior pregnancies.

Screening for GDM remains controversial. According to the 2021 U.S. Preventive Services Task Force, diabetes screening is recommended for all pregnant patients at or greater than 24 weeks of gestation. ACOG (2017a) recommends a two-step screening between 24 and 28 weeks. Screening followed by treatment can reduce the rate of pre-eclampsia, shoulder dystocia, fetal macrosomia, and fetal mortality but does not appear to reduce other adverse outcomes, such as cesarean delivery rate, birth injury, or patients' perception of their health. Currently, recommendations vary on whether and to what degree GDM screenings are needed (Table 20.7).

Because selective screening of patients with risk factors for GDM has a high sensitivity but low specificity, ACOG recommends universal screening using a two-step method. Step 1 begins between 24 and 28 weeks of gestation with a 50-g 1-hr oral glucose tolerance test (OGTT) using a venous blood sample. The 1-hr test is performed without regard to the timing of the patient's last intake. The 50-g load is usually delivered via a commercial glucose-sweetened cola-like beverage (e.g., Glucola, Trutol); alternatively, the patient may eat 28 jelly beans within a 5-minute period (USPSTF, 2013).

The results of the 1-hr test determine whether to proceed to step 2, a 3-hr OGTT using a 100-g load. The thresholds for determining a "positive" 1-hr test (130 mg/dL, 135 mg/dL, or 140 mg/dL) vary by institution, depending on the sensitivity and specificity desired. The 3-hr OGTT is usually administered after an overnight fast for at least 8 hours, but not more than 14 hours. A fasting blood sugar is obtained, and then a 100-g glucose load is given. Venous blood sugar samples are then obtained at 1, 2, and 3 hours after the glucose load. Either an elevated fasting blood sugar or two elevated values on the 3-hr OGTT is diagnostic of GDM. If only one value on the OGTT is elevated, the test may be repeated between 32 and 34 weeks of gestation (Figure 20.3 and Table 20.8).

Changes in glycated hemoglobin levels (HbA1c) lag behind changes in serum glucose by months. It is therefore not a good screen for GDM since glucose elevations often do not start to occur until after 20 weeks gestation (USPSTF, 2013). There remains no universally accepted gold standard for diagnosing GDM. The measures used in the United States were originally developed to identify pregnant patients at risk for developing diabetes but not those whose newborns were at risk for complications, such as macrosomia. Whereas various expert groups in the United States have proposed different diagnostic values and all predict to some extent newborn complication risk, there is no evidence to date to support any one diagnostic standard over others (see Table 20.8).

Table 20.7

Gestational Diabetes Screening Recommendations

Universal Screening	Risk Factor–Based Screening	No Recommendation for Screening
• American College of Obstetricians and Gynecologists • World Health Organization • Third International Conference on Gestational Diabetes • U.S. Preventive Services Task Force	• American Diabetes Association • Society of Maternal–Fetal Medicine	• Canadian Task Force on the Periodic Examination

Note: This list is not all-inclusive but rather is a sampling of organizations that support each recommendation.

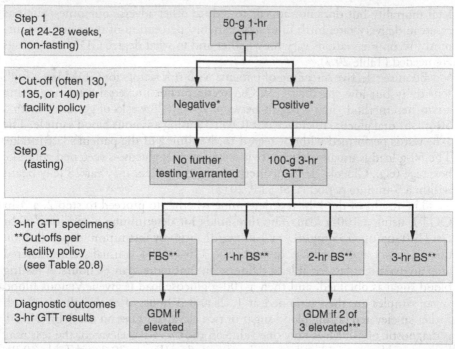

***If 1 of 3 values elevated, may repeat 3-hr OGTT at 23-24 weeks.

Figure 20.3 Oral glucose tolerance test algorithm.

Table 20.8

Three-Hour OGCT in Pregnancy (Most Common Values Used)

	National Diabetes Data Group, 1979 (Venous Plasma)	Carpenter and Coustan, 1982 (Venous Plasma)	O'Sullivan and Mahan, 1964 (Venous Whole Blood)
Fasting (mg/dL)	105	95	90
1 hr (mg/dL)	190	180	165
2 hr (mg/dL)	165	155	145
3 hr (mg/dL)	145	140	125

Note: Using a standard 100-g glucose load. Fasting and 2-hr levels are most predictive, but diagnosis requires elevation in any two or more values.

OGCT = oral glucose challenge test.

Subjective

The patient may be asymptomatic throughout the entire pregnancy or may report classic episodes of polyuria, polyphagia, or polydipsia. The patient may experience more episodes of UTIs or vaginitis; therefore, recurrent infections should signal an earlier screening for diabetes or at least a random glucose level. Prior obstetric history should be investigated for unexplained stillbirths, spontaneous abortions, unexplained preterm birth, low birthweight infant (with undiagnosed pre-existing diabetes), newborn weighing 4000 g or more, or a previous incident of major congenital abnormality. Family history should be explored for diabetes, including GDM.

Objective

Maternal age and weight should be noted because major risk factors include age older than 35 years or a pre-pregnancy weight of more than 200 pounds. Excessive weight gain during pregnancy or a fundal height greater than expected is also worrisome. The blood pressure should be noted; patients with diabetes are predisposed to hypertensive disorders, including pre-eclampsia. A retinal examination should be completed to assess for retinopathy. A urine dipstick should be evaluated for glycosuria and proteinuria.

Differential Diagnoses

Differential diagnoses include GDM, undiagnosed type 1 diabetes mellitus (DM) or type 2 DM, hyperglycemia, macrosomia, and recurrent UTI or vaginitis (not related to DM).

■ Hypertension

Hypertensive problems are among the largest problems during pregnancy. They must be identified early and treated promptly during pregnancy to ensure good maternal and neonatal outcomes. Hypertensive disorders occur in 12% to 22% of all pregnancies and are directly responsible for 16% of maternal deaths in developed countries, such as the United States. Over 7% of pregnancy deaths are related to preeclampsia and eclampsia. High blood pressure is broadly defined in four ways (Table 20.9): preeclampsia-eclampsia syndrome, chronic HTN, preeclampsia superimposed on chronic HTN, and gestational HTN. The appropriate clinical response to elevated blood pressure during pregnancy is determined by the underlying pathology rather than the actual elevation in pressure (Cunningham et al., 2018).

The diastolic pressure usually drops by an average of 10 mm Hg below nonpregnant levels by midpregnancy and then slowly returns to nonpregnant levels in the third trimester (Davidson et al., 2016). Determination of the patient's nonpregnant blood pressure is important in the evaluation of blood pressure during pregnancy, for accurate assessment.

Gestational HTN is defined as a systolic blood pressure of ≥140 mm Hg or a diastolic blood pressure of ≥90 mm Hg that occurs after 20 weeks of gestation in a patient with previously normal blood pressure. Almost 50% of patients identified with gestational HTN later develop preeclampsia. Others whose blood pressures normalize by 12 weeks postpartum without having developed eclampsia are later identified as having transient HTN (Cunningham et al., 2018).

"Preeclampsia is best described as a pregnancy-specific syndrome that can affect virtually every organ system" (Cunningham et al., 2018, p. 711).

Table 20.9	
Blood Pressure Classification in Pregnancy	
NHBPEP Classification	Description
Chronic hypertension	• Hypertension preceding conception or before the 20th week of gestation • Usually defined as blood pressure of 140/90 mm Hg or greater
Pre-eclampsia–eclampsia	• A pregnancy-specific systemic syndrome
Pre-eclampsia	• Systemic disease with hypertension accompanied by proteinuria after the 20th week of gestation in patients who were normotensive prior to pregnancy • May also be diagnosed without proteinuria if there are other systemic symptoms (e.g., thrombocytopenia, renal insufficiency, impaired liver function, pulmonary edema, cerebral or visual symptoms that are persistent)
Eclampsia	• Convulsive stage of the disease; seizures cannot be attributed to other causes
Pre-eclampsia superimposed on chronic hypertension	• Patients who are hypertensive before the 20th week of gestation who develop new-onset proteinuria • Patients with both hypertension and proteinuria before 20 weeks of gestation • Sudden increase in blood pressure in patients who previously had controlled hypertension • Patients with thrombocytopenia (less than 100,000 cells/mm³), renal insufficiency, impaired liver function, pulmonary edema, cerebral or visual symptoms that are persistent • Most often associated with the most severe maternal–fetal complications • Prognosis is much worse than for either condition alone
Gestational hypertension	• High blood pressure detected for the first time after midpregnancy, without proteinuria • Diagnosis can also be made postpartum
Transient hypertension	• Elevated blood pressure that occurs without proteinuria late in pregnancy or in the early puerperium but returns to normal by 12 weeks postpartum
Chronic gestational hypertension	• Blood pressure remains elevated beyond 12 weeks postpartum but without evidence of pre-eclampsia

From National High Blood Pressure Education Program Working Group. Working group report on high blood pressure in pregnancy. (NHBPEP Publication No. 00-3029). Washington, DC: National Heart Lung and Blood Institute, 2000.)
NHBPEP = National High Blood Pressure Education Program.

The incidence varies by race and ethnicity, with white, Hispanic, and black patients affected 5%, 9%, and 11%, respectively. Incidence is higher among nulliparas (up to 10%) than multiparas (up to 4%). Patients who develop pre-eclampsia also have a higher risk of cardiovascular disease in the future.

Subjective

As with all patients, HTN may occur without the pregnant patient's awareness. Ask about prior history of HTN and about symptoms such as headache, visual disturbances, edema, heartburn, abdominal pain, and altered mental status.

Objective

Evaluation should include the vital signs, with blood pressure measurement, weight, cardiovascular examination, ophthalmological examination, abdominal, and deep tendon reflex examination. Laboratory tests to consider include urine dipstick, urinalysis, or 24-hour urine for proteinuria; CBC and/or platelet count; and liver enzymes.

Differential Diagnoses

Differential diagnoses include chronic HTN, transient HTN, gestational HTN, pre-eclampsia, eclampsia, HELLP syndrome, disseminated intravascular coagulopathy, exacerbation of chronic renal disease, and autonomic overactivity.

■ Vaginal Bleeding

Approximately 20% to 30% of early pregnancies are complicated by vaginal bleeding (Dyne, 2015). The incidence of spontaneous abortion in clinically recognized pregnancies between 5 and 20 weeks is 11% to 22% (Cunningham et al. [2018]). Single or serial qualitative hCG levels can be helpful in evaluating vaginal bleeding during early pregnancy because the levels should double every 48 hours during the fourth to eighth weeks of gestation. In about 30% of all cases, vaginal bleeding that occurs during the second and third trimesters is of unknown etiology; however, some of the more common causes include placenta previa, abruptio placentae, uterine rupture, vasa previa, and bloody show associated with labor. Bleeding in later pregnancy is related to different concerns than in earlier pregnancy and is considered abnormal (Dyne, 2015).

Subjective

Assessment questions should be directed toward any precipitating factors of bleeding (e.g., sexual intercourse), the amount of vaginal bleeding (saturation of sanitary pads and frequency with which the pads must be changed), the quality of the vaginal bleeding (clotted versus flowing), and whether the bleeding is actually coming from the vagina or from the urethral or rectal area. The presence of low back pain, abdominal cramping, foul odor, or any passage of products of conception also should be investigated. Any history of coagulation disorders, recent antiplatelet medication use, and Rh status needs to be verified. A screening for intimate partner violence should also be done.

Objective

The vital signs should be normal for gestational age. Physical examination should concentrate on uterine size, FHTs, a pelvic examination with cervix visualization, and a digital rectal examination. Other tests that may be useful include a transvaginal ultrasound, hCG level measurement, progesterone level, wet mount, urinalysis, and stool for occult blood. CBC and coagulation studies should be considered.

Differential Diagnoses

Differential diagnoses include implantation bleeding; placenta previa; abruptio placentae; uterine rupture; early pregnancy loss; ectopic pregnancy; gestational trophoblastic disease; vaginal ectropion infection; foreign body retention; abdominal or vaginal trauma; blood dyscrasias, warts, polyps, and fibroids; and intimate partner violence.

■ Vaginal Infections

Observational studies have demonstrated an association between bacterial vaginosis and certain adverse pregnancy outcomes, such as preterm labor, preterm delivery, premature rupture of membranes, and spontaneous abortions. Bacterial vaginosis can be treated with antibiotic therapy, but cure rates are erratic and recurrences are common. There is currently conflicting evidence on whether screening and treatment of asymptomatic bacterial vaginosis in high-risk pregnant patients actually reduce the incidence of preterm delivery. The U.S. Preventive Services Task Force (USPSTF) therefore neither recommends nor discourages routinely screening these patients (USPSTF, 2020; CDC, 2011). However, the USPSTF does state that screening is not recommended in pregnant patients at low risk for preterm delivery, but treatment is appropriate for symptomatic bacterial vaginosis infections (such as with patient complaints of vaginal discharge). Trichomoniasis affects about 3% of pregnant patients; vulvovaginal candidiasis occurs in 20% of pregnant patients (Cunningham et al., 2018).

Subjective

Inquire whether there have been multiple or new sexual partners, whether sexual activity has recently been resumed, whether there has been any recent douching or antibiotic use, or whether there is a history of abnormal Papanicolaou (Pap) smears. Further assessment should explore the presence of any vaginal discharge, perineal or vaginal sores or lesions, or UTI symptoms. Worrisome symptoms include excessive, malodorous, discolored, itchy, or irritating vaginal discharge; fever; abdominal pain; dysuria; or bleeding or pain after sexual intercourse.

Objective

The examination should begin with an inspection of the external genitalia. A pelvic examination should assess for vaginal discharge, signs of vaginal infections (including herpes), and any other vaginal or cervical abnormalities. A normal saline and potassium hydroxide test (wet mount) should be conducted from secretions of the vaginal pool to check for fungal organisms, trichomonas, clue cells, and bacteria. A gonorrhea and chlamydia specimen for culture should be obtained. A nitrazine test (done to evaluate a change in the pH) or fern test should be done to evaluate for a rupture of membranes. A Pap smear should be done if it has not been done previously in the initial obstetrical evaluation to assess for dysplasia, carcinoma, or human papillomavirus.

Differential Diagnoses

Differential diagnoses include leukorrhea, vaginitis, cervicitis, gonorrhea, chlamydia, UTI, rupture of membranes, condyloma acuminatum, genital herpes, or cervical dysplasia or neoplasia.

■ Urinary Tract Infections

Urinary tract changes associated with pregnancy (e.g., pressure to the bladder, dilation of the ureters, smooth muscle relaxation) increase the risk of lower and upper UTIs, ranging from cystitis to pyelonephritis. UTIs occur in approximately 8% of pregnant patients, usually due to normal perineal organisms. Asymptomatic bacteriuria is found in 2% to 7% of pregnancies; left untreated it may cause cystitis or polynephritis, which may result in preterm labor and delivery, maternal sepsis, or even septic shock and death (Cunningham et al., 2018).

Subjective

Inquiries should be made about the presence of risk factors (frequent/recurrent UTIs, diabetes, urinary tract abnormalities, sexually transmitted infections). Inquire also about any urgency, frequency, dysuria, suprapubic pain, abnormal urinary flow pattern, discolored or malodorous urine, fever, chills, flank pain, or GI complaints.

Objective

Evaluation includes documented fever, clean catch urine, pelvic examination/wet mount (for vaginal infections), costovertebral angle or suprapubic tenderness, urine culture, CBC, and signs of shock (tachycardia, hypotension, and pallor).

Differential Diagnoses

Differential diagnoses include cystitis, pyelonephritis, asymptomatic bacteriuria, urethritis, vulvovaginitis, sexually transmitted infections, preterm labor, and renal stones.

■ Size Not Equal to Dates

A fetus may be found to be of a size that is not commensurate with normal growth rates (size not equal to dates) when the uterine size is measured and evaluated during routine prenatal visits. First-trimester uterine sizes are usually determined with bimanual examination, and size–date discrepancies are often not clinically relevant. After 20 weeks of gestation, fundal height measurements begin to correlate (within 2 cm) with gestational age. The fundus should be at the level of the umbilicus at 20 weeks of gestation, and it rises 1 cm per week until 32 weeks of gestation. False small-for-dates presentations may result from inaccurate last menstrual period dates, varying menstrual cycle lengths, improper fundal height measurement, or a fetus in a transverse lie. False large-for-dates presentations may likewise be produced by inaccurate last menstrual period dates, improper fundal height measurement, and a large amount of amniotic fluid as well as maternal obesity or short stature.

Small-For-Dates

Subjective

No subjective complaints are usually expressed by the patients; however, they may state that they do not appear as "big" as their gestational age. A 24-hour diet recall should be done.

Objective

Weight gain from prepregnancy weight should be noted. Fundal height measurements that are 3 to 4 cm smaller than the estimated gestational age during the 20- to 32-week gestational period require additional follow-up. Serial ultrasound examinations and measurements should be done for body ratios in order to plot growth velocity and to assess amniotic fluid volume.

Differential Diagnoses

Differential diagnoses include intrauterine growth restriction (either asymmetric or symmetric), which affects about 5% of the general population and as much as 10% of high-risk populations (Table 20.10); constitutionally small fetus; inaccurate pregnancy dating; improper fundal height measurement; transverse lie of the fetus, and oligohydramnios.

Large-For-Dates

Subjective

Although no subjective complaints are usually expressed, the fundal height may appear to be increased, especially in pregnant patients who are obese or short in stature. The patient may claim a "bigger" appearance than the gestational age or suggest the possibility of multiple gestations. A 24-hour diet recall should be done.

Table 20.10

High-Risk Populations for Intrauterine Growth Restriction

Associated Medical Conditions	Associated Obstetric Conditions
• Hypertension	• Pregnancy-induced hypertension
• Renal disease	• Multiple gestation
• Diabetes	• Placental abnormalities
• Lupus	• Intrauterine infections
• Sickle cell disease	• Fetal/chromosomal abnormalities
• Tobacco use; substance abuse	
• Malnutrition	
• Maternal heart disorders, especially those with decreased cardiac output	
• Thrombophilias	
• Chronic lead poisoning	

Objective

Weight gain from prepregnancy weight should be noted. Fundal height measurements that are 3 to 4 cm larger than the estimated gestational age during the 20- to 32-week gestational period require additional evaluation. Serial ultrasound examinations and measurements for body ratios should be done in order to plot growth velocity and to assess amniotic fluid volume. A serum glucose and urine dipstick should be done to evaluate for GDM.

Differential Diagnoses

Differential diagnoses include inaccurate pregnancy dating, improper fundal height measurement, fetal macrosomia, polyhydramnios, multiple gestation, uterine leiomyoma growth, molar pregnancy, GDM, and maternal obesity.

▪ Preterm Labor

Preterm labor is the onset of labor before 37 completed weeks of gestation. The accurate diagnosis of preterm labor is critical but often difficult. Among patients with regular preterm contractions, 30% resolve. Only 50% of patients hospitalized with preterm labor have preterm births. The diagnosis may be confirmed upon careful observation over a 1- to 2-hour period. Observations include assessment for regularity of uterine contractions, with cervical dilation and effacement, and/or presentation. Patients who are having persistent contractions need a cervical change of at least 1 cm, a dilatation of 2 cm or more, or a positive fetal fibronectin assay for diagnosis (AAP & ACOG, 2017b). If the diagnosis is not confirmed, but the index of suspicion remains high, it is entirely reasonable to repeat the cervical examination at a later time. Transabdominal ultrasounds and home uterine activity monitoring have also been used in an effort to identify preterm labor, but with mixed results.

Subjective

The most common complaint is contractions. The contractions should be evaluated for regularity, consistency, and location. Symptoms of preterm labor include pelvic pressure; a low, dull backache; menstrual-like cramps; a change or increase in vaginal discharge; uterine contractions that occur every 10 minutes or more frequently, with or without pain; intestinal cramping, with or without diarrhea; and contractions that do not resolve with rest and hydration. A history review should concentrate on any previous preterm labor/delivery and a determination of the gestational age. A complete review of systems should be accomplished to screen for precipitating conditions, such as cholecystitis or viral gastroenteritis.

Objective

Screening should be done for infection (urinalysis, gonorrhea, chlamydia, syphilis, group B streptococcus, bacterial vaginosis), urine specific gravity to assess for hydration status, nitrazine testing to assess for rupture of membranes, fetal fibronectin testing (should be done before a digital cervical examination), ultrasound cervical length examination, serial cervical examinations, and drug screening. Fetal fibronectin testing and cervical length evaluation both are helpful in determining likelihood of preterm labor but are not diagnostic alone (ACOG, 2018b).

Differential Diagnoses

Differential diagnoses include preterm (true) labor, false labor, maternal dehydration, infectious etiologies (either urinary, vaginal, or sexually transmitted), incompetent cervix, and premature rupture of membranes.

Summary

As stated at the beginning of this chapter, pregnancy should be considered a wellness condition and not a disease entity. Advanced practice nurses should tailor their education and interventions to the assessment of the pregnant patient and routinely reassess the clinical situation for any changes. Caring for pregnant patients is well within the advanced practice nursing model, and advanced practice nurses should know what is needed, what they can provide, and when to refer.

REFERENCES

American Academy of Pediatrics (AAP) and American College of Obstetricians and Gynecologists (ACOG). (2017). Perinatal care (8th ed.). AAP, ACOG.

American College of Obstetricians and Gynecologists (ACOG). (2017a). ACOG Practice Bulletin No. 180: Gestational diabetes mellitus. ACOG.

American College of Obstetricians and Gynecologists (ACOG). (2017b). ACOG Practice Bulletin No. 700: Methods for estimating the due date. ACOG.

American College of Obstetricians and Gynecologists (ACOG). (2018a). ACOG Practice Bulletin No. 196: Thromboembolism in pregnancy. ACOG.

American College of Obstetricians and Gynecologists (ACOG). (2018b). ACOG Practice Bulletin No. 217: Prelabor rupture of membranes. ACOG.

American College of Obstetricians and Gynecologists (ACOG). (2019). ACOG Practice Bulletin No. 203: Chronic hypertension in pregnancy. *Obstetrics and Gynecology 133*(1), e26–e50. https//doi.org/10.1097/AOG.0000000000003020

American College of Radiology. (2018). ACR-SPR practice guideline for imaging pregnant or potentially pregnant adolescents and women with ionizing radiation. https://www.acr.org/-/media/ACR/Files/Practice-Parameters/Pregnant-Pts.pdf

Carpenter, M. W., & Coustan, D. R. (1982). Criteria for screening tests for gestational diabetes. *American Journal of Obstetrics and Gynecology, 144*, 768–773.

Centers for Disease Control and Prevention (CDC). (2011). Diseases characterized by vaginal discharge. Retrieved August 29, 2017, from https://www.cdc.gov/std/treatment/2010/vaginal-discharge.htm

Cunningham, F. G., Leveno, K. J., Bloom, S. L., Spong, C. Y., Dashe, J. S., Hoffman, B. L., et al. (2018). *Williams obstetrics*. McGraw-Hill Education Medical.

Davidson, M. R., London, M. L., & Ladewig, P. W. (2016). *Olds maternal-newborn nursing & women's health across the lifespan*. Pearson.

Dyne, P. (2015). Bleeding during pregnancy causes, symptoms, treatment—Bleeding during pregnancy diagnosis. http://www.emedicinehealth.com/pregnancy_bleeding/page6_em.htm

Gomes, C. F., Sousa, M., Lourenco, I., Martins, D., & Torres, J. (2018). Gastrointestinal diseases during pregnancy: What does the gastroenterologist need to know? *Annals of Gastroenterology, 31*(4), 385–394. https://doi.org/10.20524/aog.2018.0264

Institute of Medicine and National Research Council Committee to Reexamine IOM Pregnancy Weight Guidelines. (2009). *Weight gain during pregnancy: Reexamining the guidelines*. Washington DC: National Academies Press. https://www.ncbi.nlm.nih.gov/books/NBK32802/

National Diabetes Data Group. (1979). Classification and diagnosis of diabetes mellitus and other categories of glucose intolerance. *Diabetes, 28*, 1039–1057.

National High Blood Pressure Education Program (NHBPEP). (2001). Working group report on high blood pressure in pregnancy. (NHBPEP Publication No. 00–3029). National Heart, Lung, and Blood Institute.

O'Sullivan, J. B., & Mahan, C. M. (1964). Criteria for the oral glucose tolerance test in pregnancy. *Diabetes, 13*, 278–285.

Sadro, C. T., & Dubinsky, T. J. (2013). CT in pregnancy. *Applied Radiology.* http://appliedradiology.com /articles/ct-in-pregnancy-risks-and-benefits

U.S. Preventive Services Task Force. (2021). Final update summary: Gestational diabetes: Screening. Accessed April 26,2022, from https://www.uspreventiveservicestaskforce.org/uspstf/recommendation /gestational-diabetes-screening

U.S. Preventive Services Task Force. (2020). Bacterial vaginosis in pregnant persons to prevent preterm delivery: Screening. Final Statement. https://www.uspreventiveservicestaskforce.org/uspstf/recommendation /bacterial-vaginosis-in-pregnancy-to-prevent-preterm-delivery-screening

Chapter 21

Assessment of the Transgender or Gender-Diverse Adult

- Kim Pickett
- Vanessa Pomarico-Denino

Transgender is a term used to describe a diverse group of individuals whose gender identity varies from the sex assigned at birth. Sex assignation at birth is based on the external genitalia visualized. In most cultures, society often classifies individuals into binary gender patterns based on the assigned sex (either "male" or "female"). Individuals with *gender dysphoria* may experience discomfort or distress related to their gender identity and assigned birth sex. However, it is important to remember that not all gender-nonconforming individuals experience gender dysphoria (World Professional Association for Transgender Health, 2012).

Transgender individuals may be assigned a male sex at birth and identify as female or be assigned a female sex at birth and identify as male. Individuals can also be more fluid in their identification, identifying as nonbinary (i.e., neither male nor female), genderqueer, or gender fluid (WPATH, 2012; Mayer et al., 2008). Moreover, gender identity and expression may vary from culture to culture, as with the "two-spirit" individuals of the First Nations and the "third-gender" individuals of India (Hemmila, 2016; Khaleeli, 2014).

Due to social stigma, transgender individuals have often encountered discrimination in multiple environments, including housing and employment, as well as in the health-care setting (Kcomt et al., 2020; Bradford et al., 2013; Kosenko et al., 2013; Poteat et al., 2013). Additionally, transgender individuals are at increased risk of being targeted for hate crimes involving verbal and physical abuse, as well as sexual violence (Stotzer, 2009). The perspectives of transgender individuals seeking care for acute and chronic medical conditions over the past several years have provided heightened awareness of instances such as refusal of care by providers, verbal abuse, and even forced care, including unnecessary examinations and psychiatric institutionalization (Kosenko et al., 2013). Lack of culturally competent care further perpetuates health disparities and leads to poor health outcomes.

For years, nurses have advocated for their patients, working toward reducing or eliminating health disparities across diverse patient populations, without regard to factors such as race, ethnicity, religious affiliation, sexual orientation, or socioeconomic status. Advanced practice nurses are in an excellent position to team-lead culturally competent health care for all patients, including individuals who express a gender identity or expression that may not be congruent with societal expectations. This chapter provides an introduction to physical examination techniques for transgender adults who seek health care, while illustrating ideas to facilitate a safe and inclusive environment for all patients, including those individuals who identify as transgender. Salient points for the history and physical are discussed, as well as special considerations as they relate to long-term health risk factors. While this chapter focuses on the adult population, a list of online resources for patients of all age groups is included for review in Boxes 21.1 and 21.2.

Box 21.1

Resources for Transgender Individuals and Health-Care Providers

Center of Excellence for Transgender Health: Primary Care Protocol For Transgender Patient Care

http://transhealth.ucsf.edu/trans?page=protocol-00-00

Resources for Transgender People

https://www.glaad.org/transgender/resources

National Center for Transgender Equality

http://www.transequality.org/

National LGBT Health Education Center: A Program of the Fenway Institute Medical Care of Transgender Persons

https://www.lgbthealtheducation.org/publication/transgender-sod/

Resources on Best Practices for Front Desk and Office Staff

https://www.lisettelahana.com/front-desk-staff-best-practices

The World Professional Association for Transgender Health (WPATH)

https://www.wpath.org/

University of Wisconsin-Milwaukee LGBT Resource Center: Gender Pronouns

https://uwm.edu/lgbtrc/support/gender-pronouns/

Box 21.2

Transgender Children and Adolescents

In 2018, the American Academy of Pediatrics (AAP) issued its first policy state-ment focusing on children and youth who identify as transgender or gender diverse. Recognizing that transgender youth often feel that they must conceal their gender identity and expression to avoid bullying and harassment and are subject to disproportionally high rates of physical violence, substance abuse and homeless-ness, the AAP encourages a gender-affirmative care model (GACM). The GACM seeks to provide an integrative experience in which medical, mental health, and social services work synergistically to provide a supportive environment using a family-centered approach wherever possible, with advocacy to promote acceptance of children against bullying and harassment due to gender expression.

Resources for parents, teachers, and schools can be found at the American Academy of Pediatrics Web site at https://www.healthychildren.org/English/ages -stages/gradeschool/Pages/Support-Resources-for-Families-of-Gender-Diverse -Youth.aspx

Prevalence of Transgender Individuals in the United States

Although information pertaining to transgender status and sexual orientation and/or gender identity (also referred to as SOGI) is not collected or reported by the United States Census Bureau, a recent meta-analysis of population-based survey data shows that the population of transgender individuals in the United States in 2016 was estimated to be 390 per 100,000 adults, or nearly 1 million adults nationally (Meerwijk & Sevelius, 2017). Although often included by default under the broader LGBTQ+ (lesbian, gay, bisexual, transgender, and queer or questioning) classification, which has been estimated to be 9 million people in the United States (Gates, 2011), it is important to know that trans-gender people may or may not identify as lesbian, gay, or bisexual (LGB). While the LGB category denotes individuals according to sexual orientation, sexual orientation is separate from gender identity and describes sexual identity and/or behavior. For example, a transgender person may identify as heterosexual, gay, queer, bisexual, or other terms (Mayer et al., 2008). While some transgender individuals may also identify with the LGBTQ+ community, not all transgen-der individuals are LGB. Current research continues to emphasize the need for health-care providers to remain aware of the unique needs and challenges of transgender individuals, which are specific to their population.

Terminology and Pronouns

Health-care providers may perceive a lack of sufficient knowledge to provide culturally competent care to transgender patients (Halloran, 2015; Poteat et al., 2013). Becoming familiar with basic terminology is an important first

Table 21.1	
Sexual Orientation and Gender Identity Terminology	
Sexual Orientation	**Gender Identity**
Straight	Cisgender
Lesbian	Transgender male
Gay	Transgender female
Bisexual	Pangender
Pansexual	Gender neutral
Gender fluid	Gender fluid
	Gender variant
	Third gender
	Two-spirit

step. Transgender individuals may identify as *trans, transgender man* or *transmasculine* (a person whose birth sex was female but who identifies as male), *transgender woman* or *transfeminine* (a person whose birth sex was male but who identifies as female), *bigender* or *genderqueer, asexual,* or *nonbinary*. People who identify as bigender or genderqueer may identify as neither male nor female, or they may identify with elements of both male and female (Bockting et al., 2013). Other nomenclature includes *male-to-female* (MTF) or *female-to-male* (FTM) (Hembree et al., 2017). The terms *queer* or *genderqueer*, which imply a historically pejorative context, may be reclaimed by some individuals as a self-descriptor. Individuals may have more than one gender identity, such as *transman* and *genderqueer*, and the descriptors for gender identity may change over time as language evolves (Kuper et al., 2012). The use of *transsexual* is no longer preferable, although it is used occasionally in older journal articles and in organization-based standards of care (WPATH, 2012). *Cisgender* is a term used to describe nontransgender individuals (Hembree et al., 2017) (i.e., those whose sense of personal identity and gender corresponds with their sex assigned at birth). As new language emerges, health-care providers should not assume what a particular identity means to an individual; if unclear, it is best to clarify with the individual during the medical visit. Table 21.1 lists terms relevant to sexual orientation or gender identity.

Creating a Welcoming Environment

It is important for advanced practice nurses to set the tone that creates an environment that will put patients at ease and allow transgender patients to feel that an office is safe and affirming in terms of their care. It is important in any office to educate all personnel, including receptionists, assistants, and all colleagues who will have any direct patient contact, on the appropriate care of transgender patients. It is imperative that all staff be properly educated on this population of patients to help understand any barriers that might inhibit patient care (Aisner et al., 2020; UCSF, 2016). In order to avoid embarrassment and distress to the patient, clinical and reception staff should anticipate the possibility that a FTM person who is perceived to be male may present for a gynecological pelvic examination. Also, there may be issues with insurance reimbursement that must be considered (WPATH, 2012). Displaying signs of LGBTQ+ acceptance, including rainbow decals; rainbow pins on identification badges, if allowed; and transgender-inclusive patient materials will demonstrate that the office is well-versed in the care of this population (Frei et al., 2019). Simply asking all patients' preferred or chosen name and pronouns upon check-in (not just those who identity as transgender or who may appear to be nonbinary or androgynous) demonstrates a message that all patients are treated equally.

It is important to avoid the use of any slang terms that are offensive and considered derogatory. Misgendering must also be avoided. *Misgendering* occurs when a person is intentionally or unintentionally referred to by a name, pronoun, or gender with which they do not identify, such as their *dead name* (the name assigned to them at birth). If an honest mistake has been made, the clinician should simply correct themselves and continue on with the visit. Profuse apologies only put the patient in a position to offer forgiveness to the person who made the mistake and may cause the patient to lose trust in the clinician (LGBTQIA Experiment, 2019). Clinicians and all staff should be mindful of every patient's preferred or chosen pronouns. It is helpful to adopt they/them/theirs pronouns until the patient reveals how they identify or to describe a patient to whom you do not want to assign a gender. It is becoming more widely acceptable for those who identify as transgender, gender nonconforming, or nonbinary to use they/them/theirs pronouns (GLAAD, 2021).

Providers should avoid treating patients as a "learning case." For example, it would be inappropriate to bring multiple staff members into the examination room to discuss the patient's gender identity or expression with them.

As with other patients, transgender patients may periodically be referred to a specialist. Establishing a network of transgender-friendly as well as transgender-educated practices in which the patient will feel welcome is often appreciated and further facilitates trust.

Avoiding Microaggressions

Microaggressions, such as intentionally referring to or calling a patient by the wrong gender repeatedly (also known as misgendering), have been reported in health-care settings and should not be tolerated. Using dehumanizing terms, such as "he-she," "she-male," "it," or "tranny," to refer to an individual is defamatory and, for obvious reasons, should never be used in any setting. However, as noted above, some previously derogatory terms, such as *queer*, have been reclaimed, so a good general rule is to follow the patient's lead in self-identifying terms.

Gender-Affirming Treatments

Transgender individuals experience higher degrees of depression and anxiety than their cisgender counterparts. Gender-affirming treatments, or treatments that facilitate consistency with the person's gender identity, are often noted to improve mental health status (Bränström & Pachankis, 2020). Gender-affirming treatment may include facial hair removal, behavioral modifications such as "binding" or "tucking," surgery, or hormonal therapy. Hormonal therapy involves suppression of the person's sex hormones and maintenance of physiological sex hormone levels for the affirmed gender (Hembree et al., 2017). Transgender individuals may choose a variety of treatments; some choose nonpharmacological and/or pharmacological treatments (i.e., both hormonal therapy and gender-confirming surgery). It is also important to note that the use of the terms "gender reassignment surgery" or "sex reassignment surgery" should be avoided due to the derogatory implication that a person's gender changes with surgery. Surgical procedures are performed so that the body matches the gender with which the patient identifies. Although these terms continue to pervade the literature, they are considered outdated and offensive (Planned Parenthood, 2021). The more appropriate and accepted terms are *gender-affirming surgery* or *gender confirmation surgery,* as these accurately describe part of the patient's transition (GLAAD, 2021). These are life-saving procedures that alleviate gender dysphoria and are just one part of a transgender person's transition journey. Be aware that some individuals do not recognize or acknowledge a gender "transition," as they have always identified with the lived gender versus the sex assigned at birth (WPATH, 2012).

If a patient chooses medication or surgical treatment, previous recommendations included a psychological evaluation and support assessment for living a "real-life experience," in which the person lives as their true gender (although during "transition," patients may at first find ease in living as their true gender in only certain settings). This recommendation is no longer considered imperative but may be considered by the clinician to ensure there are no undiagnosed, underlying psychiatric disorders that could be affected by any gender-affirming treatment. A discussion by the health-care provider of risks and side effects of treatment before beginning pharmacological treatment or surgery is imperative. If the patient has concomitant depression or an underlying mood disorder, every effort should be made to treat the condition before beginning gender-affirming treatments (Hembree et al., 2017). While individuals may not elect to have all, or any, gender-affirming treatments, descriptions of common options are listed below.

Surgery is recommended only in patients who are of age and after informed consent and in patients with an established diagnosis of gender dysphoria. For some surgeries, additional criteria may include prior treatment with hormone therapy, as well as 1 year of living as the true gender identity. Hormonal therapy is often continued, on a life-long basis, after surgery (WPATH, 2012). A comprehensive guide to hormonal treatment and surgical options can be found in the

WPATH Standards of Care (2012), available at www.wpath.org, and the Center of Excellence for Transgender Health (2016a), available at http://transhealth .ucsf.edu.

◼ Transgender Men

Transgender men, also referred to as FTM or assigned female as birth (AFAB) individuals (persons whose sex assigned at birth was female but who express a male gender identity), may elect to dress in gender-neutral clothing or in clothing that is associated with society's conventions of "male" clothing, such as sports-themed gear or a suit and tie. Binding of the breasts, which often involves compressing and wrapping breasts tightly to the chest wall using a binder, reduces the appearance of breast tissue, although it frequently induces costal pain and discomfort when the binding is tightly worn. Binding, especially when prolonged, can also lead to skin breakdown or fungal infections of the skin.

Hormonal therapy elected by transgender men provides masculinization of primary and secondary sexual characteristics. Testosterone therapy (e.g., injections, pellets, gel) is often prescribed if hormonal therapy is desired. Exogenous testosterone therapy carries the potential risks of acne, polycythemia, sleep apnea, weight gain, male pattern balding, elevated liver function tests, hyperlipidemia, reduced fertility, and in the presence of other risk factors, a possible increase in cardiovascular disease, hypertension, and diabetes. It can also cause exacerbation of underlying mood disorders (WPATH, 2012). Contraindications to testosterone therapy include pregnancy, unstable coronary artery disease, and untreated polycythemia with a hematocrit of 55% or greater (WPATH, 2012). Additionally, if the person has a history of cancer, a consultation with an oncologist is recommended before beginning treatment (WPATH, 2012). Transgender men who still have a uterus and ovaries should be educated that although testosterone stops menses, it is possible to become pregnant while taking testosterone if one is engaging in intimate relations or unprotected intercourse with penile penetration that includes contact with sperm, and that testosterone is teratogenic. The health-care provider may recommend a nonhormonal intrauterine device for pregnancy prevention. Gender dysphoria may cause some AFAB individuals to avoid engaging in any vaginal penetration. If a transmasculine person desires pregnancy, preconception counseling should be provided as testosterone therapy will need to be discontinued in order for ovulation to be reestablished (Cerelli et al., 2020).

Transgender men may also elect to pursue surgical treatment to remove breast tissue. This is commonly referred to among patients as "top surgery," which involves bilateral removal of breast tissue with male chest contouring, often accompanied by nipple grafts. It is important that the clinician not refer to this as a mastectomy as it is a completely different surgical approach. Being mindful of certain terms and descriptions that can trigger transgender individuals, it is important that the clinician document the surgery as "chest reconstruction." Listing top surgery as a mastectomy can be misleading for other clinicians, who may assume that a transgender individual has had this surgery performed for cancer. Transgender patients will appreciate the use of an acceptable term for this gender-affirming procedure. Individuals with smaller chests may be offered liposuction or "keyhole" surgery, which allows the patient to maintain their nipples as well as sensation. Additionally, further procedures, also referred to by some patients as "bottom surgery," may include a vaginectomy, salpingo-oophrectomy, complete hysterectomy, metoidioplasty (clitoral release), or phalloplasty with or without scrotal implants and/or urethral extension (Hembree et al., 2017).

■ Transgender Women

Transgender women, or MTF, or assigned male at birth (AMAB) individuals (persons whose sex assigned at birth was male but who express a female gender identity), may elect to dress in clothing that is gender neutral or in clothing associated with society's conventions of "female" clothing, such as a dress. Patients may "tuck," in which the penis and testes are physically reduced by compression so that the genitals are not visible, and/or use nonsurgical breast augmentation or padding. During the process of tucking, individuals may use adhesive or duct tape, which can cause pain, discomfort, and skin irritation. Patients should be educated that tucking can also increase the risk of infertility, testicular complaints, and urinary tract infection (Center of Excellence for Transgender Health, 2016a).

Hormonal therapies for feminization include androgen-blocking therapies (such as spironolactone), gonadotropin-releasing hormone (GnRH) agonists (such as goserelin, buserelin, and triptorelin), and/or estrogen replacement to promote facial feminization and other feminizing qualities. Patients should be made aware that hormonal therapies for transwomen carry the risks of increased incidence of electrolyte abnormalities, specifically hyperkalemia (with spironolactone) and hypotension, or if on estrogen therapy, increased risks of deep venous thrombosis (DVT) (the risk is higher with oral estrogen therapy versus estrogen delivered by transdermal patch), weight gain, gallstones, hypertriglyceridemia, reduced fertility, and possibly increased risk of cardiovascular disease and diabetes if other certain risk factors are present (WPATH, 2012). Estrogen therapy is contraindicated in patients with a history of DVT due to hypercoagulation, or end-stage liver disease, or an estrogen-sensitive neoplasm (WPATH, 2012). The provider should be cognizant of the patient who travels and the associated risk factors for DVT or pulmonary embolism.

Surgical options for transwomen include augmentation mammoplasty and/or genital reconstruction surgeries.

History and Physical Examination

■ Obtaining the History

During the social history, obtain, as with every other patient, demographic information including what the patient chooses to be called, who their support systems are, and who will make medical decisions for them, and assess for issues such as tobacco and alcohol use, substance use, or domestic violence. If not familiar with a gender-related or other term that the patient uses, ask the patient what the term means to them (Bosse et al., 2015). Gender-neutral descriptors, such as *partner* and *significant other* instead of *husband* or *wife*, should be used when possible. The medical history elicited should be focused and specific and pertain to the chief complaint. Asking unrelated information out of curiosity or as a personal learning opportunity is disrespectful, invasive, and unprofessional and should be avoided. While it is acceptable for a provider to admit that they do not know everything about transgender care, the patient should not be expected to teach the provider the basics.

The history should be congruent with the current chief complaint (WPATH, 2012). Although every issue that a transgender person presents with will not relate to their gender-diverse status (such as routine immunizations or an acute visit for an upper respiratory infection), it is essential that key components of history be assessed for health issues relating to long-term risk status. For example, gender-affirming hormonal treatments may increase certain health risks, so be certain to obtain a complete personal and family history of issues such as breast cancer, prostate cancer, cardiovascular disease, lipid disorders, migraines, or thrombotic disorders, as well as the patient's smoking status (Chipkin & Kim, 2017). Additionally, patients may travel for surgical procedures, so ask about recent travel history.

Transgender patients may have had particularly negative experiences with health-care providers and may, understandably, be guarded at first. Confidentiality and privacy are also important. If potentially sensitive medical information is needed, such as in the case of a new patient presenting for a comprehensive physical examination, preface the question group by describing how the questions are pertinent to the medical care. For example, the advanced practice nurse might say, "Now I'll ask you about some issues that I discuss with all of my patients. The information you tell me is obtained so that I can have an accurate medical history recorded. It will help me make accurate decisions about your health care and some future risk factors. The details that you choose to share are part of your confidential medical record." If the patient does not wish to provide a comprehensive history or details, they may feel more at ease divulging additional information to a trusted health-care provider as time progresses.

Another component of the medical record that remains crucial is the maintenance of an accurate medication list. Remember that patients may, in a quest to start or continue gender-reaffirming treatment or to access health care that is otherwise unobtainable, purchase over-the-counter medications or receive prescriptions from another person or provider (de Haan et al., 2015). In order to offer high-quality, safe care, review the medication list (including herbal medicines, over-the-counter medicines, and medicines that may not be prescribed to the individual) at each visit.

Physical Examination

The physical examination should be focused on medical necessity and should parallel similar examinations in cisgender patients, with awareness of the possible differences associated with gender-affirming treatment. For most complaints, a physical examination for a transgender person will not differ based on their transgender status, although there are special considerations to be aware of. Transgender patients may present at any point along the spectrum of gender-affirming treatments; the history should provide guidance for the physical examination. For example, if a transgender patient presents with otalgia, a focused history and assessment based on the chief complaint is warranted in the same manner as for a cisgender patient. If a transgender woman presents for evaluation of breast pain after gender-affirming hormonal treatment, the history and examination of the pertinent systems will vary accordingly.

It is reasonable to anticipate that transgender patients may express guarding, reluctance, or refusal to have certain body parts examined, and may avoid terminology for a body part that they reject (WPATH, 2012). Allow a designated support person to accompany the patient during the examination if desired. Save sensitive aspects of the examination, including disrobing of sensitive areas, for last. During the history, it is a good idea for clinicians to ask the patient if there are any anatomical terms that the patient may find triggering, such as breast, penis, vagina, or penetration, and if they have a preferred alternative. Then, use the preferred term while informing the patient as you conduct each step of the examination. The following sections are specific to the monitoring, screening, and assessment of transgender men and transgender women.

Transgender Men: Monitoring, Examination, and Screening

■ Monitoring

Laboratory test monitoring is conducted every 3 months for the first year of hormonal treatment, and then once or twice annually (Hembree et al., 2017). Laboratory tests to assess treatment response at regular intervals for transmen on hormonal therapy should include a complete blood count to monitor for polycythemia, liver function tests to monitor for enzyme elevation, and lipid profiles to monitor for hyperlipidemia, as well as testosterone levels. Normal physiological levels of the identified gender are the treatment goal, versus achieving supraphysiological levels (Hembree et al., 2017). Regular office visits should be conducted to assess the effectiveness of masculinization therapy (WPATH, 2012).

■ Screening

As long as the patient has breast tissue and/or a uterus, be certain to urge recommended screenings during the office visit, regardless of gender identity (Hembree et al., 2017). This may include a mammogram, a pelvic examination including a pap smear, and screenings for depression, domestic violence, tobacco use, and sexually transmitted infections (STIs). Table 21.2 summarizes breast cancer screening recommendations from three organizations. It is beneficial to ask the patient how their gender is listed on their insurance card to avoid any problems with rejection of insurance claims. Remember that, as with any other patient, the

Table 21.2

Selected Recommended Breast Cancer Screening Guidelines for Transgender Patients

Patient	UCSF Center of Excellence for Transgender Health	Fenway Health	Endocrine Society Clinical Practice Guidelines
Transgender woman with more than 5 years of hormone therapy	Biennial screening mammography beginning at age 50 years	Annual screening mammography beginning at age 50 years	Screening similar to that for cisgender women Length of hormone exposure not specified
Transgender man without top surgery (average risk)	Similar screening to that for cisgender women	Similar screening to that for cisgender women	Similar screening to that for cisgender women
Transgender man who has undergone top surgery	Clinicians should engage in dialogue with patients about unknown risks	No reliable evidence for screening Consider yearly chest examinations	Not addressed

Reprinted with permission from Parikh, U., Mausner, E., Chhor, C., Gao, Y., Karrington, I., & Heller, S. (2020). Breast imaging in transgender patients: What the radiologist should know. *RadioGraphics*, *40*(1), 13–27. https://doi.org/10.1148/rg.2020190044

patient may have sex with partners of any gender, so if birth control is necessary, be certain to address contraception and advise the use of condoms to prevent STIs. In addition, there is an increased prevalence of polycystic ovarian syndrome (PCOS) in FTM individuals, even if the patient does not use testosterone therapy. Since PCOS is associated with a higher risk of diabetes, hyperlipidemia, and endometrial and ovarian cancers, be certain to screen for PCOS and treat the associated comorbidities (WPATH, 2012).

■ Physical Examination

A patient requiring a breast examination may present with a breast binder in place. Ask the patient to remove the binder only after the history and any additional examinations are complete. Explain the examination, which should generally be performed consistent with the examination of a cisgender female patient. For patients who bind their breasts, note any skin problems such as breakdown or signs of fungal infections.

Whether for cancer screening or assessment of a complaint such as pelvic pain or vaginal bleeding, the pelvic examination of a transgender man requires modification compared with that of a cisgender woman. Reserve disrobing the area to be examined until the patient is ready to proceed. In addition to anxiety and guarding due to touching of the genitalia, gender-affirming hormonal treatment results in vaginal wall atrophy and dryness, which further complicate the examination. To minimize discomfort, the use of a lubricant and a small speculum is advised. Allow patients who are hesitant regarding use of a speculum to hold the device as you explain its purpose and use. If specimens are collected during the examination, note the prescribed use of specific hormones and the application of lubricant during the procedure on the laboratory request.

Transgender Women: Monitoring, Examination, and Screening

■ Monitoring

Laboratory monitoring should include blood pressure monitoring and electrolyte evaluation (especially if the patient is on spironolactone); lipid monitoring to assess for hyperlipidemia; and estradiol, testosterone, and prolactin levels if the patient is on estrogen (Hembree et al., 2017). Usually, laboratory tests are done every 3 months for the first year, then once or twice a year after that. Regular office visits should be conducted to assess the effectiveness of feminization therapy (WPATH, 2012). If the patient happens to be taking estrogen therapy and still uses tobacco, the patient should be strongly urged to quit smoking, as the incidence of DVT is increased when on estrogen (WPATH, 2012). Many healthcare providers will not prescribe estrogen therapy if the patient smokes, so be sure to urge smoking cessation (Chipkin & Kim, 2017).

■ Screening

Remember to conduct screenings accordingly based on anatomy at birth, if still applicable, as well as anatomy augmented by hormonal therapy. Any patient who has testes and a prostate gland, regardless of their gender identity, should be monitored for testicular or prostatic disease as is the case with any cisgender male patient (Hembree et al., 2017). Transgender women who may have undergone a vaginoplasty will still need to have regular prostate screenings as the anterior wall of the prostate is used to construct the vagina (UCSF, 2016). Transgender women should have breast screening as recommended by current guidelines (see Table 21.2). Monitor for cardiovascular risk factors and for DVTs if the patient is on estrogen therapy (Hembree et al., 2017), and teach the patient the warning signs and symptoms of a DVT; urge smoking cessation for smokers. Screen for domestic violence, depression, smoking, and STIs if applicable. If the patient has had a gonadectomy and does not continue hormonal replacement therapy after surgery, they will need to be screened with a bone mineral density test (Hembree et al., 2017). As with other patients, the patient may be in a sexual relationship with people of any gender, so recommend the use of condoms if appropriate. Asking about specific behaviors using a nonjudgmental approach will assist in determining current sexual behavior risks, which can then be used to guide decisions about testing and education.

■ Physical Examination

MTF patients may be reluctant to have sensitive body parts examined. However, the literature suggests that examination of the breasts or neovagina may be gender affirming. Those who have undergone vaginoplasty may present with complaints involving the neovagina and will require examination of the area. The neovagina, described as a "blind cuff," is more narrow and posteriorly oriented than the cisgender woman's vagina. The structure can be visualized by inserting an anoscope, removing the trocar, and inspecting the walls while withdrawing the device. If the transgender female patient employs genital tucking, inspect the overlying skin for areas of skin breakdown (UCSF, 2016; Hashemi et al., 2018).

Conclusion

Advanced practice nurses are in an excellent position to establish a framework of safe and effective, culturally competent care for all individuals, regardless of their gender identity or expression. By creating a safe environment and establishing a health-care setting based on mutual trust and respect, advanced nurse practitioners help patients of all gender expressions to feel comfortable seeking care. The information in this chapter provides an introduction to care of the transgender individual. Interested providers should refer to complete guidelines as described in the Center of Excellence for Transgender Health (2016); Hembree et al., (2017); and the World Professional Association for Transgender Health (2012). A robust opportunity exists for nurse practitioners to help educate colleagues and help reduce or eliminate health disparities currently experienced by gender-diverse individuals. A list of resources is supplied in the hope that it will provide further education and support for caregivers, families, and patients.

REFERENCES

Aisner, A., Zappas, M., & Marks, A. (2020). Primary care for lesbian, gay, bisexual, transgender, and queer /questioning (LGBTQ) patients. *The Journal for Nurse Practitioners, 16,*(4), 281–285.

Bockting, W. O., Miner, M. H., Swinburne Romine, R. E., Hamilton, A., & Coleman, E. (2013). Stigma, mental health, and resilience in an online sample of the US transgender population. *American Journal of Public Health, 103*(5), 943–951. https://doi.org/10.2105/ajph.2013.301241

Bosse, J. D., Nesteby, J. A., & Randall, C. E. (2015). Integrating sexual minority health issues into a health assessment class. *Journal of Professional Nursing, 31*(6), 498–507.

Bradford, J., Reisner, S. L., Honnold, J. A., & Xavier, J. (2013). Experiences of transgender-related discrimination and implications for health: Results from the Virginia Transgender Health Initiative Study. *American Journal of Public Health, 103*(10), 1820–1829. https//doi.org/10.2105/ajph.2012.300796

Bränström, R., & Pachankis, J. E. (2020). Reduction in mental health treatment utilization among transgender individuals after gender-affirming surgeries: A total population study. *The American Journal of Psychiatry, 177*(8), 727–734. https://doi.org/10.1176/appi.ajp.2019.19010080

Center of Excellence for Transgender Health. (2016a). *Guidelines for the primary and gender-affirming care of transgender and gender nonbinary people.* http://transhealth.ucsf.edu/protocols

Center of Excellence for Transgender Health. (2016b). *Guidelines for the primary and gender-affirming care of transgender and gender nonbinary people.* (2nd ed.). Center of Excellence for Transgender Health. Department of Family and Community Medicine University of California. http://transhealth.ucsf.edu /trans?page=guidelines-home

Cerelli, J., Ellis, S., & Fried, E. (2020). When sperm and egg aren't bedfellows: The WHNP role. Women's Healthcare. https://www.npwomenshealthcare.com/when-sperm-and-egg-arent-bedfellows-the-whnp -role-in-helping-families-conceive/in helping families conceive

Chipkin, S. R., & Kim, F. (2017). Ten most important things to know about caring for transgender patients. *The American Journal of Medicine. 130*(11), 1238–1245.

de Haan, G., Santos, G. M., Arayasirikul, S., & Raymond, H. F. (2015). Non-prescribed hormone use and barriers to care for transgender women in San Francisco. *LGBT Health, 2*(4), 313–323. https//doi.org /10.1089/lgbt.2014.0128

Frei, J., Kalensky, M., McIntosh, E., Mystkowski, J., Schwelnus, E., Shaw, B., & Thompson, H. (2019). Gender affirmation in adult primary care. *The Journal for Nurse Practitioners, 15*(10), 742–748. https//doi.org/10.1016/j.nurpra.2019.07.018

Gates, G. (2011). How many people are lesbian, gay, bisexual, and transgender? UCLA School of Law, Williams Institute. https://williamsinstitute.law.ucla.edu/wp-content/uploads/Gates-How-Many-People -LGBT-Apr-2011.pdf

GLAAD (2021). GLAAD Media Reference Guide-Transgender. 11th ed. https://www.glaad.org/reference /transgender

Halloran, L. P. A. (2015). Caring for transgender patients. *The Journal for Nurse Practitioners, 11*(9), 915–916.

Hashemi, L., Weinreb, J., Weimer, A., & Weiss, R. (2018). Transgender care in the primary care setting: A review of guidelines and literature. *Federal Practitioner, 35*(7), 30–37.

Hembree, W. C., Cohen-Kettenis, P. T., Gooren, L., Hannema, S. E., Meyer, W. J., Murad, M. H., Rosenthal, S. M., Safer, J. D., Tangpricha, V., &T'Sjoen, G. G. (2017). Endocrine treatment of gender -dysphoric/gender-incongruent persons: An Endocrine Society clinical practice guideline. *Journal of Clinical Endocrinology and Metabolism, 102*(11), 3869–3903. http://doi.org/10.1210/jc.2017-01658

Hemmila, A. (2016). Ancestors of two-spirits: Historical depictions of Native North American gender-crossing women through critical discourse analysis. *Journal of Lesbian Studies, 20*(3–4), 408–426. http://doi.org/10.1080/10894160.2016.1151281

Kcomt, L., Gorey, L. M., Barrett, B. J., & McCabe, S. E. (2020). Healthcare avoidance due to anticipated discrimination among transgender people: A call to create trans-affirmative environments. *SSM-Population Health, 11,* 100608. https://doi.org/10.1016/j.ssmph.2020.100608

Khaleeli, H. (2014). Hijra: India's third gender claims its place in law. *The Guardian.* https://www.theguardian .com/society/2014/apr/16/india-third-gender-claims-place-in-law

Kosenko, K., Rintamaki, L., Raney, S., & Maness, K. (2013). Transgender patient perceptions of stigma in health care contexts. *Medical Care, 51*(9), 819-822. http://doi.org/10.1097/MLR.0b013e31829fa90d

Kuper, L. E., Nussbaum, R., & Mustanski, B. (2012). Exploring the diversity of gender and sexual orientation identities in an online sample of transgender individuals. *Journal of Sex Research, 49*(2–3), 244–254. https:/doi.org/10.1080/00224499.2011.596954

Mayer, K. H., Bradford, J. B., Makadon, H. J., Stall, R., Goldhammer, H., & Landers, S. (2008). Sexual and gender minority health: What we know and what needs to be done. *American Journal of Public Health, 98*(6), 989–995. https://doi.org/10.2105/ajph.2007.127811

Meerwijk, E. L., & Sevelius, J. M. (2017). Transgender population size in the United States: A meta-regression of population-based probability samples. *American Journal of Public Health, 107*(2), e1–e8. https://doi.org /10.2105/AJPH.2016.303578

Parikh, U., Mausner, E., Chhor, C., Gao, Y., Karrington, I., & Heller, S. (2020). Breast imaging in transgender patients: What the radiologist should know. *RadioGraphics, 40*(1), 13–27. https://doi.org /10.1148/rg.2020190044

Planned Parenthood. (2021). *Transgender Identity Terms and Labels.* https://www.plannedparenthood.org /learn/gender-identity/transgender/transgender-identity-terms-and-labels

Poteat, T., German, D., & Kerrigan, D. (2013). Managing uncertainty: A grounded theory of stigma in transgender health care encounters. *Social Science and Medicine, 84,* 22–29. https://doi.org/10.1016 /j.socscimed.2013.02.019

Stotzer, R. L. (2009). Violence against transgender people: A review of United States data. *Aggression and Violent Behavior, 14*(3), 170–179.

The LGBTQIA Experiment. (2019). *What is misgendering?* https://lgbtqexperiment.com/2019/06/17 /what-is-misgendering/

University of California, San Francisco. (2016). *Guidelines for the Primary and Gender-Affirming Care of Transgender and Gender Nonbinary People.* UCSF Transgender Care. https://transcare.ucsf.edu/guidelines

World Professional Association for Transgender Health. (2012). *Standards of care for the health of transsexual, transgender, and gender nonconforming people.* Accessed May 5, 2018, from http://www.wpath.org/site _page.cfm?pk_association_webpage_menu=1351&pk_association_webpage=3926

Chapter 22

Older Patients

• Lisa Byrd

T he comprehensive assessment of older individuals requires an understanding of the physiological changes of normal aging and the complex interplay among those changes, disease, and functional status. Every person ages differently. Some 80-year-old patients are very healthy, and some 65-year-old patients have chronic disease and/or functional decline or cognitive decline. The key to promote healthy aging is to screen for problems and maintain abilities.

Performance of screening assessments may need to be personalized to meet the person's abilities and level of frailty and the setting in which the assessment occurs. Finally, some well-recognized "syndromes" that either present in unusual ways or are inadequately addressed in the typical clinical encounter require diligent investigation to promote independence and prevent functional decline in older patients. All of these factors contribute to the complexity of the comprehensive geriatric assessment and strengthen the support for a multidisciplinary approach in geriatric care.

This chapter addresses these issues by focusing on the concept of functional assessment, from its basic components to highly integrated aspects of role functioning, using the hierarchical model developed by the National Institute on Aging (NIA) (2003). The model, illustrated in Figure 22.1, provides a holistic view of the individual and a guide to management options. Functional assessment is a performance-based approach that explores how disease affects the individual; it is a useful concept in many ways. For example, in the case of older patients who have little disease but whose ability to function independently is significantly affected, the clinician is prompted to address management options that provide support to the individual and family in order to prevent or delay disease while maintaining as much independence as possible. Conversely, in older patients who have significant comorbidities and who have adapted to their disease burden and remain independent, a functional assessment supports management options to allow for continued role functioning as long as possible.

A functional assessment determines the degree to which individuals can perform those activities that enable them to live independently. The activities

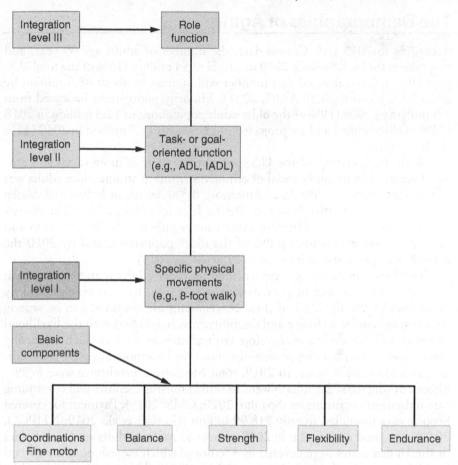

Figure 22.1 Model of a hierarchy of function. See also Box 22.1. (Adapted from National Institute on Aging. [2003]. The measurement of physical functioning in older adult populations [Report of meeting held on December 12, 2003].)

of daily living (ADLs) are dependent on basic components of specific physical movements that result in coordination and fine motor control, allowing such movements as those required to grasp a fork or spoon. Specific movements are then required to take the grasping of the spoon to a goal-oriented activity, namely, eating a meal. A higher level of integration of the physical movements involved in eating with cognitive capability provides the basis for shopping for groceries, preparing a meal, or planning a holiday dinner for a larger family (see Fig. 22.1). Degradation in the ability to perform any or all of these tasks results in greater dependence on others and may lead to a need for a change in living circumstances. Dependence among older patients has implications for society as a whole, owing to the demographic shift that has been occurring in most of the developed countries of the world.

The Demographics of Aging

According to 2019 U.S. Census data, the number of adults age 65 years and older increased by 32% since 2010 to a total of 54 million (16% of the total U.S. population); it is estimated that number will increase to about 88.5 million by 2050 (U.S. Census, 2020; AARP, 2021). Minority populations increased from 7.5 million in 2008 (19% of the older adult population) to 12.3 million in 2018 (23% of older adults) and are projected to increase to 27.7 million in 2040 (34% of older adults).

With the "graying" of the U.S. population, there is more racial and ethnic diversity. The minority racial or ethnic distribution among older adults was 9% African American, 5% Asian American, 0.5% American Indian and Alaska Native, and 0.1% Native Hawaiian/Pacific Islander (ACL, 2020). The fastest-growing minority is the Hispanic American population. In 2017 Latino and Hispanic Americans made up 8% of the older population, and by 2060 the percentage is projected to increase to 21% (ACL, 2019).

The fastest-growing age segment among older adults is those older than 100 years. The number of centenarians is projected to increase eightfold by 2050 (Stepler, 2016). Most of these centenarians are considered to be among the most vulnerable to frailty and disability, which, coupled with the likelihood that they will live alone and therefore require support services (such as nursing home care), has caused dire predictions about the enormous stress on the Medicare and Medicaid systems. In 2019, total Medicare expenditures were $799.4 billion, of which $172.2 billion went to skilled nursing facilities and continuing care retirement communities (Spanko, 2020; CMS, 2019). Payment for covered hospice care amounted to only $18.99 billion (Gumaer et al., 2019; NHPCO, 2019). The good news is that in 2019, almost 53 million adults age 65 and older in the United States were covered by Medicare, which is pushing more toward health screening and preventive care (CMS, 2021). This increase in the older population is occurring worldwide, and the projected socioeconomic impact on societies for providing health-care services to older adults is of great concern to researchers, policymakers, and providers.

There are 2.4 million older adults who identify as lesbian, gay, bisexual, or transgender (LGBTQ+) (APA, 2021). LGBTQ+ older adults experience unique economic and health disparities disproportionately compared to older individuals affected by poverty and physical or mental health conditions. This population has experienced a lifetime of unique stressors associated with being a minority and is potentially more vulnerable to neglect and mistreatment in the health-care setting. LGBTQ+ populations may face dual discrimination owing to age and sexual orientation or gender identity.

As the number of frail and dependent older patients increase, a concomitant rise in the proportion of those who are disabled will occur. Based on 2020 census data, 40% of older adults reported some degree of disability; some of these disabilities interfered with functional capacity and required caregiver assistance to accomplish basic ADLs (CDC, 2020a). Associated with these ADL limitations is the need for home and community-based or institutional services, some of which may be covered by Medicare. However, daily care for some older individuals is most often provided by family members (11% of the time) or paid out of pocket by the individuals or family. About 1.3 million older adults reside in nursing homes, about half of whom are age 85 and older (CDC, 2021a). The level of services required will largely be determined by psychosocial and economic factors along with medical necessity, all of which should be determined through a comprehensive and perhaps multidisciplinary patient assessment. It is important to remember that aging is a life process that in and of itself does not inevitably produce functional decline.

The Approach to the Assessment of Older Individuals

Older individuals are characterized by their heterogeneity; therefore, clinicians must adapt their approaches on the basis of the setting (e.g., outpatient, inpatient, home), the presenting complaint, the capabilities or limitations of the individual, and the goals for care for the individual patient in that situation. In general, an older individual will have more physical complaints, more comorbidities, more medication usage, and longer medical and surgical histories than will a younger person. Information about childhood immunizations may not be relevant, such as for those born before childhood immunizations were developed, and information about family history may be incomplete with no way to obtain the information. Certain components of the past history will be more relevant, such as occupational history; military service in wartime; environmental exposures; and functional changes in sensory, physical, or cognitive abilities over time. Lifestyle issues, such as habits, driving ability, nutrition, social support networks, and sleep and elimination patterns require particular attention. Advanced care planning, particularly advanced health-care directives and designation of durable power of attorney for health-care decisions, should be addressed with regular opportunities for discussion of changing priorities and status of significant members of the family (e.g., death of the spouse who was the designated decision maker for health care). Losses, including loss of function (physical or mental) and altered independence, as well as the loss of friends and family, become more frequent with aging. It is important to provide opportunities to discuss and allow for grieving of such losses as frequently as possible during routine health-care encounters.

The approach to the physical examination of older adults will not differ greatly from standard examination techniques presented in this text. Some tests of functional ability are not routinely considered in the usual examination of the adult; those are presented in the various sections that follow. With older adults who are debilitated, it is important to focus the examination and reduce extraneous activities and distractions. Whenever possible, begin the examination with maneuvers that can be accomplished with patients in their current position. For example, when the patient arrives to the examination seated in a wheelchair, check vital signs, heart rate, extremities, or anything else that can be done in the seated position first. If a patient's ability to transfer from the wheelchair is in question, observe the transfer, taking note of need for assistance to move or to balance before the patient becomes fatigued. The exertion of getting onto the examination table could fatigue an individual enough to preclude optimal performance. Likewise, perform all supine or standing examinations together to preserve the patient's stamina. A reordering of the sequence of the examination should be done in a logical and thoughtful manner. See Chapter 23 for assessment of patients with limited mobility.

Attend to the safety of the older person by removing obstructions, providing adequate lighting, and standing near the individual to prevent falls. Turn off background music or television if possible, and speak clearly, facing the person at eye level, to facilitate good communication. Be aware that glare off windows and other shiny surfaces can cause discomfort and can compromise vision during interviewing and testing.

The Physiology of Aging

A common adage indicates that aging changes consist of about one-third disease, one-third disuse, and one-third normal aging. The relationships among these three factors are important but often difficult to define. Although chronological aging does produce change in biochemical processes, actual function is remarkably well maintained in humans. Unless the individual experiences the effects of chronic disease or a devastating physiological event, most of the impact of the changes occurring during the aging process relates to decreased physiological reserve; very little of the impairment seen among older populations is due to actual physiological changes. It is probably more helpful to view aging as a continuum upon which physiological and pathological processes seem to vary infinitely within a given population.

Table 22.1 lists the major physiological changes associated with aging and the known or postulated impacts those changes have on functional or disease states. Some of these changes are easily detected, such as the age-related attrition of oocytes in the ovaries that leads to the loss of female reproductive ability. Other changes are much less obvious, such as the loss of nephrons in the kidney that may affect the ability to excrete drug metabolites. Loss of female reproductive ability is inevitable after a certain age, whereas loss of nephrons is much more complex and variable. Although the loss of nephrons may be a given, the effect of that loss on an individual's function may vary considerably, depending on other factors, such as disease states (e.g., hypertension, diabetes) and other physiological variables (e.g., intracellular fluid volume). Interactive effects from physiological changes, such as the effect of declining levels of estrogen production following menopause on bone remodeling, complicate the picture. Thus, geriatric assessment is most effective when it is focused on functional impact rather than on disease states. Functional assessment allows the variability that occurs with the complex relationships among disease, disuse, and physiology to remain secondary to the development and implementation of a treatment plan.

Table 22.1

Physiological Changes of Aging and Their Impacts

Physiological Change	Functional and Clinical Impact
Skin: 20% thinning of dermal and epidermal layers; slower cell reproduction with decreased epidermal proliferation and collagen flexibility; changes in elastic fiber network becoming less elastic	Increased skin fragility and cell irregularity; increased sensitivity for contact irritation/dermatitis; increased susceptibility to infection; decreased skin elasticity; increased wrinkling and dryness; uneven pigmentation with occurrence of aging spots
Redistribution of fat less deposits in extremities and increased deposits in the truncal region; decreased amount of subcutaneous fat	Sagging of skin especially around the eyes; decreased fat pads: less on the soles of feet may change gait or ability to ambulate; fat distributions shifts, making joints more prominent
Decreased sebaceous and eccrine gland activity; loss of hair pigment	Decreased rate of nail growth by 20%; hair growth slows; decreased ability to sweat may lead to poor temperature regulation with potential hyperthermia; hair thins and has an increased tendency to be gray
Proprioception: Increased threshold for pressure and touch; decreased vibratory sense in feet and toes; decreased thermal sensitivity	Potential for injury due to balance issues and decreased ability to sense heat or cold; decreased ability to detect pressure at fingertips leading to dropping objects more readily
Eyes: Increased translucency and flattening of cornea; thickening and rigidity of choroid and iris; decreased production of aqueous humor; decreased mass of ciliary muscle; decreased number of rods, cones, and ganglion cells; increased yellowing and density, with decreased elasticity of lens; liquefaction of vitreous body	Slower accommodation to light intensity; yellowing of the lens leads to impaired color discrimination—some colors (blues, greens, purples) less distinguishable while others (yellows, oranges, red) are accentuated; decreased night vision acuity that affects night driving; blurring and changes in visual acuity; pupils slower to react to light and require more light to trigger (older eyes require 20% more lighting to see accurately); floaters and light flashes increase; increased incidence of presbyopia, eye dryness, cataract development, and glaucoma; eyes more vulnerable to infection
Ear: Tympanic membrane is thinner and less resilient with sclerotic changes; ossicles become calcified and stiffer; pinna widens, elongates, and stiffens; less oil production leads to drier cerumen	Some degree of impaired auditory function; decreased sensitivity to high-frequency tones (presbycusis); increased incidence of cerumen impactions acting as a barrier to sounds; ears may appear larger
Oral cavity: Decreased salivation, decreased ability to digest starches, diminished number of olfactory cells, and decreased ability to sense thirst	Decreased sensitivity to taste (sweet and salty initially followed by sour and bitter); decreased sense of smell; food preferences change; dryer oral mucosa with recession in gumline and teeth more brittle with increased incidence of cavities, broken teeth, and tooth loss; decreased protection of teeth and tongue from bacteria; increased tendency for dehydration and undernutrition
Pulmonary system: Enlargement of alveolar duct; decreased elastic recoil; decreased lung volumes; decreased number of cilia; increased size and stiffening of trachea and bronchi with increased dead space; increased calcification of chest wall; decreased cough reflex, forced vital capacity, forced expiratory volume per second, and forced expiratory flow; increased residual volume, functional residual capacity, and residual volume/total lung capacity	Altered pulmonary function; potential change of lung expansion due to thoracic kyphosis; decreased sensitivity to changes in levels of oxygen and carbon dioxide; diminished number of alveoli; increased sensitivity to environmental irritants; decreased ability to clear inhaled irritants; increased incidence of pulmonary infections with slower recovery, increased incidence of COPD, emphysema, and effects of asthma

(cont. on page 742)

Table 22.1

Physiological Changes of Aging and Their Impacts—cont'd

Physiological Change	Functional and Clinical Impact
Cardiac system: Increased size and weight of heart and vessels; increased thickness of the left ventricular posterior wall and aorta; decreased early diastolic closure rates of mitral valve; sclerotic changes of cardiac valves; decreased response to beta-adrenergic stimulation	Slight decrease in cardiac output; heart rate slower to increase with exercise, diminished myocardial contractile efficiency, diminished maximal oxygen uptake and responsiveness to catecholamines; increased systolic pressure, left ventricular ejection time, and pre-ejection period, stroke volume with progressive exercise not as responsive; increased ectopic cardiac pacemaker activity; murmurs and S_4 heart sounds more common; orthostatic blood pressure changes may occur; increases in systolic and diastolic pressures
Gastrointestinal changes: Decreased production of saliva, gastric juices' acidity changes (including intrinsic factor, peptic and hydrochloric acids); decreased gastric motility; increased mucosal and muscle atrophy; decreased size and activity of liver, hepatocytes, secretory acini and islets of Langerhans; decreased splenic blood flow	Decreased absorption of vitamins B_{12} and D; decreased carbohydrate absorption; decreased protein, iron, and folic acid digestion; increased need for pressure to trigger the swallowing reflex, potentially leading to increased incidence of choking; delayed gastric emptying and maldigestion; impaired fat absorption; decreased drug metabolism and hepatic protein synthesis; diminished glucose tolerance
Kidney: Decreased number of glomeruli, decreased number of nephrons, decreased filtration of blood with diminished glomerular filtration rate as much as 30% to 40%; thickened tubular membranes and fatty degeneration; sclerosis or stiffening and narrowing of renal vasculature; decreased elasticity and expandability and compressibility of detrusor; decreased bladder sensation	Slower or decreased clearance of medications and other waste products via kidneys; diminished urine concentrating capacity; decrease in glomerular filtration rate, slight increase in blood urea nitrogen, yet the creatinine may not change; decreased creatinine clearance; smaller bladder capacity; increased urinary frequency and post-void residual volume; increased incidence of urinary incontinence in females; increased urinary outflow obstruction in males with hesitancy, weaker urine stream, incomplete bladder emptying, urinary frequency, and nocturia
Endocrine: Decreased secretion TSH and T_4, insulin, rennin, aldosterone, ACTH, growth hormone; decreased response to TRH, ACTH	Laboratory values may change and must be interpreted carefully; increased fatigue; weight gain; stress response is lessened
Musculoskeletal: Decreased bone mass, size, and number of muscle fibers; lean body mass lessened and increased fat accumulation	Increased incidence of thoracic kyphosis, more so in postmenopausal patients due the decreases in estrogen levels; increased incidence of osteopenia, osteoporosis, and microfractures; decreased lean body mass and total body water; increased vulnerability to fractures, balance issues, and gait problems
Sleep: Decreased sleep efficiency; changes in total sleep time (usually decreased or broken up sleep); increased sleep latency; easier arousal during sleep; decreased REM latency and total REM sleep	Increased time to fall asleep; more time in bed waiting to fall asleep; sleep disturbances due to nocturia, pain, or other issues; earlier awakening; more daytime napping; decreased sleep efficiency; no increase in daytime sleepiness; increased incidence of obstructive sleep apnea with periodic hypoxia

ACTH = adrenocorticotropic hormone; COPD = chronic obstructive pulmonary disease; REM = rapid eye movement; T4 = thyroxine; TRH = thyrotropin-releasing hormone; TSH = thyroid-stimulating hormone.
  Data from Alessi, 2000; Blair, 1990; and Cotter & Strumpf, 2002.

Functional Assessment

Within the context of health assessment, functional assessment provides an alternative perspective on the health status of an individual. In the traditional model of health assessment taught in nurse practitioner programs, the focus is on the clinical diagnosis and the development of sound diagnostic reasoning. This approach assumes that a reason for the patient's presenting symptoms can be identified and an intervention can be instituted to cure or manage the problem so that the individual returns to their baseline level of functioning (Box 22.1). Although some conditions are reversible in older persons, many are not; thus, the focus of the assessment needs to be on maximizing the older patient's function and maintaining or improving well-being.

In clinical trials, the effects of interventions on functional ability are frequently measured and reported as indicators of quality of life. The domains of quality-of-life indicators encompass physical, emotional, spiritual, and psychosocial measures; many instruments have been developed for the purpose of measuring various indicators (Besdine, 2019; Gerety, 2000). Many of these measures are self-reported; however, with assessment of older individuals,

---

Box 22.1

Functional Model Integration Levels

Basic Components. The basic components of this model are viewed as functional units that form the building blocks of a series of increasingly complex functional tasks. The basic components include strength, balance, coordination, flexibility, and endurance.

Specific Physical Movements. These are movement sequences that can be achieved by the integration of two or more basic components. Examples of specific physical movements include carry, reach, bend, stoop, transfer, chair rise, and walk.

Task- or Goal-Oriented Activities. This level requires all of the physical movements plus varying degrees of cognitive ability to conceptualize the task and follow through to achievement of the goal. Examples of these more complex tasks or activities include the ADLs (bathing, grooming, dressing, and toileting) and IADLs (shopping, managing money or medications, using the telephone, and doing laundry).

Role Function. This is the highest level of integration and the most difficult to assess because of its complexity. In the older patient, occupational activities might be replaced by volunteer activities; however, some older patients remain fully engaged in productive occupational activities until they die. This level of integration of functional abilities implies wide-ranging engagement in life, which can occur even in the presence of serious physical disability (e.g., amyotrophic lateral sclerosis, quadriplegia, multiple sclerosis) in younger as well as older people.

---

caregiver reports and direct observations are commonly used to obtain a more accurate assessment. Moreover, measured domains frequently overlap, and it may be difficult to separate the effects that emotional function or intellectual function have on physical function. One way to overcome some of these measurement dilemmas is to use standardized performance-based measures that integrate basic components of a movement and provide the opportunity to observe a patient performing a task or a goal-oriented function. This is the basis for the hierarchical model of function depicted in Figure 22.1.

■ Measures of Function

Two scales are commonly used to measure functional ability: Physical Activities of Daily Living (Box 22.2) and Instrumental Activities of Daily Living (IADLs; Box 22.3) (Lawton & Brody, 1969). Although both scales are relatively crude, they have been largely accepted as adequate for determining the need for assistive services and for classifying the level of dependency and care required, either at home or in institutional settings. Both instruments are scored according to the level of independence in performance of the task, and they both provide snapshots of a person's ability to live independently. Most health professionals

---

Box 22.2

Physical Self-Maintenance Scale (Activities of Daily Living [ADLs])

In each category, circle the item that most closely describes the person's highest level of functioning and record the score assigned to that level (either 1 or 0) in the blank at the beginning of the category.

A. Toilet

1. Care for self at toilet completely; no incontinence	1
2. Needs to be reminded, or needs help in cleaning self, or has rare (weekly at most) accidents	0
3. Soiling or wetting while asleep more than once a week	0
4. Soiling or wetting while awake more than once a week	0
5. No control of bowels or bladder	0

B. Feeding

1. Eats without assistance	1
2. Eats with minor assistance at meal times and/or with special preparation of food, or helps in cleaning up after meals	0
3. Feeds self with moderate assistance and is untidy	0
4. Requires extensive assistance for all meals	0
5. Does not feed self at all and resists efforts of others to feed him or her	0

C. Dressing

1. Dresses, undresses, and selects clothes from own wardrobe	1
2. Dresses and undresses self, with minor assistance	0

Box 22.2

Physical Self-Maintenance Scale (Activities of Daily Living [ADLs])—con'd

3. Needs moderate assistance in dressing and selection of clothes   0
4. Needs major assistance in dressing, but cooperates with efforts of others to help   0
5. Completely unable to dress self and resists efforts of others to help   0

D. Grooming (neatness, hair, nails, hands, face, clothing)

1. Always neatly dressed, well-groomed, without assistance   1
2. Grooms self adequately with occasional minor assistance (e.g., with shaving)   0
3. Needs moderate and regular assistance or supervision with grooming   0
4. Needs total grooming care but can remain well-groomed after help from others   0
5. Actively negates all efforts of others to maintain grooming   0

E. Physical Ambulation

1. Goes about grounds or city   1
2. Ambulates within residence on or about one block distant   0
3. Ambulates with assistance of (check one) a ( ) another person, b ( ) railing, c ( ) cane, d ( ) walker, e ( ) wheelchair   0
   1. Gets in and out without help
   2. Needs help getting in and out
4. Sits unsupported in chair or wheelchair but cannot propel self without help   0
5. Bedridden more than half the time   0

F. Bathing

1. Bathes self (tub, shower, sponge bath) without help   1
2. Bathes self with help getting in and out of tub   0
3. Washes face and hands only, but cannot bathe rest of body   0
4. Does not wash self but is cooperative with those who bathe him or her   0
5. Does not try to wash self and resists efforts to keep him or her clean   0

For scoring interpretation and source, see note following the next instrument.
Scoring interpretation:

For ADLs, the total score ranges from 0 to 6, and for IADLs, from 0 to 8. In some categories, only the highest level of function receives a 1; in others, two or more levels have scores of 1 because each describes competence that represents some minimal level of function. These screens are useful for indicating specifically how a person is performing currently. When they are also used over time, they serve as documentation of a person's functional improvement or deterioration.

Box 22.3

Instrumental Activities of Daily Living (IADLs) Scale

In each category, circle the item that most closely describes the person's highest level of functioning and record the score assigned to that level (either 1 or 0) in the blank at the beginning of the category.

A. Ability to Use Telephone

1. Operates telephone on own initiative; looks up and dials numbers	1
2. Dials a few well-known numbers	1
3. Answers telephone but does not dial	1
4. Does not use telephone at all	0

B. Shopping

1. Takes care of all shopping needs independently	1
2. Shops independently for small purchases	0
3. Needs to be accompanied on any shopping trip	0
4. Completely unable to shop	0

C. Food Preparation

1. Plans, prepares, and serves adequate meals independently	1
2. Prepares adequate meals if supplied with ingredients	0
3. Heats and serves prepared meals or prepares meals but does not maintain adequate diet	0
4. Needs to have meals prepared and served	0

D. Housekeeping

1. Maintains house alone or with occasional assistance (e.g., heavy-work domestic help)	1
2. Performs light daily tasks such as dishwashing and bed-making	1
3. Performs light daily tasks but cannot maintain acceptable level of cleanliness	1
4. Needs help with all home maintenance tasks	1
5. Does not participate in any housekeeping tasks	0

E. Laundry

1. Does personal laundry completely	1
2. Launders small items; rinses socks, stockings, etc.	1
3. All laundry must be done by others	0

F. Mode of Transportation

1. Travels independently on public transportation or drives own car	1
2. Arranges own travel via taxi but does not otherwise use public transportation	1
3. Travels on public transportation when assisted or accompanied by another	1

Box 22.3

Instrumental Activities of Daily Living (IADLs) Scale—cont'd

4. Travel limited to taxi or automobile with assistance of another   0
5. Does not travel at all   0

G. Responsibility for Own Medications

1. Is responsible for taking medication in correct dosages at correct time 1
2. Takes responsibility if medication is prepared in advance in
   separate dosages   0
3. Is not capable of dispensing own medication   0

H. Ability to Handle Finances

1. Manages financial matters independently (budgets, writes checks,
   pays rent and bills, goes to bank); collects and keeps track of income 1
2. Manages day-to-day purchases but needs help with banking, major
   purchases, etc.   1
3. Incapable of handling money   0

Scoring Interpretation: For ADLs the total score ranges from 0 to 6 and for IADLs, from 0 to 8. In some categories, only the highest level of function receives a 1; in others, two or more levels have scores of 1 because each describes competence that represents some minimal level of function. These screens are useful for indicating specifically how a person is performing currently. When they are also used over time, they serve as documentation of a person's functional improvement or deterioration.

accept the goal-oriented activities depicted in Figure 22.1 as minimal criteria for independent functioning in the modern world. It is important to remember that functional ability can be regained in certain circumstances, at least to a certain degree (e.g., following a stroke). The Hartford Institute for Geriatric Nursing has resources, including teaching videos, on how to use many of these assessment tools.

For well older patients, the 10-Minute Screener for Geriatric Conditions is a useful tool for general practice (Bluestein & Rutledge, 2006). This brief screening tool (Table 22.2) addresses vision, hearing, leg mobility, urinary incontinence, nutrition and weight loss, memory, depression, and physical disability. Using a combination of subjective and objective measures, the 10-Minute Screener covers all the basic ADL and IADL functions in a manner that fits well within the outpatient examination. A positive screen requires further evaluation, in some cases by a specialist or a geriatric specialist.

Table 22.2

10-Minute Screener for Geriatric Conditions

Problem	Screening Measure	Positive Screen
Vision	Two parts: Ask: "Do you have difficulty driving or watching television or reading or doing any of your daily activities because of your eyesight?" If yes, then: Test each eye with Snellen chart while patient wears corrective lenses (if applicable)	Yes to question and inability to read 20/40 on Snellen chart
Hearing	Use audioscope set at 40 dB; test hearing using 1,000 and 2,000 Hz	Inability to hear 1,000 or 2,000 Hz in both ears, or inability to hear frequencies in either ear
Leg mobility	Time the patient after asking: "Rise from the chair. Walk 20 feet briskly, turn, walk back to the chair, and sit down."	Unable to complete task in 15 sec
Urinary incontinence	Two parts: Ask: "In the past year, have you ever lost your urine and gotten wet?" If yes, then ask: "Have you lost urine on at least 6 separate days?"	Yes to both questions
Nutrition, weight loss	Two parts: Ask: "Have you lost 10 lb over the past 6 months without trying to do so?" Weigh the patient	Yes to the question or weight <100 lb
Memory	Three-item recall	Unable to recall all items after 1 min
Depression	Ask: "Do you often feel sad or depressed?"	Yes to the question
Physical disability	Six questions: "Are you able to . . ." " . . . do strenuous activities like fast walking or bicycling?" " . . . do heavy work around the house, like washing windows, walls, or floors?" " . . . go shopping for groceries or clothes?" " . . . get to places out of walking distance?" " . . . bathe, either a sponge bath, tub bath, or shower?" " . . . dress, like putting on a shirt, buttoning and zipping, or putting on shoes?"	No to any of the questions

Reprinted from Moore, A. A., Siu, A. L. (1996). Screening for common problems in ambulatory elderly: Clinical confirmation of a screening instrument. *American Journal of Medicine, 100*(4), 440. Copyright 1998, with permission from Excerpta Medica, Inc.

▪ Measures of Cognitive Function

In primary care settings, assessment of cognitive function is often not thoroughly examined. Whether due to lack of time or lack of experience with appropriate screening measures, most clinicians in primary care fail to recognize early signs of cognitive impairment. Medicare includes assessment of cognitive function as a required assessment in the annual wellness visits for Medicare Part B patients (CMS-MLN, 2021). While the NIA has not endorsed any specific screening tool, clinicians should be alert for any early signs or symptoms of cognitive impairment (e.g., problems with memory or language) (NIA, 2021). Routine screening for dementia in adults in whom cognitive impairment is not suspected is not recommended at this time due to a lack of evidence to support the benefit (U.S. Preventive Services Task Force [USPSTF], 2020; Hughes, 2014). Rather than home screening tests for dementia, the Alzheimer's Association recommends basic screening for language disturbances and memory problems (both recent and remote memories) within a context of a comprehensive assessment by a competent health-care provider. The screening results determine the need for further assessment of cognitive decline.

In the primary care setting, three issues leading to avoidance of cognition screening may be paramount. First, the time required for testing cognition may interfere with time requirements to attend to medical problems. Second, the sensitivity and specificity of various instruments for testing cognition is an important consideration. Third, clinicians may lack experience performing these assessments and nonstandard approaches can make a difference in the findings. Therefore, clinicians should be familiar with several possible American Geriatric Society (AGS) instruments and determine which is most appropriate for use in their own settings. (Teaching videos of experienced clinicians performing several types of cognition and dementia assessments are available on the Dementia Friendly America Web site [dfamerica.org]).

One instrument that holds promise for rapid screening in primary care is the Mini-Cog test; it takes 2 to 4 minutes to administer, has good sensitivity (76%–99%) and specificity (89%–96%), and has been validated in primary care (Li et al., 2018; Harvan & Cotter, 2006). The test includes registration and recall of three words/items and the ability to draw a clock face with hands representing a specified time. Copies of the Mini-Cog form and scoring criteria are free online.

The Montreal Cognitive Assessment (MoCA) is the most sensitive instrument for detecting mild cognitive impairment and is recommended by Hartford Institute for Geriatric Nursing. The MoCA Test Web site (mocatest.org) contains detailed instructions and normative data for this test in 35 languages.

If cognitive impairment is detected with a brief screening, the clinician should use judgment to determine whether a more extensive cognitive assessment is warranted. A referral may be made to a trained neurocognitive specialist who would complete a more thorough examination. Many cognitive tests are aimed at evaluating cognitive function, which measures short- and long-term (i.e., remote) memory, as well as orientation to time and place, registration, attention and calculation, recall, naming, repetition, comprehension, reading, writing, and drawing. Historically, the Mini Mental Status Examination (MMSE) has been used as a cognitive assessment tool in the older population. Almost all cognitive testing has been compared to this 30-item gold standard of mental health assessment tools. The MMSE is no longer in the public domain but is available for purchase only to qualified health-care professionals through Psychological Assessment Resources on the PARINC Web site (parinc.com).

Whenever there is a question of cognitive impairment, screening for depression is warranted. Depression as well as anxiety may have an atypical presentation, mimicking a dementia presentation, but it can also coexist with dementia. The most commonly used instrument to screen for depression is the Geriatric Depression Scale (GDS; Box 22.4). Originally, the GDS contained 30 items, but a shorter 15-item version (Short GDS) has comparable results.

Box 22.4

Geriatric Depression Scale (GDS, Short Form)

Choose the best answer for how you felt over the past week.

1. *Are you basically satisfied with your life?*   yes/**no**
2. *Have you dropped many of your activities and interests?*   **yes**/no
3. *Do you feel that your life is empty?*   **yes**/no
4. *Do you often get bored?*   **yes**/no
5. *Are you in good spirits most of the time?*   yes/**no**
6. *Are you afraid that something bad is going to happen to you?*   **yes**/no
7. *Do you feel happy most of the time?*   yes/**no**
8. *Do you often feel helpless?*   **yes**/no
9. *Do you prefer to stay at home, rather than going out and doing new things?*   **yes**/no
10. *Do you feel you have more problems with memory than most?*   **yes**/no
11. *Do you think it is wonderful to be alive now?*   yes/**no**
12. *Do you feel pretty worthless the way you are now?*   **yes**/no
13. *Do you feel full of energy?*   yes/**no**
14. *Do you feel that your situation is hopeless?*   **yes**/no
15. *Do you think that most people are better off than you are?*   **yes**/no

Score 1 point for each bolded answer. Cutoff: normal (0–5); above 5 suggests depression.

Source: Courtesy of Jerome A. Yesavage, MD. For 30 translations of the GDS, see https://web.stanford.edu/~yesavage/GDS.html

For additional information on administration and scoring, refer to the following references:

1. Sheikh, J. I., & Yesavage, J. A. (1986). Geriatric Depression Scale: Recent evidence and development of a shorter version. *Clinical Gerontology, 5*, 165–172.

2. Feher, E. P., Larrabee, G. J., & Crook, T. H., 3rd. (1992). Factors attenuating the validity of the Geriatric Depression Scale in a dementia population. *Journal of the American Geriatrics Society, 40*(9), 906–909.

3. Yesavage, J. A., Brink, T. L., Rose, T. L., Lum, O., Huang, V., Adey, M., Leier, V. O. (1983). Development and validation of a geriatric depression rating scale: A preliminary report. *Journal of Psychiatric Research, 17*(1), 37–49.

The presentation of depression in the older patient may be atypical, with fatigue and somatic symptoms predominating; therefore, traditional criteria (i.e., *DSM-V*) for diagnosis of depression may not apply. Although routine screening for depression in older adults is often overlooked, it should be routinely performed since older adults make up 13% of the U.S. population but account for 20% of all suicide deaths (MHA, 2021), and depression is difficult to detect in older adults (U.S. Preventive Services Task Force, 2013).

Anxiety can also have an atypical presentation in older patients, making it more difficult to diagnose. Anxiety is one of the most common psychiatric complaints throughout the lifespan and affects 10% to 20% of the older population (GMHF, 2021). Anxiety may lead to other problems by increasing isolation, decreasing independence, worsening physical health, and increasing mortality. Older patients with anxiety may be less observant, possibly developing a type of tunnel vision and diminished ability to hear, understand, or retain instructions and information. Anxiety screening tools are listed in Box 22.5. The clinician should inquire about certain symptoms of anxiety, which may trigger further evaluation. Common examples of anxious behaviors include rapid speech; restlessness and/or inability to sit still; and repetitive, purposeless movements such as rocking, pill-rolling of the fingers, and tapping of foot. The anxious person may exhibit exaggerated or blunted mood; the inability to maintain an organized conversation or thoroughly answer questions; or uncooperative, hostile, guarded, or suspicious behaviors.

Box 22.5

Anxiety Scales

Beck Anxiety Inventory:

https://res.cloudinary.com/dpmykpsih/image/upload/great-plains-health
-site-358/media/1087/anxiety.pdf

Geriatric Anxiety Inventory-Short form (GAI-SF):

http://http://gai.net.au/

State-Trait Anxiety Inventory (STAI):

http://oml.eular.org/sysModules/obxOml/docs/ID_150/State-Trait-Anxiety
-Inventory.pdf

Hamilton Anxiety Scale:

https://dcf.psychiatry.ufl.edu/files/2011/05/HAMILTON-ANXIETY.pdf

Hospital Anxiety Inventory:

https://www.svri.org/sites/default/files/attachments/2016-01-13/HADS.pdf

---

Loneliness and Social Isolation

Loneliness and social isolation affect nearly 25% of older adults (CDC, 2020b). Older adults are more likely to live alone, experience loss of family and friends, suffer from chronic illness, have decreased social support nearby, be unable to independently travel, and have hearing loss. Research studies have shown increases in the following consequences of social isolation:

- premature death from all causes
- risk of developing dementia
- risk of heart disease and stroke
- rates of depression, anxiety, and suicide
- risk of death, hospitalization, and emergency department visits among heart failure patients

The CDC recommends that clinicians periodically assess patients who may be at risk and connect them to community resources for any needed assistance. Those at risk include vulnerable older adults, including immigrants, LGBTQ+ populations, minorities, and victims of elder abuse (CDC, 2020a).

Annual Wellness Examination

Annual wellness visits (AWVs) are highly encouraged by Medicare for older individuals. These are a benefit covered by their Part B insurance, and many insurance carriers often will reduce the older patient's premiums if an AWV is conducted on an annual basis (CMS-MLN, 2021). The initial wellness visit, referred to as the "Welcome to Medicare" preventive visit, may be conducted only within the first 12 months an individual becomes covered by Medicare Part B (CMS-MLN, 2021). This initial visit includes a review of the individual's medical and social history as well as a review of preventive services, including the following:

- Review and update of medical and surgical history, reconciliation of medication lists, identifying other providers involved in the patient's care, and summarizing the patient's acute care needs
- Certain screenings, vaccinations, and referrals for other care, if needed
- Height, weight, and blood pressure measurements
- Calculation of body mass index (BMI)
- Vision test
- Review of potential risk for depression and level of safety
- Social history screening for tobacco, alcohol, and illicit drug use
- Inquiry regarding advanced directives and information on having one implemented

After the initial year an older patient is enrolled in Medicare Part B, AWVs are suggested. The intent of the annual visit is to develop or update a personalized prevention plan of care designed to help prevent disease and disability based on the individual's current health and risk factors. A health risk assessment should be completed by the patient to assist in developing a personalized prevention plan to help promote health and safety. The visit will include:

- Review of the medical, social, and family history
- Development or updating of a list of current providers, diagnoses, and medications
- Height, weight, blood pressure, and other routine measurements
- Personalized health advice
- A list of risk factors and treatment options identified through screening

This visit is covered once every 12 months providing at least 11 full months have passed since the last wellness visit. Table 22.3 depicts the elements of the Annual Wellness Examination.

The Atypical Presentation of Common Conditions

The atypical presentation of common illnesses is a hallmark in geriatric care. The most common symptoms that may herald the onset of infection include cognitive changes, changes in the level of ADL or IADL abilities, decreased appetite, weight loss over a short period of time, or sudden onset of urinary incontinence. Even those patients who are already debilitated may exhibit a measurable decline in function from baseline. The following two case studies compare the presentations of illness for a simple urinary tract infection in two patients, one age 23 years and the other 83 years. The cases contrast the clinical reasoning processes used to arrive at a diagnosis.

CASE 1. Linda M. is a 23-year-old woman, gravida 0, who presents with a 24-hour history of severe dysuria, frequency, and urgency. Her symptoms began approximately 8 hours after sexual intercourse with her longtime male partner, with whom she has had a monogamous relationship for the past 2 years. She denies fever, flank pain, anorexia, or malaise. The last normal menstrual period began 2 weeks ago. She has been on a triphasic oral contraceptive for the past 4 years and has regular menstrual cycles every 28 days lasting 2 to 3 days without intermenstrual spotting or discharge. She denies vaginal discharge, odor, itching, or irritation. Although she has never had similar symptoms in the past, her sister has a long history of cystitis, so Linda attributes these symptoms to a urinary tract infection. She is otherwise in good health; does not smoke, drink alcohol, or take other drugs; and takes no medications other than her oral contraceptives and an occasional ibuprofen for headaches.

Physical signs include normal vital signs, mild suprapubic tenderness, and sensation of increased urgency with palpation over the bladder. There is no costovertebral angle tenderness. A clean-voided midstream urine sample reveals clear, straw-colored urine without obvious blood; dipstick analysis is positive for leukocyte esterase and nitrites.

Table 22.3

Elements of Annual Wellness Examinations

Screening	Required Elements
Review the risks for depression, including current or past issues regarding mood disorders	Use any approved depression screening tool
Functional abilities and safety screening	• Ability to successfully perform ADLs and IADLs • Fall risk • Hearing impairment • Home safety
History	Update medical and surgical history, any medical events which have occurred, allergies, and any other health-care providers
Assessment	**Required Elements**
Physical examination	• Height, weight, blood pressure, basic metabolic index • Other routine assessments as deemed appropriate based on medical and health history
Cognitive assessment	Assess cognition based on direct observation with consideration of information from the family and/or caregivers
Counseling	**Required Elements**
Written plan for screening (e.g., suggested screening over the next 5 or 10 years)	Basic written screening schedule: • Age appropriate preventive care • Recommendations from the United States Preventive Services Task Force (USPSTF) (e.g., screenings for breast cancer, cervical, prostate, or colon cancer; osteoporosis; and adequacy of pain management, if applicable) The Advisory Committee on Immunization Practices recommendations (e.g., influenza, pneumonia, shingles, and tetanus), individual's health risk assessment, health status, and health screening assessment
List of risk factors and conditions for which the primary, secondary, or tertiary interventions are recommended	• Any mental health conditions or any risk factors or conditions identified through an IPPE • A list of treatment options and their associated risks and benefits
Personalized health advice and referral as appropriate to health education or preventive counseling	• Community-based lifestyle interventions to reduce health risks and promote self-management and wellness • Fall prevention • Nutrition • Physical activity • Tobacco-use cessation • Weight loss

Adapted from: CDC (2017b), Bluestein et al. (2017).

For additional information on Medicare preventive services, http://www.cms.gov/Outreach-and-Education/Medicare-Learning-Network MLN/MLNProducts/PreventiveServices.html

CASE 2. Mary T. is an 83-year-old woman who has resided in a long-term care facility for the past 12 months. She has mild dementia of the Alzheimer's type; osteoporosis with a history of right femoral neck fracture status post–internal fixation and pinning 1 year ago; stage C congestive heart failure well controlled on a diuretic and a beta blocker; osteoarthritis of hands, knees, and low back; and a history of stage 1 breast cancer treated 10 years ago with lumpectomy and radiation. Functionally at baseline, Mary requires assistance with ADLs and IADLs and supervision for medications; she uses a walker and requires assistance to ambulate outside her room, but in her room she is able to get to the toilet or her chair without assistance with use of her walker; she is normally continent of urine and stool with an occasional episode of enuresis; she requires assistance with bathing and grooming; her appetite is good, and she feeds herself and eats with others in the dining room; her usual mental status is mild dementia, and she is alert, pleasant, and participates in many activities in the facility.

The nurse practitioner was called to the facility to see Mary for a sudden change in her condition, which began approximately 12 hours earlier. The nursing assistant on the evening shift reported that she did not eat any of her dinner and seemed more confused than usual. During the night, she was incontinent of urine three times, soaking the bed each time. When the charge nurse assessed her on rounds in the morning, Mary was very lethargic, did not know her name or where she was, could not respond appropriately to any questions, and became quite agitated when the nurse attempted to auscultate her heart and lungs. There had been no recent change in her medication regimen. Her vital signs were normal, and she was afebrile. There had been no change in her weekly weights, and her bowel movements had been regular. By the time the nurse practitioner arrived, Mary was very agitated, shouting and crying out for her dead husband; was trying to get out of her bed; and had been put in adult diapers, which were saturated with urine and stool. Her skin was warm and dry without any obvious lesions or erythema, her color was pale, and she was inconsolable and unable to respond coherently to any questions. Although the cardiac auscultation was less than ideal, the nurse practitioner did not appreciate any extra sounds or murmurs. Lung sounds were somewhat diminished at the bases bilaterally, but the lungs were clear to auscultation otherwise, although again, the examination was hampered by Mary's agitation. The abdominal examination was also unremarkable.

■ Case Analysis

Nurse practitioners can feel comfortable treating a patient such as Linda M. with a telephone consultation. Her symptoms do not suggest any complicating factors, and although the urine dipstick for leukocyte esterase is cost-effective with good sensitivity (75% to 96%) and specificity (94% to 98%), treatment without an examination or urinalysis is an acceptable option (Esherick, Clark, & Slater, 2013). In contrast, when faced with the situation of Mary T., the nurse practitioner must perform a more extensive examination in a timely manner, including at least a urinalysis and, if needed, a culture and sensitivity on a catheterized urine specimen, a complete blood count with differential, pulse oximetry if available, and possibly even a chest radiograph; blood cultures are rarely useful except in atypical presentations to validate empirical treatment or when systemic symptoms are present in a patient who is unable to provide adequate history (Godbole et al., 2020).

The differential diagnosis for an older patient with a sudden change in condition includes infectious processes, most commonly involving the lungs, skin, and gastrointestinal or urinary tracts; cardiac decompensation; drug toxicity; fecal impaction; and occult trauma from an undocumented fall or injury. With such a varied differential, a comprehensive examination is essential, and a thorough knowledge of the patient and the environment is more likely to guide the process of clinical reasoning. In the case of Mary T., the nurse practitioner examined the skin for obvious cellulitis; reviewed the record for changes in medication, weight, and stool pattern; and examined the heart, lungs, and abdomen for obvious signs of cardiac decompensation and pain. Armed with knowledge of the patient's previous level of function and the meager clinical findings, the nurse practitioner will prioritize the differential diagnoses with the following considerations.

Although Mary T. has Alzheimer's disease, a sudden worsening of cognitive status or level of consciousness is not characteristic of the progression of dementia and usually indicates what is commonly referred to as *delirium* (Box 22.6). Delirium is a reversible condition frequently caused by infection (Table 22.4). According to the nurse practitioner's chart review, Mary is not on any new medications or any medications likely to cause toxicity; there is a fairly stable record of normal bowel movements, so impaction or gastroenteritis are not the likely culprits; and there was no recent weight gain, which is common in worsening congestive heart failure, although another weight should be obtained to compare with the most recent one. When a patient resides in an institution, the environment is a strong consideration in the analysis of the problem. In this case, there had been no recent outbreak of upper respiratory infection or influenza in the facility, so pneumonia is unlikely to be the cause. Tachypnea of greater than 25 breaths per minute, not seen in the case of Mary T., is one of the few physical findings with a positive predictive value (90%) for pneumonia, although pulse oximetry is helpful in absolutely ruling out pneumonia as a source of infection (Balogun & Philbrik, 2013). The physical examination did not reveal any other possible sources of sepsis, such as skin infections. The

---

Box 22.6

Decision Support: Cognitive Impairment

When there is a suspicion of delirium as a cause of cognitive impairment, the Confusion Assessment Method (CAM) is the most widely used and accurate algorithm, with a sensitivity of 46% to 100% and specificity of 90% to 95% when applied by trained health-care professionals (Francis, 2000). Delirium is present if there is an acute onset and fluctuating course, plus inattention, plus either disorganized thinking or altered level of consciousness. The findings of inattention, disorganized thinking, and altered level of consciousness can be demonstrated by the MMSE and a trained caregiver's or professional's observations.

Table 22.4

Differentiating Dementia, Depression, and Delirium in the Older Patient

Characteristic	Dementia	Depression	Delirium
Onset	Insidious	Insidious or precipitated by an event	Acute
Duration	Months–years	Months–years	Hours–days
Fluctuations	No or occasional due to stress	Some, may feel worse in the morning	Prominent with abnormal day/night cycles
Affect	Labile	Flat	Variable
Alertness	Normal or lethargic	Normal or lethargic	Highly variable from lethargy to agitation
Attention	Normal to progressively abnormal inattention	Normal to mildly distracted	Prominently abnormal, fluctuates
Orientation	Impaired but may be close to correct	Normal	Usually abnormal, may fluctuate
Memory	Abnormal	Normal	Normal when registers
Speech/language	Anomic or worse	Normal to slightly slowed	Dysarthric/misnaming
Speech content	Empty or sparse	Normal	Confused or incoherent
Perceptual	Normal to moderately abnormal	Normal	Hallucinations common

sudden onset of complete incontinence in a patient who has been mostly continent could be due to either the cognitive changes attendant to delirium or an infection in the urinary tract. Several urinary pathogens, most notably some of the strains of *Escherichia coli*, have a direct irritative effect on bladder mucosa and can cause incontinence.

Clinical and laboratory findings that support a diagnosis of urinary tract infection include an elevated white blood cell count higher than $14,000/mm^3$ or a left shift; pyuria on the microscopic urinalysis of greater than 10 white blood cells per high-power field; or a positive leukocyte esterase test. The absence of pyuria is equally significant in that it provides a negative predictive value approaching 100% and is therefore more useful in excluding the diagnosis of urinary tract infection (Balogun & Philbrik, 2013; Bentley et al., 2001). Additionally, clinical practice guidelines suggest that in 77% of episodes of functional decline in long-term-care residents, infection is the cause, and the most frequent site of such infection is the urinary tract (55%). Taking all of this into consideration, urinary tract infection is the most likely diagnosis for Mary at this point.

It is clear from this case analysis that a simple urinary tract infection can cause widespread and rapid physical decline in frail older persons, particularly those who are institutionalized. The assessment process is much more involved and less focused when there is an atypical presentation, which is common among older patients regardless of whether they reside in long-term care or present to the emergency department from home. Adequate treatment of the underlying infection should resolve the delirium, and the patient should return to baseline functioning.

Geriatric Syndromes

There is no commonly accepted definition or list of "geriatric syndromes." There is, however, some agreement about their common characteristics. Geriatric syndromes tend to be multifactorial in nature, have vague or atypical presentations, progress so as to result in frailty, are often interrelated, and display some degree of iatrogenesis or medical error. In short, they are often precipitated by a convergence of events that cause a cascade of further problems and end in a serious change of health status. Case 2 in the preceding section is an example of the geriatric syndrome of delirium, which was precipitated by a urinary tract infection and led to urinary incontinence. It is not unusual for such a situation to progress rapidly to additional adverse events: a fall as the patient attempts to climb out of bed, malnutrition and dehydration owing to the loss of appetite and the presence of infection, and skin breakdown resulting from the constant presence of urine on the perineal and coccygeal areas. Many of the geriatric syndromes are adverse events that occur as a result of immobility and hospitalization or inappropriate prescribing of medications; such syndromes require systems interventions to improve or change outcomes. Among these are seven syndromes—bladder control issues, sleep problems, delirium, dementia, falls, osteoporosis, and weight loss—and these are considered iatrogenic events. These types of consequences are often labeled as "medical errors" because they are largely preventable in older hospitalized patients (Wu, Bellantoni, & Weiner, 2020; Health in Aging, 2015).

The reasons older adults fall are diverse and include affective disorders and psychiatric conditions, cardiovascular diseases, infectious and metabolic conditions, musculoskeletal disorders, neurological conditions, sensory abnormalities, and iatrogenic situations such as functional decline resulting from hospitalizations or following procedures and side effects or adverse effects caused by medications and therapies.

It is important that nurse practitioners have a basic understanding of the risk factors, causes, and clinical presentations of geriatric syndromes and routinely assess for factors that may be amenable to intervention beyond the medical issues. Prevention is particularly important in managing geriatric syndromes both in the hospitalized and in the community-residing older patient. For example, falls in the home can be prevented with a thorough evaluation of any senior who reports a single fall or who demonstrates an unsteady gait; an appropriate intervention should be instituted for any problems detected.

Falling in an older individual can lead to injuries that can be detrimental to a person's health and independence and could lead to death (e.g., death caused by a head injury). After a person recovers from a fall, there could be posttraumatic

Box 22.7

Fear of Falling Scales

Activities-Specific Balance Confidence (ABC) Scale

The 16-item ABC can be self-administered or administered via personal or by phone or video interview. The tool prompts adults to rate their confidence that they will lose their balance or become unsteady in the course of daily activities. Available: https://sites.temple.edu/rtassessment/files/2018/10/Activities-Specific-Balance -Confidence-ABC-Scale.pdf

Falls Efficacy Scale (FES)

FES is a 10-item rating scale to assess confidence in performing daily activities without falling.
Available: https://www.sralab.org/sites/default/files/2018-08/Falls-Efficacy -Scale.pdf

---

anxiety with worry that another fall will occur. Fear of falling tools are clinically useful. Two are summarized in Box 22.7.

Details of the fall provide direction for further investigation. Date, time, and location of the fall provide important clues, as does detail about what the patient was experiencing before the fall. Ask about the presence of dizziness, blurred vision, weakness, palpitations, and a sensation of faintness preceding the fall and an awareness or lack thereof of the sensation of falling in an effort to uncover possible medical reasons for the fall. The get-up-and-go test is a simple screening measure that takes only minutes and can be conducted by trained staff. Instruct the patient to stand up from a seated position without using the patient's arms or the chair arms for support, walk a few feet away, turn around and return to the chair, and sit down again without using any support. If the examiner observes any instability or difficulty with this test, further evaluation of gait and balance is required.

Using the example of falls again, a home safety evaluation that includes questions about lighting, clutter on floors, footwear, bathroom configuration, stairways, sidewalks, and the availability of help in the case of a fall can focus attention on areas where safety can be improved to prevent falls. A useful tool that can be completed by patients or their families is available online in the Falls Toolkit from the Practicing Physicians Education in Geriatrics (2006) (U.S. Department of Veteran's Affairs, 2019). In the case of patients who frequently fall, a home visit by a nurse or physical therapist is very helpful when determining what risk factors are modifiable. When patients fall in hospitals or long-term care facilities, similar attention to environmental and other system factors that increase risk has been shown to reduce falls by as much as 30% (Cameron et al., 2018; Tsilimingras et al., 2003). Owing to the multifactorial nature of falling, interventions are most successful when they go beyond a simple plan to treat medical risk factors. A multidisciplinary approach that includes patient and family education, training in gait and balance, strengthening exercises, nutrition counseling, behavior modification, and elimination of environmental hazards has been found to be most successful.

Pressure ulcers are another common condition that is preventable both in the home and in institutional settings. Tissue trauma occurs when soft tissue is compressed between a bony prominence and a hard or rough surface or when shearing of the skin occurs with movement such as sliding a patient across bed sheets. The trauma produces visible change of the skin, ranging from a mild erythema or discoloration to deep ulceration down to bone. The important point to remember when assessing individuals who are immobile and dependent in ADLs as well as those being cared for at home is to include the caregivers in the process and to use it as a teachable opportunity. Ask about caregivers' knowledge of the importance of keeping skin clean and dry and their ability to move, transfer, and position the patient. Remind caregivers that an older adult who is not moving or turning independently should be repositioned every 2 hours to prevent pressure ulcer development. Support for caregivers is a crucial part of geriatric care and one that is often forgotten in clinical practice. Provide links to caregivers for access to educational services as well as additional aging services, such as respite care, caregiver support groups, and social service guides to help families cope with the burden of caregiving.

Frailty has been suggested for inclusion as a geriatric syndrome. It is characterized by age-associated declines in physiological reserve and function across multiple organ systems, leading to increased vulnerability for adverse health outcomes. Frailty can be defined as a distinct clinical syndrome meeting three or more of the following criteria: weakness, slowness, low level of physical activity, self-reported exhaustion, and unintentional weight loss (Chen et al., 2014). The physiological process of chronic inflammation likely directly and indirectly plays a major role in the development of a frailty syndrome, a cascade of problems due to the interrelated function of multiple body systems (e.g., musculoskeletal, endocrine, hematological). Attention should include risk assessment and prevention of adverse health effects. Currently, management of frail older patients includes exercise to improve physiological reserves and comprehensive interdisciplinary assessment to identify potential problems and develop a realistic expectation of probable outcomes.

The Assessment of Physical Activity Readiness

Older adults are increasingly turning to exercise for socialization and fitness and this trend should be supported to improve strength and balance. The question always arises, how much screening and assessment should be conducted prior to initiating an exercise program? A screening tool utilized by many health-care professionals is the PAR-Q+, a four-page document that contains a range of questions to identify any possible restrictions or limitations on activity levels and exercise participation. The older adult answers the seven questions on page 1 of the PAR-Q+. If the answer is no to all seven questions, the individual is cleared for unrestricted physical activity participation following the general physical activity guidelines for healthy asymptomatic populations. If the participant answers yes to one or more of the questions, the individual is required to complete pages 2 and 3 of the PAR-Q+ (Bredin et al., 2013). These guidelines could serve as a screening tool in primary care for older adults who are just beginning an exercise program; however, it is important to remove barriers to exercise whenever possible for those who wish to begin exercising at any age.

The Assessment of Driving Safety

Most people rely on personal transportation, such as driving an automobile, as the most convenient and efficient mode of transportation for obtaining medical services, groceries, and other necessities of life, as well as for maintaining social contact with friends, families, and organizations, such as a church or place of employment. The need to drive might be related to a lack of public transportation as well as to a sense of independence associated with driving that many seniors are reluctant to relinquish. The ability of an older individual to drive safely is dependent on several factors, which need to be considered in a comprehensive assessment of that individual. Drivers 65 years and older account for 15% of the total driving population yet account for 7% of all automobile accidents and 25% of all fatal crashes, making unsafe driving among the older population a significant and growing public health problem (IIHS, 2021; American Medical Association [AMA], 2010).

■ Driving Safety: General History

At least one or two questions about driving should be included in the comprehensive history of any older adult. Questions might be as simple as "Do you drive an automobile?" "Have you changed your driving patterns recently?" or "Are there any situations in which you feel uncomfortable driving?" Many seniors voluntarily restrict their driving when they recognize a feeling of discomfort with, for example, driving after dark or driving on high-speed highways. In addition, families might express concerns about the ability of a senior to drive safely with such comments as "He's had a couple of near misses with the car recently" or "No one will ride with her anymore because it's too scary." Comments from family members should always be addressed with both the family and the patient. It is important to remember that increasing chronological age is not an indicator of an inability to drive safely.

■ Focused History

Another screening option for driving safety is to give all older patients the questionnaire "Am I a Safe Driver?" (included in the AGS 2019 *Clinician's Guide to Assessing and Counseling Older Drivers* and freely available on the National Highway Traffic Safety Administration Web site). Positive responses can provide a starting point for a more comprehensive evaluation of driving safety. The AGS

Box 22.8

Medications That Might Affect Driving Ability

1. Alcohol
2. Anticholinergics
3. Anticonvulsants
4. Antidepressants
   a. Bupropion
   b. Mirtazapine
   c. Monoamine oxidase (MAO) inhibitors
   d. Selective serotonin reuptake inhibitors (SSRIs)
   e. Tricyclic antidepressants (TCAs)
5. Antiemetics
6. Antihistamines
7. Antihypertensives
8. Antiparkinsonians
9. Antipsychotics
10. Benzodiazepines and other sedatives/anxiolytics
11. Muscle relaxants
12. Narcotic analgesics
13. NSAIDs
14. Stimulants
15. Cannabis

resource on safe driving contains other useful resources for practice, state licensing and reporting laws, and ways to encourage safe driving as well as cessation of driving in certain individuals.

Certain medical conditions or medications should be red flags to the nurse practitioner as areas for exploration of medically impaired driving. Obvious acute events include myocardial infarction, stroke, brain injury, syncope, vertigo, seizures, delirium, or recent surgery. Other chronic conditions include those that affect vision, cognition, strength, mobility, and uncontrolled diabetes mellitus. The most common offending medications are listed in Box 22.8. Any new medication has the potential to affect driving ability temporarily; thus, patients should be cautioned to restrict driving at least temporarily until the response to the new medication is known.

■ Habits

Alcohol consumption is known to impair driving ability in any driver and may be an even greater concern among older persons. Ask specifically about the type, quantity, and timing of drinking behavior, and verify with an independent observer if possible.

■ Physical Assessment for Driving Ability

The AGS guidelines provide useful information on appropriate physical examination techniques to validate medical recommendations about driving ability; however, the report cautions that there are currently no tests that predict crash risk in the older population. These tests focus on vision, cognition, and motor function and can be integrated into the routine examination. Begin with a general observation of the patient, including orientation and alertness, general appearance, stability of gait, and interactive ability, looking specifically for signs of depression, dementia, delirium, motor instability, or generalized weakness. Vision is responsible for 95% of driving-related inputs (AGS, 2019), and vision testing should at least include tests for visual acuity and assessments of visual fields. Although contrast sensitivity is an important factor in the ability to distinguish objects against a background, currently there are no validated clinical measures for this dimension of vision. Decreased accommodation also contributes to discomfort with driving at night and is easily tested but not easily quantified.

Cognition is the most complex variable to test in the driving safety assessment. The ability to drive the car and navigate from one point to another requires many complex cognitive skills: crystallized and working memory, awareness-alertness and ability to stay focused, visual perception and processing, visuospatial skills, and executive skills (AGS, 2019). These skills are not adequately tested on the MMSE; therefore, supplemental tests specific to the higher executive functions are suggested, such as the clock-drawing test and the trail-making test (available on the NHTSA Web site). There are specific criteria for scoring each of these additional tests as well as clear directions for their administration. Research has demonstrated that the trail-making test, part B, is a reasonable predictor of "at-fault" crashes in older drivers (NHTSA, 2021; Staplin et al., 2003). It is possible that a patient with mild dementia according to the MMSE could still score well enough on these supplemental tests to continue driving. The problem arises when the dementia progresses and those afflicted fail to recognize that they have become unsafe drivers. This usually results in family members being forced to take away the driving privilege and/or request the assistance of the nurse practitioner or other professionals.

Motor ability testing involves testing range of motion in the neck, motor strength in both upper limbs and the right lower limb, and trunk stability and balance. Adequate range of motion of the neck without excessive pain or hesitation is essential for checking behind and to the sides of the car. Often a patient with a lack of central vision owing to macular degeneration can still drive safely if the peripheral vision is intact and the ability to turn the head quickly allows adequate scanning of the street and traffic situations. Although adequate range of motion is difficult to quantify, it is rarely the sole reason for restriction of driving. Upper limb strength is essential for steering, and the lower right limb is usually the one used for acceleration and braking. Strength should be graded on a scale of 0 to 5, with 4 to 5 signifying adequate strength against at least some resistance. Adaptive technologies in some automobiles may compensate for less than adequate strength in one or more areas. The rapid pace walk is specifically suggested (AGS, 2019) as a good predictor of driving safety. In this test, the patient is timed walking as swiftly as possible along a 10-foot path marked on the floor both away from and returning back toward the examiner. A cane can be used, but this should be noted on the chart. A completion time of greater than 9 seconds indicates a possible need for intervention.

■ Resources

Many states now have safe-driving programs for at-risk drivers that provide further testing and driver rehabilitation. Testing might include on-road tests or computerized simulations of driving situations. Some vision problems can be corrected with lenses or other medical interventions, although a referral might be needed to an ophthalmologist or low-vision specialist. Automobiles that are easier to drive, have controls in more convenient locations, better visibility, back-up cameras and night vision mirrors; and are fully automatic rather than manual may compensate for restricted movement and strength, allowing an older person to continue driving for longer. Restricting driving to familiar locations, daylight hours, low-traffic situations, and good weather may also suffice in some situations. The AGS (2019) strongly recommends against the use of a "copilot" to allow unsafe drivers to continue driving, although this practice has been accepted by some state driver-licensing agencies. Even the best and most observant copilots might not have time to alert the driver to a potential hazard, and the driver might not respond quickly enough to avoid a crash.

Addressing patient and family concerns about safe driving for an older individual is one of the most common issues in clinical practice. It is incumbent on nurse practitioners to know the laws in the state where they practice regarding reporting medically unsafe drivers; reporting guidelines vary across the country. Besides reporting or referring questionably safe drivers for further evaluation, it is important to help patients and their families plan for a transition to a nondriving status because everyone who drives will stop driving one day. Make both local and national resources available for patients facing this dilemma (Box 22.9). Open the dialogue at every opportunity with patients and their families to monitor changes and the need for further interventions. Incorporate an awareness of the need for and an ability to accomplish an evaluation of an older person for safe driving.

Habits

Alcohol consumption is known to impair coordination and can lead to falls or other injuries. Ask specifically about the type, quantity, and timing of drinking behavior. Inquire regarding any complications caused by alcohol use such as mood disorders, health issues, falls, effects on the person's ability to perform daily activities, and other consequences such as gastritis or accidents in a motor vehicle. Identification of alcohol dependence or alcohol abuse requires further investigation.

Use of tobacco products as in cigarette smoking, cigar smoking, tobacco chewing, dipping, or vaping can lead to lung disease and cancer as well as various

---

Box 22.9

Resources for Safe Driving

AARP 55 ALIVE Driver Safety Program

1-888-227-7669, https://www.aarp.org/auto/driver-safety/

American Automobile Association (AAA) Foundation for Traffic Safety

1-800-993-7222, www.aaafoundation.org

AAA Safe Driving for Mature Operators Program

Call your local AAA club to find a class near you.

National Safety Council Defensive Driving Course

1-800-621-7619, https://www.nsc.org/safety-training/defensive-driving

Driving School Association of the Americas

1-800-270-3722, www.thedsaa.org

---

other health conditions. It can also contribute to safety concerns, including risk of burns or fire.

Use of controlled substances to manage anxiety, insomnia, and pain on a routine basis can lead to dependence and addiction as well as cause other problems such as falling. Opioid dependence and addiction have become a major concern due to the high potential to cause death. Cannabis or marijuana is becoming more common as states move toward legalizing its use either with a prescription for medical necessity or as a recreational drug. Screening for use of any of these substances is essential, as well as screening for use of nonprescription substances that have potential for abuse.

Polypharmacy

Polypharmacy is commonly referred to as taking five or more medications daily. Most older patients take at least five medications daily. Forty percent of older individuals take 5 to 9 medications, and 18% take 10 or more medications on a daily basis (Fixen, 2019). Each medication has intended effects and adverse effects and can interact with other medications. The combined effects lead to increased utilization of health care with increases in emergency department visits, increased hospitalizations, increased costs of care, and increased morbidity and mortality.

The Beers Criteria were developed by the AGS in 1991 and have been updated every 3 years since 2012 to include newer medications. This list makes recommendations on medications that may be inappropriate for older adults. The recommendations grade the medications into categories: medications that should be avoided in all older patients, medications that should be avoided in older patients with certain conditions, and medications that can be utilized with caution in certain circumstances. These recommendations assist the clinician in determining whether a medication is appropriate in a given situation.

Head, Eyes, Ears, Nose, and Mouth

Specific attention should be directed toward those organs that affect functional ability: the eyes, ears, and mouth directly affect one's ability to see, hear, and eat. There are some particular points to remember when assessing these systems:

- An examination of the eyes should always include measuring ocular pressure to rule out glaucoma, which is a serious cause of blindness and is more common with aging; corneal arcus, which could be a sign of hyperlipoproteinemia; screening for close and distance vision, particularly when there are questions related to driving or medication-taking ability; dilating the pupil to examine the retina for macular degeneration, a common cause of blindness in the older population; and screening for cataracts, also increasingly common with age. Referral to an optometrist or an ophthalmologist is ideal and may be covered by Medicare and other insurance depending on the diagnosis. An annual vision examination is recommended. Older patients with a diagnosis of diabetes should have a retinal examination at least every 2 years, annually or more often if abnormalities such as diabetic retinopathy are identified (Holland, 2020).
- Examination of the ears should include carefully inspecting and removing cerumen impactions, which are a common cause of hearing loss. A reliable screening test for hearing is the whisper test, which is performed by standing behind the patient at a distance of 24 to 36 inches, having the patient cover one ear, and having the patient repeat the words whispered by the examiner. In addition to the whisper test, screening with an audioscope at 40 dB and testing both ears using 1,000 and 2,000 Hz provides reasonable sensitivity (94%) and specificity (72%) in community-dwelling populations (Lycke et al., 2018). Referral to an audiologist is ideal, although many seniors do not have the ability to pay for hearing aids, and in some cases hearing aids do not help with speech discrimination.
- Examination of the mouth should include a thorough inspection of the teeth as well as the oral mucosa. Ill-fitting or missing dentures and loose teeth can severely affect an older person's ability to chew and eat sufficient food to maintain adequate nutrition. Referral to a dentist is ideal; however, many seniors without dental insurance do not have the ability to pay for dental services or replacement dentures.

Neuromuscular System

Specific attention should be directed toward gait and mobility, which greatly affect functional ability and predict a person's risk of falling. Beyond the usual examination of range of motion and strength, there are several specific tests to measure performance that can be incorporated into an examination:

- The timed get-up-and-go test should be administered to all patients who have experienced a fall, who feel unsteady on their feet with standing or walking, or who report difficulty with strenuous activities, such as fast walking, heavy housework, shopping, or climbing stairs. It is easy to perform and takes very little additional time during the examination. Place a chair in an unobstructed location and instruct the patient to rise from the seated position, walk 20 feet, turn, walk back to the chair, and sit down. Time this activity with a stopwatch. In populations that cannot complete the task in 15 seconds or less, research has shown a strong correlation (0.6–0.8) with other measures of gait and balance (CDC, 2017).

- Contributors to pathologic gait include foot or joint pain, weakness, sensory impairment, bone and joint abnormalities, and an impaired neurological system (Webster & Darter, 2019). The Tinetti Performance-Oriented Mobility Assessment (POMA) scale is a more sensitive and specific test of gait, balance, and mobility. The gait and mobility components of the POMA include opportunities to evaluate the initiation of gait, adequacy of step length and height, step and path symmetry and continuity, and ability to turn and pick up speed. Balance is tested by observing immediate standing balance; balance during tandem, one-leg, heel, and toe standing; and a nudge to the sternum or tug from behind. The POMA is sensitive and reproducible and can be used to measure improvement over time; thus, it is often used in clinical trials of exercise interventions.

- The functional reach test is another useful test for upper extremity function that correlates well with an increased risk for falls and dependence (Williams et al., 2017). Give the patient the following instructions: Stand with your feet hip-width apart and your dominant side next to but not touching a wall. Extend the arm closest to the wall, parallel to the floor at shoulder height with fingers extended. Now reach forward as far as you can, bending at the waist, but do not lift your heels off the floor. The examiner measures the distance in centimeters from the back of the shoulder to the tip of the middle finger in the "normal reach" position and again in the "forward reach" position. Differences greater than 25 cm are a significant predictor of falls and increased dependence in ADLs and IADLs.

Nutritional Assessment

According to Dwyer et al. (2019) and Kaiser et al (2010), nutritional deficiencies are a common problem among older adults. The overall rate of nutritional deficiencies is 40%, with rates varying depending on setting: 5.8% for community-dwelling older adults, 38.7% in hospital settings, 13.8% in nursing homes, and 50.5% in rehabilitation settings. Older adults with low levels of serum albumin (below 3.0) on hospital admission show an increased risk of mortality, but the death rate is substantially reduced with a higher calorie intake according to Cabrerizo et al. (2015). Undernourishment among institutionalized older adults increases mortality rates and places discharged individuals at risk for serious malnutrition, which then predisposes the older adult to frailty, dependence, and long-term care placement.

One of the key factors for tracking malnutrition is measuring and recording patients' heights and weights and then calculating the basic metabolic index. The formula for calculating BMI is the same for older people as for any other population. A BMI of less than 21 or a total body weight of less than 100 pounds is an indicator of a high risk for protein–energy malnutrition. Although a lot of attention is devoted to undernutrition, obesity—defined as a BMI of greater than 30, or 20% greater than ideal body weight—is also an independent risk factor for functional decline in the older person. Women have a higher prevalence of functional decline than men at the upper end of the BMI categories (three times greater risk at a BMI of greater than 35) independent of the usual factors, such as depression and polypharmacy (Zhu et al., 2018; Jensen & Friedmann, 2002).

Most adults overestimate their height and underestimate their weight on self-report; height is a particular problem because adults tend to lose 1 inch of height every 20 years after age 35 to 40. The following are some tips to ensure accurate height and weight measures in difficult situations:

- Measurement of standing height is also difficult to estimate if there is any degree of kyphosis. If kyphosis is suspected, ask the patient to stand with the back and head against the wall. If the head does not touch the wall, measure and record that distance; greater than 2 cm distance indicates some degree of kyphosis, which may influence measured height.
- It is difficult to accurately measure height in older adults who cannot safely stand. Estimates of actual adult height can be made with either a wingspan or knee-to-heel measurement, although accuracy varies by gender, ethnicity, and age.
- For residents of long-term care facilities, always use the same scale for the same patient. Document what the patient is wearing, and always weigh in that same state when possible.
- For amputees, add the following percentages of the weight obtained on the scale prior to calculating the BMI: below knee 6%, at knee 9%, above knee 15%, arm 6.5%, arm below elbow 3.6%.

Nutrition screening can be accomplished by asking patients to complete diet records or food frequency questionnaires or by screening for other risk factors, such as those in the Nutrition Screening Initiative. The Nutrition Screening Initiative (Posner et al., 1993) is appropriately used with older persons and provides a screening tool with support documentation online. For residents in long-term care facilities, the Mini Nutritional Assessment on the MNA Web site is the best validated instrument for screening.

Useful laboratory measures that indicate protein–energy malnutrition or potentially poor outcomes in hospitalized older adults include a serum albumin level below 3.4 g/dL and total cholesterol below 160 mg/dL. An albumin level below 3.0 g/dL significantly increases an older person's risk for death.

Dehydration is common in the older person and has serious consequences. The average fluid intake for community-dwelling older persons is less than 1,000 mL per day. Thirst is not a reliable indicator of the need for fluids, and most older individuals need reminders to drink fluids. The best method for monitoring hydration status is with the blood urea nitrogen/creatinine ratio; anything greater than 20:1 is highly suggestive of dehydration.

The type and amount of food and fluids strongly influence the occurrence of constipation among older adults. The prevalence of constipation is about 30% among the older population regardless of their state of health. With a decrease in gastrointestinal motility and fluid intake, a tendency to eat easily digestible foods (i.e., less fibrous), and the common use of medications that are constipating, special attention should be directed toward the prevention of constipation. Additionally, older adults frequently use laxatives; routine laxative use occurs with more than 50% of residents in long-term care facilities. Besides causing great discomfort, constipation can lead to fecal impaction, which can be life-threatening.

Chronic Medical Conditions

The overall determination of an older patient's health includes assessment of all conditions and disease processes. Identifying any and all diagnoses and how the diagnosis impacts the individual's physical and psychological health as well as functional abilities will have significant impact upon the goals for health and lifestyle choices for the individual.

Advance Care Planning

Discussions about individual preferences for limits on medical intervention should be initiated long before an older patient becomes incapable of making their wishes known; such discussions should also be a routine part of primary care practice (Waller et al., 2019; Kass-Bartelmes & Hughes, 2003). All states recognize and provide guidelines for some type of official document that outlines an individual's care preferences. Nurse practitioners should become familiar with these documents and make them available to their patients or provide referrals to a service that can facilitate this process. Most of the time, patients make these decisions with their family members; however, it is not uncommon for families to disagree on the patients' decisions for their health-care directives. Patients who are cognitively intact should be allowed to choose how their health should be directed, based on their wishes. For nurse practitioners who care for residents of long-term care facilities, family discussions and case conferences are a useful way to assist in resolving any issues of disagreement.

To make good decisions, patients need to feel comfortable asking questions about death, dying, and medical interventions. They also need to be assured that having an advance care directive does not mean they will be abandoned by the health-care team. Decisions reached at any point are never irreversible; in fact, advance care decisions should be revisited at least annually and whenever a significant change in the patient's condition or the family's situation has occurred. Nurse practitioners can play a significant role in educating patients and their families about the realities of cardiopulmonary resuscitation, tube feedings, artificial ventilation, and other invasive procedures by giving factual and unhurried explanations. If the patient does not have a living will, designation of a person to serve as the power of attorney should be determined—the

---

Box 22.10

Decision Support: CPR Survival

Cardiopulmonary arrest occurring outside of a hospital setting has shown that less than 10% of patients survive. Research suggests that 40% percent of patients who receive cardiopulmonary resuscitation (CPR) after experiencing cardiac arrest in a hospital setting initially survived after being resuscitated, but only 10% to 20% survive long enough to be discharged from the hospital (AHA, 2021). Murphy and colleagues (1994) interviewed 287 older patients (mean age 77 years) in a geriatrics practice about their wishes to undergo CPR following a cardiac arrest during an acute illness. Before learning the facts about the probability of survival to discharge for older patients, 41% opted for CPR. After learning the probability of survival (10% to 17%), only 22% opted for CPR; of that number, only 6% older than age 85 would choose to undergo CPR in the same conditions. Using a scenario of having a chronic illness and choosing CPR when there was a life expectancy of 1 year or less, only 11% opted for CPR before learning the probability of survival to discharge after CPR declines to 0% to 5%; after the discussion, the number decreased to 5%. Prognostic information, when given during a discussion of decisions related to end-of-life choices, has a significant influence on older adults' decisions.

---

designation could be a medical power of attorney to make medical decisions and/or a legal power of attorney to make legal and financial decisions. Most people have only seen optimal outcomes after heroic efforts at resuscitation portrayed in the media; the realities of likely or average outcomes need to be addressed in order for individuals to make decisions consistent with their own values and wishes (Box 22.10).

Conclusion

The assessment of older individuals requires a thorough understanding of physiology, awareness of the patient's environment, good communication skills, avoidance of ageist thinking, and good critical-thinking ability—plus time and patience. It is often the lack of time that leads to problems. Sufficient time to perform some of the additional tests of functional ability and to talk with family and caregivers is optimal. Ideally, home assessments can be made in cases of a concern about safety and the ability to function independently. A multidisciplinary team approach facilitates management of complex situations and affords older patients and their families the best opportunities for maximizing health and quality of life.

REFERENCES

AARP. (2021). Researchers call for road improvements geared to older drivers. https://www.aarp.org/auto/trends-lifestyle/info-2018/older-drivers-road-issues-fd.html ACL. (2019). Minority Aging. Retrieved June 3, 2021 from https://acl.gov/aging-and-disability-in-america/data-and-research/minority-aging

AHA. (2021). Out-of-Hospital Chain of Survival. https://cpr.heart.org/en/resources/cpr-facts-and-stats/out-of-hospital-chain-of-survival

Alessi, C. (2000). Sleep. In D. Osterweil, K. Brummel-Smith, & J. Beck (Eds.), *Comprehensive geriatric assessment*. McGraw-Hill.

American Medical Association. (2010). *Physician's guide to assessing and counseling older drivers* (2nd ed.). American Medical Association. https://www.nhtsa.gov › nti › older_drivers › pdf

APA. (2021). American Psychological Association. Growing Mental and Behavioral Health Concerns Facing Older Americans. https://www.apa.org/advocacy/health/older-americans-mental-behavioral-health

Balogun, S., & Philbrik, J. (2014). Delirium, a symptom of UTI in the elderly: Fact or fable? A systematic review. *Canadian Geriatric Journal, 17*(1):22–26.

Bentley, D. W., Bradley, S., High, K., Schoenbaum, S., Taler, G., & Yoshikawa, T. T., (2001). Practice guideline for evaluation of fever and infection in long-term care facilities. *Journal of the American Geriatrics Association, 49*(2), 210–222.

Besdine, R. (2019). Quality of Life in Older People. Merck Manual (Online). https://www.merckmanuals.com/professional/geriatrics/aging-and-quality-of-life/quality-of-life-in-older-people

Blair, K. A. (1990). Aging: Physiological aspects and clinical implications. *Nurse Practitioner, 15*(2), 14–16, 18, 23, 26–28.

Bluestein, D., Diduk-Smith, R., Jordan, L., Persaud, K., & Hughes, T. (2017). Medicare annual wellness visits: How to get patients and physicians onboard. *Family Practice Management, 24*(2), 12–16.

Bluestein, D., & Rutledge, C. M. (2006). Perceived health and geriatric risk stratification: Observations from family practice. *Canadian Family Physician, 52*(5), 626–627.

Bredin, S., Gledhill, N., Jamnik, V., & Warburton, D. (2013). PAR-Q+ and ePARmed-X+: New risk stratification and physical activity clearance strategy for physicians and patients alike. *Canadian Family Physician. 59*(3): 273–277.

Cabrerizo, S., Cuadras, D., Gómez-Busto, F., Artaza, I., Martín Ciancas, F., & Malafarina, V. (2015). Serum albumin and health in older people: Review and meta analysis. *Maturitas. 81*(1), 17–27. https://doi.org/10.1016/j.maturitas.2015.02.009

Cameron, I., Dyer, S., Panagoda, C., Murray, G., Hill, K., Cumming, R., Kerse, S., & Cochran Bone, Joint and Trauma Group. (2018). Interventions for preventing falls in older people in care facilities and hospitals. *Cochran Database Systematic Review.* https://www.ncbi.nlm.nih.gov/pmc/articles/PMC6148705/

CDC. (2017a). Assessment/Timed Up & Go. https://www.cdc.gov/steadi/pdf/TUG_test-print.pdf

CDC. (2017b). Older persons' health. Retrieved from https://www.cdc.gov/nchs/fastats/older-american-health.htm

CDC. (2020a). Disability & Health Promotion. Disability Impacts All of Us. https://www.cdc.gov/ncbddd/disabilityandhealth/infographic-disability-impacts-all.html

CDC. (2020b). Loneliness and Social Isolation Linked to Serious Health Conditions. https://www.cdc.gov/aging/publications/features/lonely-older-adults.html

CDC. (2021a). Nursing Home Care. https://www.cdc.gov/nchs/fastats/nursing-home-care.htm

CDC. (2021b). The state of mental health and aging in America. Depression as a Public Health Issue. https://www.cdc.gov/aging/pdf/mental_health_brief_2.pdf

Chen, X., Mao, G., & Leng, S. (2014). Frailty syndrome: An overview. *Clinical Interventions in Aging, 9,* 433–441.

CMS. (2019). NHE Fact sheet. Retrieved March 3, 2021 from https://www.cms.gov/Research-Statistics-Data-and-Systems/Statistics-Trends-and-Reports/NationalHealthExpendData/NHE-Fact-Sheet#:~:text=Medicare%20spending%20grew%206.7%25%20to,31%20percent%20of%20total%20NHE

CMS. (2021). Medicare beneficiaries at a glance. https://www.cms.gov/Research-Statistics-Data-and-Systems/Statistics-Trends-and-Reports/Beneficiary-Snapshot/Downloads/Bene_Snaphot.pdf

CMS-MLN. (2021). Medicare Wellness Visits. https://www.cms.gov/Outreach-and-Education/Medicare-Learning-Network-MLN/MLNProducts/preventive-services/medicare-wellness-visits.html

Cotter, V., & Strumpf, N. E. (2002). Advanced practice nursing with older adults: Clinical guidelines. New York: McGraw-Hill.

Dwyer, J., Gahche, J., Weiler, M., Arensberg, M. B. (2019) Screening community-living older adults for protein energy malnutrition and frailty: Update and next steps. *Journal of Community Health, 45,* 640–660. https://link.springer.com/article/10.1007/s10900-019-00739-1

Esherick, J., Clark, D., & Slater, E. (2013). *CURRENT practice guidelines in primary care.* Lange Medical Books.

Fixen, D. (2019). 2019 AGS Beers criteria for older adults. *Pharmacy Today, 25*(11), 42–54.

Gerety, M. (2000). Health status and physical capacity. In D. Osterweil, K. Brummel-Smith, & J. Beck (Eds.), *Comprehensive geriatric assessment*. McGraw-Hill.

GMHF. (2021). Geriatric Mental Health Foundation: Anxiety and Older Adults: Overcoming Worry and Fear, https://www.aagponline.org/index.php?src=gendocs&ref=anxiety

Godbole, G. P., Cerruto, N., & Chavada, R. (2020). Principals of assessment and management of urinary tract infections in older adults. *Geriatric Therapeutics Review, 50*(3), 276–283. https://doi.org/10.1002/jppr.1650

Gumaer, D. (2019) What are the emotional needs of the elderly? Griswald Home Care. Retrieved June 3, 2021 from https://www.griswoldhomecare.com/blog/2019/december/what-are-the-emotional-needs-of-the-elderly-/

Harvan, J. R., & Cotter, V. T. (2006). An evaluation of dementia screening in the primary care setting. *Journal of the American Academy of Nurse Practitioners, 18*(8), 351–360.

Health in Aging. (2015). *A guide to geriatric syndromes.* Retrieved June 4, 2018, from https://www.healthinaging .org/tools-and-tips/tip-sheet-guide-geriatric-syndromes-common-and-often-related-medical-conditions

Holland, K. (2020). What you should know about diabetes and eye exams. Healthline. Retrieved April 16, 2021 from https://www.healthline.com/health/diabetes/diabetic-eye-exam

Hughes, S. (2014). USPSTF: No to routine screening for cognitive impairment. *Annals of Internal Medicine.* http://www.medscape.com/viewarticle/822581

IIHS. (2021). Older Drivers. Retrieved April 16, 2021, from https://www.iihs.org/topics/older-drivers

Jensen, G. L., & Friedmann, J. M. (2002). Obesity is associated with functional decline in community -dwelling rural older persons. *Journal of the American Geriatrics Society, 50*(5), 918–923.

Kaiser, M. J., Bauer, J. M., Rämsch, C., Uter, W., Guigoz, Y., Cederholm, T., Thomas, D. R., Anthony, P. S., Charlton, K. E., Maggio, M., Tsai, A. C., Vellas, B., Sieber, C. C., & the Mini Nutritional Assessment International Group. (2010). Frequency of malnutrition in older adults: A multinational perspective using the mini nutritional assessment. *Journal of the American Geriatrics Society, 58*(9), 1734–1738.

Kass-Bartelmes, B. L., & Hughes, R. (2003). Advance care planning: Preferences for care at the end of life. *Research in Action, 12.* Retrieved November 30, 2013, from www.ahrq.gov/research/findings/factsheets /aging/endliferia/index.html

Lawton, M. A., & Brody, E. M. (1969). Assessment of older people: Self-maintaining and instrumental activities of daily living. *Gerontologist, 9*(3), 179–186.

Li, X., Dai, J., Zhao, S., Liu, W., & Li, H. (2018). Comparison of the value of Mini-Cog and MMSE screening in the rapid identification of Chinese outpatients with mild cognitive impairment. *Medicine, 97*(22):e10966.

Lycke, M., Lefebvre, T., Cool, L., Van Eygen, K., Boterberg, T., Schofield, P., & Debruyne, P. (2018). Screening methods for age-related hearing loss in older patients with cancer: A review of the literature. *Geriatrics, 3*(3), 48.

Mental Health Association (MHA). (2021). Depression in Older Adults: Mental Health in Older Adults. https://www.mhanational.org/depression-older-adults

Moore, A. A., & Siu, A. L. (1996). Screening for common problems in ambulatory elderly: Clinical confirmation of a screening instrument. *American Journal of Medicine, 100*(4), 440.

Murphy, D. J., Burrows, D., Santilli, S., Kemp, A. W., Tenner, S., Kreling, B., & Teno, J. (1994). The influence of the probability of survival on patients' preferences regarding cardiopulmonary resuscitation. *New England Journal of Medicine, 330*(8), 545–549.

National Institute on Aging. (2003). The measurement of functioning in older adult populations (Report of meeting held on December 12, 2003). Retrieved from http://www.nia.nih.gov/sites/default/files/d7/meeting -report_19.pdf (accessed May 4, 2022)

NHCPO. (2019). A re-envisioned report on hospice access and usage in the U.S. Retrieved March 10, 2021, from https://www.nhpco.org/nhpco-releases-updated-edition-of-hospice-facts-and-figures-report/#:-:text=At %2098.2%20percent%2C%20Routine%20Home,percent%20and%2021%20percent%20respectively

NHTSA. (2021). Assessing and Counseling Older Drivers. https://one.nhtsa.gov/people/injury/olddrive /OlderDriversBook/pages/Chapter3.html

NIA. (2021). Dementia Resources For Health Professionals: Assessing Cognitive Impairment in Older Patients. https://www.nia.nih.gov/health/assessing-cognitive-impairment-older-patients

Posner, B. M., Jette, A. M., Smith, K. W., & Miller, D. W. (1993). Nutrition and health risks for the elderly: Nutrition Screening Initiative. *American Journal of Public Health, 83*(7), 972–978. https://www.ncbi .nlm.nih.gov/pmc/articles/PMC1694757/pdf/amjph00531-0046.pdf

Spanko, A. (2020). Spending growth on nursing home care falls far behind home health, hospitals. *Skilled Nursing News.*

Staplin, L., Lococo, K., Gish, K., & Decina, L. (2003). *Model driver screening and evaluation program: Final technical report volume II: Maryland pilot older driver study.* Department of Transportation and Highway Safety, Document # 809 583. Retrieved from https://www.nhtsa.gov/sites/nhtsa.gov/files/vol1scr.pdf.

Stepler, R. (2016). World centenarian population projected to grow eightfold by 2050. Pew Research Center. https://www.pewresearch.org/fact-tank/2016/04/21/worlds-centenarian-population-projected-to-grow -eightfold-by-2050/

Tsilimingras, D., Rosen, A. K., & Berlowitz, D. (2003). Patient safety in geriatrics: A call for action. *Journal of Gerontology: Biological Sciences and Medical Sciences, 58A*(9), 813–819.

U.S. Census. (2020). 65 and Older Population Grows Rapidly as Baby Boomers Age. Release number CB20-89. https://www.census.gov/newsroom/press-releases/2020/65-older-population-grows.html

U.S. Department of Veteran's Affairs. (2019). VHA National Center for Patient Safety: Fall toolkit. https://www.patientsafety.va.gov/professionals/onthejob/falls.asp

USPSTF. (2020). Cognitive impairment in older adults, Screening. https://www.uspreventiveservicestaskforce .org/uspstf/recommendation/cognitive-impairment-in-older-adults-screening

Waller, A., Sanson-Fisher, R., Nair, B., & Evans, T. (2019). Are older and seriously ill inpatients planning ahead for future medical care? *BMC Geriatrics. 19*, 212.

Webster, J., & Darter, B. (2019). *Principles of normal and pathological gait* (pp. 49–62). Elsevier Publishing.

Williams, B., Brandon Allen, B., Hu, Z., True, H., Cho, J., Harris, A., Fell, N., & Sartipi, M. (2017). Real time fall risk assessment using Functional Reach Test. *International Journal of Telemedicine & Applications.* https://www.ncbi.nlm.nih.gov/pmc/articles/PMC5259990/

Wu, S., Bellantoni, M., & Weiner, J. (2020). Geriatric syndrome risk factors among hospitalized postacute Medicare patients. *The American Journal of Managed Care, 26*(10).

Zhu, J., Xiang, Y., Cai, H., Li, H., Gao, Y., Zheng, W., & Shu, X. (2018). Associations of obesity and weight change with physical and mental impairments in elderly Chinese people. *Maturitas, 108*, 77–83.

Chapter 23
Persons With Disabilities

- Mary Jo Goolsby

P ersons with disabilities (PWD) comprise a large and diverse population. Over 56 million persons in the United States have at least one disability. The percentage of U.S. adults age 18 years and older reporting mobility, hearing, and vision disabilities in 2018 was 12.4%, 5.9%, and 5.0%, respectively (CDC, n.d.). PWD are more likely to face health care–related physical and communication barriers (Bauer et al., 2016). They are less likely to have a regular source of health care, and they may have unmet needs, including cancer screenings and vaccinations, and are more likely to have poor outcomes associated with conditions such as breast cancer due to delays in diagnosis (CDC, 2013; Horner-Johnson et al., 2014).

Issues related to the timeliness and quality of health care experienced by PWD have been addressed by policymakers at the state and federal levels. For instance, Healthy People 2020 set and met a goal for the proportion of adults with disabilities who experience delays in receiving primary and episodic preventive care due to barriers to decrease from the baseline of 49.5% to 44.6%. The Americans with Disabilities Act (ADA) requires that PWD receive health care equivalent to that available to others without disabilities (U.S. Department of Justice, 2010, 2014).

This chapter focuses on strategies to proactively promote readiness to perform each component of the physical examination properly, even when patients present with significant disabilities. The emphasis is on the subset of PWD that involves physical disabilities impacting a patient's mobility (persons with physical disabilities, or PWPD) and those with sensory deficits affecting communication.

Persons With Physical Disabilities (PWPD)

Consider the range of patients whose mobility limitations could challenge the ability to adequately examine them. These patients include individuals of all ages with conditions such as muscular dystrophy, cerebral palsy, stroke, spinal cord injury, and different forms of arthritis, as well as persons with recent acute limiting injuries or conditions. In spite of the ADA requirement for PWPD to receive care equivalent to that received by others, practice sites and clinicians often are ill-prepared to conduct necessary examinations when PWPD present. Faced with the complexity of working around these limitations, clinicians sometimes selectively omit components of the examination or conduct them on a seated patient in the absence of a wheelchair scale, height-adjustable examination table, or staff trained to assist PWPD in transferring to the examination table (Graham & Mann, 2008; Lagu et al., 2013; Morrison et al., 2008; Pharr, 2014). However, many components of the physical examination and diagnostic studies cannot be completed while a patient is seated. These include comprehensive assessment of cardiac murmurs, breast examination, percussion and palpation of abdominal structures, and the gynecological or perineal examination.

In order to provide equivalent care to PWPD, planning is required. Before starting the examination or encounter, discuss with the PWPD strategies to enable a careful examination—they are the experts on the level of assistance and accommodations needed in undressing and dressing, transferring, and positioning. Only when this is accomplished will the accuracy of the examination be optimized.

The physical examination for a PWPD often begins with accurate measurement of weight and vital signs. A wheelchair-accessible scale is a necessary piece of equipment for PWPD who cannot stand briefly to be weighed. In clinical decision-making, avoid the temptation to rely on a self-reported weight as a substitute for weighing persons who require a wheelchair; the PWPD may not have had access to a wheelchair scale elsewhere, and the reported weight is unlikely to be accurate. PWPD with conditions limiting mobility or those lacking tolerance in the upper extremities may require an alternative method of measuring blood pressure, for example, measuring radial or lower extremity blood pressure.

The visit should be coordinated so that the PWPD is seen in a room with a height-adjustable examination table that can be accessed from either side, depending on the patient's need. If the patient requires examination in a reclining posture, this will ensure the appropriate examination can be accomplished without having to move to another room. Of course, if the needed examinations do not require the PWPD to lie down, then there is no need to use the examination table.

Height-adjustable examination tables should lower to 17 to 20 inches, allowing for an easier transfer from wheelchair to table. For the patient's safety, staff should be available to assist in the transfer, as needed. The examination table should also be equipped with handrails or grips to assist the PWPD in transferring and positioning, as well to prevent a fall from the table. As needed, ask a staff person to remain during the examination to assist with any balance or repositioning needs. While PWPD may be accompanied by a friend or family member, this individual cannot be required to assist during the examination or to stay in the examination room, unless the patient so requests.

Prior to assisting the PWPD onto the examination table, discuss what is intended—the transfer to the examination table as well as the position(s) expected during the examination. Confirm what will help make the examination feasible and tolerated, optimizing comfort and maintenance of the position needed. For example, it may help to have positioning devices such as pillows or rolled or folded blankets available. Patients prone to spasticity, contractions, or pain may require slow and gentle supported movements. If a Foley catheter or other device is in place, plan to secure it to avoid dislodgement during the transfer and examination. Establish how the patient will communicate the need to slow or stop the examination; remember to observe the patient's facial expressions and body language to be sensitive to discomfort associated with the examination.

The pelvic examination is among the most challenging for PWPD. The following figures (Fig. 23.1–Fig. 23.5) depict alternatives for the traditional lithotomy position. As shown in Figure 23.5, if the patient cannot be positioned on an examination table, an alternative, such as a bed or mat, may be used. When a pillow can be placed beneath the buttocks to elevate the pelvic area while using an alternative position, the speculum can often be inserted in the

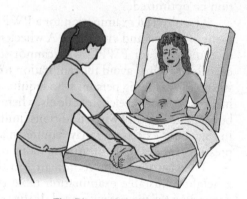

Figure 23.1 Diamond-shaped position
(Smeltzer & Sharts-Hopko [2005] and ACOG [n.d.]).

The Diamond-shaped position

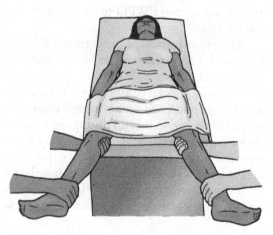

Figure 23.2 V-shaped position
(Smeltzer & Sharts-Hopko [2005] and
ACOG [n.d.]).

The V-shaped position

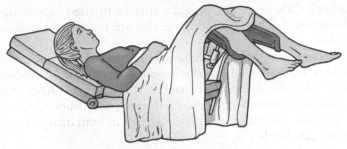

The OB Stirrups position

Figure 23.3 OB stirrups position (Smeltzer & Sharts-Hopko [2005] and ACOG [n.d.]).

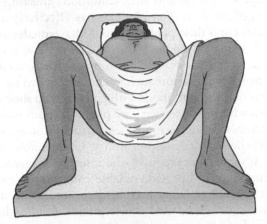

The M-Shaped position

Figure 23.4 M-Shaped position (Smeltzer & Sharts-Hopko [2005] and ACOG [n.d.]).

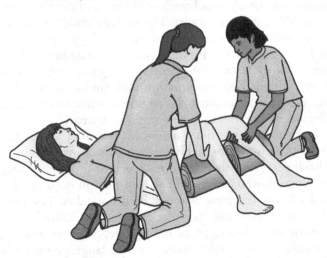

Figure 23.5 Use of positioning aids (Smeltzer & Sharts-Hopko [2005] and ACOG [n.d.]).

normal manner. Otherwise, the speculum may be inserted "upside down" with the handles upward. These positions are also appropriate for examination of male genitalia.

Two excellent resources to guide individualized care for women with physical disabilities are available from the American Congress of Obstetricians & Gynecologists (ACOG, n.d.) and Smeltzer & Sharts-Hopko (2005). The ACOG resource provides an extensive tutorial on the laws and issues related to the care of PWPD that lays a foundation for effective care of both men and women with diverse health-care needs.

Persons With Sensory Deficits

The ADA also requires that persons with conditions affecting communication are able to communicate with their clinicians as effectively as those without disabilities. Clinicians and their practices should have predetermined means to communicate with patients who are blind or deaf or have a speech disability. There are a number of options available to support these communications, and planning should be based on factors such as the anticipated nature, complexity, length, and content of communications with patients. You should always consult the patient to learn what aid or service they prefer in communicating.

Even when another person accompanies a patient during the visit, effective communication is the practice's responsibility. Companions cannot be relied upon unless it is at the patient's request, the interpreter agrees, and you determine that the interpreter will provide reliable communication (i.e., is able to understand the terminology being used and communicate impartially). For example, children should not be used as interpreters. Adults who may be biased or otherwise prejudiced in some way (e.g., a spouse when concern involves domestic abuse, a companion uncomfortable with the nature of the discussion) should not be used as interpreters.

For patients who are blind or have low vision, staff members can be trained and made available to serve as a reader. The reader should be able to read forms and material accurately using appropriate terminology, without inserting any bias—through taking shortcuts, for instance. They must be equally able to then record a patient's written response when necessary (e.g., write-in responses on a history form). Alternatively, information also can be conveyed or requested through large print (or a computer/digital screen when larger format is appropriate), by Braille, or by prerecording in an audio format.

When a patient is deaf or has a significant hearing loss, solutions for conducting a history, counseling, or otherwise communicating include using printed material or having a system that supports speech-to-text conversion during the interchange. A person who can record any information imparted in an accurate and impartial manner can serve as a qualified notetaker. The notes can then be used so that the patient can "see" the clinician's verbalized communication (i.e., questions or instruction) and, as appropriate, can serve as a reference after the visit. For patients who prefer signing, a sign language interpreter familiar with appropriate terminology is helpful in interpreting signing to the clinician and speech to the patient.

Speech disabilities can make it difficult for the patient's needs to be understood. For patients with speech disabilities, determine whether the patient uses a communication board or other device to support communication. When a speech disability affects your understanding, always ask the patient to repeat necessary details or questions and allow time for the patient to speak slowly without feeling rushed or becoming frustrated. Provide writing implements and ask the patient to write out words or phrases that are not understood.

Summary

Throughout this text, the content has focused on the development of skills and knowledge necessary to accurately conduct patient assessments and interpret the findings. Only by thoughtful planning will this knowledge be extended to the growing population of PWD.

REFERENCES

American Congress of Obstetricians and Gynecologists (ACOG). (n.d.). Interactive site for clinicians serving women with disabilities. Retrieved August 14, 2018, from http://www.acog.org/About-ACOG/ACOG-Departments/Women-with-Disabilities/Interactive-site-for-clinicians-serving-women-with-disabilities

Bauer, S. E., Schumacher, J. R., Hall, A. H., Marlow, N. M., Friedel, C., Scheer, D., & Redmon, S. (2016). Disability and physical and communication-related barriers to health care related services among Florida residents: A brief report. *Disability and Health Journal, 9*(3), 552–556.

Centers for Disease Control and Prevention, National Center on Birth Defects and Developmental Disabilities, Division of Human Development and Disability. Disability and Health Data System (DHDS) (n.d.) Data [online]. Retrieved January 20, 2021, from https://dhds.cdc.gov

Centers for Disease Control and Prevention. (2013). People with disabilities: What healthcare professionals can do to be accessible. https://www.cdc.gov/ncbddd/disabilityandhealth/documents/pd_hcprof_can_do.pdf

Graham, C., & Mann, J. (2008). Accessibility of primary care physician practice sites in South Carolina for people with disabilities, *Disability and Health Journal, 1*(4), 209–214.

Healthy People. (n.d.). 2020. Topics & objectives: Disability and health. https://www.healthypeople.gov/2020/topics-objectives/topic/disability-and-health

Horner-Johnson, W., Dobbertin, K., Lee, J., Andresen, E., & the Expert Panel on Disability and Health Disparities. (2014). Disparities in health care access and receipt of preventive services by disability type: Analysis of the Medical Expenditure Panel Survey. *Health Services Research, 49*(6), 1980–1999.

Lagu, T., Hannon, N., Rothberg, M., Wells, A., Green, K., Windom, M., Dempsey, K. R., Pekow, P. S., Avrunin, J. S., Chen, A., & Kindenauer, P. K. (2013). Access to subspecialty care for patients with mobility impairment: A survey. *Annals of Internal Medicine, 158*(6), 441–446.

Morrison, E., George, V., & Mosqueda, L. (2008). Primary care for adults with physical disabilities: Perceptions from consumer and provider focus groups. *Family Medicine, 40*(9), 645–651.

Pharr, J. (2014). Accommodations for patients with disabilities in primary care: A mixed methods study of practice administrators. *Global Journal of Health Science, 6*(1), 23–32.

Smeltzer, S., & Sharts-Hopko, N. (2005). *A provider's guide for the care of women with physical disabilities and chronic conditions.* North Carolina Office on Disability & Health.

U.S. Department of Justice. (2010). ADA requirements: Access to medical care for individuals with mobility disabilities. https://www.ada.gov/medcare_ta.htm

U.S. Department of Justice. (2014). ADA requirements: Effective communication. https://www.ada.gov/effective-comm.pdf

Symptoms Index

Abdomen
abdominal pain, 348
constipation, 379–380
diarrhea, 373
epigastric pain, 355
gastrointestinal bleeding, 388
jaundice, 384
left upper quadrant pain, 353
nausea and vomiting, 367
pelvic pain, 366
right and left lower quadrant pain, 359
right upper quadrant pain, 349
suprapubic pain, 366

Breasts
breast mass, 326
breast pain, 329
male breast enlargement or mass, 337
nipple discharge, 332
skin lesions of the nipple and areola, 336

Cardiac System
acute and subacute bacterial endocarditis, 290
chest pain/chest pressure, 264
difficulty breathing and shortness of
    breath, 286
elevated blood pressure, 280
elevated lipids, 283
heart murmur, 270
palpitations or arrhythmia, 260

Ear
aural fullness, 217, 218
decreased hearing or hearing loss, 210
ear discharge (otorrhea), 207–208
ear pain (otalgia), 202
tinnitus (ringing in the ears), 217

Eye
double vision, 186
eye discharge, 183
eyelid problems, 188
eye pain, 180
ptosis, 184
reddened eye, 173
visual disturbances, 166

Female Reproductive System
abnormal Pap test, 488
abnormal uterine bleeding, 490
amenorrhea, 494
dysmenorrhea, 498
infertility, 504
labial lesions, 484
mass and/or swelling at introitus, 475
ovarian cancer, 500
sexual dysfunction, 502
vaginal discharge, 478

Genitourinary System
anuria, oliguria, and renal failure, 408
asymmetric prostate, 411
asymptomatic microscopic
    hematuria, 410
decreased force of stream or spraying with
    urination, 424
difficulty urinating, 422
dysuria, 417
elevated prostate-specific
    antigen, 411
flank pain and renal colic, 401

Index